PHYSICAL THERAPY RESEARCH

Principles and Applications

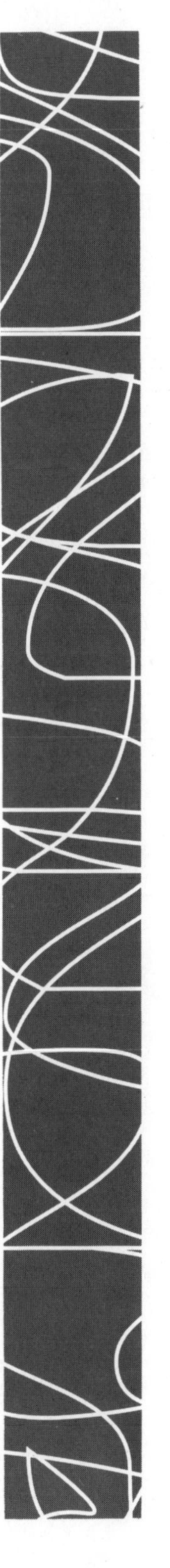

PHYSICAL THERAPY RESEARCH

Principles and Applications

Elizabeth Domholdt, PT, EdD
Krannert Graduate School of Physical Therapy
University of Indianapolis
Indianapolis, Indiana

W.B. SAUNDERS COMPANY
A Division of Harcourt Brace & Company
Philadelphia London Toronto
Montreal Sydney Tokyo

W.B. SAUNDERS COMPANY
A Division of
Harcourt Brace & Company

The Curtis Center
Independence Square West
Philadelphia, Pennsylvania 19106

Library of Congress Cataloging-in-Publication Data

Domholdt, Elizabeth

Physical therapy research: principles and applications /
Elizabeth Domholdt.

p. cm.

ISBN 0–7216–3611–X

1. Physical therapy—Research. I. Title.

[DNLM: 1. Physical Therapy. 2. Research. WB 25 D668p]

RM708.D66 1993

615.8′2′072—dc20

DNLM/DLC 92–13390

PHYSICAL THERAPY RESEARCH
Principles and Applications

ISBN 0–7216–3611–X

Copyright © 1993 by W. B. Saunders Company.

All rights reserved. No part of this publication may be reproduced or transmitted in any form or by any means, electronic or mechanical, including photocopy, recording, or any information storage and retrieval system, without permission in writing from the publisher.

Printed in the United States of America.

Last digit is the print number: 9 8 7 6 5

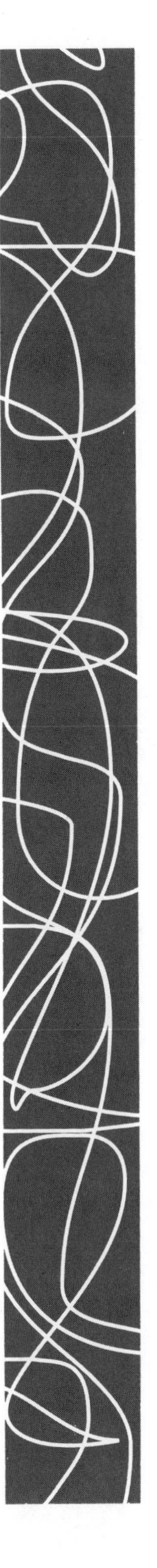

PREFACE

Research in physical therapy has never been more dynamic. More physical therapists with doctoral preparation are conducting research than ever before, there are numerous peer-reviewed journals related to physical therapy, and there is a foundation that funds physical therapy research. Physical therapy research has also never been more sophisticated or diverse. It ranges from quantitative experimental research on the effects of physical therapy modalities on physiologic function to qualitative descriptive research giving a sociological perspective to the work of physical therapists. In a single issue of a journal, a physical therapist may encounter data analysis techniques from repeated measures analysis of variance, to celeration line approaches for single subject research designs.

This textbook was designed to capture this diversity and complexity to enable physical therapists and students to apply research principles as they read the literature and design and implement studies. Physical therapists and physical therapy students are intelligent, motivated individuals who deserve to have research presented to them in a rigorous but straightforward manner, made relevant through the use of examples from the physical therapy literature.

The text is divided into two major parts: principles and applications. The first 15 chapters present the principles of research, including fundamentals of theory and ethics, design, measurement, and data analysis. The final 5 chapters present guidelines for the application of the principles, including chapters on finding and evaluating the literature, planning and implementing research, and publishing and presenting the results. Figures, tables, and examples from the physical therapy literature are included to illustrate the sometimes complex and abstract concepts that underlie research.

No project of this magnitude can be completed without the assistance of many others. A generous sabbatical policy at the University of Indianapolis gave me six uninterrupted months in which to work on the text. Once I was back from sabbatical, my faculty colleagues respected my writing days and tolerated what I hope was relatively benign neglect of some administrative tasks. Several classes of students used a first draft of this material as their textbook. I thank them for both their patience with rough material and typographic errors and their frank feedback, which helped make this a better book. I thank Karen Horwood, Anita Burrell, Brian Overbeck, PT, MS, and Cindi Wooden, PT, MS, current and former students, for many hours spent photocopying references and proofreading chapters.

Several colleagues read portions of the text for content and clarity. Julia Sheffield, PT, MS, and Candy Conino, PT, gave input from the entry-level and postprofessional student perspectives, respectively. Mark Reinking, PT, MS, gave excellent feedback from the perspective of a clinician. Ann Marriner-Tomey, RN, PhD, provided feedback on the theory chapter; Christine Guyonneau, MLS, reference librarian at the University of Indianapolis, did the same for the chapter on locating the literature. Ann Clawson, PT, MS, reviewed the sample manuscript in Appendix F—as she has done for some of my actual manuscripts in the past. Janet Wigglesworth, PhD, reviewed the chapters on measurement and data analysis. I appreciate the willingness of these colleagues to devote their time and expertise to make this a better text. The responsibility for any remaining inaccuracies is mine, however.

Margaret Biblis, my editor at Saunders, got me fired up about writing this text and provided consistent encouragement during the past two years. Dave Prout, a developmental editor, provided gentle feedback about each chapter and was always just a phone call away when I had a question.

Finally, I have to thank my husband, Gary Shoemaker, for all he adds to my life. Throughout our marriage he has lovingly tolerated my preoccupation with work and accepts that there is always another project just around the corner.

Elizabeth Domholdt
Indianapolis, Indiana

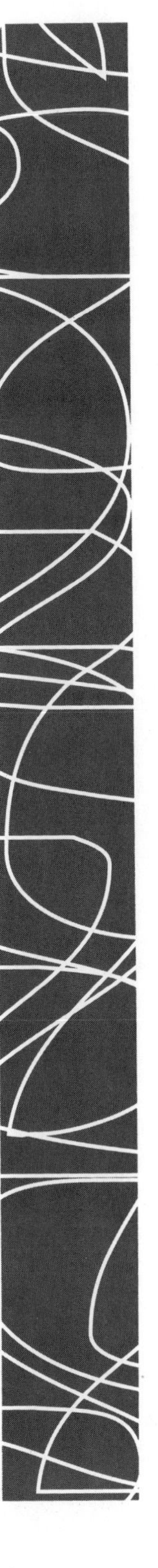

CONTENTS

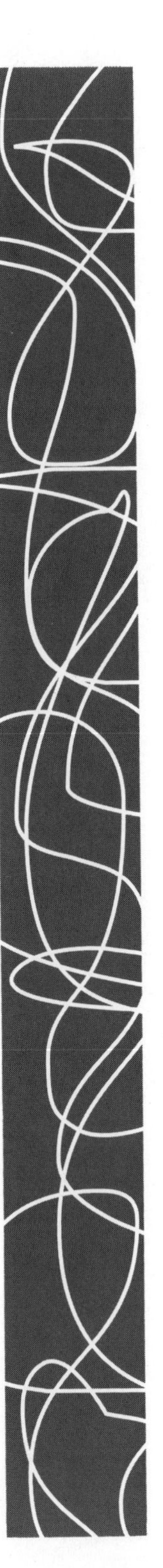

SECTION ONE

RESEARCH FUNDAMENTALS

CHAPTER 1

Research in Physical Therapy

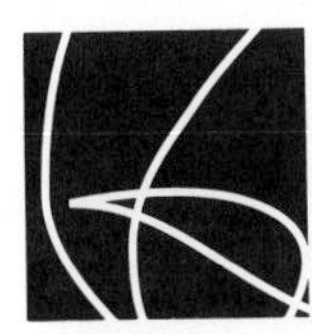

Research in physical therapy has different meanings for different people. To some, it represents the essence of the profession—the way to determine whether what we do as physical therapists makes a difference. To others, it represents a challenging intellectual exercise regardless of its relation to clinical practice. To still others, it is a course or project they are required to complete to obtain an academic degree.

This introductory chapter defines research, examines reasons for and barriers to implementing physical therapy research, offers strategies for overcoming barriers to research in physical therapy, and puts physical therapy research into a historical context. After this foundation is laid, the rest of the book presents the principles needed to understand research and suggests guidelines for the application of those principles in the interpretation and implementation of research.

DEFINITIONS OF RESEARCH

Research has been defined by almost every person who has written about it. Charles Franklin Kettering, engineer and philanthropist, had this to say:

> Research is a high-hat word that scares a lot of people. It needn't. . . . it is nothing but a state of mind—a friendly, welcoming attitude toward change. . . . It is the problem-solving mind as contrasted with the let-well-enough-alone mind. It is the composer mind instead of the fiddler mind. It is the "tomorrow" mind instead of the "yesterday" mind.[1(p91)]

Others have characterized research as "akin to detective work or puzzle solving."[2(pix)]

Eugene Michels, Otto Payton, and Dean Currier, three physical therapists who have written widely on research in physical therapy, all emphasize the organized, systematic nature of research.[3–5(p4)] Three important characteristics about research emerge from these different views: research challenges the status quo, research is creative, and research is systematic.

Research Challenges the Status Quo

Sometimes the results of research support current clinical practices; other times, the results point to areas of treatment that are not effective when put to a systematic test. But whether or not research leads to a revision of currently accepted principles, the guiding philosophy of research is that it challenges the field. Is this treatment effective? Is it more effective than another treatment? Would this person recover as quickly without physical therapy? Is physical therapy management superior to pharmacological or surgical management for a given condition?

Walker and colleagues[6] challenged the physiological basis of high-voltage pulsed current when they studied its effect on blood flow to the gastrocnemius muscle complex. Griffin and associates[7] also challenged the use of high-voltage pulsed current, in a more clinically oriented study of its effect on hand volume for patients with chronic hand edema. Whereas no blood flow changes were found in the first study, clinically important changes in hand volume were found after the high-voltage treatment in the second study. Thus, these two challenges to the status quo resulted in support for a current clinical procedure but questioned the underlying mechanism of action of the modality. Research is about making these kinds of challenges, in the hope that what we currently do will be supported, but with the willingness to change our practice when it is not.

Research Is Creative

Rothstein believes that many physical therapists are quick to accept an authoritarian view of physical therapy: "Our teachers and our texts tell us how it should be, and we accept this in our eagerness to proceed with patient care."[8] Researchers, however, are creative individuals who move past the authoritarian teachings of others and look at physical therapy in a different way. For example, most physical therapists who work with patients who have had a stroke or amputation strive for these patients to exhibit as symmetric a gait pattern as possible. Winter, a biomechanist, was creative enough to ask whether a symmetric gait is the most efficient gait for an individual with unilateral dysfunction:

> At the outset, the author would be cautious about gait retraining protocols which are aimed at improved symmetry based on nothing more than an idea that it would automatically be an improvement. It is safe to say that any human system with major structural asymmetries in the neuromuscular skeletal system cannot be optimal when the gait is symmetrical.[9(p362)]

Researchers thrive on the creative intellectual processes that lead to the development of new ways of conceptualizing their discipline. The creative aspects of physical therapy research are emphasized in Chapter 2, which presents information about the use of theory in physical therapy, and Chapter 4, which provides a framework for the development of research problems.

Research Is Systematic

Much of physical therapists' clinical knowledge is anecdotal, or is passed on through "ecclesiastical succession"[5(p3)] from prominent therapists who teach a particular treatment to eager colleagues or students. Anecdotal claims for the effectiveness of treatments are colored by the relationship between the physical therapist and patient and do not provide control of factors other than treatment that may account for changes in a patient's condition.

In contrast, research is systematic. It attempts to isolate treatment effects from other influences that are not ordinarily controlled in the clinic setting. Much of this text is devoted to the systematic principles that underlie research methods: Chapters 5 through 9 cover research design, Chapters 10 through 12 discuss measurement in physical therapy, and Chapters 13 through 15 introduce data analysis.

PURPOSE OF THIS TEXT

The purpose of this book is to provide physical therapists with a framework for understanding and applying the systematic processes of research. As with other fields of study, research is ever changing, and a text can represent research thought only at a particular point in time. This text however, does present both traditional research methods and emerging approaches. Just as physical therapy researchers must question their beliefs about physical therapy, they must be willing to question their ideas about research.

Learning about research in physical therapy can be challenging. First, one must develop a diverse set of skills in statistics, research design, and writing. At the same time these new skills are being mastered, one is challenging the status quo by questioning the conventional wisdom of the profession. The combination of trying to learn new material while simultaneously challenging previously held beliefs can engender frustration with the new material and doubt about one's previous learning. Some physical therapists are unable to cope with such uncertainty and retreat to anecdotes and ecclesiastical succession as the basis for their work in physical therapy. Others delight in the intellectual challenge of research and create for themselves a professional life that balances the use of practical treatment strategies with clinical research that tests the assumptions under which they deliver physical therapy care.

This text is designed to encourage delight rather than retreat. It does so through the use of many figures and tables to illustrate abstract concepts. In addition, most of the principles are made relevant to physical therapists through the use of examples from research related to the profession.

REASONS FOR DOING RESEARCH IN PHYSICAL THERAPY

There are at least four reasons for doing physical therapy research:

1. To establish a body of knowledge for physical therapy,
2. To determine the efficacy of physical therapy treatments,
3. To provide development opportunities for physical therapists, and
4. To improve patient care in physical therapy.

Body of Knowledge

The body-of-knowledge rationale for physical therapy research is related to the concept of a profession. The characteristics of a profession have been described by many authors but include several common elements. Houle divided the characteristics of a profession into three broad groups: conceptual, performance, and collective identity (Table 1–1).[10] One of

TABLE 1–1. Characteristics of a Profession[a]

CONCEPTUAL CHARACTERISTIC
Establishment of a central mission
PERFORMANCE CHARACTERISTICS
Mastery of theoretical knowledge
Capacity to solve problems
Use of practical knowledge
Self-enhancement
COLLECTIVE IDENTITY CHARACTERISTICS
Formal training
Credentialing
Creation of a subculture
Legal reinforcement
Public acceptance
Ethical practice
Penalties
Relations to other vocations
Relations to users of service

[a]List developed from Houle CO. *Continuing Learning in the Professions.* San Francisco, Calif: Jossey-Bass Publishers; 1981.

the critical performance characteristics is mastery of the theoretical knowledge that forms the basis for the profession.

Physical therapists have been accused of being beggars and borrowers of information from anatomy, physiology, kinesiology, psychology, and physical education, rather than being creators of our own body of knowledge:

> Physical therapy has a soft underbelly because its science is in disarray. This disarray leaves it open to attacks against its inadequacies—attacks from medicine, attacks from government, challenges from fiscal agencies, and questions from the consuming public.[11(p1070)]

One response to this accusation has been to propose the development of a new science, *pathokinesiology*, the science of abnormal movement. Another response is to assert that the disarray in physical therapy research is common to all applied professions that borrow knowledge from the basic arts and sciences. For example, medicine borrows from anatomy and physiology, and law borrows from logic and philosophy.

Whether one believes that a new science is needed or that the existing sciences can be applied, what physical therapists must do is concentrate on developing systematic ways of testing the means by which we meet the physical therapy needs of our clients. We need to document what we do; how we do it; what effect it has on our clients; and what effect it has compared with no treatment, other physical therapy techniques, or other health care approaches. It is through research that we can systematically develop a body of knowledge about physical therapy, irrespective of whether we believe this body of knowledge to be pathokinesiology or the application of basic sciences to those with functional limitations.

Efficacy of Physical Therapy

The second major rationale for performing research in physical therapy is to determine the efficacy of physical therapy treatments. The desire for such documentation can be motivated by concern for the well-being of clients, by the desire to be viewed as a legitimate profession by other health professionals, or by the need to ensure that we obtain appropriate reimbursement for the services we provide. In 1990, a major insurer in Indiana stopped paying for hot packs and ultrasound given in the same treatment session.[12] There was an outcry from physical therapists—doesn't everyone know that hot packs are superficial heaters and ultrasound is a deep heater? Aren't the differing physiological effects reason enough to justify their combined use? Apparently not. Although there are physiological data to support different levels of heating of the two modalities,[13, 14] experts who reviewed the literature related to hot packs and ultrasound failed to identify studies that support the use of the combined modalities over either one individually. Perhaps third-party payers are justified in questioning the use of the combined treatment until physical therapists establish whether it is more effective than either treatment alone.

Professional Development of Physical Therapists

A third reason for research in physical therapy is to provide intellectual challenges and professional development for physical therapists. In a time when there are more applicants than there are available spaces in physical therapy programs, those who become physical therapists are bright and motivated. Therapists of such caliber require continuing intellectual challenges to remain in the profession; research can provide such challenges.

Improvements in Patient Care

The fourth reason for research in physical therapy is perhaps the most important one: improving patient care. When we know what has or has not been supported by research, we can make intelligent decisions about which clinical procedures to use with our clients. For example, Wessling and coworkers[15] found that a combined program of static stretch and ultrasound produced greater range-of-motion gains than did static stretch alone. Therapists with a good knowledge base in research will be able to critique Wessling and coworkers' article to determine whether they believe the results can be applied to the clinical situations in which they work. Chapter 17 presents guidelines for evaluating research literature.

Unfortunately, there is evidence that research results are not often incorporated into clinical practice.[16] The reasons for this nonutilization are thought to be a negative perception of science, an unwillingness to put clinical beliefs on the line, the formality and jargon of research communication, the lack of emphasis on research in educational programs, and a preference for personal observations. Physical therapists have a professional responsibility to move past these reasons and become regular consumers of the research literature.

BARRIERS TO RESEARCH IN PHYSICAL THERAPY

Although most physical therapists recognize the importance of research, many obstacles to physical therapy research are documented. Figure 1–1 shows the obstacles that were identified by more than 50% of the respondents in a 1980 study of California physical therapists.[17] These obstacles include lack of familiarity with research methodology, lack of statistical support, lack of funding, and lack of time. A fifth obstacle to physical therapy research was the concern for ethical use of animals or humans in research activities.[3, 18]

Lack of Familiarity with the Research Process

Research is sometimes viewed as a mysterious process that occupies the time of an elite group of physical therapists who cannot be bothered with actually delivering patient care. The language of research and data analysis is specialized, and those who have not acquired the vocabulary are understandably intimidated when it is spoken. The goal of this book is to demystify the process by clearly articulating the knowledge base needed to understand and implement research.

There is no agreement on the best way to acquire research skills. Entry-level programs

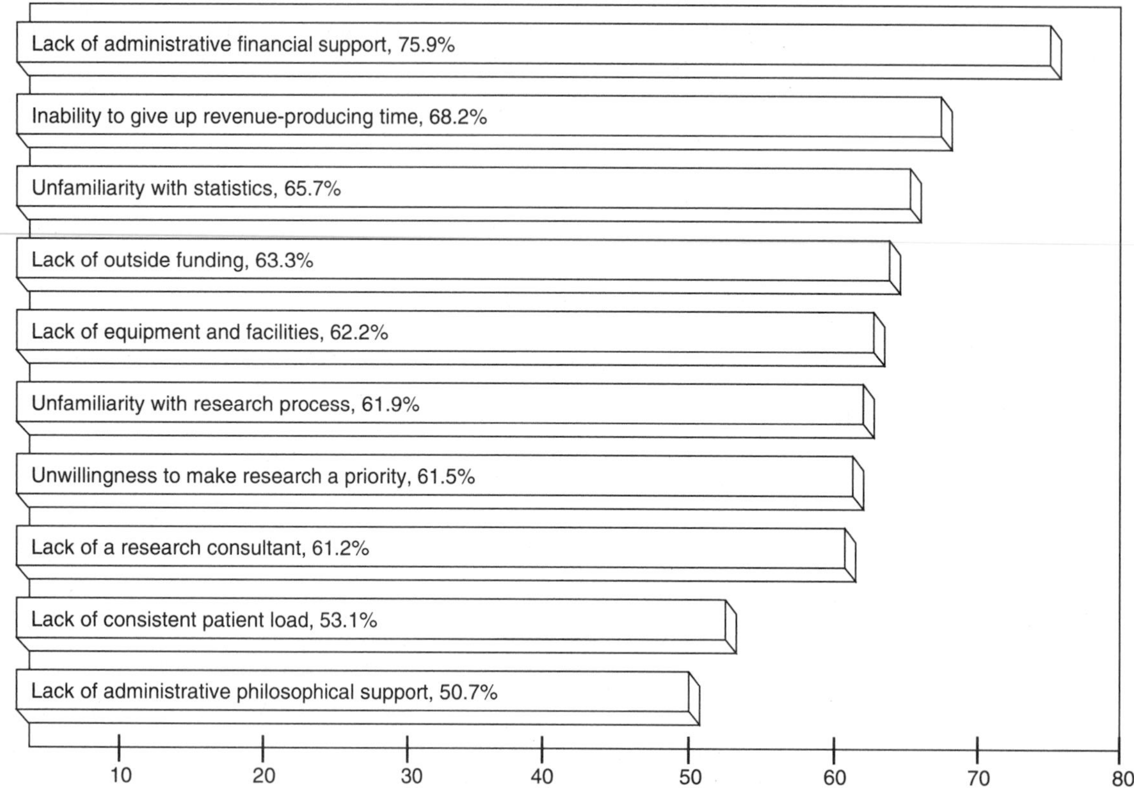

FIGURE 1–1. Barriers to research. Compiled from data presented in Ballin AJ, Breslin WH, Wierenga KAS, Shepard KF. Research in physical therapy: philosophy, barriers to involvement, and use among California physical therapists. *Phys Ther*. 1980;60:888–895.

in physical therapy have diverse patterns of research education: Some require completion of individual research projects, some require group projects, some require that student research complement ongoing faculty projects, and some require only that students acquire skills in critiquing the literature.[19] For therapists who did not acquire a sufficient research background through their entry-level education, participation in continuing education workshops on research or pursuit of advanced degrees can fill in the gaps. Whatever method of familiarization is chosen, a critical element seems to be working with others to share new ideas and insights about research.[20, 21]

Lack of Statistical Support for Research

The second major barrier to research is lack of statistical support. Even those who become familiar enough with the research process to implement research often need assistance with statistical analysis. This book provides the reader with the conceptual background needed to understand most of the statistics reported in the physical therapy research literature.[22] A conceptual background does not, however, provide an adequate theoretical and mathematical basis for the selection and computation of a given statistic on a particular occasion. Thus, most researchers require the services of a statistician at some point in the research process. Guidelines for working with statisticians are provided in Chapter 19.

Lack of Funds for Research

A third barrier to research is lack of funding. Because research is not a revenue-producing activity like patient care or teaching, administrators find it difficult to provide clinicians or faculty members with the time they need to implement a study. In addition, research has many direct costs: equipment, computer time, statistical and engineering consultants, clerical time, production and travel for presentation of the research at conferences, and figure and photographic production for publication of the research. Funding sources for physical therapy research are discussed in Chapter 18.

Lack of Time

A fourth barrier to research in physical therapy is lack of time. Tasks with firm deadlines are given higher priority than research, which usually has only those deadlines that are self-imposed by the researchers. Although physical therapy students have a strong motivation to complete research projects required for graduation, conversion of the academic paper into a journal article suitable for publication becomes a low priority once the student enters clinical practice.[18] The immediate time pressures placed on physical therapy clinicians and academicians may lead to postponement or abandonment of research ideas. One solution to this problem is to design studies that are relatively easy to integrate into the daily routine of a physical therapy practice. Chapters 5, 6, and 9 present a variety of research designs suitable for implementation in a clinical setting.

Ethical Concerns About the Use of Human or Animal Subjects

The fifth barrier to research implementation is ethical concern about the use of either animals or humans as research subjects. Physical therapists who choose to study animal models must follow appropriate guidelines for the use, care, and humane destruction of animal subjects. Physical therapists who use human subjects in their research must balance the risks of the research against the potential benefits from the results. Chapter 3 examines ethical considerations in research in detail; Chapter 18 provides guidelines for working with the committees that work with researchers to ensure the rights of research subjects.

OVERCOMING BARRIERS TO RESEARCH IN PHYSICAL THERAPY

Given these barriers, how do physical therapists promote research in the profession? Several strategies have been described by physical therapists who have implemented successful programs to promote clinical research in three different settings: a major teaching hospital,[23] a rehabilitation hospital,[24] and an orthopedic clinic.[25] A prerequisite to developing a strategy is strong administrative support for research. Meaningful research cannot be conducted if administrators are not willing to provide the time, funds, and means for their staff to obtain research expertise.

One strategy to ensure research development is to have a research coordinator or a research committee.[23–25] The coordinator is someone with expertise in research who can work with other therapists to develop their skills and knowledge. The committee helps make decisions about which of several possible projects will enable the clinic to best meet its mission.

A second strategy is to provide educational opportunities about research for staff members. This has been done by employing a consultant to work with staff members,[24] sponsoring continuing education courses,[24] or providing in-service education.[25]

A third strategy is to provide therapists time away from patient care to engage in research.[23, 25] Even when research is designed for smooth implementation in the clinical setting, researchers need considerable time before and after data collection to plan and summarize a project. The time-consuming process of finding and evaluating the literature (Chapters 16 and 17) to define a sound research problem grounded in the work of others is crucial to the eventual usefulness of a project. In addition, the researcher needs time to produce written and oral presentations of the research (Chapter 20) so that the results can be used to benefit patients and advance the base of knowledge in physical therapy.

A fourth theme is doing collaborative research with others who have the needed resources. Collaboration between physical therapy clinicians and physical therapy faculty at nearby universities has been reported.[25] In addition, personal communication with therapists at two of the clinics referred to in this section (P. Cebulski, University of Michigan, 1990; J. Seto, Kerlan-Jobe Orthopedic Clinic, 1990) reveals that they are collaborating on research with physicians. Physical therapists work in concert with other professionals to deliver quality care; we should not be afraid of collaboration in research efforts to refine that care.

HISTORY OF RESEARCH IN PHYSICAL THERAPY

In 1960, Catherine Worthingham, a leader in physical therapy, called for physical therapists to give attention to developing the body of knowledge of physical therapy through research.[26] Eight years later, Eugene Michels, a well-known physical therapy researcher, identified a credibility gap in that physical therapists were not sufficiently sophisticated in research methods and noted that the profession was in crucial need of more and better clinical research.[27] In 1975, Helen Hislop, in her prestigious Mary McMillan lecture, explained one reason that the clinical science of physical therapy is developing slowly:

> After fifty years, the science of physical therapy is entering its infancy. A great difficulty in developing the clinical science of physical therapy is that we treat individual persons, each of whom is made up of situations which are unique and, therefore, appear incompatible with the generalizations demanded by science.[11(p1076)]

In 1989, Rothstein, a physical therapist and editor of *Physical Therapy*, challenged physical therapists with the fact that we still know so little about the core techniques of the profession:

> Although we have begun to develop a body of research literature in physical therapy, we still lack a body of clinical literature. . . . We have no collective body of knowledge about how long it takes for even our simplest treatments to have a beneficial effect on some of the most straightforward conditions.[28(p796)]

These statements from the past 30 years might lead one to believe that no progress has been made in articulating and testing the body of knowledge of physical therapy. This is deceptive because part of the character of research is that when one question is answered, several more spring up. Thus, the profession's appetite for research should be insatiable, and apparently is, if the consistent cry for more research is any indication.

The history of research in physical therapy can be traced by examination of the goals of professional associations, the standards of educational programs, the development of vehicles for the publication of research reports, and support for research funding in the discipline. The objective of the American Women's Physical Therapeutic Association (now the American Physical Therapy Association [APTA]), as defined in its first constitution of 1921, was "to establish and maintain a professional and scientific standard for those engaged in the profession . . . to disseminate information by the distribution of medical literature and articles of professional interest."[29(p5)] Today, one of the objectives of the APTA is to "improve the art and science of physical therapy including practice, education, and research."[30(p880)] The Canadian Physiotherapy Association has also established research as one of its highest priorities.[31]

As educational programs for physical therapists developed, the profession began to establish its own criteria for such educational programs. In 1974, the APTA House of Delegates adopted accreditation criteria for physical therapist education programs that required both that faculty be involved in scholarly pursuits and that students be able to use research principles to critically analyze research findings.[32] Current accreditation criteria maintain the expectation that students be able to critically evaluate the literature and have added the expectation that students participate in research activities.[33] The relatively recent development of doctoral education programs in physical therapy also points to the increased legitimacy of research in physical therapy.[34]

Scholarly publications in physical therapy have mirrored the increasing interest in research in physical therapy. The Chartered Society of Physiotherapists in Great Britain published its first volume of *Physiotherapy* in 1915. *Physical Therapy*, the journal of the APTA, was first published in 1921 as the *PT Review*. After the lead that medicine and nursing had provided for many years, the 1980s saw the rise of various specialty journals in physical therapy: The *Journal of Orthopaedic and Sports Physical Therapy* began in 1979, *Physical and Occupational Therapy in Pediatrics* was launched in 1980, and *Physical Therapy and Occupational Therapy in Geriatrics* followed shortly thereafter. The *Journal of Physical Therapy Education* was developed in 1986, and in 1989 the *Journal of Pediatric Physical Therapy* was launched. Chapter 16 includes a list of many journals relevant to physical therapists.

Financial support of research is another indication of the value that is placed on research activities. The Foundation for Physical Therapy, founded in 1979, awarded almost $150,000 in clinical research grants and almost $200,000 in doctoral scholarships during the 1989–1990 year.[35] Physical therapists have also been successful in securing funds from corporate and government sources (Chapter 18).

Although the refrain to increase and improve physical therapy research seems to continue from one generation of therapists to the next, this review shows that the professional association and its components place more emphasis on research than ever before, the educational standards for physical therapists include criteria related to research, doctoral programs in physical therapy exist, the number of journals related to physical therapy research has increased during the last decade, and external funds for physical therapy research are available from several sources. Yes, the barriers to research are significant. Yes, identifying and using the available resources require initiative and energy. Still, there is much to be gained in taking that initiative and overcoming the barriers that prevent physical therapists from testing and substantiating their practice.

SUMMARY

Research is the creative process by which professionals systematically challenge their everyday practices. Developing a body of physical therapy knowledge, documenting the efficacy of physical therapy research, providing professional development for physical therapists, and improving patient care are reasons for conducting physical therapy research. Barriers to research are lack of familiarity with the research process, lack of statistical support, lack of funds, and concern for the ethics of using animals and humans as research subjects. Strategies that have worked to overcome the barriers to clinical research include developing research coordinator positions and research committees; educating physical therapists about research; providing therapists time away from patients to conduct clinical research; and forming collaborative research relationships among physical therapists, physicians, and other professionals, health care institutions, and universities. Although the need for research within a discipline should never be satisfied, the profession of physical therapy has made progress in research, as shown by its educational standards, expansion of research journals in physical therapy, and funding for physical therapy research.

References

1. Kettering CF. "Research" is a high-hat word. In: Boyd TA. *Prophet of Progress*. New York, NY; EP Dutton and Co Inc; 1961:91.
2. Oyster CK, Hanten WP, Llorens LA. *Introduction to Research: A Guide for the Health Science Professional*. Philadelphia, Pa: JB Lippincott Co; 1987.
3. Michels E. Evaluation and research in physical therapy. *Phys Ther*. 1982;62:828–834.
4. Payton OD. *Research: The Validation of Clinical Practice*. 2nd ed. Philadelphia, Pa: FA Davis Co; 1988:10.
5. Currier DP. *Elements of Research in Physical Therapy*. 3rd ed. Baltimore, Md: Williams & Wilkins; 1990.
6. Walker DC, Currier DP, Threlkeld AJ. Effects of high voltage pulsed electrical stimulation on blood flow. *Phys Ther*. 1988;68:481–485.
7. Griffin JW, Newsome LS, Stralka SW, Wright PE. Reduction of chronic posttraumatic hand edema: a comparison of high voltage pulsed current, intermittent pneumatic compression, and placebo treatments. *Phys Ther*. 1990;70:279–286.
8. Rothstein JM. Clinical literature. *Phys Ther*. 1989;69:895. Editorial.
9. Winter DA, Sienko SE. Biomechanics of below-knee amputee gait. *J Biomech*. 1988;21:361–367.
10. Houle CO. *Continuing Learning in the Professions*. San Francisco, Calif: Jossey-Bass Publishers; 1981.
11. Hislop HJ. The not-so-impossible dream. *Phys Ther*. 1975;55:1069–1080.
12. Blue-Cross, Blue Shield of Indiana. *Provider Update*. Jan-Feb 1990;1:3.
13. Michlovitz SL. Biophysical principles of heating and superficial heat agents. In: Michlovitz SL, ed. *Thermal Agents in Rehabilitation*. 2nd ed. Philadelphia, Pa: FA Davis Co; 1990:94.
14. Ziskin MC, McDiarmid T, Michlovitz SL. Therapeutic ultrasound. In: Michlovitz SL, ed. *Thermal Agents in Rehabilitation*. 2nd ed. Philadelphia, Pa: FA Davis Co; 1990:144.
15. Wessling KC, DeVane DA, Hylton CR. Effects of static stretch versus static stretch and ultrasound combined on triceps surae muscle extensibility in healthy women. *Phys Ther*. 1987;67:674–679.
16. Bohannon RW, LeVeau BF. Clinicians' use of research findings: a review of literature with implications for physical therapists. *Phys Ther*. 1986;66:45–50.
17. Ballin AJ, Breslin WH, Wierenga KAS, Shepard KF. Research in physical therapy: philosophy, barriers to involvement, and use among California physical therapists. *Phys Ther*. 1980;60:888–895.
18. Walker JM. Research in pathokinesiology—what, why and how. *Phys Ther*. 1986;66:382–385.
19. Chambliss T. *Research Education in Physical Therapy: Standards, Goals, and Methods in Entry-Level Programs*. St Louis, Mo: Washington University; 1990. Thesis.
20. Bennett KJ, Sackett DL, Haynes RB, Neufeld VR, Tugwell P, Roberts R. A controlled trial of teaching critical appraisal of the clinical literature to medical students. *JAMA*. 1987;257:2451–2454.
21. Linzer M, Brown JT, Frazier LM, DeLong ER, Siegel WC. Impact of a medical journal club on house-staff reading habits, knowledge, and critical appraisal skills. *JAMA*. 1988;260:2537–2541.
22. Zito M, Bohannon RW. Inferential statistics in physical therapy research: a recommended core. *Journal of Physical Therapy Education*. 1990;4(1):13–16.

23. Vraciu JK, Darnell RE. Making clinical research a reality. *Phys Ther*. 1982;62:35–39.
24. Ritch JM. Starting research in a clinical setting. *Clinical Management in Physical Therapy*. 1981;1(3):7–10.
25. Morrissey MC, Kanda LT, Brewster CE. Development of a clinical physical therapy research program. *Phys Ther*. 1987;57:1110–1114.
26. Worthingham C. The development of physical therapy as a profession through research and publication. *Phys Ther*. 1960;40:573–577.
27. Michels E. On closing the credibility gap. *Phys Ther*. 1968;48:1081–1082.
28. Rothstein JM. *Phys Ther*. 1989;69:796. Editorial.
29. American Women's Physical Therapeutic Association. Constitution. *Phys Ther*. 1921;1:5.
30. American Physical Therapy Association. Bylaws. *Phys Ther*. 1989;69:880.
31. Dean E. Research the right way. *Clinical Management in Physical Therapy*. 1983;3(4):29–33.
32. *Essentials of an Accredited Educational Program for the Physical Therapist*. Alexandria, Va: American Physical Therapy Association; 1974.
33. Commission on Accreditation in Physical Therapy Education. *Evaluative Criteria for Accreditation of Education Programs for the Preparation of Physical Therapists*. Alexandria, Va: American Physical Therapy Association; 1990.
34. Soderberg GL. The future of physical therapy doctoral education. *Journal of Physical Therapy Education*. 1989;3(1):15–19.
35. Foundation for Physical Therapy. 1989/90 Report. *Progress Report of the American Physical Therapy Association*. September 1990;19(8):11.

CHAPTER 2

Theory in Physical Therapy Research

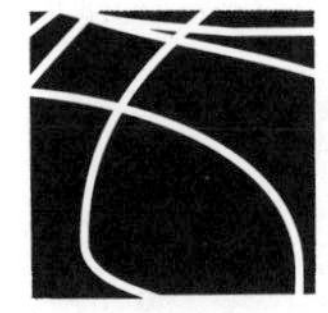

All of us have had ideas, and we may have dubbed some of these ideas theories. An instructor, after conducting an uninspired class on a beautiful spring day, may theorize that the level of interest in class discussion is inversely related to the outside environmental conditions. The students, on the other hand, may theorize that their interest in the outside conditions is inversely related to the enthusiasm and organization of the instructor!

When do ideas about the nature of the world become theories? What distinguishes theory from other modes of thought? Is theory important to an applied discipline such as physical therapy? The purpose of this chapter is to answer these questions by defining theory and some closely related terms, categorizing theories on the basis of scope, and examining the relationship among theory, research, and practice.

DEFINITIONS OF THEORY

Theories are, by nature, abstractions. Thus, the language of theory is abstract, and there are divergent definitions of theory and its components. Three basic elements of the different definitions of theory are discussed: level of restrictiveness, tentativeness, and testability.

Level of Restrictiveness

Fawcett and Downs,[1] in their text on the relationship between theory and research, reviewed several definitions of theory and categorized them by their level of restrictiveness. The level of restrictiveness of a theory is related to the way in which the theory can be used. To illustrate the differences between the levels of restrictiveness, a simplistic example about hemiplegia is developed throughout this section of the chapter. This example is not meant to be a well-developed theory; it is merely an illustration based on a clinical entity that most physical therapists should have encountered at some point in their professional education or practice.

Least Restrictive Definition. The least restrictive definition of theory is that of Stevens: "A theory is a statement that purports to account for or characterize some phenomenon."[2(p1)] This definition is least restrictive because it requires description of only one phenomenon. Thus, following Stevens's definition, the statement, "Patients with hemiplegia have difficulty ambulating, eating, and reading," is a simple form of theory because it characterizes [difficulty ambulating, eating, and reading] a phenomenon [patients with hemiplegia]. This simplest form of theory is referred to as *descriptive theory* because it describes only the phenomenon of interest.

Descriptive theories may be further classified as either *ad hoc theories* or *categorical theories*. The statement, "Patients with hemiplegia have difficulty ambulating, eating, and reading," presents an ad hoc collection of characteristics of patients with hemiplegia. An ad hoc list is not exhaustive; it is merely a list of possible characteristics. The statement about difficulty ambulating, eating, and reading in no way implies that these traits are the only difficulties experienced by patients with hemiplegia.

Contrast the ad hoc list with the statement, "The deficits experienced by patients with hemiplegia may be either motor, sensory, or functional." This example is a categorical descriptive theory because it implies that all the deficits experienced by a patient with hemiplegia can be classified into one of these three categories. In the ad hoc example, discovery of another type of difficulty (i.e., speaking) would not invalidate the theoretical statement because the list was not meant to be exhaustive. In the categorical example, discovery of another classification of deficits (i.e., cognitive) would require revision of the theory because the categories listed were meant to be exhaustive.

Moderately Restrictive Definition. Kerlinger has advanced a more restrictive definition of theory: "A theory is a set of interrelated constructs (concepts), definitions, and propositions that present a systematic view of phenomena by specifying relations among variables, with the purpose of explaining and predicting the phenomena."[3(p9)] Several terms Kerlinger used to define theory need definition themselves.

First, although Kerlinger's definition implies that constructs and concepts are similar, Kerlinger and others distinguish between the two. A *concept* has been defined as a "word or collection of words expressing a mental image of some phenomenon."[1(p16)] Concepts are generally thought to be observable. Thus, "joint range of motion" is a concept that can be observed by measuring joint motion with a goniometer. A *construct* "refers to a property that is neither directly nor indirectly observed"[1(p18)] and has been "deliberately and consciously invented or adopted for a special scientific purpose."[3(p27)] Thus, according to this definition, constructs are more abstract than concepts. "Motivation" and "social support" are examples of constructs; direct measurement of the constructs themselves is impossible because levels of motivation and social support can only be inferred from individual and family behaviors.

Although some authors recognize a distinction between concepts and constructs, others use the terms interchangeably. Even those who make the distinction recognize that the boundaries between concept and construct are not clear. Because of the blurred distinction between the two terms, they are used interchangeably within this text.

Second, a *proposition* is "a statement about

a concept or the relationship between concepts."[1(p14)] The term *hypothesis* is sometimes used interchangeably with *proposition,* as in Kerlinger's definition that a hypothesis is "a conjectural statement of the relation between two or more variables."[3(p17)] The hallmark of Kerlinger's definition of theory, then, is that it must specify relationships among concepts.

Our statement about patients with hemiplegia would need to be developed considerably before Kerlinger would consider it to be theory. Such a developed theory might read like this: "The extent to which hemiplegic patients will have difficulty ambulating is directly related to the presence of flaccid paralysis, cognitive deficits, and balance deficits and is inversely related to prior ambulation status." This is no longer a simple description of several characteristics of hemiplegia; this is a statement of relationships between concepts.

Researchers who prefer the most restrictive definition of theory (discussed later) may consider descriptions at this moderately restrictive level to be *conceptual frameworks* or *models*. Polit and Hungler, for example, were careful to distinguish between theory and less well articulated conceptual frameworks in nursing.[4]

Theory that meets Kerlinger's definition is known as *predictive theory* because it can be used to make predictions based on the relationships between variables. If the four factors in our hypothetical theory about hemiplegic gait were found to be good predictors of eventual ambulation outcome, therapists might be able to use information gathered at admission to predict long-term ambulation status.

Most Restrictive Definition. The most restrictive definition reviewed by Fawcett and Downs was that of Homans: "Not until one has properties, and propositions stating the relations between them, and the propositions form a deductive system—not until one has all three does one have theory."[5(p812)] This is the most restrictive definition because it requires both relationships among variables and a deductive system.

Deductive reasoning goes from the general to the specific and can take the form of if–then statements. To make our hypothetical theory of hemiplegic gait meet this definition, we would need to add a general gait component to the theory. This general statement might read, "Human gait characteristics are dependent on muscle power, skeletal stability, proprioceptive feedback, balance, motor planning, and learned patterns." The specific deduction from this general theory of gait is the statement, "In patients with hemiplegia, the critical components that lead to difficulty ambulating independently are presence of flaccidity (muscle power), impaired sensation (proprioceptive feedback), impaired perception of verticality (balance), cognitive difficulties (motor planning), and prior ambulation status (learned patterns)." In an if–then format, this theory might read as follows:

1. *If* normal gait depends on intact muscle power, skeletal stability, proprioceptive feedback, balance, motor planning, and learned patterns, and
2. *if* hemiplegic gait is not normal,
3. *then* patients with hemiplegia must have deficits in one or more of the following areas: muscle power, skeletal stability, proprioceptive feedback, balance, motor planning, and learned patterns.

This theory forms a deductive system by advancing a general theory for the performance of normal gait activities and then examining the elements that are affected in hemiplegic patients. Figure 2–1 presents this theory schematically. The six elements in the theory are central to the figure. In the absense of pathology, normal gait occurs, as shown above the central elements. In the

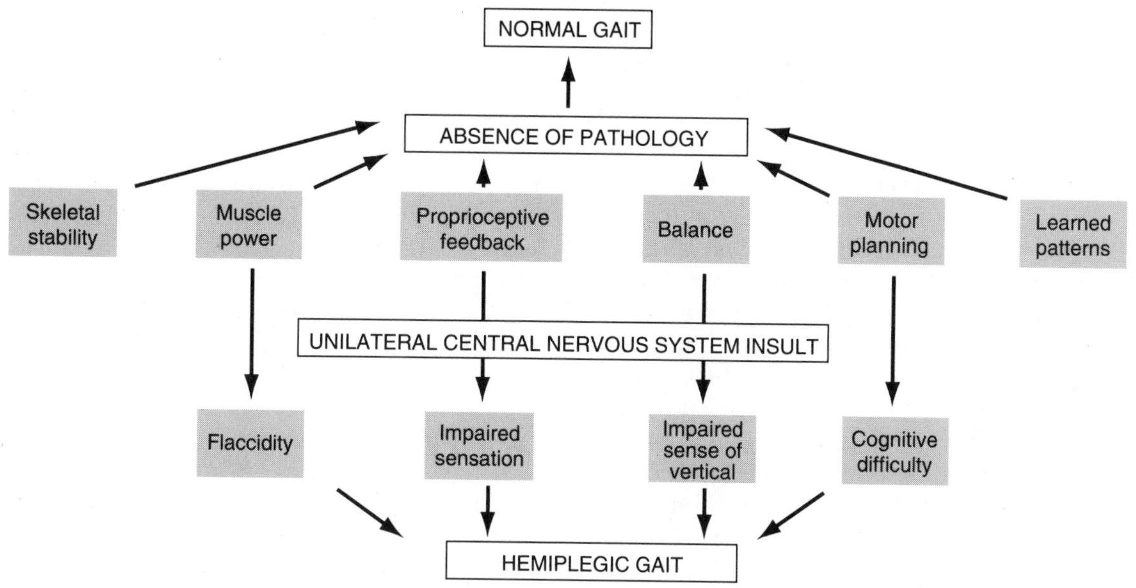

FIGURE 2–1. Diagram of the factors thought to cause hemiplegic gait.

presence of pathology, the elements are altered and an abnormal gait results, as shown below the gait elements.

With a deductive system in place, theory can begin to be used to explain natural phenomena. *Explanatory theory* looks at the why and how questions that undergird a problem. The hypothetical explanatory theory about gait begins to explain ambulation difficulty in terms of six elements needed for normal gait. Of course, explanations can always go deeper: Why do patients with hemiplegia experience balance disorders? How are proprioception and balance related? This spiral of ever more specific explanations is what drives the entire research process: Each time one question is answered, a series of other questions appears to take its place. Table 2–1

TABLE 2–1. Level of Restrictiveness in Theory Definitions

	Level of Restrictiveness		
	Least	***Moderate***	***Most***
Definition	Account for or characterize phenomena	Specify relationships between constructs	Specify relationships and form a deductive system
Purpose	Description	Prediction	Explanation
Comments	Subdivided into ad hoc and categorical theories	Sometimes referred to as conceptual frameworks or models	Can take the form of if–then statements

summarizes the distinctions between the definitions and purposes of theories that meet the different levels of restrictiveness.

Tentativeness of Theory

The second element of the definition of theory is the tentativeness of theory. The tentative nature of theory is emphasized in the following description from an American Physical Therapy Association (APTA) document:

> Theory is a body of interrelated principles, concepts, and constructs that presents a systematic view of phenomena in a manner acceptable at the time to the sciences that study the phenomena. Theory is a formalization of people's beliefs of why things work or why phenomena occur. The formalization makes theory testable by scientific method.[6(p92)]

A unique feature of this characterization is the idea that theory is not absolute, but that it is a view that is acceptable, at the time, to the scientists studying the phenomenon. For example, the idea that the sun revolved around the earth (geocentric theory) suited its time. It was also a useful theory:

> It described the heavens precisely as they looked and fitted the observations and calculations made with the naked eye. . . . It fitted the available facts, was a reasonably satisfactory device for prediction, and harmonized with the accepted view of the rest of nature. . . . Even for the adventurous sailor and the navigator it served well enough.[7(p295)]

However, the small discrepancies between the geocentric theory and the yearly calendar were troublesome to Renaissance astronomers and led to the development of the current heliocentric theory, that the earth revolves around the sun. Perhaps a later generation of scientists will develop different models of the universe that better explain the natural phenomena of the changing of days and seasons. Natural scientists do not assume an unchangeable objective reality that will ultimately be explained by the perfect theory; there is no reason for physical therapy researchers to assume that their world is any more certain or ultimately explainable than the natural world.

Testability of Theory

Another element of the APTA characterization of theory is that theory is testable. Krebs and Harris[8] believe that testability is the *sine qua non* (an indispensable condition) of theory. Thus, theory needs to be formulated in ways that allow the theory to be tested. Theories cannot be proved true because one can never test them under all the conditions under which they might be applied. In addition, if testing shows that the world behaves in the manner predicted by a theory, this does not prove that the theory is true; other rival theories might provide equally accurate predictions. Theories can, however, be proved false by a single instance in which the predictions of the theory are not borne out.

For example, if one can accurately predict the discharge ambulation status of patients with hemiplegia based on tone, sensation, perception, and cognition, then the theory is consistent with the data. However, rival theories might predict discharge ambulation status just as well. A behaviorally oriented therapist might develop a theory that predicts discharge ambulation status as a function of the level of motivation of the patient and the extent to which the therapist provides immediate rewards for gait activities. If the behavioral theory accurately predicts discharge ambulation status of patients with hemiplegia as well as the other theory, it

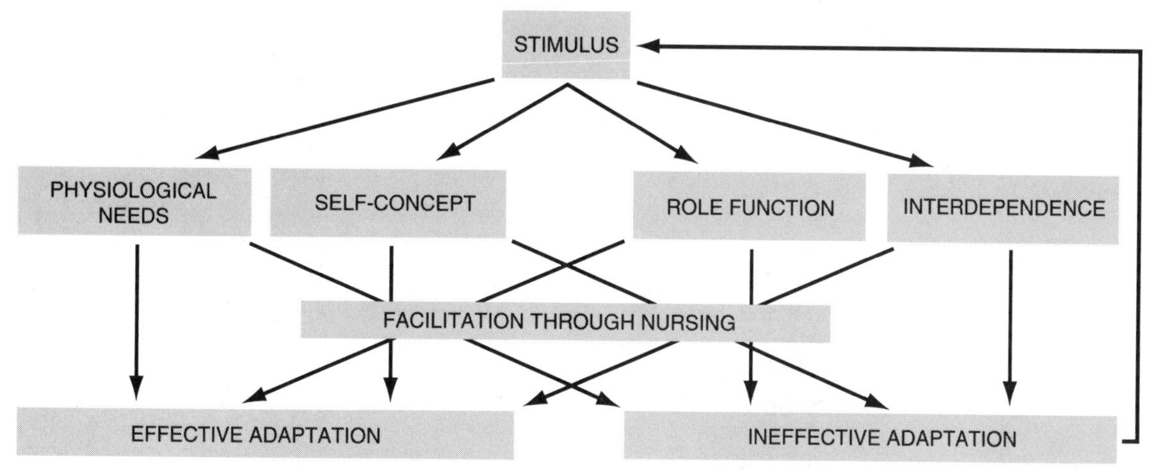

FIGURE 2–2. Simplified diagram of the Roy adaptation model of nursing.

would also be consistent with the data. Neither theory can be proved in the sense that it is true and all others are false; both theories can, however, be shown to be consistent with available information.

Definition of Theory Used in This Text

Because the APTA characterization of theory presented earlier in the chapter is moderately restrictive (it does not require a deductive system), it is appropriate to the current level of theory development in physical therapy. Because the definition also includes the important tentativeness and testability concepts, this characterization of theory guides the remainder of this chapter and this book. In addition, the terms *theory, conceptual framework,* and *model* are used interchangeably.

SCOPE OF THEORY

Theories have been classified by different researchers in terms of their scope. Fawcett and Downs[1(p55)] classified theories as either grand or middle-range theories. To illustrate what is meant by these two different scopes, examples of each type are described.

Grand Theory

Grand theories provide broad conceptualizations of phenomena. The grand theory level is far better represented in the nursing literature than in the physical therapy literature. Thus, examples from both nursing and physical therapy are provided below to illustrate grand theory.

An Example of Grand Theory in Nursing. One of several grand theories in nursing is the Roy adaptation model, which was developed from several psychological and sociological frameworks. This model assumes that people are biopsychosocial beings who adapt to stimuli using one of four subsystems, or adaptive modes: physiological needs, self-concept, role function, and interdependence.[9] The goal of nursing is to facilitate the adaptation process along the health/illness dimension of

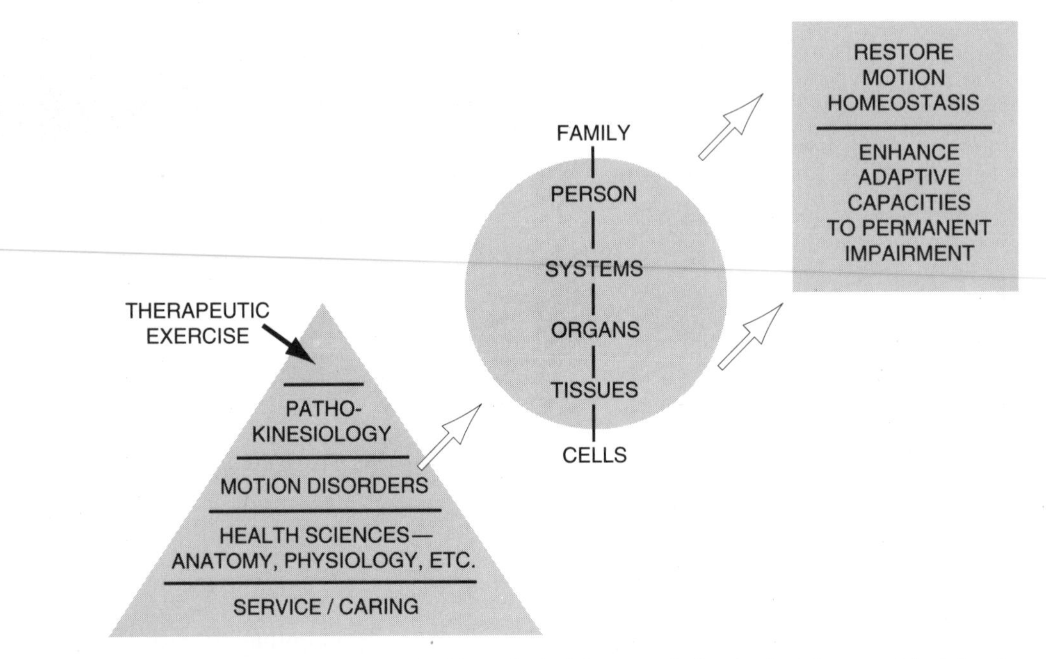

FIGURE 2–3. Interpretation of Hislop's pathokinesiological framework for physical therapy. The triangle represents the structure of physical therapy, the circle a hierarchy of systems affected by physical therapy, and the square the goals of physical therapy. Adapted from Hislop HJ. The not-so-impossible dream. *Phys Ther.* 1975;55:1073,1075. Reprinted from *Physical Therapy* with the permission of the American Physical Therapy Association.

life.[10] Note that this description of the Roy adaptation model is skeletal and is presented for illustrative purposes only; in-depth discussions of this model can be found in the references cited. Figure 2–2 presents a simplified schematic of Roy's adaptation model.

A nurse who is caring for a patient who has just undergone a below-knee amputation might elevate the patient's residual limb to control edema, a physiological factor. The nurse might discuss the patient's altered body image, a self-concept factor. The nurse might discuss how the amputation may affect the patient's leisure activities, a role function factor. Finally, the nurse might facilitate discussion about the patient's need to accept assistance with lawn care, an interdependence factor. One criticism of Roy's model is that the four adaptive modes are not distinctly different from one another. In the example presented here, one could argue that body image, leisure activities, and ability to complete usual chores all relate to self-concept. Physical therapy might also be conceptualized as facilitation of adaptive responses to functional deficits. Roy borrowed ideas from psychologists and sociologists to develop her model; physical therapy theorists could do the same and adapt the Roy model to their discipline.

Examples of Grand Theory in Physical Therapy. Hislop's[11] conceptual model of pathokinesiology and movement dysfunction as the basis for physical therapy is one of few works in physical therapy that can be classified as grand theory. This model looks at physical therapy using the overarching phenomena of movement disorders (others prefer to use the term *movement dysfunction*) and pathokinesiology (the application of anatomy and physiology to the study of abnormal hu-

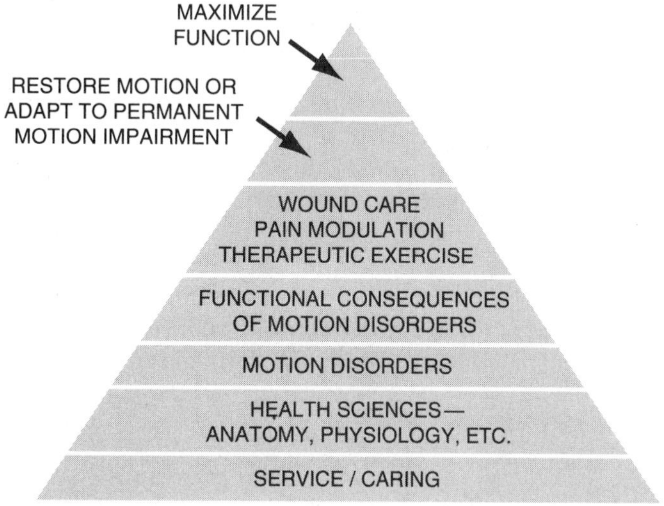

MAXIMIZE FUNCTION

RESTORE MOTION OR ADAPT TO PERMANENT MOTION IMPAIRMENT

WOUND CARE
PAIN MODULATION
THERAPEUTIC EXERCISE

FUNCTIONAL CONSEQUENCES OF MOTION DISORDERS

MOTION DISORDERS

HEALTH SCIENCES— ANATOMY, PHYSIOLOGY, ETC.

SERVICE / CARING

FIGURE 2–4. Model of a functional framework for physical therapy.

man movement). Figure 2–3 is an interpretation of Hislop's formulation of the pathokinesiological basis for physical therapy. Physical therapy is viewed as a triangle with a base of service values supplemented by science, focusing on treatment of motion disorders through therapeutic exercise based on the principles of pathokinesiology. In this theory, physical therapy is viewed as affecting motion disorders related to four of six components of a hierarchy of systems ranging from the family to the cellular level. The goal of physical therapy is to either restore motion homeostasis or enhance adaptation to permanent impairment. Although the pathokinesiological model has been adopted by many within the profession, others caution against turning pathokinesiology into a "buzzword."[12] Purtilo was particularly articulate in her caution to physical therapists:

> The concept of pathokinesiology surely will become chillingly vacuous or be reduced to simply a shrill slogan if physical therapists neglect to engage in a diligent search for its roots and appropriate shape in today's practice of physical therapy.[13(p374)]

An alternative conceptualization of physical therapy might be termed the "functional framework" for physical therapy. Figure 2–4 presents a schematic conceptualization of such a functional framework. The first three elements of the seven-tiered triangle are identical to those of Hislop, and the goal of restoring normal motion or adapting to permanent impairment is also hers.[11(p1073)] This conceptualization differs from Hislop's, however, in that it emphasizes that the functional consequences of movement disorders precipitate the need for physical therapy, it recognizes therapeutic exercise as only one of several types of interventions, and it recognizes function as a higher goal than motion. A named science such as pathokinesiology is not created; this model accepts that professions may legitimately base themselves on the applications of existing sciences.

Which grand theory of physical therapy is correct, Hislop's pathokinesiology model or the functional framework introduced here? The answer is that neither needs to be correct but each must be useful. The purpose of grand theory is to provide broad conceptualizations of a phenomenon, in this case physical therapy. Each theory should be critically evaluated in terms of the extent to which it accurately describes physical therapy and provides a framework for study of phenomena within physical therapy. Different researchers will find that one or the other theory provides a better framework for the questions they wish to ask about physical therapy. Stevens wrote of the folly of adhering to one nursing theory:

> The next obstacle to understanding and developing nursing theory . . . is the great press for a universal, unitary nursing theory. . . . Imagine what we would think of the field of psychology were it to dictate that each of its practitioners be Freudian. Indeed, it is the conflict and diversity among theories that account for much of the progress in any discipline. A search for conformity is an attempt to stultify the growth of a profession.[2(ppxii–xiii)]

Physical therapists need not choose between the pathokinesiological and functional frameworks. What they must do is analyze, develop, and use these theories to enhance their understanding of physical therapy.

Middle-Range Theory

Middle-range theories are more specific than grand theories; they address individual problems and issues, rather than trying to place an entire discipline into a single theoretical context. Two examples of middle-range theory in physical therapy are presented below: theories of muscle strength augmentation with electrical muscle stimulation and a model of the etiology and treatment of chronic ankle instability.

Muscle Strengthening with Electrical Stimulation. Delitto and Snyder-Mackler[14] have presented two middle-range theories about muscle strengthening with percutaneous electrical stimulation. The two theories were developed to explain the results of research on muscle strengthening with electrical stimulation. On the basis of research reports documenting the effectiveness of neuromuscular electrical stimulation, Delitto and Snyder-Mackler advanced two opposing theories to explain the mechanism for the increases in strength: overload and differential recruitment. They then proposed how these two theories could be tested and the types of results that would be found if either theory were operating.

Figure 2–5 is a schematic presentation of research results that would support each theory. The overload theory predicts that muscle performance improvements achieved with electrical stimulation or with exercise should be parallel at all training intensities because electrical stimulation and voluntary exercise place similar functional overloads on muscles. The differential recruitment theory predicts that differences in improvement of muscle performance between high-intensity electrical stimulation and high-intensity exercise will be small, but that differences in improvement of muscle performance between low-intensity electrical stimulation and low-intensity exercise will be great. The physiological basis advanced for this difference is the differential recruitment of muscle fibers in voluntary and electrically elicited contractions. At low intensities, slow-twitch fibers are recruited volitionally. At high intensities, both slow-twitch and fast-twitch fibers are recruited volitionally. With electrically elicited contractions, fast-twitch fibers are recruited first, regardless of intensity of training. Thus, high-intensity electrically stimulated contractions and high-intensity volitional contractions are similar in that they both involve recruitment of fast-twitch fibers. At low intensities, the two types of contractions are quite different in that the volitional low-intensity contraction recruits

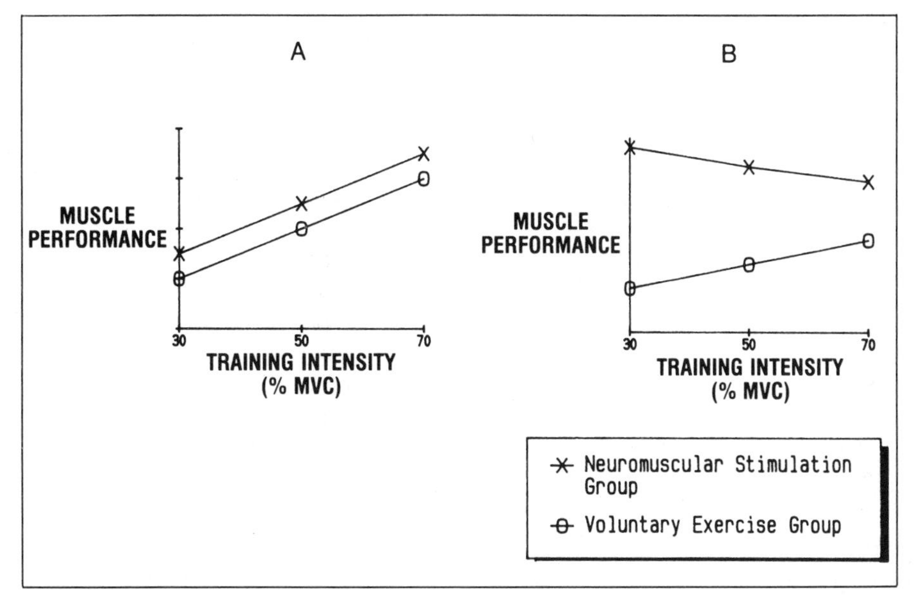

FIGURE 2–5. Competing theories of muscle strength augmentation using percutaneous electrical stimulation. MVC, maximal voluntary contraction. From Delitto A, Snyder-Mackler L. Two theories of muscle strength augmentation using percutaneous electrical stimulation. *Phys Ther.* 1990;70:163. Reprinted from *Physical Therapy* with the permission of the American Physical Therapy Association.

slow-twitch fibers and the electrically elicited contraction recruits fast-twitch fibers. Hence the supposition that differences between volitional and electrically induced contractions are greatest at lower training intensities.

These two theories of muscle strengthening fit the most restrictive definition of theory. Each describes relationships between concepts (the primary concepts being muscle performance, training intensity, and type of exercise). Each has a deductive system that moves from the general (patterns of fiber recruitment) to the specific (improvements in muscle performance). And each can be stated in if–then language: *If* muscle strengthening in the two modes works through a general overload principle, *then* the following results will be seen. The theories are obviously explanatory; they provide physiological rationales for differences between strength increases with each exercise type. These two theories can be tested as suggested by Figure 2–5; they can also provide a framework for further studies of neuromuscular electrical stimulation.

Etiology and Treatment of Chronic Ankle Instability. Lentell and associates[15] reported the results of a study in which their primary purpose was to determine whether peroneal muscle weakness and clinically detectable balance deficits were present in individuals with chronic ankle instability. A secondary purpose was to determine the extent to which peroneal muscle weakness and balance deficits were related in individuals with chronic ankle instability. The background information cited by the authors indicated that three causative factors are frequently given for chronic ankle instability: anatomic instability, peroneal muscle weakness, and proprioceptive deficits. In the discussion section of the article, the authors noted that there are three mechanisms of support for any joint:

osseous configuration, ligamentous restraints, and muscular restraints.

Figure 2–6 presents two schematic drawings, with differing levels of complexity, of how the general support mechanisms can be applied to the ankle and how treatment might proceed based on identified deficits. The question marks on part A illustrate the two portions of the theory tested by Lentell and associates: (1) Are proprioceptive deficits and muscle weakness characteristic of unstable ankles? and (2) Are muscle weakness and proprioceptive deficits related in chronically unstable ankles? This conceptualization meets the most restrictive definition of theory because it has a deductive system: If all joints depend on bony, ligamentous, and muscular restraints for stability, and if loss of one or more of these supports causes instability, then loss of one or more of these supports in the ankle should cause ankle instability.

The benefit of a theoretical framework is that it suggests areas for further research in a way that an isolated study cannot. A schematic diagram of a theory may also reveal gaps in one's thinking. In the development of Figure 2–6 based on information presented in Lentell and associates' article, it became apparent that there was initially no proposed treatment factor that directly corresponded to the anatomic instability factor (Figure 2–6A). Therefore, orthotic stabilization was added (Figure 2–6B). In addition, straight lines from problems to treatments seemed limited. Perhaps, for example, strength beyond that found in normal ankles can contribute to functional stability in the absence of anatomic stability. This idea of compensatory treatment led to the additions of the diagonal arrows in Figure 2–6B.

Table 2–2 presents a range of possible study topics suggested by the elaboration of a theory about chronic ankle instability. An entire research career could be built around testing the elements of this theory. Each subsequent project would either confirm portions of the theory or lead to refinements of the hypothesized relationships.

TABLE 2–2. Research Suggested by the Ankle Instability Model

Anatomic instability
- What are the bony relationships of the unstable ankle in weight bearing?
- Are heel-off and push-off different for normal ankles and unstable ankles?

Proprioceptive deficits
- Does proprioception differ between once-sprained ankles and unstable ankles?
- Do unstable ankles show deficits on multiple measures of proprioception?
- Do unstable ankles have both open- and closed-chain proprioceptive deficits?

Muscle weakness
- Can muscle weakness of unstable ankles be demonstrated in closed-chain testing?
- How do unstable ankles perform on functional muscle strength tests?
- Is endurance of unstable ankle musculature different from that of normal ankle musculature?
- Do muscles other than peroneals contribute to ankle instability?

Relationships among support factors
- Are anatomic stability and proprioceptive deficits related?
- Are anatomic stability and muscle weakness related?
- To what extent are strength and proprioceptive deficits related?

Treatment questions
- Can orthotic stabilization substitute for any of the three support factors?
- Can strengthening beyond normal levels aid stability?
- Does proprioceptive training decrease the frequency of giving way?

RELATIONSHIP AMONG THEORY, RESEARCH, AND PRACTICE

Theory is important because it allows researchers to place questions into logically related clusters and provides a basis for developing ongoing lines of inquiry, as illustrated in the examples earlier. Figure 2–7 presents a schematic drawing showing the relationship among theory, research, and

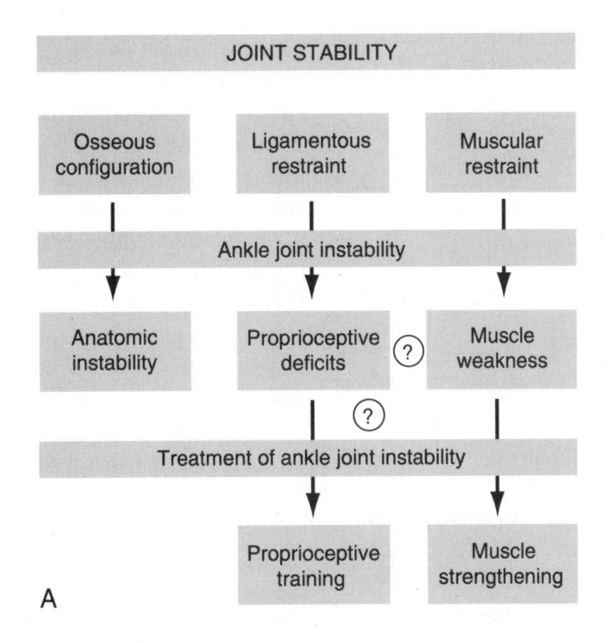

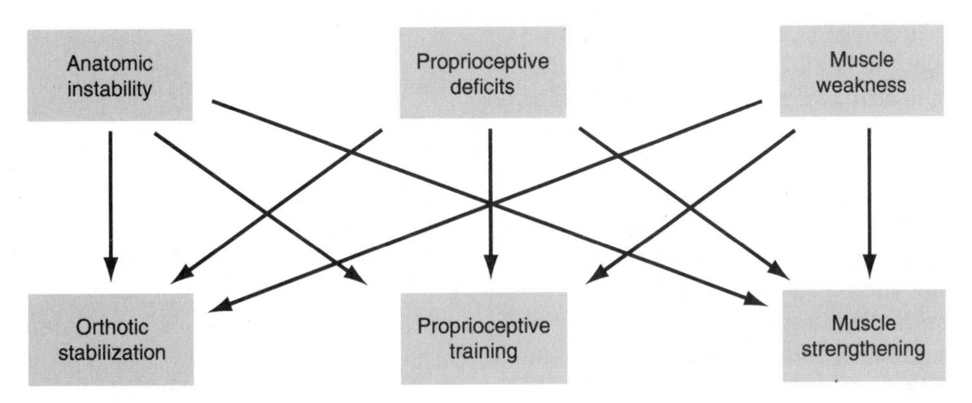

FIGURE 2–6. Diagram of the theory that underlies the etiology and treatment of chronic ankle instability. *A*. A simple theory, as extracted from Lentell GL, Katzman LL, Walters MR. The relationship between muscle function and ankle stability. *Journal of Orthopaedic and Sports Physical Therapy*. 1990;11:605–611. The question marks in *A* represent the relationships tested in that study. *B*. A detailed expansion of the lower portion of *A*, as suggested by the missing elements in *A*.

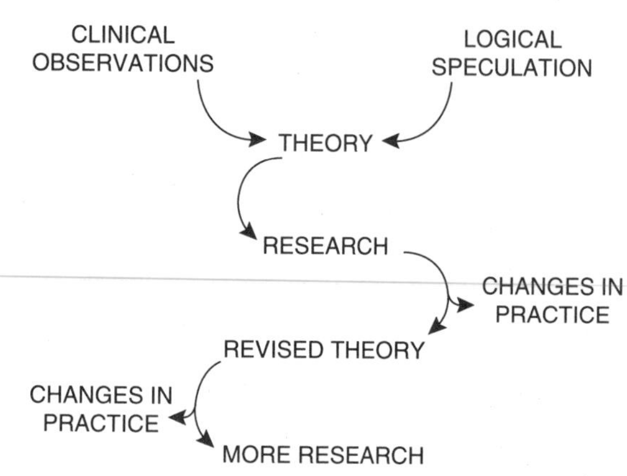

FIGURE 2–7. Relationship of theory, research, and practice.

clinical practice. Theory is developed through either clinical observations and experiences (i.e., "It seems to me that patients who pay for their own therapy are more compliant with home exercise than those whose insurance companies cover the cost") or logical speculation (i.e., "If pain is related to the accumulation of metabolic byproducts in the tissues, then modalities that increase local blood flow should help reduce pain").[16]

Theory is then tested formally through research. On the basis of the research results, the theory is either confirmed or modified, as are the clinical practices that are based on the theory. If the research itself was conducted with a clinical population using the types of treatments that can be easily implemented in actual practice, then clinicians may change their practices based on the research results themselves. If the research was conducted with animals, with normal human subjects, or using techniques not directly applicable to the clinic, then the results will not be directly applicable to the clinical setting. Instead, the research results may lead to modification of the theory, and modification of the theory may in turn lead clinicians to rethink the ways in which they treat their patients.

SUMMARY

Theory in physical therapy can be defined according to level of restrictiveness, tentativeness, and testability. The different levels of theory are used for description, prediction, and explanation. Theories are also differentiated on the basis of scope. Grand theories attempt to place a large body of work into a unified framework and are represented by Roy's[9] adaptation model of nursing and Hislop's[11] pathokinesiological framework for physical therapy. Middle-range theories address specific problems and are represented by Delitto and Snyder-Mackler's[14] theories of electrically stimulated muscle strength augmentation and Lentell's[15] implied theory of the etiology and treatment of chronic ankle instability. Theory, research, and practice are related by the development of theory through clinical observation or logical speculation, through research that tests theories, and through revisions of theory and clinical practice based on research results.

References

1. Fawcett J, Downs FS. *The Relationship of Theory and Research.* Norwalk, Conn: Appleton-Century-Crofts; 1986.
2. Stevens BJ. *Nursing Theory: Analysis, Application, Evaluation.* 2nd ed. Boston, Mass: Little, Brown & Co; 1984.
3. Kerlinger FN. *Foundations of Behavioral Research.* 3rd ed. Fort Worth, Tex: Holt, Rinehart & Winston Inc; 1986.
4. Polit DF, Hungler BP. *Nursing Research: Principles and Methods.* 3rd ed. New York, NY: JB Lippincott Co; 1987:85.
5. Homans GC. Bringing men back in. *American Sociological Review.* 1964;29:809–818.
6. Board of Directors Policy 11–88–40–160. Alexandria, Va: American Physical Therapy Association; 1990:92–94.
7. Boorstin DJ. *The Discoverers.* New York, NY: Random House; 1983.
8. Krebs DE, Harris SR. Elements of theory presentations in physical therapy. *Phys Ther.* 1988;68:690–693.
9. Roy C. The Roy adaptation model. In: Riehl JR, Roy

C, eds. *Conceptual Models for Nursing Practice*. New York, NY: Appleton-Century-Crofts; 1974:135–144.
10. Blue CL, Brubaker RM, Fine JM, Kirsch MJ, Papazian KR, Riester CM. Sister Callista Roy adaptation model. In: Marriner-Tomey A, ed. *Nursing Theorists and Their Work*. 2nd ed. St. Louis, Mo: CV Mosby Co; 1989:325–344.
11. Hislop HJ. The not-so-impossible dream. *Phys Ther*. 1975;55:1069–1080.
12. Rothstein JM. Pathokinesiology—a name for our times? *Phys Ther*. 1986;66:364–365.
13. Purtilo RB. Definitional issues in pathokinesiology—a retrospective and look ahead. *Phys Ther*. 1986;66:372–374.
14. Delitto A, Snyder-Mackler L. Two theories of muscle strength augmentation using percutaneous electrical stimulation. *Phys Ther*. 1990;70:158–164.
15. Lentell GL, Katzman LL, Walters MR. The relationship between muscle function and ankle stability. *Journal of Orthopaedic and Sports Physical Therapy*. 1990;11:605–611.
16. Tammivaara J, Shepard KF. Theory: the guide to clinical practice and research. *Phys Ther*. 1990;70:578–582.

CHAPTER 3

Research Ethics

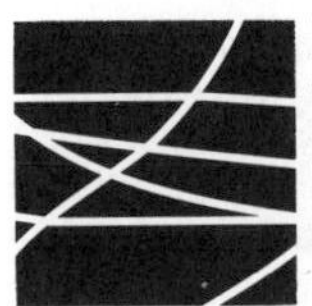

Ethical principles provide a basis for making decisions about personal and professional conduct. Professional groups often formalize ethical principles into codes of ethics that apply general ethical principles to specific practices of professionals.[1] For example, the American Physical Therapy Association (APTA) *Code of Ethics* for the physical therapist provides guidelines for therapist–patient interactions, for interprofessional relations, and for relationships with external parties such as health care insurers and equipment manufacturers.[2] In addition to codes of ethics for clinical practice, various organizations, including the APTA, have developed more specific ethical guidelines for the conduct of research.[3–6]

The existence of these specialized guidelines indicates that there are fundamental differences between practice and research and that these differences have ethical implications. The purpose of this chapter is to articulate ethical principles important to the conduct of research. After the boundaries between physical therapy practice and research are delineated, the basic moral principles to guide action in both areas are presented. Examples of these moral principles in action are given for everyday life, treatment situations, and research settings. A special case of the moral principle of autonomy—informed consent—is then examined in detail. Following this, the specific application of the moral principles to research is illustrated through discussion of several widely used research codes of ethics. Finally, the risks of research to subjects are detailed.

BOUNDARIES BETWEEN PRACTICE AND RESEARCH

Every relationship between the physical therapist and the patient is predicated on the principle that the physical therapist can render services that are likely to benefit the patient. The roles, relationships, and goals in the treatment milieu are vastly different from those in the research setting. In the research setting, the physical therapist becomes an investigator rather than a practitioner; the patient becomes a subject. The patient seeks a practitioner, who may or may not decide to accept the patient for treatment; the investigator seeks potential subjects, who may or may not agree to participate in the proposed research. The patient's goal is improvement; the investigator's goal is development of knowledge.

When accepted physical therapy care is delivered in the context of interaction between the physical therapist and the patient, it is clear that the intent of the episode is therapeutic. When an innovative treatment technique is tested on a group of normal volunteers, it is clear that the intent of the episode is knowledge development. However, when a new technique is administered to a clinical population, the distinction between treatment and research becomes blurred. If the physical therapist views each participant as a patient, then individualized treatment modifications based on each patient's response would be expected. In contrast, if the physical therapist views each participant as a subject, then standardization of treatment protocols is often desirable. Protecting subjects from the risks of participating in research requires that one be able to distinguish research from practice. The National Commission for the Protection of Human Subjects of Biomedical and Behavioral Research, in its *Belmont Report*, developed a definition of research that makes such a distinction:

> Research (involving humans) is any manipulation, observation, or other study of a human being . . . done with the intent of developing new knowledge and which differs in any way from customary medical (or other professional) practice. . . . Research may usually be identified by virtue of the fact that [it] is conducted according to a plan.[7(pp6,7)]

Three main elements of this definition warrant careful consideration: intent, innovation, and plan.

The *Belmont Report* definition recognizes that a fundamental difference between practice and research is that the two entities have different intents. Practice goals relate to individual patients. Research goals relate to the development of new knowledge. Because of these disparate goals, different levels of protection from risk are needed for patients and subjects.

Health care rendered to an individual is always presumed to have some probability of benefit. When deciding whether to undergo a particular treatment, a patient will evaluate its risks against its potential benefits. In contrast, research on human subjects is often of no benefit to the individual who assumes the risk of participation, although subsequent patients benefit from the application of the new knowledge. Some projects fall in a gray zone between research and practice. In this zone, innovative therapies with potential benefits are tested, providing both potential individual benefits and new knowledge.[7]

The second element of the *Belmont Report* definition is that the procedure differs in some way from customary practice. Simply reporting the treatment results of a series of patients who have undergone standard shoulder reconstruction rehabilitation would not be considered research. Because the treatment given is not innovative, the patients do not need special protection; the risk of being a patient whose results happen to be reported is no different from the risk associated with the treatment. Note, however, that if standard treatment calls for isokinetic testing every four weeks, but the group in the series is tested every week, this would now be classified as research. The risks of repeated isokinetic testing, however minimal, are different from the risks of standard treatment alone. An implication of this component of the *Belmont Report* definition is that innovative therapies should be considered research and conducted with appropriate research safeguards until they can be shown to be effective and are adopted as accepted or customary practice.

The third element that distinguishes research from practice is that research generally is conducted according to a plan. This implies a level of control and uniformity that is usually absent from clinical practice.

MORAL PRINCIPLES OF ACTION

All professionals, including physical therapists, deal with complex, specialized issues for which the correct course of action may not be clear. Thus, professionals tend to be guided not by a rigid set of rules, but by general principles that demand that each practitioner assess a given situation in view of those principles and make decisions accordingly.

Although the decisions one makes as a professional differ from one's personal decisions, the underlying principles are the same. This is the case whether one is acting as a practitioner seeing a patient or as an investigator studying a subject: The content of practice and research decisions may differ, but the underlying principles remain the same. Before presenting the ethical principles for the conduct of research, it is therefore appropriate to lay a groundwork of moral principles of action. Four major principles are discussed: nonmaleficence, beneficence, utility, and autonomy. Examples from daily life, practice, and research are given to illustrate these principles.

The Principle of Nonmaleficence

The principle of nonmaleficence states that "we ought to act in ways that do not cause needless harm or injury to others."[9(p33)] In addition, the principle implies that we should not expose others to unnecessary risk. In daily life this means that one should not rob people at knifepoint in the subway or drive while intoxicated. People with backyard pools need to have them fenced properly to protect curious children from accidental drowning. Society levels civil and criminal penalties against members who violate the principle of nonmaleficence.

For physical therapy clinicians, nonmaleficence means that one should neither intentionally harm one's patients nor cause unintentional harm through carelessness. Suppose that a therapist is seeing a frustrating patient, one who demands much of the therapist but does not comply with home exercises to increase shoulder range of motion. The therapist decides to "teach the patient a lesson," being deliberately vigorous in mobilization techniques to make the patient "pay" for not following directions. This action would violate the principle of nonmaleficence; the regimen was intentionally sadistic, not therapeutic.

The practice of physical therapy does, however, require that we expose patients to various risks in order to achieve treatment goals. We cannot guarantee that no harm will come to patients in the course of treatment: They may fall, they may become sore, their skin may become irritated. However, fulfilling the principle of nonmaleficence means that we have to exercise due care in the practice of our profession. Due care requires the availability of adequate personnel during gait activities, planned progression of exercise intensity, and monitoring of skin condition during procedures.

In conducting research, we also must avoid exposing subjects to unnecessary risk. The risks of research are described in detail later in this chapter. In general, though, the principle of nonmaleficence requires that we refrain from research that uses techniques we know to be harmful, and that we terminate our research if harm becomes evident. Although the risks of harm as a consequence of research can be great, there is also harm associated with *not* conducting research. If research is not performed to assess the effects of physical therapy, then patients may be exposed to time-consuming, expensive, or painful treatments that may be ineffective or harmful. When the effects of a treatment are unknown, it is necessary to place someone at risk to systematically assess those effects. The researcher's job is to minimize these necessary risks.

The Principle of Beneficence

The principle of beneficence states that "we should act in ways that promote the welfare of other people."[9(p35)] Not only should we not harm them, but we should attempt to help them. A daily example of the principle of beneficence is the person who goes grocery shopping for a homebound neighbor.

The professional–client relationship is based on the principle of beneficence. Patients would not come to a physical therapist if they did not believe the therapist could help them. The extent of beneficence required is not always clear, however. Occasionally working beyond one's usual hours to provide transfer training to a family member who cannot attend during normal clinic hours is a reasonable expectation of a professional. Never taking a vacation out of a sense of duty to one's patients is an unreasonable expectation.

The principle of beneficence presents conflicts for researchers. As noted previously, the individual subject who assumes the risks of the research is unlikely to be the recipient of any benefit from the research project. Individuals who agree to be in a vigorous early-movement group following anterior cruciate ligament surgery take the risk that the reconstructed ligament may stretch or tear. They may, however, benefit from a shorter rehabilitation time if the new regimen does not lead to failure. The researcher–subject relationship puts immediate beneficence aside for the sake of new knowledge, knowledge that should allow clinicians to establish beneficent relationships with future patients.

The Principle of Utility

The principle of utility states that "we should act in such a way as to bring about the greatest benefit and the least harm."[9(p37)] If a family has limited financial resources, they need to make utility decisions. Should funds be spent on health insurance or life insurance? Which is potentially more devastating financially, an enormous hospital bill or loss of the primary earner's income? The answer that would bring about the most potential benefit and the least risk of harm varies from family to family. If a clinic cannot accommodate all the patients who desire appointments on a given day, decisions about who receives an appointment should focus on who will benefit most from immediate treatment and who will be harmed least by delayed treatment. One would hope that national health care funding decisions would be made on the basis of utility. Which would bring about the greatest benefit and the least harm, funding for prenatal care or funding for neonatal intensive care treatment for premature infants?

Regarding the conduct of research, the principle of utility can guide the development of research agendas. Which projects will contribute most to the advancement of patient care in physical therapy? Which projects involve risks that are disproportional to the amount of beneficial information that can be gained? Should a funding agency support a project that would assess the effects of different stretching techniques on later injury in recreational athletes, or a project that would develop new movement initiation techniques for patients with Parkinson's disease? The former project has the potential to reduce lost work days for large numbers of full-time employees; the latter has the potential to prevent or delay the institutionalization of small numbers of patients with the disease. Knowing about the principle of utility does not make allocation decisions easy!

The Principle of Autonomy

The principle of autonomy states that "rational individuals should be permitted to be self-determining."[9(p41)] Suppose that your elderly mother owns and lives alone in a house that badly needs a new roof. She says that it doesn't rain often, that it only leaks in the formal dining room, and that she won't live long enough to get her money's worth out of a new roof. Your respect for her autonomy indicates that you should respect her decision to determine whether her roof will be repaired.

However, your sense of utility dictates that since the house is your mother's primary financial asset and may be used to pay for eventual health care for her, she will benefit from the preservation of the structural stability of that asset, even if you must violate her autonomy by hiring a roofer yourself. This violation of the principle of autonomy "for someone's own good" is known as paternalism.

Autonomy issues in patient treatment and research revolve around the concept of informed consent. Informed consent is an essential component of the research process and is therefore discussed in detail in the following section.

INFORMED CONSENT

Informed consent requires that patients or subjects give permission for treatment or testing and that they be given adequate information to make educated decisions about undergoing the treatment or test. Four components are required for a patient to make a truly autonomous decision on whether to participate in health care or research: disclosure, comprehension, voluntariness, and competence.[10]

Disclosure. Information about treatment or research is needed before a patient or subject can make an informed decision from among several treatment options. Disclosure of treatment details should include

- the nature of the condition,
- the long-term effects of the condition,
- the effects of not treating the condition,
- the nature of available treatment procedures,
- anticipated benefits of any procedures,
- the probability of actually achieving these benefits, and
- potential risks of undergoing the procedure.

Time commitments related to the treatment should be detailed, as should cost of the treatment. For patients, the physical therapist usually provides this information verbally. The therapist explains the evaluative procedures to the patient, proceeds with an evaluation if the patient agrees, and then outlines the planned course of treatment to the patient. The patient may determine that the time needed for treatment is not worth the anticipated benefit and may not proceed with treatment.

For research subjects, disclosure of research details involves many of the same information items, depending on the nature of the research. Because research is usually not for the immediate benefit of the participant, more formal protection of the research subject is required than is needed for the patient. Thus, information about research risks and potential benefits should be written.

Comprehension. Disclosing information is not enough, however. The practitioner or researcher must ensure that the patient or subject comprehends the information given. Physical therapists who are sensitive to the comprehension issue describe procedures in lay language, prepare written materials that are visually appealing, provide ample time for explaining procedures and answering questions, and allow ample time before requiring a participation decision.

Voluntariness. The clinician or researcher also needs to ensure the voluntariness, or freedom from coercion, of consent. If free health care is offered in exchange for participation in a research study, will a poor family's decision to participate be truly voluntary? If a wife stands over her husband in the examining room and says he'd be a fool not to go ahead with surgery, can we know that the decision is truly his? When a physical therapist requests that patients participate in a study and ensures them that their care will not suffer if they choose not to participate, is it unreasonable for the patients to feel coerced based on the presumption that there might be subtle consequences of not participating? Practitioners and researchers need to be sensitive to real or perceived coercive influences faced by their patients or subjects.

Competence. Competence is the final component of informed consent. One must determine whether potential patients or subjects are legally empowered to make decisions for themselves. Consent from the legal guardian must be sought for minor children. If a legal guardian has been appointed for a mentally ill person, a mentally retarded person, or an incompetent elderly person, then consent must be sought from this party. When conducting research with populations where such "proxy" consent is required, the researcher should also consider the views of the subjects themselves. This should be done especially if it appears that they can make informed decisions about participation even though they do not have the legal power to do so. Suppose that a physical therapist wishes to study the differences between in-class and out-of-class therapy for public school children with cerebral palsy. If out-of-class therapy has been the norm, a child who voices a preference for out-of-class treatment should probably not be required to be a member of the in-class group even though the child's parents have given permission for him or her to be assigned to either group.

The opposite problem occurs when a group is legally empowered to make decisions but the characteristics of the group make informed consent meaningless. For example, at state institutions for developmentally disabled adults, many of the residents may not have legal guardians and are therefore legally entitled to make their own decisions about participation in many activities. They might therefore consent to participate in a research project, but their consent would not be informed.

RESEARCH CODES OF ETHICS

The general moral principles of action discussed earlier become formalized when they are developed into codes of ethics to guide the practice of various professionals. There are four codes of ethics that can provide physical therapy researchers with guidance on ethical issues. The first of these is the Nuremberg Code, developed in 1949 as a reaction to Nazi atrocities in the name of research.[4] The second is the World Medical Association's Declaration of Helsinki, developed in 1964 and modified in 1975.[5] The third is the U.S. Department of Health and Human Services (DHHS) regulations that govern research conducted or funded by the DHHS.[6] The fourth is the *Integrity in Physical Therapy Research* document adopted by the APTA in 1987.[3] The Nuremberg, Helsinki, and DHHS documents are reproduced in their entirety in Levine's *Ethics and Regulation of Clinical Research*.[8] The APTA Ethics and Research Document is reprinted as Appendix A of this text.

Seven distinct ethical themes can be gleaned from these documents; most are present in at least two of the four documents. The themes are informed consent, whether the research design justifies the study, avoidance of suffering and injury, risks commensurate with potential benefit, independent review of research protocols, integrity in publication, and explicit attention to ethics.

Informed Consent Is Obtained

One principle common to all the documents is that the individual must voluntarily consent to participate in the research. The responsibility for ensuring the quality of consent is with the individual who "initiates, directs, or engages in"[4] the experiment. This means that the very important issues of consent should be handled by an involved researcher. Using clerical staff to distribute and collect informed consent forms does not meet this requirement. In addition to securing the consent of their human research participants, researchers should treat animal subjects humanely[3] and respect the environment[5] in the course of their research.

The Design Justifies the Study

A link exists between research methodology and research ethics: "The experiment should be so designed . . . that the anticipated results will justify the performance of the experiment."[4] The implication is that it is not appropriate to expose humans to risks for a study that is so poorly designed that the stated purposes of the research cannot be achieved. This, then, is essentially a utility issue: Why expose people to risk if the probability of benefit is low?

Suffering and Injury Are Avoided

Avoidance of suffering and injury is a nonmaleficence concern. Risks can be avoided through careful consideration during the design of a study and by careful protection of physical safety and prevention of mental duress during the implementation of the study. A concern in the design phase of a study might be how to quantify safely the effects of exercise on the quadriceps femoris muscle. The researchers might consider using various histological, strength, radiological, or girth measures to document change. The final decision about which measures to use would depend both on the specific research questions and on which measures are likely to cause the least amount of suffering or injury.

Safety issues during research implementation would arise if one were evaluating the gait of patients with hemiplegia when walking on a treadmill. Adequate personnel to act as spotters and to monitor blood pressure and electrocardiographic changes would be needed.

Privacy during evaluation and treatment and confidentiality of results can also be considered here as an issue of prevention of mental suffering. Seemingly innocuous portions of the research protocol may be stressful to the subject. For example, a protocol that requires documentation of weight may be acceptable to a subject if the measure is taken and recorded by only one researcher. The same subject may be extremely uncomfortable with a protocol in which the body weight is recorded on a data sheet that accompanies the subject to five different measurement stations for viewing by five separate researchers.

A final component of the safety issue is that the researcher must terminate the study, or an individual's participation in the study, if injury or harm becomes apparent. For example, if a high proportion of patients fall while on the treadmill, the entire study should be stopped. If an isolated patient exhibits a troublesome electrocardiograph while on the treadmill, his or her participation should be stopped, although the study may proceed without this patient.

Risk Is Commensurate with Potential Benefit

High-risk activities can be justified only if the potential for benefit is also great. Levine noted that researchers are usually quick to identify potential benefits of their research, without always considering carefully all the potential risks to participants.[7] Because of the subtle nature of many risks and the duty of researchers to minimize and consider all risks, a detailed analysis of the risks associated with research is presented later in this chapter.

Study Is Independently Reviewed

Adequate protection of human subjects requires that a body independent of the researcher review the protocol and assess the level of protection afforded to the human subjects. The generic name for such an independent body is an *institutional review board* (IRB). The IRB's charge is to examine research proposals to ensure that adequate safety and confidentiality are provided for human subjects, that the elements of informed consent are present, and that the risks of the study are commensurate with the potential benefits. The nature of these committees and the procedures for putting the principles of informed consent into action are discussed in Chapter 18.

Publication Integrity Is Maintained

Researchers need to ensure the accuracy of reports of their work, should not present others' work as their own, and should acknowledge any financial support or other assistance received during the conduct of a research study. Chapter 20 provides specific guidelines for determining who should be listed as a study author and how to acknowledge the participation of those who are not authors.

Explicit Attention Is Given to Ethics

Researchers need to give explicit attention to ethical principles when they design, implement, and report their research. They should act to change research projects for which they are responsible if ethical problems arise or should dissociate themselves from projects if they have no control over unethical acts.[3] For example, assume that a physical therapist is collecting data in a study that is under the direction of a physician. If the therapist believes that patient consent is being coerced, he or she should ask the physician to change the consent procedure, discuss his or her concerns with the institutional review board that approved the study, or refuse to participate further if no change occurs.

RISKS OF RESEARCH TO SUBJECTS

Much of the discussion in this chapter has been related in some way to risk–benefit analysis. The risks of research can be categorized as physical, psychological, social, and economic.[7] Each category is described, and examples from the physical therapy literature are presented when available.

Physical Risks

The physical risks associated with some research are well known. When a particular risk is known, subjects should be informed of its likelihood, severity, duration, and reversibility. Methods for treating the physical harm should also be discussed, if appropriate. If a strengthening study uses isokinetic equipment to provide an overload stimulus to hamstring musculature, participants need to know that almost all subjects will develop delayed muscle soreness, that it will peak 24 to 48 hours after exercise, that it typically dissipates within one week,[11] and that ice and stretching may decrease pain.[12] A higher risk procedure, such as an invasive muscle biopsy, might include the risk of infection. Participants should receive information about signs and symptoms of infection and procedures to follow if infection occurs.

A more subtle form of physical risk is the effect of not receiving treatment. Subjects who agree to receive an experimental treatment may be asked to discontinue a treatment of known effectiveness in favor of a treatment with unknown benefits and risks. Subjects who are placed in a control group are often deprived of the benefits of the accepted treatment for the condition in question. A report by Snyder-Mackler and colleagues provides an example of a study in which discontinuance of accepted treatment was not considered acceptable by the IRB of one of the hospitals at which the study took place.[13] This was resolved by having the control group receive traditional physical therapy and the experimental group receive both traditional physical therapy and the helium–neon laser irradiation that was the modality under study.

The risks of research may be population specific. For example, treatments such as the use of ultrasound over epiphyseal plates have relatively low risk for adults but may have high risks for children.[14] When delineating the risks of participation in a given study, researchers must consider whether the procedures they are using pose special risks to the population they are studying.

The physical risks of an intervention are not always known or may not become apparent for long periods of time. For example, the use of "twister" cables in the treatment of rotational hip deformities is now thought to cause femoral anteversion; this risk was not known when twisters were originally used.[15] Researchers must always consider whether the potential benefit of a study is proportional to its long-term or hidden risks.

Psychological Risks

Although physical therapy researchers naturally focus on the physical risks of their research, they must also consider psychological risks. Subject selection that requires normality can cause psychological harm to those identified as abnormal. Subjects who receive an experimental treatment may lie awake nights wondering what untoward effects they may experience. Subjects in the hypothetical study of the anterior cruciate ligament described earlier in this chapter may experience guilt if their reconstruction fails and the need for a second reconstruction disrupts family or work life. Researchers must carefully consider ways to minimize the psychological risks to participants in their studies.

Social Risks

The major social risk to individual research subjects is the breach of confidentiality. For example, a participant in a work-hardening study in which test results were classified as valid (subject exerting full effort) or invalid (subject not exerting full effort) might have difficulty gaining future employment if he or she is labeled a malingerer.

Another confidentiality concern relates to the manner in which subjects are identified for the research. Patients who receive a mailed questionnaire from a researcher performing a study not connected with their care might understandably wonder how the investigator received their name, and whether their name and address will be put to other uses.

Economic Risks

When research has a combined goal of knowledge and treatment, at least some portion of the payment for the research will be the responsibility of subjects or the subjects' health care insurers. Even if the treatment in question is not experimental, the participant may incur additional costs through lost work hours, baby-sitting fees while undergoing treatment, and transportation costs to and from the research facility.

A major source of economic risk associated with research is the cost of care related to negative outcomes of research. Levine indicated that current ethical thought is that researchers should provide compensation for untoward effects of their research.[8] He noted, though, that few centers have taken the initiative to develop a system for accomplishing this compensation.[8(p159)]

SUMMARY

The differences between practice and research demand that the participants in research receive special protection from the risks associated with research. The general moral principles of nonmaleficence, beneficence, utility, and autonomy form the foundation on which research codes of ethics are built. Informed consent requires that participation be a voluntary action taken by a competent individual who comprehends the risks and benefits of research participation as disclosed by the researcher. In addition to securing the informed consent of their subjects, researchers must ensure that the design of a study justifies its conduct, that procedures are designed to minimize risk, that risk is commensurate with potential benefits, that an independent review body has approved the conduct of the research, that integrity is maintained in publication of the research, and that careful consideration is given to all ethical concerns related to the study. The risks associated with research may be physical, psychological, social, and economic.

References

1. Freidson E. Concept of a profession. In: Abrams N, Buckner MD, eds. *Medical Ethics: A Clinical Textbook and Reference for the Health Care Professions.* Cambridge, Mass: MIT Press; 1983:46–62.
2. American Physical Therapy Association. *Code of Ethics.* Alexandria, Va: American Physical Therapy Association; 1987.
3. American Physical Therapy Association. *Integrity in Physical Therapy Research.* Alexandria, Va: American Physical Therapy Association; 1987.
4. The Nuremberg Code. *Trials of War Criminals before the Nuremberg Military Tribunals under Control Council Law No. 10, Vol 2.* Washington, DC: US Government Printing Office; 1949:181–182.
5. World Medical Association. *Declaration of Helsinki: Recommendations Guiding Medical Doctors in Biomedical Research Involving Human Subjects.* Tokyo, Japan: 29th World Assembly; 1975.
6. Department of Health and Human Services Rules and Regulations, 45 CFR 46. *Federal Register.* March 8, 1983.
7. Levine RJ. The boundaries between biomedical or behavioral research and the accepted and routine practice of medicine. In: The National Commission for the Protection of Human Subjects of Biomedical and Behavioral Research. *The Belmont Report: Ethical Principles and Guidelines for the Protection of Human Subjects of Research, Appendix Volume I.*

Washington, DC: US Government Printing Office; 1975. DHEW Publication OS 78–0013.

8. Levine RJ. *Ethics and Regulation of Clinical Research.* 2nd ed. Baltimore, Md: Urban & Schwarzenberg Inc; 1986:393–412, 425–429.
9. Munson R. *Intervention and Reflection: Basic Issues in Medical Ethics.* 3rd ed. Belmont, Calif: Wadsworth Publishing Co; 1988.
10. Sim J. Informed consent: ethical implications for physiotherapy. *Physiotherapy.* 1986;72:584–587.
11. Talag T. Residual muscle soreness as influenced by concentric, eccentric and static contractions. *Research Quarterly.* 1973;44:458–469.
12. Denegar CR. Effect of cryotherapy, transcutaneous electrical nerve stimulation and a combined treatment, alone and in conjunction with static stretching, on pain, restricted motion and strength loss association with induced muscle soreness. Charlottesville, Va: University of Virginia; 1989. Dissertation.
13. Snyder-Mackler L, Barry A, Perkins AI, et al. Effect of helium-neon laser irradiation on skin resistance and pain in patients with trigger points in the neck or back. *Phys Ther.* 1989;69:336–341.
14. Ziskin MC, McDiarmid T, Michlovitz SL. Therapeutic ultrasound. In: Michlovitz SL, ed. *Thermal Agents in Rehabilitation.* 2nd ed. Philadelphia, Pa: FA Davis Co; 1990:164.
15. Rose GK. *Orthotics: Principles and Practice.* London: William Heinemann Medical Books; 1986:52.

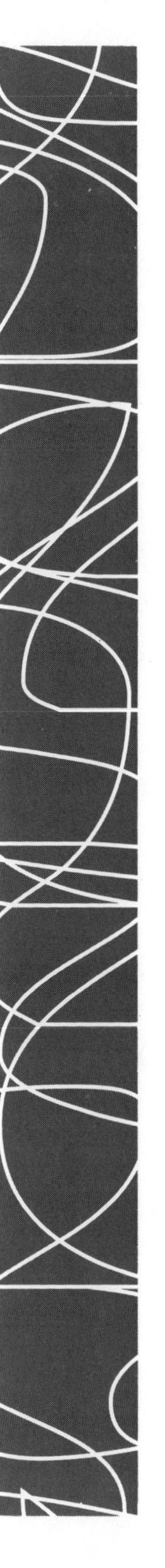

SECTION TWO

RESEARCH DESIGN

CHAPTER 4

Research Problems and Questions

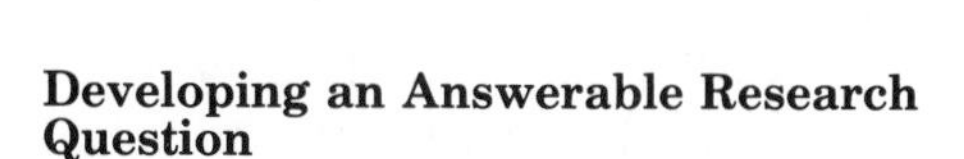

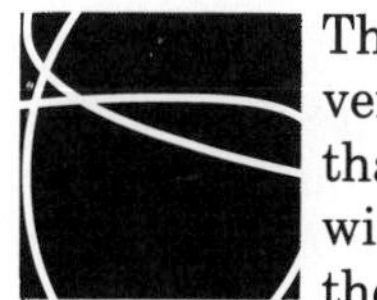

The first step in any research venture is to define the problem that is to be studied. The clarity with which a researcher views the problem at hand will greatly influence each and every subsequent step of the research process. Researchers should therefore devote a great deal of intellectual energy to developing their research problems. In this chapter, strategies for developing problems and questions are presented and criteria are offered for determining whether a question has promise as a basis for research. Hypothetical and actual research problems are used to illustrate the process of research problem and question development.

DEVELOPING AN ANSWERABLE RESEARCH QUESTION

"The challenge in searching for a research question is not a shortage of uncertainties in the universe; it is the difficulty of finding an *important* one that can be transformed into a *feasible and valid* study plan."[1(p12)] Novice researchers usually have little difficulty identifying a general topic of interest: "I want to do something with the knee" or "My interest is in cerebral palsy." From these general statements of interest, they often take a giant leap directly into asking research questions: "What is the relationship between hamstring strength and knee stability in patients with anterior cruciate ligament tears?" or "Does use of ice massage improve hip range of motion in children with spastic diplegia?"

The answers to these questions may well be important to advancing the body of knowledge in physical therapy. Moving directly from topic to question, however, does not establish that the questions are relevant to problems within the profession. This leap also fails to place the research question in a theoretical context. At the inception of a research project, researchers need to focus on *problems within the profession,* not on questions they want to answer. By focusing on problems, researchers are more likely to develop relevant questions, and their research is more likely to make meaningful contributions to the profession. The process of moving from a general topic to a specific research question involves four sets of ideas: topic identification and selection, problem identification and selection, theoretical framework identification and selection, and question identification and selection. At each step in the process, researchers must first be creative enough to generate many ideas and then must be selective enough to focus on a limited number of these ideas for further study. Figure 4–1 shows this process. Each diamond represents an expansion and contraction of ideas; the ovals represent the selection of an idea for further development. The background of the figure is the professional literature, which guides the entire problem development process.

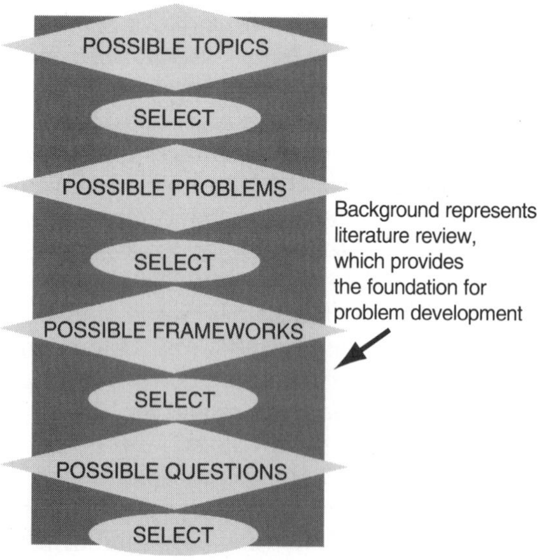

FIGURE 4–1. Development of a research problem. The diamonds represent the expansion and contraction of ideas. The ovals represent selection of an idea for further development. The shaded rectangle in the background represents the professional literature, which is the foundation on which all problems are built.

Topic Identification and Selection

As noted earlier, selection of a general topic is usually not a problem for researchers. For the few who cannot identify a general area of interest, direction should come from reading widely in the literature of the discipline until a spark of interest is found. From all the possible topics considered by a researcher, only one is selected for further study. This is the first of the four cycles of expansion (identification of many possible topics) and contraction (selection of a single topic from the many) of ideas that take place during the development of a research question. One topic is used as a comprehensive example throughout this chapter. Other examples are provided in isolated steps as necessary to illustrate the range of research problems that are available for study.

The idea for the comprehensive example was formed when a physical therapist enrolled in a research course commented that she was concerned that some physicians did not refer patients to physical therapy because of their perception that physical therapy care is very expensive. Potential topics of study within this idea are physician referral patterns, physician perceptions of physical therapy, and the cost of physical therapy. Let's study a problem related to the cost of physical therapy.

Problem Identification and Selection

After a topic is selected, it is the job of the researcher to articulate important problems related to that topic area. Problems, whether in daily life or in research, are perplexing situations without clear solutions. The purpose of research in physical therapy is to shed light on perplexing situations, or problems, within the profession. Unfortunately, many researchers fail to give much consideration to articulating the perplexing situation that their research will address. Clark believes that educational researchers often neglect the process of problem identification:

> The weakness of much of our research in education is that we have failed to take seriously the initial step in research design, that is, formulating the problem. Artists, musicians, novelists . . . all know . . . that variation in the quality of creative products is affected by the way in which the creator formulates the problem. But in education, and much of social science research, we have turned the process upside down. We concentrate on precision in methodology . . . while tolerating imprecision in problem formulation.[2]

Clark has developed a formal framework for developing research problems.[2] He suggests that researchers develop most types of problems through three statements: a principle proposition, an interacting proposition, and a speculative proposition. The *principle proposition* is a given, that is, a statement that is generally accepted. The *interacting proposition* contradicts or casts doubt on the principle proposition. The conflict between the principle and interacting propositions creates the perplexing situation that is the research problem. The *speculative proposition* lists possible causes for the problem. The generation of speculative propositions is a creative effort that begins the process of placing the problem in a theoretical context. The three propositions can be thought of as the "given," the "however," and the "because" statements within a research problem.

Clark has provided a typology of 13 different types of contradictions or conflicts that can form research problems.[2] Of these, the ones that are most relevant to physical therapy research include conflicting evidence; knowledge, action, theory, or policy conflicts; and knowledge voids.

Conflicting Evidence. A conflicting-evidence problem exists when formal evidence about a phenomenon is inconsistent. For example, several authors have documented peroneal muscle weakness in patients with chronic ankle instability. *However*, Lentell and associates were unable to document peroneal muscle weakness in their sample of people with chronic ankle instability.[3] This conflicting evidence may have occurred *because* different authors have used different definitions of chronic ankle instability; because Lentell and associates may have used insensitive measures of strength within their study; because inappropriate comparisons have been made to the "normal" side, which may be weakened from decreased activity; or because strength has been measured inappropriately in nonfunctional open-kinetic-chain positions.

Knowledge–Knowledge Conflict. The conflict here is between different types of knowledge. In the following example, the conflict is between experiential knowledge and formal knowledge. Kendall stated that overstretched musculature is weaker and shortened musculature stronger than musculature at a neutral length.[4] An imbalance in muscle length and strength about a joint is thought to lead to postural deviations. *However*, DiVeta and colleagues found no relationship between position of the scapula and muscular forces produced by middle trapezius and pectoralis minor muscles.[5] This discrepancy between experiential knowledge and formal knowledge may have occurred *because* DiVeta and colleagues did not study a sufficient range of altered muscle lengths, because measuring tools were not sensitive enough to detect differences in strength, because subjects reset their muscles to more effective lengths before initiating maximal contractions, because the range of neutral length is greater than previously imagined, or because there is in fact no relationship between the variables studied.

Policy–Action Conflict. In this type of conflict, there is a discrepancy between professional actions and internal or external rules. Because health care decisions are often influenced by state, federal, or third-party payer policies, this type of conflict arises frequently in physical therapy practice. For example, Public Law 99–457 requires that early intervention programs include an individualized family service plan. *However*, Cochrane and associates found that entry-level and postprofessional curricula in physical therapy provide little information about working with families.[6] This policy–action conflict may arise *because* curricula are slow to adjust to any policy change, because physical therapy educators believe that students need to master patient treatment skills and can acquire other skills when they graduate, because graduates perform well in this area and thus no formal education is needed, because clinical experiences in the physical therapy curriculum provide the needed familiarity with this area, or because material on interaction with family is integrated throughout curricula and was not accurately documented in the study.

Knowledge Void. This type of problem is less confrontational than the others, because there is a void rather than a conflict. Because of the void, the speculative proposition may be self-evident: The void exists because nobody has bothered to conduct research in this area. The speculative proposition may also focus on why and how the principle proposition was established, and why it remains despite lack of supporting evidence. For example, treatment three times per week is a common pattern of outpatient physical therapy delivery, irrespective of the nature of the patient problem or the treatment techniques used. *However*, the benefits of this treatment frequency over other treatment frequencies have not been established. The three-time-per-week frequency may have originally developed *because* theories of muscle strengthening require alternating periods of work and rest, because therapists believe that patients require moderate amounts of time between appointments to assimilate information before receiving additional direction from the therapist, because of a paternalistic view that patients require regular follow-up to ensure compliance with an exercise program established by the therapist, or because practice patterns may reflect an unconscious conformation to the norms set by peers. This knowledge void is the problem that is developed throughout the rest of the chapter.

Sources of Research Problems. As shown by the examples just presented, a problem cannot be defined until the researcher knows what is or is not known about the topic area of interest. The first three problems depended on information presented in the professional literature; the fourth problem was based on lack of information in the literature.

Once researchers define their topic of interest, they must familiarize themselves with the professional literature related to that topic. A review of the literature can identify the conflicts and voids that form the basis for problem development. How to find the relevant literature and synthesize the results from many studies into a conceptual review of the literature is discussed in Chapters 16 and 17.

Theoretical Framework Identification and Selection

Once a problem is selected, it needs to be placed into a theoretical framework that will allow it to be viewed in relation to other works. The literature review that one conducts to establish the problem is likely to be fairly narrowly focused on the topic at hand. In contrast, the theoretical grounding provides a much broader perspective from which to view the problem.

The first phase of theoretical grounding is defining and selecting the *macrostructure* for the study.[7] This is the third cycle of expansion (identification of possible frameworks) and contraction (selection of a framework) of ideas within the problem development process. The researcher should examine the speculative propositions he or she developed earlier for potential approaches to studying the problem. The problem we've chosen to develop throughout this chapter, the treatment-frequency problem, can be viewed from a physiological perspective (the speculation that periods of work and rest are needed for muscle strengthening), from an educational perspective (the speculations that time is needed to assimilate information and that regular reinforcement is needed from the therapist), or from a sociological perspective (the speculation that practitioners are simply conforming to group norms).

Sometimes a researcher is drawn to a particular macrostructure because of his or her previous interests or education; other times the researcher needs to read widely in several areas in order to settle on a macrostructure that seems most promising for further study. For the treatment-frequency problem, let's take the educational perspective as the framework for our study. Readings in the area of patient education focus on adult learning principles, specifically, the Knowles model of adult learning. The model states that the adult learner is characterized by (a) self-directedness, (b) past experiences, (c) readiness to learn, (d) task-centered orientation to learning, and (e) internal motivators.[8] The Knowles model also has implications for the role of the teacher. It indicates that when working with learners with the aforementioned five characteristics, the teacher should act as a facilitator of the learning process rather than an authoritative presenter of information. Because the speculative propositions to our treatment-frequency problem focus on the need for reinforcement from the therapist (related to the self-directedness concept within the Knowles model) and on time needed to assimilate information (related to the readiness to learn concept within the Knowles model), the Knowles model appears to provide a useful macrostructure for the study.

With the macrostructure in place, the second phase of the theoretical grounding of the problem—development of the *microstructure*—can now proceed. The researcher constructs the microstructure by combining the topic and problem with the theoretical framework, specifying the relationships between the variables.

For our treatment-frequency problem, the general topic area is the cost of physical therapy care and the central concepts of the problem are treatment frequency and benefits. The central concepts of Knowles's adult model of learning are the learner characteristics of self-directedness, past experiences, readiness to learn, task-centered orientation to learning, and internal motivators. The final relevant concept is the role of the therapist, which corresponds to the role of the teacher in Knowles's adult learning model.

Thinking about the relationships between these factors might yield a model such as that presented in Figure 4–2. In Part A, an adult learning model of treatment frequency is proposed. When therapists treat patients who exhibit high levels of the adult learner characteristics, they act as facilitators of self-care, see patients infrequently, and realize high benefits at low costs. When therapists treat patients who exhibit low levels of the adult learner characteristics, they deliver care directly, see patients frequently, and realize

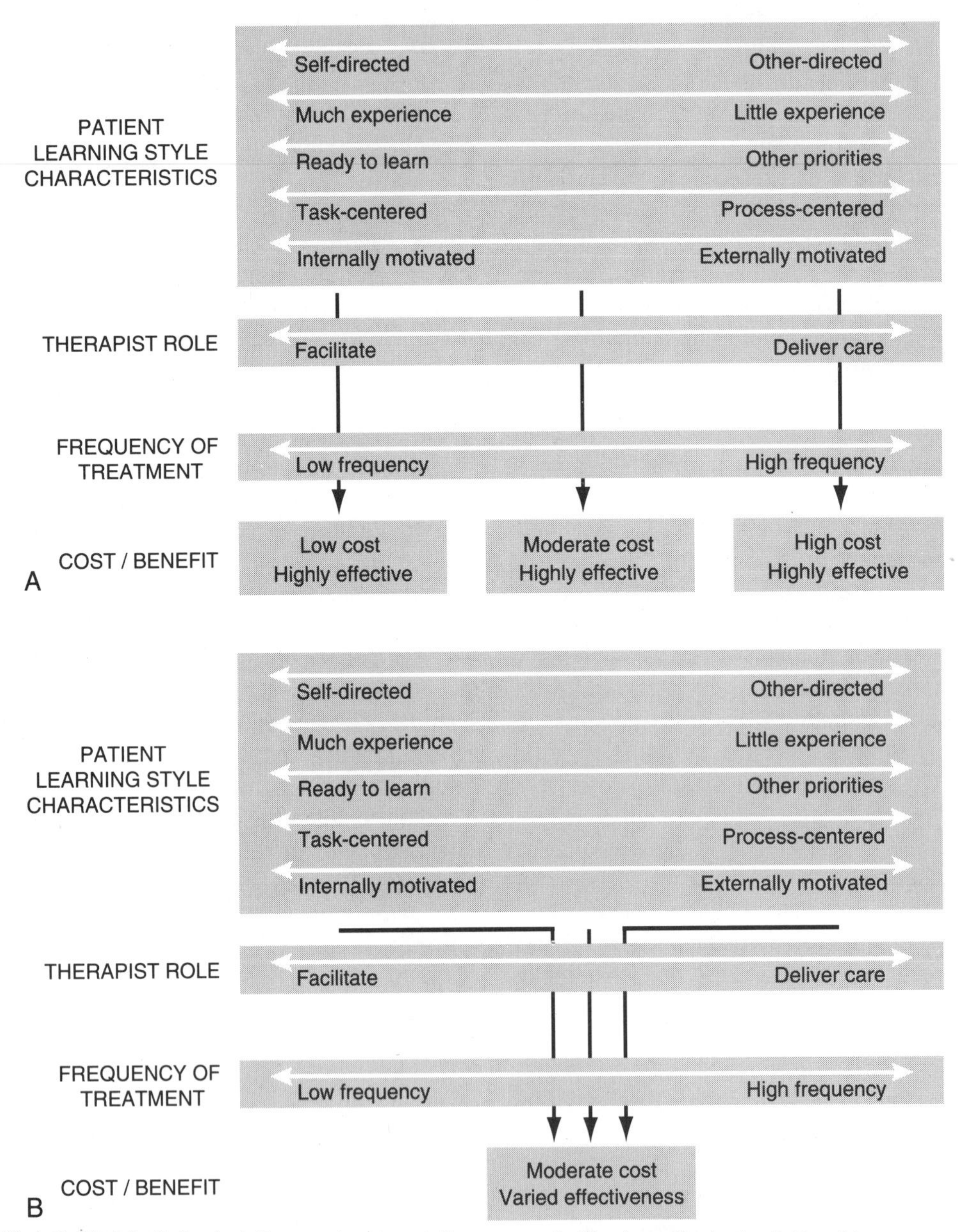

FIGURE 4–2. Model of physical therapy treatment frequency. *A*. The hypothesized relationships among variables when an adult learning model is in place. Therapist role, treatment frequency, and cost match the patient's learning needs. *B*. The hypothesized relationships among variables when a routine treatment frequency model is in place. Therapist role, treatment frequency, and cost are constant, regardless of the patient's learning needs.

high benefits at high costs. In this model, the benefits of therapy are uniform, but the costs vary based on the characteristics of the patients.

In Part B of Figure 4–2, a routine model of treatment frequency is proposed. In this model, therapists assume the same role regardless of patient learning characteristics, see all patients at an intermediate frequency, and achieve inconsistent results. In this model, the cost of therapy is uniform, but the benefits vary based on whether the routine treatment provides enough care to meet the needs of individual patients.

Question Identification and Selection

Once the problem is identified and placed in a theoretical perspective, the researcher must develop the specific questions that will be studied. This is done through the fourth cycle of expansion (identification of many possible questions) and contraction (selection of a limited number of questions for study) of ideas within the problem development process. The model of treatment frequency diagrammed in Figure 4–2 generates the following questions:

1. Do therapists vary treatment frequency on the basis of the learning characteristics of their patients?
2. Do therapists vary their style of treatment on the basis of the learning characteristics of their patients?
3. Do therapists vary their style of treatment on the basis of the specified frequency of treatment?

Others could be generated, but three are enough to demonstrate the types of questions suggested by the model. Let's select the third question for study. Some researchers prefer to state the purpose of their study as a question; others prefer to state their purpose as an *objective*, which takes the form of a declarative sentence; and still others prefer to state a *hypothesis*, which predicts a particular result. The third question restated as an objective would read, "The purpose of this study is to determine whether therapists exhibit different treatment styles in response to different specified treatment frequencies."

A *research hypothesis* is a statement that specifies relationships among variables. It requires the investigator to make predictions about the outcome of the study. The research hypothesis is usually different from the *null hypothesis*, which is a statistical hypothesis (discussed in Chapter 13). The third question rewritten as a research hypothesis based on the adult learning model would read, "We hypothesize that therapists will adopt a more facilitatory care style when frequency of treatment is limited to once a week and a more direct care style when frequency of treatment is specified as three times per week."

Researcher preferences and expectations about the study outcomes will determine whether the research question is framed as a question, an objective, or a hypothesis. In some areas of inquiry, the knowledge void is so great that the researcher is not willing to make predictive hypotheses. In such instances, a question or objective is the appropriate way to state the purpose of the research.

Research Methods Identification and Selection

Only after the research question is determined can the investigator begin to consider which research methods are appropriate to answer the question. Several distinctions can be made between different classes of research. The broadest distinction is between experimental and nonexperimental research. Experimental research involves controlled ma-

.lation of subjects; nonexperimental arch does not.

esearch can also be categorized into types ɘd on two dimensions of interest: the purɘ of the research and the timing of data ection. There are three broad purposes of ɘarch: *description*, analysis of *relationps*, or analysis of *differences* between ›ups or treatments. There are two levels to ɘ time dimension: *retrospective*, in which ɘ researcher uses data collected before the search question was developed, and *proective*, in which the researcher completes ıta collection after the research question is ɘveloped.[9]

A 3 × 2 matrix of research types can be enerated, as shown in Figure 4–3. This figıre also shows that the nonexperimental deıigns appear in all the cells within the ma;rix, but the experimental designs are limited to just one of the cells within the matrix. This reflects the limitation imposed by controlled manipulation as the criterion for experimental research. Experimental designs are discussed in detail in Chapter 5, and nonexperimental designs are discussed in Chapter 6.

Our treatment-frequency problem could be approached in experimental or nonexperimental ways. A nonexperimental study would analyze the relationship between treatment style and frequency. Assume that we have access to a treatment-style inventory (a questionnaire) that rates therapist behaviors and gives a score of 100 for a totally facilitatory care style and a score of 0 for a totally direct care style. On the basis of Knowles's adult learning model, we would hypothesize an inverse relationship between variables such that when treatment frequency is high the treatment inventory score will be low, and when treatment frequency is low the treatment inventory score will be high. Relationship analysis does not require manipulation of therapists or patients; it requires only measurement of the relevant variables and analysis of the relationship between them.

An experimental study of our treatment-frequency problem would require manipulation of treatment frequency and measurement of treatment style. In one of several possible experimental designs, one group of therapists would be selected for study. Half of their patients would receive treatment once a week; the other half would receive treatment three times per week. Treatment sessions would be monitored to determine whether the treatment-style inventory scores were higher when therapists were treating the once-a-week group than when they were treating the three-times-a-week group.

	TIMING OF DATA COLLECTION	
PURPOSE	Retrospective	Prospective
Description	Nonexperimental	Nonexperimental
Analysis of relationships	Nonexperimental	Nonexperimental
Analysis of differences	Nonexperimental	Nonexperimental Experimental

FIGURE 4–3. Matrix of research types.

CRITERIA FOR EVALUATING RESEARCH PROBLEMS

While proceeding through the steps of research problem development, the researcher is faced with several selection decisions. Which topic, problem, or question should be studied? Which research approach to the question should be adopted? Cummings and associates believe that a good research problem is feasible, interesting, novel, ethical, and relevant;[1(p14)] the acronym FINER can be used to remember these five characteristics.

The Study Is Feasible

Feasibility should be assessed in terms of availability of subjects, equipment and technical expertise, time, and money. For example, if a therapist wishes to study the differences between two electrical stimulation bicycle ergometry programs for patients with spinal cord injury, he or she needs to have access to adequate numbers of patients who are willing to participate in a lengthy study. If the phenomenon of delayed muscle soreness is to be studied, subjects who are willing to experience soreness must be found.

Physical therapy researchers need to be realistic about the technical resources available to them. If a therapist wishes to study hindfoot movement during ambulation in different types of footwear, then motion analysis equipment is required. If the proper equipment is not available, then another problem should be selected for study.

Researchers often underestimate the time needed to complete a research study. Physical therapy students usually have a time limitation for degree completion, so they must develop their research questions in light of that limitation. Physical therapy clinicians must view research in light of the varied demands on their time. As noted in Chapter 1, lack of time is a significant impediment to clinical research. Rather than decide that research in general is not feasible, clinicians need to develop research questions that can be answered within the time constraints of their clinics.

Financial resources needed to conduct research must also be considered. Direct costs such as equipment, postage, and printing must be met. Personnel costs may include salaries and benefits for the primary investigator, data collectors, secretaries, statisticians, engineers, and photographers. If there are no funds for statisticians and engineering consultants, then complex experimental designs with highly technical measures should not be attempted.

The Problem Is Interesting

The research question must be of interest to the investigator. Physical therapy is a broad profession, and physical therapy research is in its infancy. Given these two facts, there should be no reason for physical therapy researchers to study questions that do not whet their intellectual appetites. Research can be an exciting venture, but several steps along the way are tedious and time consuming. The researcher must be interested in the question to be motivated to get through the drudgery to reach the discovery.

The Problem Is Novel

Good research adds to knowledge. However, novice researchers are often unrealistic in their desire to be totally original in what they do. Novel research problems are designed to either confirm or refute previous findings, extend previous findings, or provide new findings.[1(p14)] Many aspects of physical therapy are not well documented, so novel research ideas abound.

The Problem Can Be Studied Ethically

An ethical study is one in which the elements of informed consent can be met and the risks of the research are in proportion to the potential benefits of the research, as described in Chapter 3. In the rehabilitation literature, for example, there are no studies comparing a comprehensive rehabilitation program with a program consisting of no rehabilitation services for patients who have had cerebral vascular accidents. Such a protocol would be considered unethical because a totally untreated control group would be at risk for developing complications of bedrest or requiring extended care. Researchers overcome this ethical concern by comparing different levels of rehabilitation services rather than completely depriving some patients of such care.

The Question Is Relevant

When developing research questions, physical therapists need to answer an important relevancy question: "Who cares?" If the first phase of the problem development process was taken seriously, the researcher should be able to provide a ready answer to that question. If the researcher skipped that phase and generated a research question without knowing how it related to a problem within the profession, then the question may not be relevant to physical therapy practice. Relevant physical therapy research questions are grounded in day-to-day problems faced by physical therapists.

SUMMARY

The research problem development process involves selection of a topic of interest, a problem within the profession, a theoretical framework for the study, and one or more specific questions related to the problem as conceptualized through the theoretical framework. Only after these four steps have been completed should the researcher begin to consider the various research methods that could be used to answer the questions. Good research problems are feasible, interesting, novel, ethical, and relevant.

References

1. Cummings SR, Browner WS, Hulley SB. Conceiving the research question. In: Hulley SB, Cummings SR, eds. *Designing Clinical Research.* Baltimore, Md: Williams & Wilkins; 1988.
2. Clark DL. Worksheet A—Statement of the Problem. Unpublished material. Charlottesville, Va: School of Education, University of Virginia; 1990.
3. Lentell GL, Katzman LL, Walters MR. The relationship between muscle function and ankle stability. *Journal of Orthopaedic and Sports Physical Therapy.* 1990;11:605–611.
4. Kendall FP, McCreary EK. *Muscles: Testing and Function.* 3rd ed. Baltimore, Md: Williams & Wilkins; 1983:270–272.
5. DiVeta J, Walker ML, Skibinski B. Relationship between performance of selected scapular muscles and scapular abduction in standing subjects. *Phys Ther.* 1990;70:470–476.
6. Cochrane CB, Farley BG, Wilhelm IJ. Preparation of physical therapists to work with handicapped infants and their families: current status and training needs. *Phys Ther.* 1990;70:372–380.
7. Clark DL. Worksheet C—Logical Structure: A Perspective on the Study. Charlottesville, Va: School of Education, University of Virginia; 1990.
8. Knowles MS. Introduction: the art and science of helping adults learn. In: Knowles MS, ed. *Andragogy in Action.* San Francisco, 1984:12.
9. Tietjen GL. *A Topical Dictionary of Statistics.* New York, NY: Chapman & Hall; 1986:125.

CHAPTER 5

Experimental Research

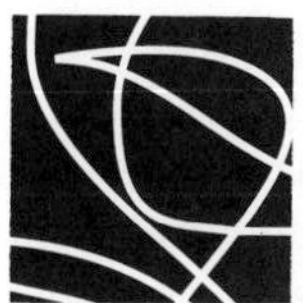

Experimental research, as defined in Chapter 4, is characterized by controlled manipulation of variables by the researcher. In this chapter, experimental designs are described in detail, to provide readers with a sense of the diversity and complexity of research designs presented in the physical therapy literature. The chapter is divided into four major sections. The two hallmarks of experimental research—manipulation and control—are discussed, followed by explanations of single-factor and multiple-factor research designs. Although some evaluation of the relative merits of the different designs is incorporated in this chapter, a complete discussion of the problems, or sources of invalidity, associated with both experimental and nonexperimental designs is deferred until Chapter 7.

Even though this chapter on design is presented separately from earlier chapters on problem development and later chapters on data analysis, recognize that these three phases of the research process are, in fact, inseparable. The research problem influences the design, and the design influences the analysis.

MANIPULATION

The essential characteristic of experimental research is controlled manipulation of variables by the researcher, and the purpose for doing experimental research is to determine whether the manipulation caused some change in the subjects under study. Any experimental design must include controlled manipulation of at least one variable, which is termed the *independent variable*, or the *factor*. The effect of manipulation of the independent variable is determined by variations in some measure of interest, called the *dependent variable*. This section of the chapter presents examples of manipulated and nonmanipulated variables, discusses interpretation of experimental research results, and presents examples of independent and dependent variables in simple and complex research studies.

Manipulation of Variables

The specification that manipulation be controlled distinguishes experimental designs from nonexperimental reports of clinical outcomes. However, determination of whether controlled manipulation has occurred is more complicated than might be imagined. In some experiments, controlled manipulation is obvious. For example, King and associates measured pain threshold in a group of normal subjects, applied a standardized treatment to acupuncture points, and then remeasured pain threshold.[1] Treatment to the acupuncture point was the manipulation, and the standardization of the treatment lent a great deal of control to the experiment.

However, some nonexperimental research studies appear to be experimental because an independent variable takes several values within the study. Closer examination reveals that although an independent variable is present, it has not been manipulated in a controlled manner by the researcher. There are four general categories of nonmanipulated independent variables: (1) The manipulation was retrospective, (2) the variable is inherently nonmanipulable, (3) the variable could have been manipulated but was not, and (4) the independent variable is an integral part of the measurement of the dependent variable.

Manipulation Is Retrospective. Consider a case in which a therapist reviews the initial and discharge range-of-motion measurements reported in the clinical records of his or her last 20 patients with low back pain who received heat and exercise. This type of study is retrospective because the researcher seeks to answer a question by examining data that were collected before the question was developed. When the data are collected before the question is developed the researcher has little or no control over the actual implementation of the treatment, the outside activities of the patients, or the technique of measuring range of motion. Even though the heat and exercise are manipulations, this example does not meet the controlled-manipulation criterion and is considered a nonexperimental study.

The Variable Is Nonmanipulable. A common example of a nonmanipulable independent variable is subject age. Researchers cannot change the age of subjects who present themselves for study; they can only group subjects according to age. This type of a variable is called an *attribute* or a *classification* variable. When a grouping is made on the basis of some attribute, and not through random assignment, it is called a *block*.

The Researcher Chooses Not to Manipulate. Sometimes a variable can be manipulated but is not. For example, Sinaki and Offord studied the relationship of physical activity and back muscle strength to bone mineral density in postmenopausal women.[2] It is possible to manipulate the variable physical activity. For example, subjects could be randomly assigned to two groups: One group of women would participate in a weight-bearing exercise program for 18 months, and the other group would maintain a sedentary lifestyle during the same period of time. A study that manipulated physical activity in this manner would be an experimental study. Sinaki and Offord, however, did not *manipulate* physical activity. They merely *measured* the physical activity, back muscle strength, and bone mineral density of postmenopausal women, and examined the relationships among the variables. Despite the potential for manipulation of the variable physical activity, the researchers chose to study the problem nonexperimentally, without manipulation.

The Independent Variable Is a Component of the Dependent Variable. Sometimes an inherent part of the measurement of a dependent variable is treated as an independent variable. With the increasing sophistication of measurement tools in physical therapy comes that ability to vary aspects of the measurement itself. For example, isokinetic testing can occur at varying speeds, anterior–posterior displacement of the tibia on the femur can be measured under different stress levels, and grip strength can be measured at different handle positions on a dynamometer.

An example of this alteration of the measurement tool is found in Hageman and associates' study of the effects of speed and limb dominance on isokinetic testing of the knee.[3] In this study, the quadriceps femoris and hamstring muscles of both legs of participants were tested at 30°/s and 180°/s on an isokinetic dynamometer. Speed and limb dominance were the independent variables; torque and torque:body weight ratio were the dependent variables. Limb dominance is an inherently nonmanipulable factor. The nature of the speed-of-testing variable is not quite as clear-cut. Certainly the researchers placed different demands on participants by testing them first at a slow speed, then at a faster speed. However, the manipulation of the speed of testing is so closely tied to the measurement of the dependent variable that it is difficult to consider it a separate experimental manipulation.

When the only manipulation that occurs is an inherent part of the measurement of the dependent variable, the research should be considered nonexperimental. However, an important distinction must be made between the use of certain equipment for testing versus training purposes. If speed is manipulated as part of a training program, then the study becomes experimental. If one group of subjects participates in a four-week isokinetic exercise program at 30°/s, and another group exercises at 180°/s, then the independent variable becomes speed of training. Manipulating the speed of training is an experimental approach; manipulating only the speed of testing is a nonexperimental, descriptive approach.

Interpretation of Experimental Research

Experimental research occurs when the researcher manipulates a variable or variables in a controlled fashion. Nonexperimental research describes existing phenomena, without alteration through manipulation. Although one type of research is not inherently superior to the other, interpretation of research results differs depending on the methods of study, and thus it is important that readers of the literature be able to distinguish between experimental and nonexperimental studies.

In particular, the presence of controlled manipulation enables researchers to draw *causal conclusions* about the variable under study, although the strength of the conclusions depends on the level of control in the research study. For example, Rikli and McManis studied the effects of three different exercise conditions (general aerobic exercise, aerobic exercise plus upper body weight training, and no exercise) on bone mineral content in three groups of postmenopausal women.[4] They assigned each woman to one of the three groups and monitored her participation in the appropriate conditioning class for 10 months. They found that the exercising groups had increased bone mineral content compared with the nonexercising control group. The controlled manipulation of activity level allowed them to conclude that the exercise programs caused the change in bone mineral content.

In contrast, Sinaki and Offord's nonexperimental study of the relationships among physical activity, back muscle strength, and bone mineral content can only lead to the conclusion that physical activity is related to changes in bone mineral content, not necessarily the cause of them.[2] Uncontrolled factors such as diet or body weight might be equally plausible explanations of differences in bone mineral content among subjects. Without controlled manipulation, no causal conclusions can be drawn.

Identification of Independent and Dependent Variables

Contemporary experimental researchers in physical therapy frequently examine several different manipulated factors in the same study. Unfortunately, research reports do not always explicitly identify the number and character of the independent variables in the study. In this section of the chapter, three research reports are dissected to make explicit the number and character of the independent variables studied. A report of experimental research will never make sense to readers unless they understand the factors of interest within the study. A *variable* is some characteristic that takes different forms within a study. In contrast, a *constant* takes only one form within a study. If the differences between range-of-motion values for men and women are studied, then sex is a variable. If range-of-motion values for women only are studied, sex is a constant.

According to Kerlinger, "an *independent variable* is the *presumed* cause of the *dependent variable*, the *presumed* effect."[5(p32)] An independent variable is also sometimes called a *factor*. By definition, in experimental research at least one independent variable, or factor, must be manipulated by the investigator. Additional nonmanipulated variables such as age or sex may also be studied as components of experimental research.

Analysis of Research Titles. The first indication of whether a study is experimental or nonexperimental is found in the title of the research article. When the title contains the phrase "the effects of" or refers to a specific effect that was found, the study was likely experimental.

In addition to providing clues about the nature of the research, the article title presents preliminary information about the independent and dependent variables. Preliminary identification of the independent and dependent variables in the three research reports we are examining in this chapter is presented in Table 5–1, based solely on the information contained in the title of each article.[6–8]

Levels of the Independent Variable. A full description of each independent variable includes the *levels* of the independent variable. The levels of the independent variable are the forms that the independent variable takes within the study. The three articles whose titles are listed in Table 5–1 demonstrate what is meant by levels of the independent variable. As you will see, the studies are more complex than their titles alone indicate.

Identification of the independent variable in the first study, Burr and associates' research on bone loading, is straightforward.[6] The design is diagrammed in Figure 5–1. There was one independent variable, group. There were two levels of group: loaded, which was the experimental treatment, and sham loaded, which was the control treatment. An apparatus was used to load the right hindlegs of the three experimental-group rabbits with their own body weight. The three control-group rabbits maintained normal activity in their cages. The dependent variables were

TABLE 5–1. Independent and Dependent Variables in Three Research Article Titles

Title	Independent Variable	Dependent Variable
"Lower Extremity Loads Stimulate Bone Formation in the Vertebral Column: Implications for Osteoporosis"[6]	Lower extremity loading	Bone formation
"Effects of a Developmental Physical Therapy Program on Oxygen Saturation and Heart Rate in Preterm Infants"[7]	Physical therapy	Oxygen saturation Heart rate
"Effects of High Voltage Pulsed Electrical Stimulation on Blood Flow"[8]	Electrical stimulation	Blood flow

four bone remodeling measures (osteons/mm^2, percent surface bone formation, resorption spaces/mm^2, and intracortical porosity) measured in each of nine locations (right tibia, left tibia, right humerus, left humerus, L_6, L_1, T_{12}, T_1, and C_7). Thus, 36 dependent measures (4 measures × 9 locations) were collected for each rabbit.

The second example, a study of a developmental physical therapy program for preterm infants, is considerably more complex than the bone development study. As diagrammed in Figure 5–2, Kelly and associates observed infants while resting, during administration of a treatment consisting of six activities, and during a recovery period after the treatment.[7] Three of the activities were administered when the infants were in a sidelying position, and three were administered with the infants in a supported sitting position; all six were administered in a random order. The first independent variable was phase. The phase variable had seven levels: baseline, early intervention, middle intervention, late intervention, early recovery, middle recovery, and late recovery. If you read the article, you will see that 44 measurements of heart rate and 44 measurements of oxygen saturation were actually taken over time for each subject within the study. Why then wasn't the inde-

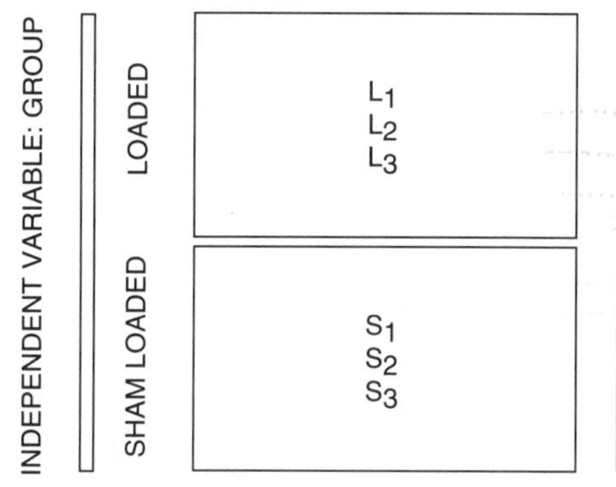

FIGURE 5–1. Study of bone loading in rabbits. One independent variable was used, with posttest measures only. Thirty-six dependent measures were taken on each of the three rabbits in each group. L, loaded; S, sham loaded. (Experimental design presented in Burr DB, Martin RB, Martin PA. Lower extremity loads stimulate bone formation in the vertebral column: implications for osteoporosis. *Spine*. 1983;8:681–686.)

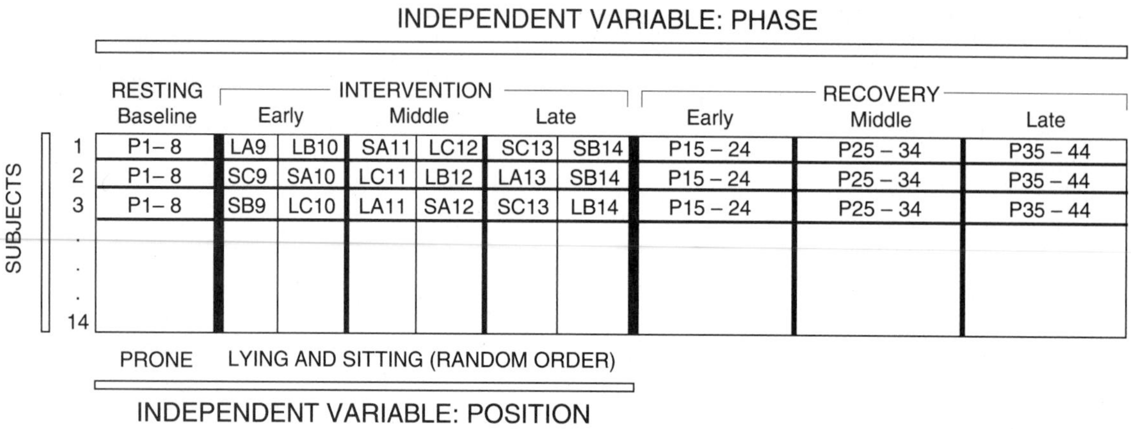

INDEPENDENT VARIABLE: PHASE

SUBJECTS	RESTING	INTERVENTION						RECOVERY		
	Baseline	Early		Middle		Late		Early	Middle	Late
1	P1–8	LA9	LB10	SA11	LC12	SC13	SB14	P15–24	P25–34	P35–44
2	P1–8	SC9	SA10	LC11	LB12	LA13	SB14	P15–24	P25–34	P35–44
3	P1–8	SB9	LC10	LA11	SA12	SC13	LB14	P15–24	P25–34	P35–44
.										
.										
.										
14										
	PRONE	LYING AND SITTING (RANDOM ORDER)								

INDEPENDENT VARIABLE: POSITION

FIGURE 5–2. Study of developmental physical therapy for 14 preterm infants. Two independent variables were used, phase and position. Forty-four measures of O_2 saturation and heart rate were taken for each infant. Infants were placed in one of three positions: P, prone; S, supported sitting; and L, side-lying. During the intervention phase, three activities (A, B, and C) were administered in each of the positions, in a random order. Thus, for example, the first infant might have received the first activity in the side-lying position before the ninth measurement was taken (LA9); the second infant might not have received the same activity until before the thirteenth measurement was taken (LA13). (Experimental design presented in Kelly MK, Palisano RJ, Wolfson MR. Effects of a developmental physical therapy program on oxygen saturation and heart rate in preterm infants. *Phys Ther*. 1989;69:467–474.)

pendent variable really time, with 44 levels? Because it would be very difficult to conceptualize 44 levels of the variable time, the authors collapsed the 44 levels into the more manageable 7 levels, which they referred to as "phase." The dependent variables of interest in each phase, then, were the average of the heart rate measurements and the average of the oxygen saturation measurements taken during that phase.

The second independent variable in Kelly and associates' study was position. This variable had three levels: prone position (during baseline), sidelying position (during intervention), and supported sitting (during intervention). Note that the authors were not interested in the interrelationship between position and phase; if they had been, they would have needed to design the study so that each position would have been implemented in each phase. Each subject received the six different activities in a different sequence of intervention. The dependent measures used to assess the effects of position were the mean of the heart rate and oxygen saturation measures taken when subjects were prone during the baseline, the mean of the measures taken when subjects were in the sidelying position, and the mean of the measures taken when subjects were in a supported sitting position.

In the third example, Walker and associates studied blood flow responses to electrical stimulation.[8] Their study adds another layer of complexity to the identification of independent variables, as diagrammed in Figure 5–3. Subjects were assigned to one of three groups: stimulation, exercise, or rest. Each subject rested, exercised, or was stimulated at two different intensities: 10% and 30% of maximum voluntary contraction torque of the right plantar flexor muscle. Measurements of blood flow, heart rate, systolic blood pressure, and diastolic blood pressure were taken at three different times at each intensity: before intervention, at the midpoint of intervention,

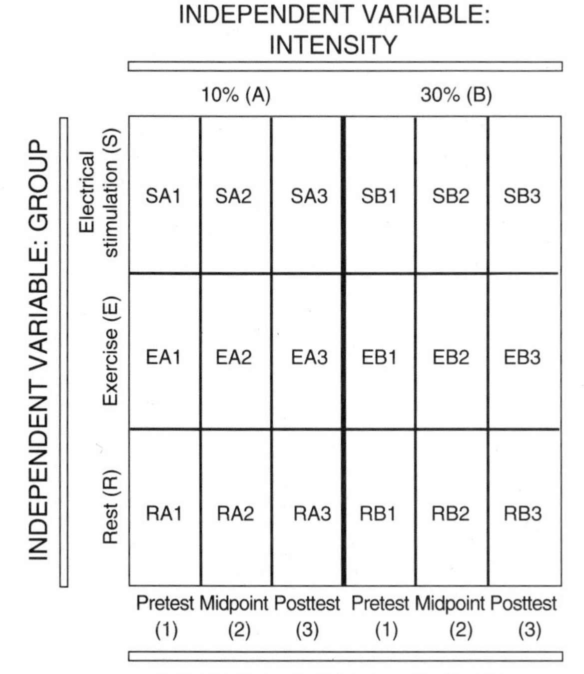

FIGURE 5–3. Study of blood flow responses to rest (R), voluntary exercise (E), and electrical stimulation (S) at different intensities and times. Each group was measured at each intensity and time. (Experimental design presented in Walker DC, Currier DP, Threlkeld AJ. Effects of high voltage pulsed electrical stimulation on blood flow. *Phys Ther.* 1988;68:481–485.)

and at the conclusion of the intervention. There were three independent variables in this study: group, intensity, and time. The group variable had three levels: rest, voluntary exercise, and electrical stimulation. The intensity variable had two levels: 10% and 30% of maximum voluntary contraction torque. The time variable had three levels: pretest, midtest, and posttest. Shorthand notation for this design would be that it was a 3 × 2 × 3 design. These three factors were all *crossed* with one another in that each level of each factor occurred with each of the other factors. The authors were interested not only in the effects of each variable alone, but also in the interrelationships among the three factors.

From the hypothetical and real examples presented in this section of the chapter, readers should now be able to differentiate between experimental and nonexperimental research on the basis of whether a controlled manipulation has occurred. Having determined that a research report is indeed representative of experimental research, the reader should also be able to identify the names and levels of the independent variables within those experimental studies.

CONTROL

Experimental research can be divided into true experimental and quasiexperimental categories based on the level of control present in the study. True experiments are characterized by high levels of control. This control takes the form of at least two separate groups of subjects, with random assignment of subjects to groups. The term *randomized clinical trial* is used frequently to describe health care research that is truly experimental in nature.[9]

Quasiexperimental research is characterized by less control than true experimental research, and this lesser degree of control of the experimental situation is achieved either with a single subject group, whereby subjects act as their own controls, or by using multiple groups to which subjects are not randomly assigned. Some authors believe that quasiexperimental studies are inferior designs that should only be used when a true experimental study is not feasible.[10, 11] Some authors even classify quasiexperimental designs as nonexperimental research.[9]

There are two problems with such strong differentiation between true experimental and quasiexperimental research. First, the value of quasiexperimental research designs in which subjects are used as their own controls is underestimated. There are many clinical research questions for which single-group, quasiexperimental designs are ideal; several are presented throughout this chapter. Second, the ability of true experimental designs to capture the complexity of the clinical situation is overestimated. True experiments are far more controlled than the daily practice of physical therapy, and the results of such experiments may apply only to similarly controlled situations.[12] In this text, then, the term *experimental research* is used to refer to both truly experimental and quasiexperimental designs.

In any type of experimental study, some level of control must be present. Six types of control are common: control of implementation of the independent variable, control of subject selection and assignment, control of extraneous variables related to the experimental setting, control of extraneous variables related to the subjects, control of measurement of the dependent variable, and control of information given to subjects and researchers.

Implementation of the Independent Variable

In controlling the independent variable, the investigator must develop a rationale to govern the implementation of the variable and a mechanism to monitor the implementation. In a study of the effect of heat and exercise on range of motion of the low back, the implementation of the heat and exercise would need to be systematized in some way. Does "heat" mean hot pack, ultrasound, or diathermy? If a hot pack is used, should packs of the same size be used on all patients, or should there be flexibility to accommodate patients of different sizes? Should heating continue until a certain skin temperature has been reached for a certain period of time?

Feinstein described two general research philosophies that influence how these implementation decisions are made: fastidiousness and pragmatism.[12] Fastidious researchers seek precise control over all aspects of implementation, believing that the ability to draw causal conclusions is jeopardized by variations in treatment implementation. Pragmatic researchers seek closer simulation of clinical environments, believing that research results are most useful when the experimental setting reflects the vagaries of the clinical setting. Both approaches are acceptable, but the limitations of both approaches need to be acknowledged by researchers. Fastidious researchers must acknowledge the limited clinical applicability of their work; pragmatic researchers must acknowledge their limited ability to draw causal conclusions from their work.

Selection and Assignment of Subjects

The second control component is control over the selection of subjects for the study and assignment of subjects to groups within the study. First, criteria for selection of individuals to be included in the study must be determined. In our hypothetical study of low back range of motion, many subject selection questions would arise. Should both men and women be studied? What age groups are appropriate for study? Does it make any difference whether the patient is being seen for a first episode of back pain or for a chronic condition that has recently flared up? Those who prefer fastidious designs tend to define selection criteria narrowly and therefore study relatively homogeneous groups. Those who prefer pragmatic designs develop broader selection criteria and therefore study relatively heterogeneous groups.

Once the criteria for admission to the study are determined, actual admission of individuals to the study must proceed. Random selection of a limited number of subjects from a larger subject pool is the best way to control for a variety of subject factors by maximizing the probability that any extraneous factors in the sample are present in the proportions actually found in the overall population. An in-depth discussion of sampling is presented in Chapter 8.

Extraneous Variables in the Experimental Setting

The third component of control is control over the experimental setting. *Extraneous*, or *confounding*, variables are factors other than the independent variables that may influence the dependent variables. Control of extraneous variables includes, for example, keeping the temperature, lighting, time of day of testing, and the like constant to rule out differences in these factors as possible explanations for any changes in the dependent variable.

Extraneous Variables Related to Subjects

Control of extraneous variables related to the subject is the fourth means of control within experimental design. Researchers usually attempt to hold factors other than the independent variable constant for all subjects or groups. In this way, extraneous variables are controlled because they will affect all subjects or groups equally. In our hypothetical study of low back range of motion, one extraneous variable might be the level of analgesic, antiinflammatory, or antispasmodic medication being taken by subjects. A fastidious approach to the research problem would require tight control over medication; a pragmatic approach would permit greater variability from subject to subject.

The use of a randomly assigned control group, in and of itself, is a powerful tool that balances extraneous variables throughout the experimental groups. If a randomly assigned, untreated control group is used in the study of low back range of motion, controlling the medications taken by subjects may not be necessary. The process of randomization increases the chance (but does not guarantee) that any medication effects will be balanced across the treatment and control groups.

In studies with only one group, control of extraneous variables must be achieved through means other than a control group. If one were to study a single group of patients after cerebral vascular accident to determine the effect of proprioceptive neuromuscular facilitation on gait velocity, it would be important to establish that changes were the result of treatment and not the normal healing process (maturation). One way to control for the effect of maturation would be to take weekly velocity measurements of all patients and admit into the study only those who had several weeks of stable velocity measures.

A second common way to control extraneous variables is to use the same subjects for all levels of the independent variable. This only works if the effect the researcher is measuring is thought to be short-lived. Brooks and associates studied the effect of electrode alignment (longitudinal versus horizontal) on quadriceps femoris muscle torque generated during electrical stimulation.[13] Because the short-term application of electrical stimulation should not cause permanent alterations in torque-generating capacity, an ideal way to control extraneous subject factors is to use a *repeated measures*, or *repeated treatment*, design, whereby subjects act as their own controls and receive all experimental conditions. In addition, repeated treatment designs require fewer subjects and may require less time for setup and preparation because the number of subjects is reduced.[14]

The repeated measures design, however, introduces its own set of extraneous variables related to the administration of multiple treatments. If one of the electrode placements is always given last, fatigue may reduce the torque generated by that placement. Conversely, familiarity with the electrical stimulation unit may lead to greater relaxation of antagonist muscles and greater torque production by the agonist during the second placement. One way to control the effects of familiarization with equipment or procedures is to schedule one or more training sessions with subjects prior to actual data collection.

Another way to control fatigue and learning in a repeated measures design is by randomizing, or *counterbalancing*, the order of presentation of the experimental conditions (that is, half the subjects get the longitudinal placement first and half get the horizontal placement first). This becomes problematic when more than two levels of treatment are present. If there are three levels (A, B, and C) of the independent variable, there are six possible presentation orders (3!—that is, 3 factorial, or $3 \times 2 \times 1 = 6$): ABC, ACB, BAC, BCA, CAB, and CBA. With four levels, the number of permutations increases to 24 ($4! — 4 \times 3 \times 2 \times 1 = 24$). With six levels, there are 720 possible orders ($6! — 6 \times 5 \times 4 \times 3 \times 2 \times 1 = 720$). Random assignment of subjects to all available orders in a study with six levels of an independent variable would require a minimum of 720 subjects. To obviate the need for so many subjects, a sampling of orders can be used.

There are two basic strategies for selecting treatment orders in a repeated measures design with several levels of the independent variable. These two strategies are illustrated by the four repeated treatments that Condon and Hutton used in their study of stretching procedures for the soleus.[15] The four stretching methods were static stretch, hold relax, agonist contraction, and hold relax–agonist contraction. The first strategy is to randomly select an order and then rotate the starting position, as shown in Figure 5–4A. In a random start with rotation, each condition appears at each position in the rotation equally often. One-fourth of the subjects would be randomly assigned the order in the first row; one-fourth, the order in the second row; and so on.

RANDOM ORDER WITH ROTATION

Presentation position			
1st	2nd	3rd	4th
SS	HC	HR	AC
HC	HR	AC	SS
HR	AC	SS	HC
AC	SS	HC	HR

A

LATIN SQUARE

Presentation position			
1st	2nd	3rd	4th
SS	HC	HR	AC
HC	AC	SS	HR
AC	HR	HC	SS
HR	SS	AC	HC

B

FIGURE 5–4. Selection of presentation orders from many possibilities. With four levels of the independent variable (SS, static stretch; HC, hold relax–agonist contraction; HR, hold relax; AC, agonist contraction), there are 24 (4!) possible orders. **A.** Selection of four orders through random ordering of the first row, and through rotation of orders for the remaining rows. The highlighted condition, AC, illustrates that each level is represented at each presentation position in a systematic way through rotation. **B.** Selection of four orders through generation of a Latin square. The highlighted condition, AC, illustrates that each level is represented at each presentation position in a random way that also ensures that each condition precedes and follows each other condition only once.

The second strategy is to use a *Latin square*

technique. The Latin square technique ensures not only that each condition appears at each position equally often, but also that each condition precedes and follows every other condition equally often. Thus, a Latin square has a greater level of randomization than does a random start with rotation. A sample Latin square is shown in Figure 5–4B. Condon and Hutton did in fact use a Latin square to determine the order of presentation of the four stretching techniques in their study.[15] Rules for the formation of a Latin square can be found in several texts.[16–18]

Measurement Variation

The fifth component of experimental control is control of the measurement techniques used to provide data for the experiment. Reliability and validity of measurements used in experiments are critical to the ability to draw conclusions from the data. Sound experimental design includes pilot testing of the measures to be used to ensure that each measure is reproducible. If multiple raters are used in the study, a pilot study to ensure the interrater reliability of measures is essential. Chapters 10 through 12 are devoted to measurement theory, research designs that evaluate reliability and validity of measurement tools, and critical examination of measures commonly employed in physical therapy research.

Information Received by the Subject and Researcher

The final means of control in experimental designs is control of the information given to the subject and the researcher during the course of the study. Placebo effects, subject expectations, and researcher expectations may all result in changes in the dependent variable that are unrelated to the implementation of the independent variable. Three means of information control are commonly used to limit these effects: incomplete information, subject blinding, and researcher blinding.

Incomplete Information. Sometimes subjects are given incomplete information about the purpose of the study to control any effects that their expectations about the experimental results would cause. For example, Montgomery studied the effect of lumbar posture on forward head position, but did not want subjects to know the specific dependent variable of interest.[19] The lumbar posture variable had two levels, created by having each subject positioned with a back-rest cushion to facilitate lumbar flexion and a different cushion to facilitate lumbar extension, with the order of presentation of the cushions randomly determined. When Montgomery obtained informed consent from participants, she stated only that she wished to study postural relationships. When she measured forward head position she also took sham measurements of neck rotation. In this way the true measure of interest was disguised from the subject.

With an innocuous intervention such as using cushions, there is no ethical problem in withholding the specific purpose of the study. However, study of higher risk procedures requires complete disclosure of purpose and risks so that subjects can make an informed decision about participation.

Subject Blinding. A second means of controlling information is to withhold information about which of several treatments a patient is receiving. In many procedures in physical therapy, patient blinding is not possible because of the nature of the procedures themselves. Subjects in Montgomery's lumbar position study were aware of size differences between the two cushions. Subjects in our hypothetical low back range-of-motion study would obviously be able to distinguish between a heat/exercise program and a manual therapy approach to treatment of low back pain.

When the treatment is a physical modality, subjects may be partially blinded to which physical modalities they are receiving. For example, subjects may be told that they may or may not feel a heat sensation with ultrasound treatment; the control group may then receive placebo or sham ultrasound, whereby the machine is not plugged in or the intensity is not turned on. Ethical treatment of research subjects requires that they be informed of the possibility of receiving a placebo treatment.

Researcher Blinding. A third means of controlling information is to blind the researcher to the group membership of, or treatment received by, the subjects. In this way the experimenter's expectations about the outcome of the study are controlled.

Researcher blinding was implemented in Montgomery's study of lumbar position.[19] The cushion was placed by a research assistant, and the subject was draped so that when Montgomery was taking the forward head position measurements, she was unaware of which cushion was in place. In modality studies, three investigators may be used: One sets up the equipment, one administers the treatment, and one takes the measurements. Only the first investigator knows which subjects have received a treatment and which have received a placebo.

A study in which either the subject or the researcher is blind to the treatment administered is termed a *single-blind* study. A study in which both subject and researcher are blinded is termed a *double-blind* study. Deyo and associates studied the effectiveness of blinding techniques with transcutaneous electrical nerve stimulation.[20] After completion of a double-blind study, they asked subjects to indicate whether they believed their units were working properly and asked researchers to indicate which subjects they believed had functioning units. They found that both subjects and researchers guessed correctly more often than would have been predicted by chance, indicating only partial success of the blinding procedure. They hypothesized that the lack of full blinding was due to sensory differences between real and sham therapy and to unintended communication between the subjects and researchers.

Implementation of the treatment, extraneous variables in the setting, extraneous subject variables, selection and assignment of subjects, measurement techniques, and information given to subjects and researchers must all be controlled in an experimental design. In the next section of this chapter, experimental designs are examined from a structural standpoint—that is, looking at the number of variables, the levels of variables, and the relationship of variables to one another. However, even the most sophisticated of structural designs will fail if the control elements listed above are not in place.

SINGLE-FACTOR EXPERIMENTAL DESIGNS

Single-factor experimental designs have one independent variable. Although multiple-factor experimental designs, which have more than one independent variable, are becoming increasingly common, single-factor designs remain an important part of the physical therapy literature. In 1963 Campbell and Stanley published what was to become a classic work on single-factor experimental design: *Experimental and Quasi-Experimental Designs for Research*.[10] Their slim volume diagrammed 16 different experimental designs and outlined the strengths and weaknesses of each. Such a comprehensive catalogue of single-factor designs cannot be repeated here, but several of the more commonly observed designs are illustrated by studies from the physical therapy literature. It should be noted that some of the studies presented included secondary purposes that involved an additional independent variable. If readers go to the research reports themselves, they will find that some of the studies are more complex than would be assumed from reading this chapter.

Pretest–Posttest Control-Group Design

The first design example is the pretest–posttest control-group design. This design is also referred to as a randomized clinical trial. In addition, this is an example of a *between-subjects design* because the differences of interest are those differences that occur between subject groups. The Campbell and Stanley notation for the pretest–posttest control-group design is as follows:[10(p13)]

R	O	X	O
R	O		O

The Os represent observation, or measurement. The X represents an intervention, or manipulation. The Rs indicate that subjects were assigned randomly to the two groups.

In clinical research, the pretest–posttest control-group design is often altered slightly, as follows:

R	O	X_1	O
R	O	X_2	O

This alteration is often made in order to deal with clinical populations ethically. If the researcher does not wish to withhold treatment altogether, one group receives a typical treatment, and the other group receives the experimental treatment.

Sims performed a simple experiment using a pretest–posttest control-group design that contrasted a typical position used in the clinic with an alternative position.[21] He noted that in clinical practice, many physical therapists treat ankle edema by administering modalities with the ankle in a dependent position. As a first step to studying the relationship between position and edema, Sims placed normal subjects in one of two positions and evaluated ankle volume after 20 minutes in the position. Fifty subjects were randomly assigned to either the supine–elevation group or the sitting–dependent group. This design would be termed a *reversed treatment design* because both groups were expected to change, with the effects of one treatment expected to be in the opposite direction from those of the other.[11(p76)] This is in contrast to a typical control-group design, in which the experimental group is expected to change and the control group is expected to remain the same.

Other variations on the pretest–posttest control-group design include taking more than two measurements and using more than two treatment groups. An example of both variations is found in Griffin and associates' study of reduction of chronic posttraumatic hand edema with high-voltage pulsed current, intermittent pneumatic compression, or placebo treatments.[22] The notation for this design would be as follows:

R	O	O	X_1	O
R	O	O	X_2	O
R	O	O		O

Patients were randomly assigned to the stimulation, compression, or placebo group. The placebo group received sham high-voltage stimulation. The first measure (prerest) was taken when the patient arrived at the clinic. The second measure (postrest) was taken after subjects rested for 10 minutes with their arm positioned at the level of the heart. This rest period was used to control for the possible effects of varied hand positions prior to coming to the clinic for treatment. The third measure (posttreatment) was taken after the conclusion of treatment.

Posttest-Only Control-Group Design

A second common design is the posttest-only control-group design. Researchers use this design when they are not able to take pretest measurements, and therefore the posttest is the only basis on which to make judgments about the effect of the independent variable on the dependent variable. This design is also a between-subjects design. The Campbell and Stanley notation for this design is as follows:[10(p25)]

R	X	O
R		O

An example of this design is found in Draper's study of electromyographic biofeedback and recovery of quadriceps femoris muscle function following anterior cruciate ligament surgery.[23] She compared peak quadriceps torque ratios (operative limb:nonoperative limb peak torque) between a group who received a 12-week program of traditional therapy and a group who received a 12-week program of traditional therapy augmented by electromyographic biofeedback. In this study, pretest measures of quadriceps torque would not be accurate because of the pain and dysfunction associated with an acutely reconstructed knee. Therefore, only posttest measures were taken. Because subjects were randomly assigned to groups, it is assumed (but not guaranteed) that the randomization procedure balanced any extraneous variables across the two groups.

Single-Group Pretest–Posttest Design

The Campbell and Stanley notation for the single-group pretest–posttest design is as follows:[10(p7)]

O X O

An example of this design is seen in Yarkony and associates' study of rehabilitation outcomes in patients with complete thoracic spinal cord injury.[24] In this study, paraplegic patients were assessed with a functional measure at admission and discharge from a rehabilitation center. The independent variable was rehabilitation and had two levels: before rehabilitation and after rehabilitation. Patients showed significant improvements in the dependent measure from admission to discharge. This design did not control for the possibility that patients would make similar functional gains without a formal rehabilitation program. To control for this possibility, a study comparing inpatient rehabilitation with no rehabilitation would need to be conducted. As noted in Chapter 3, ethical concerns about withholding treatment would prevent such a study from being conducted.

Nonequivalent Control-Group Design

The nonequivalent control-group design is used when a nonrandom control group is available for comparison. The Campbell and Stanley notation for this design is as follows:[10(p47)]

O X O
\- - - - - - - - - -
O   O

The dotted line between groups indicates that subjects were not randomly assigned to groups. Amundsen and colleagues studied the effects of a group exercise program on various physiological variables in elderly women.[25] Five women completed pretests and posttests but were unable to participate in the training sessions, 19 attended fewer than half of the twice weekly sessions, and 14 completed at least half of the sessions. Comparisons were made between the 14 regular attendees (exercise group) and the 5 untrained women (control group). This nonrandom assignment to groups did not control for extraneous factors that might explain different results between the two groups.

Another approach to the nonequivalent control-group design is the use of cohorts for the experimental groups. The term *cohort* is generally used to refer to any group; a more specific use of the term refers to groups of individuals who follow each other in time. A cohort approach would be a convenient way to study the effects of a planned curriculum change on first job performance of physical therapy students. The last class, or cohort, who studied under the old curriculum would form the control group; the class, or cohort, who were exposed to the curricular innovation would form the experimental group.

Time Series Design

The time series design is used to establish a baseline of measurements before initiation of treatment to either a group or an individual. When a comparison group is not available, it becomes important to either establish the stability of a measure before implementation of treatment or document the extent to which the measure is changing solely as a function of time. The Campbell and Stanley notation for the time series design is as follows:[10(p37)]

O O O O X O O O O

The number of measurements taken before, after, or even during the intervention varies depending on the nature of the study. Time series designs can be applied to either group or individual studies. If it is important to assess changes over many time intervals, any of the two or more group designs can be modified by use of additional measurements before or after treatment.

Kelly and associates' study of the effects of a developmental physical therapy program on oxygen saturation and heart rate in a group of preterm infants,[7] discussed earlier in this chapter and diagrammed in Figure 5–2, is an example of a group time series design. Measurements of oxygen saturation and heart rate were taken every minute during a baseline phase during which infants were in the prone position. These eight baseline measures provided a good yardstick against which the six intervention measurements could be compared. Thirty measures taken after the treatment were used to establish the pattern of recovery to baseline physiological values.

Application of a time series design to an individual subject is termed a *single-subject design*. The single-subject design is not to be confused with a "case study." The single-subject design is prospective in nature, and in it many extraneous variables are controlled. Single-subject designs are considered in detail in Chapter 9.

Repeated Measures or Repeated Treatment Designs

Repeated measures designs are widely used in health science research. The term *repeated measures* means that the same subjects are measured under all the levels of the independent variable. In this sense, any of the pretest—posttest designs can be considered a repeated measures design because each subject is measured at both levels (before and after treatment) of the independent variable. The *repeated treatment* design is a type of repeated measures design in which each subject receives more than one actual treatment. The repeated measures designs are also referred to as *within-subject* designs because the effect of the independent variable is seen within subjects in a single group rather than between the groups.

As discussed earlier in the chapter, Brooks and associates studied differences in quadriceps torque output with horizontal versus longitudinal placement of electrical stimulation electrodes.[13] The 35 subjects each received electrical stimulation with horizontal *and* longitudinal electrode placement. The repeated treatment design controlled for many extraneous factors because the same subjects were used for all the treatment conditions. However, as noted earlier, the use of repeated treatments creates a new set of extraneous factors related to fatigue and learning. These factors must be controlled by counterbalancing the order of administration of the treatments.

MULTIPLE-FACTOR EXPERIMENTAL DESIGNS

Multiple-factor experimental designs are used frequently in physical therapy research. Because of their widespread use, it is essential that physical therapists have command of the language and concepts related to multiple-factor designs. This section of the chapter is divided into several subsections. After a discussion of the basic research questions that would prompt a researcher to develop a multiple-factor design, some common multiple-factor designs are presented.

Questions That Lead to a Multiple-Factor Design

Researchers usually design multiple-factor experiments because they are interested not only in the individual effects of the multiple factors on the dependent variable, but also in the effects of the interaction between the multiple factors on the dependent variable. For example, say we wished to conduct a study to determine the effects of different physical therapy programs (heat/exercise, manual therapy, and home program) on low back range of motion in patients with low back pain. We could start by selecting 60 patients for study and randomly assigning them to one of the three groups. The first independent variable would be type of treatment, or group. Say two therapists are going to provide the treatments. We might wonder whether one therapist might simply get better results than the other therapist, regardless of the type of treatment provided. A second independent variable, then, is therapist. If therapist is added as a second independent variable, a third question must also be asked in this design: Is one therapist more effective with one type of treatment and the other therapist more effective with another type of treatment? In other words, is there an interaction between type of treatment and therapist? It is the study of interaction that clearly differentiates a multiple-factor experimental design from a single-factor design.

Factorial Versus Nested Designs

The Type of Treatment × Therapist design developed above is a factorial design. In a *factorial design,* the factors are crossed, meaning that each level of one factor is combined with each level of each other factor. This simply means that each treatment group has members who are exposed to each therapist, and each therapist is exposed to members of each treatment group. This design is diagrammed in Figure 5–5. Group is one variable, with three levels: heat/exercise, manual therapy, and home program. Therapist is the second variable, with two levels: A and B. There are six cells in the design, formed by crossing the two factors. In this example, assume there is an equal number, say 20, of subjects in each cell. The assigned therapists measure lumbar flexion at two weeks postinjury, implement the appropriate program to each subject, and measure lumbar

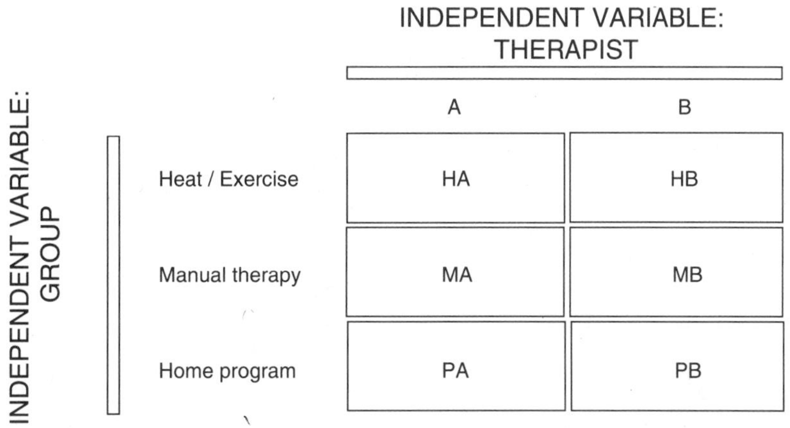

INDEPENDENT VARIABLE: GROUP	INDEPENDENT VARIABLE: THERAPIST A	B
Heat / Exercise	HA	HB
Manual therapy	MA	MB
Home program	PA	PB

FIGURE 5–5. Two-factor, 3 × 2 factorial design. The notation within each cell shows the combination of the two independent variables. For example, HA indicates that individuals within this cell received the heat/exercise treatment from Therapist A.

flexion at six weeks postinjury. The dependent variable is the difference in range of motion from two weeks to six weeks postinjury.

Figure 5–6 shows a hypothetical set of data and a graph of the data. Part A shows that Therapist A is superior overall to Therapist B (the overall mean for Therapist A is a 40° improvement in range of motion; the overall mean for Therapist B is 30°), regardless of the type of treatment being delivered. The home program (overall mean is 45°) is superior overall to the manual therapy and heat/exercise programs (overall means are 35° and 25°, respectively), regardless of which therapist was delivering the treatment. In this example, there is no interaction between treatment and therapist. The home program is the superior treatment, regardless of therapist, and Therapist A gets superior results, regardless of the treatment given. This lack of interaction is shown graphically by the parallel lines in Part B between therapists for the three treatments. A concise way to summarize these results is to say there are *main effects* for both type of treatment and therapist, but no interaction between type of treatment and therapist.

Figure 5–7 presents a different set of data. In this instance, Part A shows that there are no overall differences in treatments (mean improvement for each treatment, regardless of therapist, is 30°) and no overall differences in therapist results (mean improvement for each therapist, regardless of treatment, is 30°). However, there is a significant interaction between treatment and therapist. Part B shows that Therapist A achieved better results using a home program and Therapist B achieved better results using heat/exercise. Both obtained intermediate results using manual therapy. A concise way of summarizing these results is to say there are no main effects for either type of treatment or therapist, but there is an interaction between type of treatment and therapist. If we had studied only the different treatment types without examining the second factor, therapists, we would have concluded that there were no differences between these treatments. The two-factor study allows us to come to a more sophisticated conclusion: Even though there are no overall differences between the treatments and therapists studied, certain therapists are considerably more effective when using certain treatments.

Nested designs occur when not all the factors cross one another. For example, we could

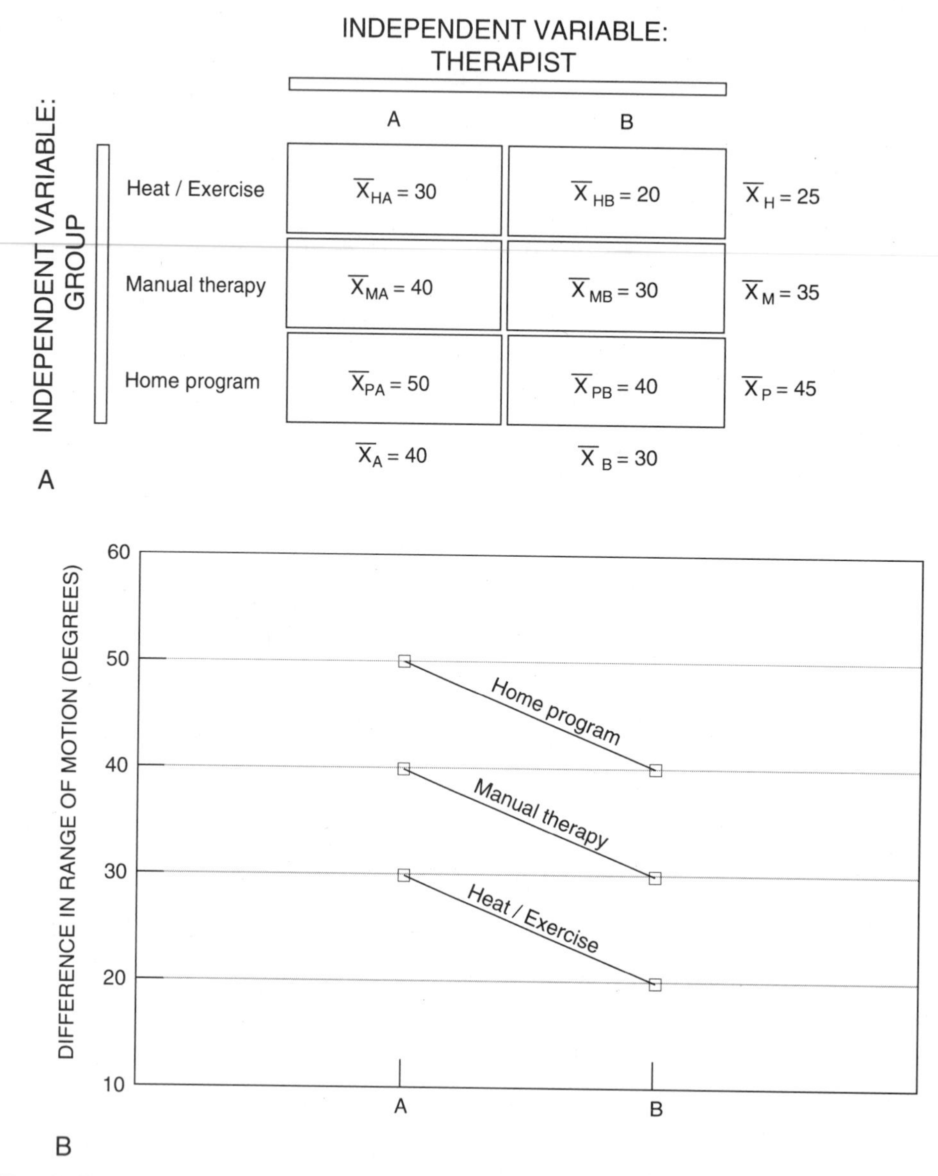

FIGURE 5–6. Example with no interaction. **A.** Sample data. The notations within the cells represent the mean scores for subjects for each combination. The means in the margins are the overall means for the column or row. **B.** Graph of sample data. Parallel lines indicate that there is no interaction between therapist and treatment.

make the example above more complex by adding some additional therapists and an additional clinic. The treatment variable remains the same: It has three levels—heat/exercise, manual therapy, and home program. Perhaps there are two competing clinics in town—one has a clientele with varied diagnoses, and the other specializes in spine disorders. This is a second independent variable, with two levels: general and specialty clinics.

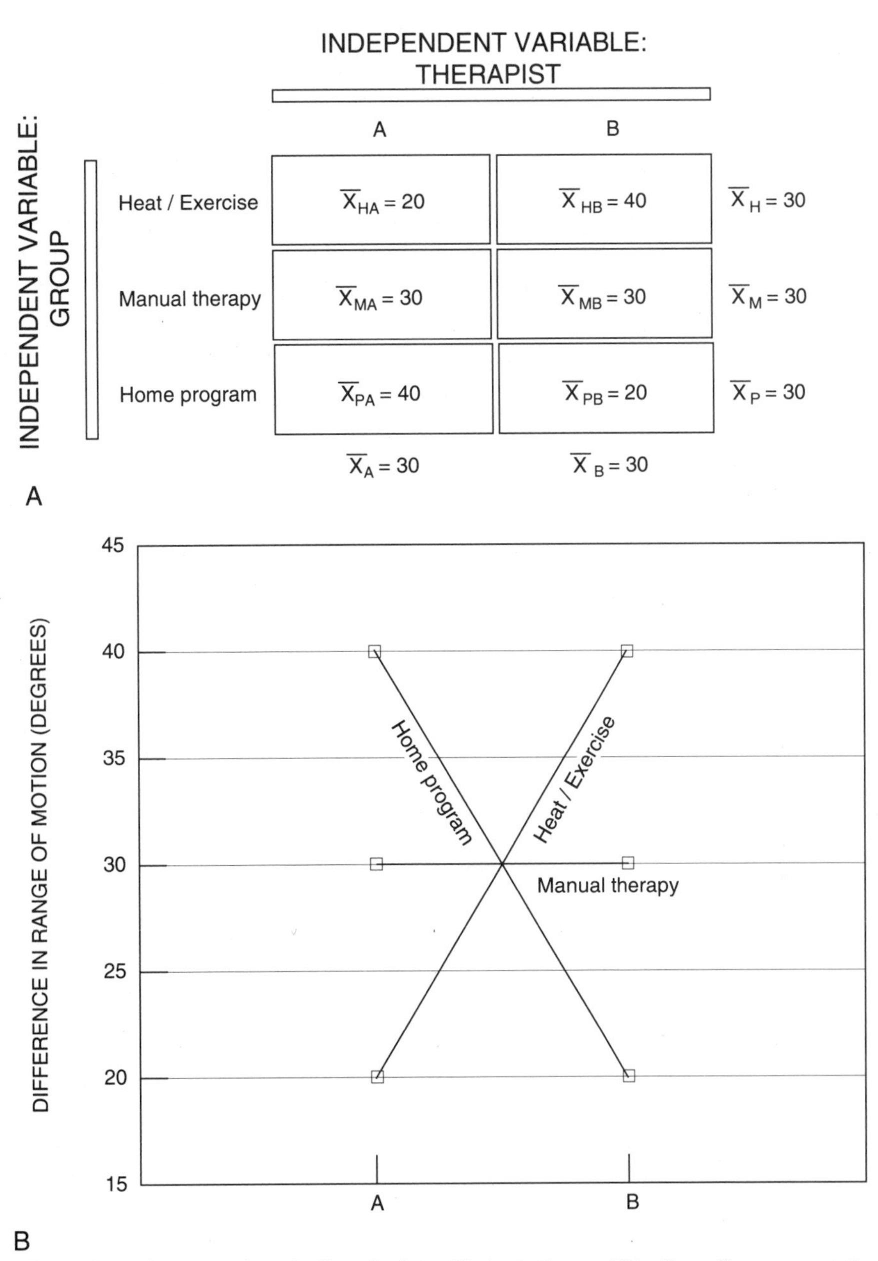

FIGURE 5–7. Example with interaction. **A.** Sample data. The notations within the cells represent the mean scores for subjects for each combination. The means in the margins are the overall means for the column or row. **B.** Graph of sample data. Nonparallel lines indicate an interaction between therapist and treatment.

One research question might be whether patient outcomes at the two clinics are different. The research question of whether different therapists achieve different results remains. This could be studied by using three different therapists at each clinic. Because there are different therapists at each clinic, the therapist variable is nested within the clinic variable. Figure 5–8 presents a schematic view of this hypothetical design in which treatment and clinic are crossed and therapist is nested within clinic.

Completely Randomized Versus Randomized-Block Designs

The Treatment × Therapist example just presented could also be termed a *completely randomized design* because type of treatment and therapist assignment were both manipulable variables and subjects were assigned randomly to both treatment group and therapist.

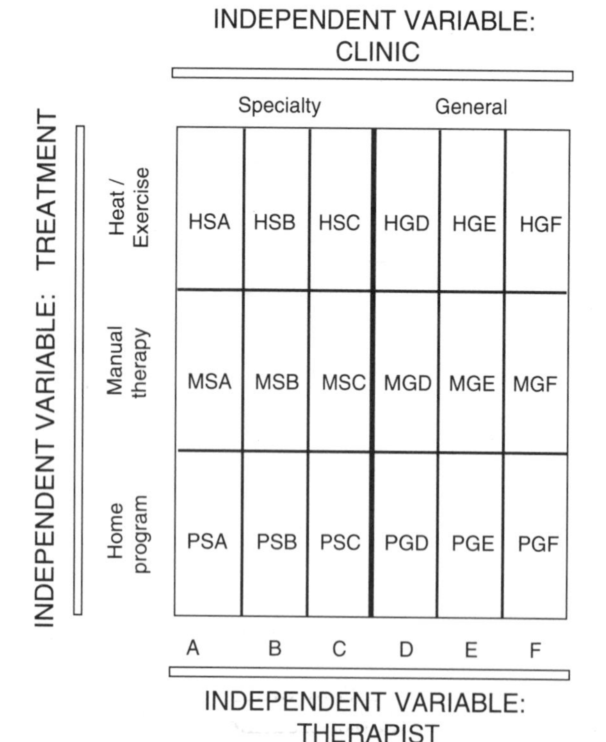

FIGURE 5–8. Schematic diagram of three-factor, nested design. Treatment (H, M, P) and clinic (S, G) are crossed factors. Therapist (A–F) is nested within clinic.

Sometimes a *randomized-block design* is used, in which one of the factors of interest is not manipulable. If, for example, we had wanted to look at the factors sex and treatment, then sex would have been a classification or attribute variable. Subjects would be placed into blocks on the basis of sex and then randomly assigned to treatments. Condon and Hutton's study of four stretching methods, discussed earlier in the chapter, used sex as a blocking factor.[15]

Between-Subjects, Within-Subject, and Mixed Designs

The Treatment × Therapist example could also be termed a *between-subjects design* for both factors. Different subjects were placed into each of the six cells of the design. The research questions related to differences between groups who received different treatments and between groups who had different therapists.

In a *within-subject* design, one group of subjects receives all levels of the independent variables. Stern used a within-subject design to study dexterity and grip strength with and without four different wrist orthoses. For the dependent variable grip strength, there were two independent variables: orthotic condition (five levels: Each subject was tested without the orthosis and with each of four different wrist orthoses) and session (three levels: Each subject was tested with each orthotic condition on three different days). Both independent variables in this study were repeated measures factors, making this a within-subject design.

A *mixed*, or *split-plot, design* contains a combination of between-subjects and within-

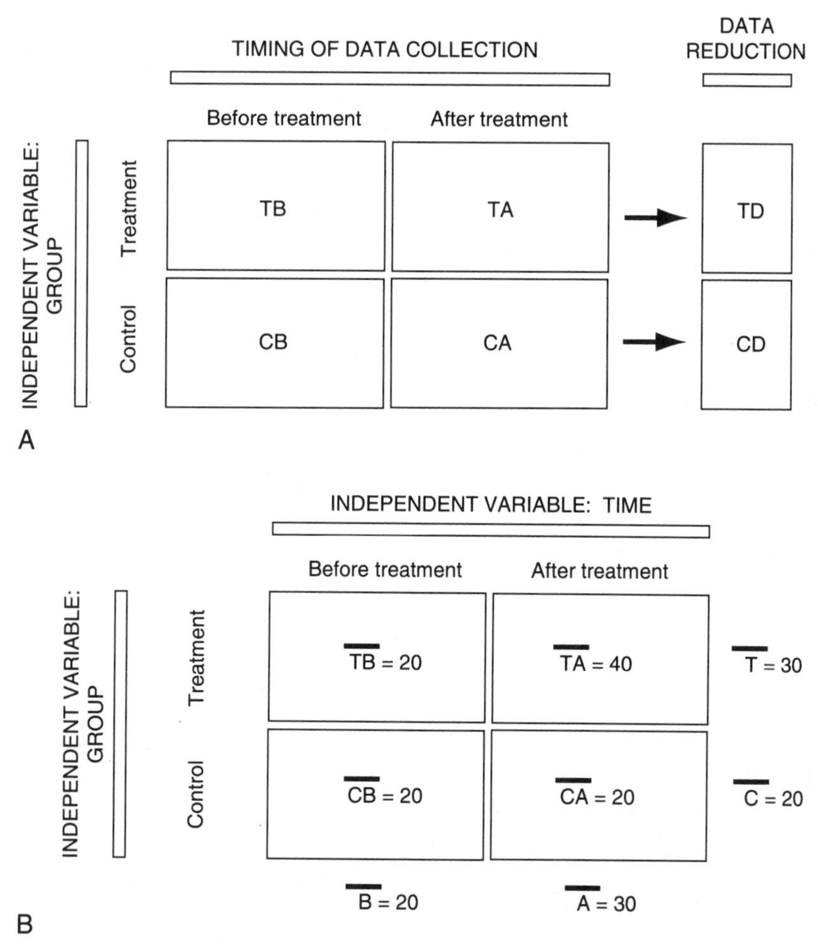

FIGURE 5–9. One- and two-factor approaches to the pretest–posttest control-group design. **A.** One-factor approach using group as the independent variable and range-of-motion difference scores (D) as the dependent variable. **B.** Two-factor approach using group and time as independent variables and range-of-motion score as the dependent variable. Sample data, with cell and margin means, are included.

Illustration continued on following page

subject factors. Condon and Hutton's study of stretching techniques represents such a mixed design.[15] Subjects were blocked according to sex, a between-subjects factor. Each subject received all four stretching techniques, making technique a within-subject factor. Each subject also received three trials with each stretching technique, making trial a within-subject factor as well.

In a common mixed design, the familiar single-factor, pretest–posttest, control-group design is treated as a two-factor design. Figure 5–9A shows how a pretest–posttest control-group design can be handled as a single-factor study by using the pretest–posttest difference as the dependent variable. If the data are not reduced to difference scores, then the before- and after-treatment measures can be viewed as a second independent variable, time. In this two-factor mixed design, group

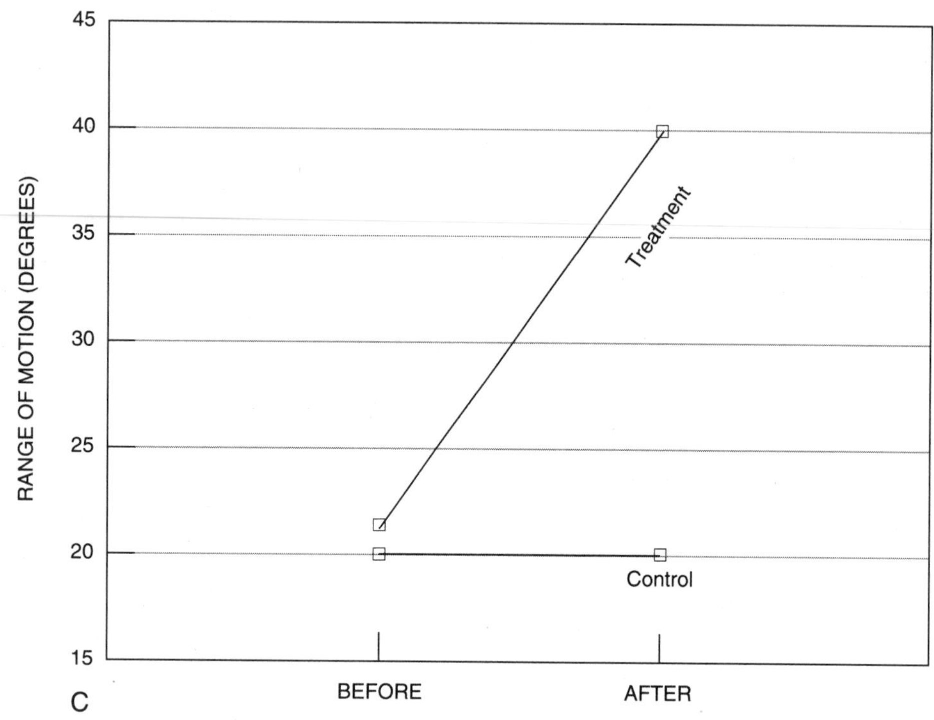

FIGURE 5–9 *Continued* **C.** Interaction with two-factor approach. Nonparallel lines between treatment and control groups indicate a Group × Time interaction.

is the between-subjects factor and time is the within-subject factor. This approach is diagrammed in Figure 5–9B.

In the pretest–posttest control-group design, the main effects are not of inherent interest because the presence of the control group reduces the size of the main effects. For example, the "after" column in Figure 5–9B shows that there is a 20° difference in range of motion between the treatment and control groups after treatment. The main effect for treatment, however, looks at overall differences in treatment, regardless of the time of measurement. Looking at the means in the right margin, we see that there is only a 10° main effect for treatment. The same can be seen for the variable time. If we compare the before- and after-treatment means for the treatment group, we see that there is a 20° increase in range of motion after treatment. The main effect for time, however, looks at overall differences in the time periods, regardless of group. Looking at the means in the lower margin, we see that there is only a 10° main effect for time. Both main effects are blunted by the presence of the control group. Therefore, when the pretest–posttest control-group design is handled as a two-factor mixed design, the real item of interest is the interaction between time and treatment. Figure 5–9C graphs this interaction and shows clearly that whereas the control group remains the same across time periods, the treatment group shows dramatic increases in range of motion.

SUMMARY

Experimental research is characterized by controlled manipulation of variables by the researcher. Researchers can achieve control by uniformly implementing the independent variable, selecting and assigning subjects randomly, eliminating extraneous variables from the experimental setting, limiting extraneous variables related to subjects, ensuring the reliability of measurements of the dependent variable, and limiting the information provided to themselves and to subjects. Single-factor experimental designs are those in which the researcher manipulates only one variable. Multiple-factor research designs are those in which the researcher studies more than one variable and is interested in the interactions among variables.

References

1. King CE, Clelland JA, Knowles CJ, Jackson JR. Effect of helium-neon laser auriculotherapy on experimental pain threshold. *Phys Ther.* 1990;70:24–30.
2. Sinaki M, Offord K. Physical activity in postmenopausal women: effect on back muscle strength and bone mineral density of the spine. *Arch Phys Med Rehabil.* 1988;69:277–280.
3. Hageman PA, Gillaspie DM, Hill LD. Effects of speed and limb dominance on eccentric and concentric isokinetic testing of the knee. *Journal of Orthopaedic and Sports Physical Therapy.* 1988;10:59–65.
4. Rikli RE, McManis BG. Effects of exercise on bone mineral content in postmenopausal women. *Research Quarterly for Exercise and Sport.* 1990; 61:243–249.
5. Kerlinger FN. *Foundations of Behavioral Research.* 3rd ed. Fort Worth, Tex: Holt, Rinehart & Winston Inc; 1986.
6. Burr DB, Martin RB, Martin PA. Lower extremity loads stimulate bone formation in the vertebral column: implications for osteoporosis. *Spine.* 1983; 8:681–686.
7. Kelly MK, Palisano RJ, Wolfson MR. Effects of a developmental physical therapy program on oxygen saturation and heart rate in preterm infants. *Phys Ther.* 1989;69:467–474.
8. Walker DC, Currier DP, Threlkeld AJ. Effects of high voltage pulsed electrical stimulation on blood flow. *Phys Ther.* 1988;68:481–485.
9. Norton BJ, Strube MJ. Making decisions based on group designs and meta-analysis. *Phys Ther.* 1989;69:594–600.
10. Campbell DT, Stanley JC. *Experimental and Quasi-Experimental Designs for Research.* Chicago, Ill: Rand McNally College Publishing Co; 1963.
11. Oyster CK, Hanten WP, Llorens LA. *Introduction to Research: A Guide for the Health Science Professional.* Philadelphia, Pa: JB Lippincott Co; 1987:70.
12. Feinstein AR. An additional basic science for clinical medicine, II: limitations of randomized trials. *Ann Intern Med.* 1983;99:544–550.
13. Brooks ME, Smith EM, Currier DP. Effect of longitudinal versus transverse electrode placement on torque production by the quadriceps femoris muscle during neuromuscular electrical stimulation. *Journal of Orthopaedic and Sports Physical Therapy.* 1990;11:530–534.
14. McGuigan FJ. *Experimental Psychology: Methods of Research.* 5th ed. Englewood Cliffs, NJ: Prentice Hall; 1990:231–232.
15. Condon SM, Hutton RS. Soleus muscle electromyographic activity and ankle dorsiflexion range of motion during four stretching procedures. *Phys Ther.* 1987;67:24–30.
16. Shaughnessy JJ, Zechmeister EB. *Research Methods in Psychology.* 2nd ed. New York, NY: McGraw-Hill Publishing Co; 1990:217.
17. Winer BJ. *Statistical Principles in Experimental Design.* 2nd ed. New York, NY: McGraw-Hill Publishing Co; 1971:685–691.
18. Kirk RE. *Experimental Design: Procedures for the Behavioral Sciences.* Belmont, Calif: Wadsworth Publishing Co; 1968.
19. Montgomery CA. Effect of lumbar position on forward head posture. Master's research project. Indianapolis, Ind: University of Indianapolis; 1990.
20. Deyo RA, Walsh NE, Schoenfeld LS, Ramamurthy S. Can trials of physical treatments be blinded? The example of transcutaneous electrical nerve stimulation for chronic pain. *Am J Phys Med Rehabil.* 1990;69:6–10.
21. Sims D. Effects of positioning on ankle edema. *Journal of Orthopaedic and Sports Physical Therapy.* 1986;8:30–33.
22. Griffin JW, Newsome LS, Stralka SW, Wright PE. Reduction of chronic posttraumatic hand edema: a comparison of high voltage pulsed current, intermittent pneumatic compression, and placebo treatments. *Phys Ther.* 1990;70:279–286.
23. Draper V. Electromyographic biofeedback and recovery of quadriceps muscle function following anterior cruciate ligament reconstruction. *Phys Ther.* 1990; 70:11–17.
24. Yarkony GM, Roth EJ, Meyer PR, Lovell LL, Heinemann AW. Rehabilitation outcomes in patients with complete thoracic spinal cord injury. *Am J Phys Med Rehabil.* 1990;69:23–27.
25. Amundsen LR, DeVahl JM, Ellingham CT. Evaluation of a group exercise program for elderly women. *Phys Ther.* 1989;69:475–483.
26. Stern EB. Wrist extensor orthoses: dexterity and grip strength across four styles. *Am J Occup Ther.* 1991;45:42–49.

CHAPTER 6

Nonexperimental Research

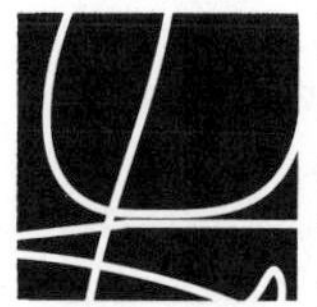

In contrast to experimental research, nonexperimental research does not involve manipulation of variables. Kerlinger noted that "in the nonexperimental research situation, . . . control of the independent variables is not possible. Investigators must take things as they are and try to disentangle them."[1] In nonexperimental studies, then, the researcher examines records of past phenomena, documents existing phenomena, or observes new phenomena unfolding. The label "*non*experimental" implies an unfavorable comparison with research that meets the controlled-manipulation criterion for "experimental" research. This is an unfortunate implication. Nonexperimental research is exceedingly important within the physical therapy literature. A review of articles in the 1989 volume of *Physical Therapy* shows that two-thirds of the research articles report the results of nonexperimental studies.

Because nonexperimental research does not have to fit a rigid definition like controlled manipulation, the variety of nonexperimental designs is greater than that of experimental designs. There are nonexperimental research designs to fit every research type in the Purpose × Time matrix presented in Figure 4–3.

The purpose of this chapter is to provide the reader with a view of the diversity of nonexperimental research designs. This is done by providing examples of nonexperimental research articles that fit into each of the six cells of the matrix of research types. As in earlier chapters, the pertinent portion of each study is reviewed; readers who go to the literature to review these studies will find that some are more involved than would be assumed just from reading this chapter. Problems with the various research designs are alluded to in this chapter, but a complete discussion of the problems associated with each design is deferred until Chapter 7.

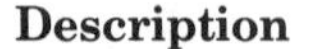

Description
Retrospective descriptive research
Prospective descriptive research

Analysis of Relationships
Retrospective analysis of relationships
Prospective analysis of relationships

Analysis of Differences
Retrospective analysis of differences
Prospective analysis of differences

DESCRIPTION

The purpose of descriptive research is to document the nature of a phenomenon through the systematic collection of data. In this text, a study is considered descriptive if it either provides a snapshot view of a single sample measured once or involves measurement and description of a sample several times over an extended period of time. The former approach is said to be *cross-sectional*; the latter is referred to as *longitudinal*.

In most descriptive studies, many different variables are documented. For the most part, though, there is no presumption of cause or effect. Thus the distinction between independent and dependent variables is not usually made in reports of descriptive research. As is the case with all three research purposes that make up the matrix of research types, a distinction can be made between prospective and retrospective descriptive research designs.

Retrospective Descriptive Research

The purpose of retrospective descriptive research is to document past events. The description of the past may be of inherent interest, may be used to evaluate the present against the past, or may be used to make decisions in the present based on information from the past. The common denominator among research studies of this type is the reliance on archival data. *Archives* are "records of documents recounting the activities of individuals or of institutions, governments, and other groups."[2] Archival data may be found in medical records, voter registration rosters, newspapers and magazines, telephone directories, meeting minutes, television news programs, and a host of other sources. The information found in archival records is subjected to content analysis by the researcher.[3] *Content analysis* is a painstaking process that involves operational definition of the variables of interest and a system for determining whether the record being examined contains an example of the desired variable.

Assume that we wish to study patterns of use of transcutaneous electrical nerve stimulation (TENS) in a particular physical therapy department in the 15-year period from 1975 to 1990. We have a hunch that when a new treatment modality comes along, therapists use it somewhat indiscriminately, then go through a period of disillusionment in which they seldom use it, and then settle into a period of relatively stable use of the modality. We decide to test this hypothesis about modality adoption patterns by examining medical record information on TENS use. Our first decision might be which patients to include in this review.

Assume that we decide that any patient with a pain diagnosis would be eligible to be reviewed for the study, and one relevant factor would be the percentage of pain patients who received TENS during each year of the study. Patients with diagnoses of low back, knee, or pelvic pain would clearly fit this description. But what about those with diagnoses such as cervical radiculopathy, acute ankle sprain, and partial-thickness burn that describe painful conditions without the use of the word *pain?* Such provisional decisions about content analysis are made before beginning a pilot data extraction project. On the basis of the pilot study, more definitive decisions about classification criteria can be made before the study itself is begun.[4]

Archival records are generally classified as either primary or secondary sources. *Primary sources* are original documents that provide firsthand information from the author. *Secondary sources* are interpretations of primary ones. Thus the information in secondary sources may suffer from bias, inaccuracy, and selective reporting from the primary sources.

For example, a journal article is a primary source of information about the study being described. The literature review portion of the article is a secondary source of information, being colored by the interpretations of the journal article author.

Individuals who use archival data should use primary sources whenever possible. When one is conducting a chart review, a laboratory printout of cardiac enzyme levels would be considered a primary source; the discharge summary information would be considered a secondary source of information. If cardiac enzymes are an important part of a chart review, one should search for the original laboratory report rather than relying solely on the information in the discharge summary.

Once archival data are assembled, researchers need to subject them to two types of scrutiny: external criticism and internal criticism. *External criticism* is concerned with the authenticity of the records. *Internal criticism* is concerned with whether the records are accurate and the interpretation unbiased.[5]

An example of retrospective descriptive research is Wolf and associates' study of prosthetic rehabilitation of elderly patients with bilateral amputations.[6] The researchers determined the functional level of each patient exclusively by retrospective analysis of the medical records of an amputee clinic. They found that all patients who had bilateral below-knee amputations without major cardiovascular complications were fitted with prostheses and used them successfully.

When patients are followed in a formal setting such as an amputee clinic, there is a good chance that uniform records exist on each patient. Imagine the difficulty you would have obtaining this information if all patients were followed by their own physicians. Some physicians might not document any functional information, and those who do might use different definitions for function. In addition, abilities that patients demonstrate in the clinic setting may not correspond to those at home. If a patient who has had an amputation walks the length of a corridor with prostheses on the day he or she is at the clinic, but only uses the prostheses for cosmetic purposes at home, is the chart notation "Independent with prostheses" an accurate description of function? Would the surgeon who performed the amputations unconsciously exaggerate patient ability with the prostheses? These two questions are examples of internal criticism of the records.

A combined retrospective and prospective approach to data collection was used by Tator and Edmonds to study spinal injuries to hockey players.[7] These Toronto-based health professionals had noticed what they believed to be an increase in spinal injuries to hockey players in the early 1980s. To confirm whether their impression was correct, they studied the problem formally, using both archives (retrospective information) and interviews (prospective information) to gather data. In the winter of 1982 they sent a questionnaire to neurosurgeons, orthopedic surgeons, and physiatrists throughout Canada asking for information on spinal injuries to hockey players that had occurred in the previous 18 months. The questionnaire was the method used to gain access to the archives of the physicians in question. Physicians were to provide patient ages and initials and date and place of injury so that duplicate information on single patients could be deleted.

Tator and Edmonds's study is an example of *epidemiological research*. Epidemiology is the study of disease, injury, and health in a population. The purposes of epidemiological research are to (1) document the incidence of disease or injury, (2) determine causes for the disease or injury, and (3) develop mechanisms to control the disease or injury.[8(p3)] The retrospective component (the questionnaires) of Tator and Edmonds's study accomplished the first purpose of epidemiological research, documenting the incidence of spinal injuries in hockey players. The second purpose of epidemiological research was accomplished by interviews of the injured players. In the interviews, Tator and Edmonds were able to obtain information about the specific conditions under which the injuries occurred, information that was not readily available in the physician records.

Another research approach that uses retrospective descriptive methods is *historical research*. The purpose of historical research is to document past events because they are of inherent interest or because they provide a perspective that can guide decision making in the present. An example of historical research in physical therapy is the study of direct-access legislation patterns by Taylor and Domholdt.[9] These patterns were determined by obtaining records from several archival sources: the laws themselves, state records that documented the sequence of events surrounding attempts to pass direct-access legislation, and newsletters from different states. In addition to the retrospective data, information was requested from individuals who were active in the states when direct-access legislation was being pursued. Like the Tator and Edmonds's study of spinal injuries to hockey players, this study combined retrospective and prospective data collection to develop a fuller description of the phenomenon under study.

Prospective Descriptive Research

Prospective descriptive research enables the researcher to control the data that are collected for the purpose of describing a phenomenon. The prospective nature of data collection makes the results of such research more believable than the results of purely retrospective studies. There are three basic methods of data collection in prospective descriptive research: observation, interview, and questionnaire.

Observation. An example of the observational method is a study by Heriza, who determined the leg movement patterns of preterm infants by videotaping them and analyzing the number of kicks and angular motions on the tapes.[10] She did this analysis at two different periods of time, when the infants were 34 to 36 and 40 weeks postgestational age. The two purposes of the research were to document the extent of movement organization in preterm infants and to determine maturational changes in kicking patterns. Another term for this type of research is *developmental*, meaning that the infants were described at more than one point in time to document the effects of the passage of time. In a developmental study such as this, time may be viewed as an independent variable and the measure of interest as the dependent variable.

Interview. The interview method of data collection was used by Brodzka and colleagues to study the long-term function of persons with bilateral below-knee amputations who were living in the inner city.[11] Subjects were identified retrospectively through review of medical records. Data collection was prospective and was accomplished through home interviews with the subjects by occupational and physical therapists. Presumably, the medical records did not contain the information the researchers believed was critical to answer their questions about the function of elderly individuals with bilateral below-knee amputations. The population being studied did not lend itself to study through a mailed questionnaire: The diabetic elderly often have visual problems that make reading difficult, and the poor elderly may have had little education, resulting in difficulties in both reading questionnaires and writing answers. In addition, the researchers were interested in these individuals' satisfaction with their abilities; answers to a questionnaire item about such a complex notion as satisfaction would likely lack the depth and breadth of answers obtained in an interview.

In comparing this prospective study of individuals with bilateral amputations with the retrospective study of individuals with bilateral amputations described earlier, we can have more confidence in the results of the prospective study because of its control over data collection. The interview method is not without hazards, however. Patients who have worked closely with the occupational or physical therapist who is interviewing them might exaggerate their use of prostheses so that they do not disappoint the therapist. Interviews with family members or observations of function can provide checks on the accuracy of interview information.

Questionnaire. The questionnaire method was used by Granick and colleagues to study curriculum content related to geriatrics in entry-level physical therapy education programs.[12] The respondents were entry-level physical therapy program directors, by definition a well-educated group whose reading and writing skills should be sufficient to respond to a questionnaire. In addition, the national sample that was desired made mailing the questionnaire far more efficient and less expensive than conducting interviews with subjects. Another advantage of a mailed questionnaire is that it can maintain the anonymity of the respondent. Chapter 19 provides specific guidelines for collecting data through questionnaires and interviews.

ANALYSIS OF RELATIONSHIPS

The second major group of nonexperimental research consists of the designs in which the primary purpose is the analysis of relationships among variables. The general format for this research is that one group of subjects is tested on several different variables and the mathematical interrelationships among the variables are studied. This type of research is sometimes called *correlational research*. The term *correlation* also refers to a specific statistical technique. Therefore, there is a temptation to consider as correlational research only those studies in which the statistical correlation technique is used. As we will see in the examples, however, analysis of relationships entails more than just statistical correlation techniques. Therefore, in this text, the term "correlation" is reserved for the statistical analysis, and the longer, but more accurate, "analysis of relationships" is used to describe a type of research.

There are several reasons why one would want to identify relationships among variables. The first is that establishing relationships among variables without researcher manipulation may suggest fruitful areas for future experimental study. Research of this type is said to have *heuristic* value, meaning that the purpose of the study is to discover or reveal relationships that may lead to further enlightenment. The value of such heuristic research is not necessarily in its immediate results, but in the direction in which it moves the researcher.

The second specific purpose for the analysis of relationships among variables is that it allows scores on one variable to be predicted on the basis of scores on another variable. In clinical practice, a strong relationship between certain admission and discharge characteristics in a group of patients who recently completed their course of treatment might allow better prediction of discharge status for future patients.

The third specific purpose of the analysis of relationships is to determine the reliability of measurement tools. Reliability is the extent to which measurements are repeatable. In clinical practice, we plan treatment on the basis of certain measurements or observations. If a therapist evaluates a new prosthesis for a patient who has had an amputation and cannot reliably determine whether the pelvis is level, she might recommend to the prosthetist that he shorten the prosthesis on Monday, lengthen the prosthesis on Tuesday, and leave it alone on Wednesday! The statistical determination of the reliability of measurements provides an indication of the amount of confidence that should be placed in such measures.

A fourth reason to analyze relationships among variables is to determine the validity of a measure. By comparing scores on a new test with those on a well-established, or criterion, test, the extent to which the tests are in agreement can be established. Reliability and validity of measurements are discussed in detail in Chapters 10 and 11.

Retrospective Analysis of Relationships

Relationships can be analyzed retrospectively through use of medical records. Two examples illustrate the range of complexity that can be found in studies of this type.

A study of the relationship between just two variables was performed by Korner-Bitensky and associates.[13] The variables of interest were the therapists' prediction of functional recovery and actual functional recovery of stroke patients. Review of medical records identified 222 patients with stroke who had been admitted to the facility during a two-year period. Medical records for 204 of these patients contained both initial therapist goals and discharge outcomes in the format required for the study. The relationship between the admitting goal and the actual discharge status for each patient was classified as accurate (if the goal matched the discharge outcome), optimistic (if the goal was higher than the actual discharge status), or pessimistic (if the goal was lower than the actual discharge status).

A more complex analysis of relationships was performed by Roehrig, who studied multiple predictors of licensing examination scores for physical therapy graduates.[14] Data collection was retrospective in that Roehrig used existing sources of data: She examined the admission records of students who had completed one physical therapy program and received permission from the students to have their licensing examination scores released to her. Nine different admission variables, such as scores on standardized aptitude tests, grade point average, interview scores, and scores on recommendation letters, were used to predict licensing examination scores.

Prospective Analysis of Relationships

Analysis of relationships is often accomplished prospectively, with concomitant control over selection of subjects and administration of the measuring tools. A typical example of research in which relationships are analyzed prospectively is Sinaki and Offord's study of the relationship among physical activity, back extensor muscle strength, and bone mineral density.[15] Although determining the extent of the relationship among these factors was of interest to the researchers, identifying the relationships does not imply that manipulation of one variable will influence the other. If there is a strong, direct, relationship between physical activity and bone mineral density, we may be tempted to conclude that an increase in physical activity will cause an improvement in bone mineral density. However, when the investigator has not subjected any variables to controlled manipulation, such causal inferences are not justified.

Prospective analysis of relationships has been used to establish the validity of a particular isokinetic torque curve pattern in predicting the presence of a tear in the anterior cruciate ligament (ACL). Stratford and associates reported that several clinical and research reports had reported that different torque curve patterns characterized different knee joint disorders.[16] In particular, "double-hump" or "rapid initial downslope" patterns were noted to be associated with ACL damage. To test the validity of the supposition that torque patterns were related to ACL damage, Stratford and associates performed isokinetic testing and arthroscopic knee examination on 30 patients with a positive history of knee trauma and clinical evidence of joint instability. The criterion, or "gold standard," measurement was the arthroscopic diagnosis.

Stratford and associates evaluated the relationship between the torque curve pattern and the arthroscopic result with the traditional epidemiological concepts of sensitivity, specificity, positive predictive value, and negative predictive value.[17, 18] Sensitivity and specificity compare correct conclusions with the new test with the results on the criterion test. The *sensitivity* of a test is the percentage of individuals with a particular diagnosis who are correctly identified as positive by the test. The *specificity* is the percentage of individuals without a particular diagnosis who are correctly identified as negative by the test. The *positive predictive value* is the percentage of individuals identified by the test as positive who actually have the diagnosis. The *negative predictive value* is the percentage of those identified by the test as negative who actually do not have the diagnosis.

These four epidemiological concepts are illustrated in Figure 6–1, which uses data from Stratford and associates' study.[16] When testing patients with ACL tears, the researchers found that the torque curve tracings had a sensitivity of 25%, meaning that

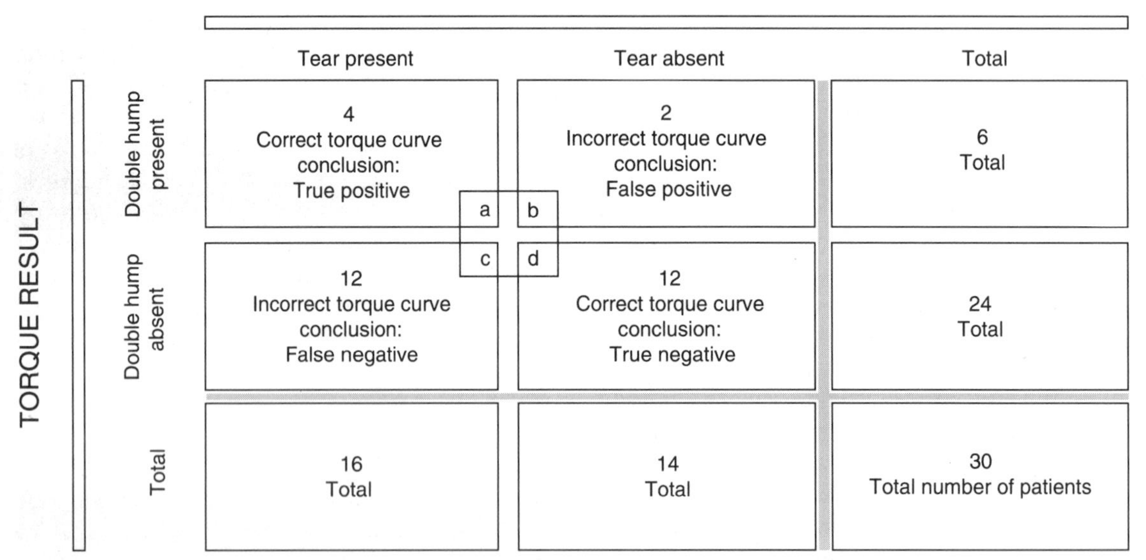

FIGURE 6–1. Illustration of traditional epidemiological concepts. Sensitivity = $a \div (a + c)$ = true positives ÷ number with tears = 4 ÷ 16 = 25%. Specificity = $d \div (b + d)$ = true negatives ÷ number without tears = 12 ÷ 14 = 86%. Positive predictive value = $a \div (a + b)$ = true positives ÷ number with characteristic torque curve pattern = 4 ÷ 6 = 67%. Negative predictive value = $d \div (c + d)$ = true negatives ÷ number without characteristic torque curve pattern = 12 ÷ 24 = 50%. (From Stratford P, Agostino V, Armstrong B, Stewart T, Weininger S. Diagnostic value of knee extension torque tracings in suspected anterior cruciate ligament tears. *Phys Ther.* 1987;67:1535. Reprinted from *Physical Therapy* with the permission of the American Physical Therapy Association.)

only 25% of the patients with ACL tears were identified by the torque curve pattern. When testing patients without ACL tears, they found that the torque curve tracings had a specificity of 86%, meaning that 14% of patients without tears had false-positive tracings that identified them as having tears. When examining torque curves with the characteristic pattern, Stratford and associates found a positive predictive value of 67%, which means that two-thirds of the patients with the characteristic pattern could be expected to actually have an ACL tear. When examining torque curves without the characteristic pattern, the researchers found a negative predictive value of 50%, which means that half of patients with negative torque curve patterns could still be expected to have ACL tears.

Whereas studies in the medical literature frequently report epidemiological data in the foregoing manner, this sort of presentation is relatively rare in the physical therapy literature today. However, it should increase in importance as physical therapists continue to critically examine the bases on which they make diagnostic and treatment decisions.

ANALYSIS OF DIFFERENCES

The general purpose of research in which differences are analyzed is to focus on whether groups or treatments are different in some reliable way. Although analysis of differences is often accomplished experimentally, there have been many nonexperimental studies in which differences were analyzed. Nonexperimental analysis of differences among groups or treatments is called *ex post facto* or *causal-comparative* research.[19] The independent variables in such studies are not manipulated but are the presumed cause of differences in the dependent variable. The *ex post facto* (after the fact) designation refers to the fact that assignment to groups is not under the control of the investigator, but rather is determined by existing characteristics of the individuals within the study. Note that *ex post facto* does not mean questions are developed after data collection; *ex post facto* designs may use either retrospective or prospective data collection.

Retrospective Analysis of Differences

Medical records provide a vast source of information about patient treatment and outcomes. When groups of patients can be identified from the medical records as having undergone different courses of treatments, it is possible to study the relationship of treatment to outcome in a retrospective manner. Three articles illustrate three different ways of developing groups in the retrospective *ex post facto* designs.

The first, by Timm, is a large retrospective study of postsurgical knee rehabilitation.[20] The medical charts of more than 5,000 patients who had undergone surgery in one calendar year were reviewed. Four groups of patients who had completed knee rehabilitation were identified by the type of program they had completed, as documented in the medical chart: no exercise, home exercise, isotonic exercise, or isokinetic exercise. Thus the groups constituted patients treated in the same time frame, but with different rehabilitation protocols.

One disadvantage of retrospective designs such as this is that nonrandom placement into groups makes it impossible to determine why a particular patient was placed in a particular rehabilitation group. For example, did those who wanted to return to athletic competition get placed in the isokinetic group, thereby giving it a bias toward motivated patients? Unless the medical records contain information about patient goals and motivation, there is no way to determine whether or not this bias occurred.

In a second retrospective *ex post facto* study, successive cohorts were studied to determine whether the Medicare prospective payment system affected use of physical therapy services by the hospitalized elderly. Holt and Winograd studied the medical records of certain patients aged 75 years or older for a period of six years.[21] The first four years of records were from patients treated before implementation of the prospective payment system; the last two years were from patients treated after implementation of the prospective payment system. The difference in patient selection between this study and Timm's study of postoperative knee rehabilitation is that answering this study question required sampling of patients from two different points in time; Timm's rehabilitation study is strengthened by its use of patients treated in a single time frame.

The third example of subject grouping within the retrospective *ex post facto* designs followed what is called the *case-control* design. In this design, a group of patients with the desired effect is identified, and then a group without the effect is identified. Presumed causes for the effects are then sought, and the proportions of patients with the causes in the two groups are compared. One example of a case-control design is Morris and associates' study of the effect of preexisting conditions on mortality in trauma patients.[22] In this study patients who died after trauma (the cases) were compared with age- and injury-matched patients who survived trauma (the controls). The incidence in both groups of 11 preexisting chronic conditions that were thought to influence survival rate after trauma was then established. The confidence that can be placed in case-control research depends in large part on the criteria used to define the case and control groups.[23, 24]

As defined in this text, retrospective research uses data collected before question development, and prospective research uses data collected after question development. Epidemiological researchers sometimes use the terms *retrospective* and *prospective* differently. Retrospective epidemiological research is research in which the researcher works backward from effect to cause and is synonymous with case-control research. Prospective epidemiological research works forward from cause to effect and is sometimes referred to as a *cohort* design. Although all three of the studies just presented relied on preexisting medical record information, epidemiologists might refer to the reports on knee rehabilitation and payment system as prospective articles because the authors worked from causes (different rehabilitation and different payment systems, respectively) to effects (success and use of physical therapy, respectively). The trauma article would be considered retrospective because the researchers started with the effect (death) and proceeded to look for causes (preexisting medical conditions). The original definitions of *prospective* and *retrospective* as related to the timing of data collection are used throughout the remainder of this text; readers should, however, be aware of the varied uses of these terms.[8(p133)]

A final example of retrospective analysis of differences among groups is a specialized research technique called *meta-analysis*. This technique provides a means to synthesize research results across several different studies.[25–28] Meta-analysis is usually undertaken when a body of research about the effectiveness of a given technique provides discrepant results. Narrative reviews of the literature are subject to the biases of the author, as noted rather humorously, but perhaps truthfully, by Glass:

> A common method of integrating several studies with inconsistent findings is to carp on the design or analysis

> deficiencies of all but a few studies—those remaining frequently being one's own work or that of one's students and friends—and then advance the one or two "acceptable" studies as the truth of the matter.[26(p7)]

Meta-analytic methods provide a quantitative way of synthesizing the results of different research studies on the same topic.

A relevant example of meta-analysis is Ottenbacher and Petersen's[25] study of the effectiveness of vestibular stimulation. Only 18 of 41 studies on vestibular stimulation were sufficiently similar in design and contained the necessary statistical information to be included in the meta-analysis. The independent variable in all studies was stimulation condition, with stimulation either absent or present. The dependent variables differed from study to study, but all were some measure of motor or reflex function. The basic concept behind meta-analysis is that the size of the differences between treatment groups (the effect size) is mathematically standardized so that it can be compared between studies with different, but conceptually related, dependent variables. More specific information about meta-analysis can be found in several educational and behavioral sciences texts, as well as in rehabilitation journals.[29–31]

Prospective Analysis of Differences

Prospective analysis of differences is the final cell of the six-cell matrix of research types. It is the only cell that is shared between the experimental and nonexperimental designs. By definition, the experimental designs must be prospective, and their purpose is to determine the effects of some intervention on a dependent variable by analyzing the differences in groups who were and were not exposed to a manipulation or the differences within a single group exposed to more than one experimental treatment. Differences between groups or within a group can also be analyzed in the absence of controlled manipulation.

An example of a nonexperimental study in which the independent variable could have been manipulated but was not is Jansen and Minerbo's comparison of early dynamic mobilization with immobilization after flexor tendon repair in the hand.[32] To make this comparison, the researchers selected subjects retrospectively by reviewing their medical records to determine who had been immobilized postoperatively and who had received early dynamic splinting. Even though the division into treatment groups was accomplished before question development, the researchers collected data themselves at four and a half months after surgery. As was the case with our other comparisons between retrospective and prospective studies, we can place more confidence in this study because prospective data analysis allowed the researchers to standardize the measures used in the study. If the study had been completely retrospective, with group assignment and dependent measures drawn from the medical chart, the uniformity of the measures would be questioned. If the study had been completely prospective, with random group assignment, treatment, and then measurement, it no longer would have been a nonexperimental study because the manipulation would have been under the control of the investigators.

An example of a nonexperimental analysis of differences in which the independent variable was inherently nonmanipulable is Shinabarger's comparison of joint mobility in adults with diabetes mellitus versus adults without diabetes mellitus.[33] She identified male subjects with diabetes mellitus of at least two years' duration and then identified a comparable group of men without diabetes mellitus. She then measured upper extremity range of motion and contrasted the average measurements of the two groups.

SUMMARY

Unlike experimental research, nonexperimental research does not require controlled manipulation of variables. Because of this permissive definition, there is a greater variety of nonexperimental research designs. Descriptive studies use retrospective or prospective data collection to characterize a phenomenon of interest. In studies that involve the analysis of relationships, researchers use prospective or retrospective data collection to measure variables, which they then analyze to make predictions or determine reliability or validity of the measures. Nonexperimental analysis of differences, or *ex post facto* research, is accomplished when a nonmanipulated variable, such as sex or age, is the only independent variable being studied.

References

1. Kerlinger FN. *Foundations of Behavioral Research.* 3rd ed. Fort Worth, Tex: Holt, Rinehart & Winston Inc; 1986:349.
2. Shaugnessey JJ, Zechmeister EB. *Research Methods in Psychology.* 2nd ed. New York, NY: McGraw-Hill Publishing Co; 1990:130.
3. Holsti OR. *Content Analysis for the Social Sciences.* Reading, Mass: Addison-Wesley; 1969.
4. Findley TW, Daum MC. Research in physical medicine and rehabilitation, III: the chart review or how to use clinical data for exploratory retrospective studies. *Am J Phys Med Rehabil.* 1989;68:150–157.
5. Isaac S, Michael WB. *Handbook in Research and Evaluation for Education and the Behavioral Sciences.* San Diego, Calif: EdITS Publishers; 1971:17.
6. Wolf E, Lilling M, Ferber I, Marcus J. Prosthetic rehabilitation of elderly bilateral amputees. *Int J Rehabil Res.* 1989;12:271–278.
7. Tator CH, Edmonds VE. National survey of spinal injuries in hockey players. *Can Med Assoc J.* 1984;130:875–880.
8. Hennekens CH, Buring JE. *Epidemiology in Medicine.* Boston, Mass: Little, Brown & Co; 1987.
9. Taylor TK, Domholdt E. Legislative change to permit direct access to physical therapy services: a study of process and content issues. *Phys Ther.* 1991;71:382–389.
10. Heriza CB. Organization of leg movements in preterm infants. *Phys Ther.* 1988;68:1340–1346.
11. Brodzka WK, Thornhill HL, Zarapkar SE, Malloy JA, Weiss L. Long-term function of persons with atherosclerotic bilateral below-knee amputation living in the inner city. *Arch Phys Med Rehabil.* 1990;71:895–900.
12. Granick R, Simson S, Wilson LB. Survey of curriculum content related to geriatrics in physical therapy education programs. *Phys Ther.* 1987;67:234–237.
13. Korner-Bitensky N, Mayo N, Cabot R, Becker R, Coopersmith H. Motor and functional recovery after stroke: accuracy of physical therapists' predictions. *Arch Phys Med Rehabil.* 1989;70:95–99.
14. Roehrig SM. Prediction of licensing examination scores in physical therapy graduates. *Phys Ther.* 1988;68:694–698.
15. Sinaki M, Offord KP. Physical activity in postmenopausal women: effect on back muscle strength and bone mineral density of the spine. *Arch Phys Med Rehabil.* 1988;69:277–280.
16. Stratford P, Agostino V, Armstrong B, Stewart T, Weininger S. Diagnostic value of knee extension torque tracings in suspected anterior cruciate ligament tears. *Phys Ther.* 1987;67:1533–1536.
17. How to read clinical journals, II: to learn about a diagnostic test. *Can Med Assoc J.* 1981;124:703–710.
18. Leaverton PE. *A Review of Biostatistics: A Program for Self-Instruction.* 2nd ed. Boston, Mass: Little, Brown & Co; 1978.
19. Gay LR. *Educational Research: Competencies for Analysis and Application.* Columbus, Ohio: Charles E Merrill Publishing Co; 1976.
20. Timm KE. Postsurgical knee rehabilitation: a five year study of four methods and 5,381 patients. *Am J Sports Med.* 1988;16:463–468.
21. Holt P, Winograd CH. Prospective payment and the utilization of physical therapy service in the hospitalized elderly. *Am J Public Health.* 1990;80:1491–1494.
22. Morris JA, MacKenzie EJ, Edelstein SL. The effect of preexisting conditions on mortality in trauma patients. *JAMA.* 1990;263:1942–1946.
23. Hayden GF, Kramer MS, Horwitz RI. The case-control study: a practical review for the clinician. *JAMA.* 1982;247:326–331.
24. Norton BJ, Strube MJ. Some cautionary comments on the use of retrospective designs to evaluate treatment efficacy. *Phys Ther.* 1988;68:1374–1377.
25. Ottenbacher KJ, Petersen P. A meta-analysis of applied vestibular stimulation research. *Physical and Occupational Therapy in Pediatrics.* 1985;5:119–134.
26. Glass GV. Primary, secondary and meta-analysis of research. *Educational Research.* 1976;5:3–9.
27. Glass GV, McGaw B, Smith ML. *Meta-Analysis in Social Research.* Newbury Park, Calif: Sage Publications; 1981.
28. Thomas JR, French KE. The use of meta-analysis in

exercise and sport: a tutorial. *Research Quarterly for Exercise and Sport.* 1989;57:196–204.

29. Cooper HM. Scientific guidelines for conducting integrative research reviews. *Review of Educational Research.* 1982;52:291–301.
30. Norton BJ, Strube MJ. Making decisions based on group designs and meta-analysis. *Phys Ther.* 1989;69:594–600.
31. Ottenbacher KJ, Biocca Z, DeCremer G, Gevelinger M, Jedlovec KB, Johnson MB. Quantitative analysis of the effectiveness of pediatric therapy: emphasis on the neurodevelopmental treatment approach. *Phys Ther.* 1986;66:1095–1101.
32. Jansen CWS, Minerbo G. A comparison between early dynamically controlled mobilization and immobilization after flexor tendon repair in zone 2 of the hand: preliminary results. *Journal of Hand Therapy.* 1990;3:20–25.
33. Shinabarger NI. Limited joint mobility in adults with diabetes mellitus. *Phys Ther.* 1987;67:215–218.

CHAPTER 7

Research Validity

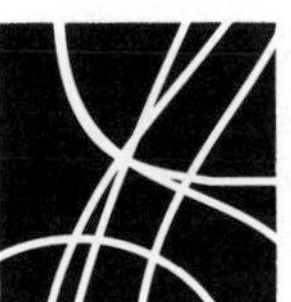

The validity of a piece of research is the extent to which the conclusions of that research are believable and useful. Cook and Campbell have outlined four types of validity, and this chapter relies to a great extent on their work.[1] When determining the value of a piece of research, readers need to ask four basic questions about the research.

1. Is the research designed so that there are few alternative explanations for changes in the dependent variable other than the effect of the independent variable? Factors other than the independent variables that could be related to changes in the dependent variable are threats to *internal validity*.
2. Are the research constructs defined and used in such a way that the research can be placed in the framework of other research within the field of study? Poor definition of constructs or inconsistent use of constructs is a threat to *construct validity*.
3. To whom can the results of this research be applied? Sampling and design factors that lead to limited generalizability are threats to *external validity*.
4. Are statistical tools used correctly to analyze the data? Irregularities in the use of statistics are threats to *statistical conclusion validity*.

The purpose of this chapter is to provide a discussion of the first three types of validity. Understanding statistical conclusion validity requires some background in statistical reasoning. Threats to statistical conclusion validity are therefore covered in Chapter 13 in the introduction to statistical reasoning. Each of the remaining three types of validity has several identifiable threats that can be illustrated either in examples from the physical therapy literature, or in examples of hypothetical research in physical therapy. For each of these threats, at least one example is presented and mechanisms for controlling the threat suggested. The chapter ends with an examination of the interrelationships between the types of validity.

INTERNAL VALIDITY

Internal validity is the extent to which the results of a study demonstrate that a causal relationship exists between the independent and dependent variables. In experimental research, the central question about internal validity is whether the treatment caused the observed changes in the dependent variable. In nonexperimental research designed to delineate differences between groups in the absence of controlled manipulation by the researcher, the question becomes whether the independent variable is a plausible cause of group differences on the dependent variable.

The general strategy that researchers use to increase internal validity is to maximize their control over all aspects of the research project. Eliminating extraneous variables through control of the experimental setting removes them as plausible causes of changes in the dependent variable. Randomized assignment of subjects to treatment groups maximizes the probability that extraneous subject characteristics will be evenly distributed across groups. If random assignment is not possible, the researcher can collect information about patient characteristics that threaten internal validity to determine whether the characteristics in question were equally represented across groups.

When developing research proposals, investigators should carefully consider each threat to internal validity to determine whether their design is vulnerable to that threat. If it is, the researchers must decide whether to institute additional controls to minimize the threat, collect additional information to document whether the threat materialized, or accept the threat as an unavoidable design flaw. There is no perfect research design, and high levels of internal validity may compromise construct or external validity, as discussed at the end of the chapter. Eleven of Cook and Campbell's threats to internal validity are important for physical therapy researchers and are discussed below.[1]

History

History is a threat to internal validity when events unrelated to the treatment of interest occur during the course of the study and may plausibly change the dependent variable. Amundsen and associates studied the effect of a group exercise program on the mean aerobic power of elderly women living in a high-rise apartment complex.[2] They used a nonrandom method to assign subjects to the experimental group and the control group. The experimental group was made up of women who participated consistently in the group exercise program, and the control group was made up of women whose schedules did not permit their attendance at the exercise sessions. Several historical events could reduce the internal validity of this, or any, study. Consider the effect on the study of an elevator malfunction in the building that required all individuals in the study to walk up at least two flights of stairs to get to their apartments during the last three weeks of the study. This hypothetical historical event, which is not under the researchers' control, would introduce another aerobic training stimulus into the study. In the absence of control, the researchers should gather information to determine how much of an effect stair climbing may have had on the results of the study.

Researchers could ask subjects to estimate the number of times per day that they climbed the stairs during the interruption in elevator service. If experimental and control subjects used the stairs with equal frequency, then the effect of the stair climbing would be uniform across the two groups, and some separation of the effects of the stair climbing versus the effects of the group exercise program could be accomplished, as shown in Figure 7–1. The hypothetical data in this figure show that the groups began the study with the same average fitness level, that the control group improved slightly, and that the experimental group improved markedly. The conclusion drawn from this data might be written in a journal article as follows:

The control group showed a 0.5 metabolic equivalent (MET) improvement in mean aerobic power at the posttest, presumably because of the unintended training stimulus of stair climbing during the last three weeks of the study. The experimental group, who also received the unintended stimulus of stair climbing, showed three times the mean aerobic power improvement of the control group. We assume that the experimental group results represent an approximately 0.5 MET improvement related to stair climbing and a 1.0 MET improvement attributable to the group exercise program.

Researchers can use three strategies to minimize the effects of history: planning, use of a randomly selected control group, and description of unavoidable historical events. In experimental studies, careful planning by

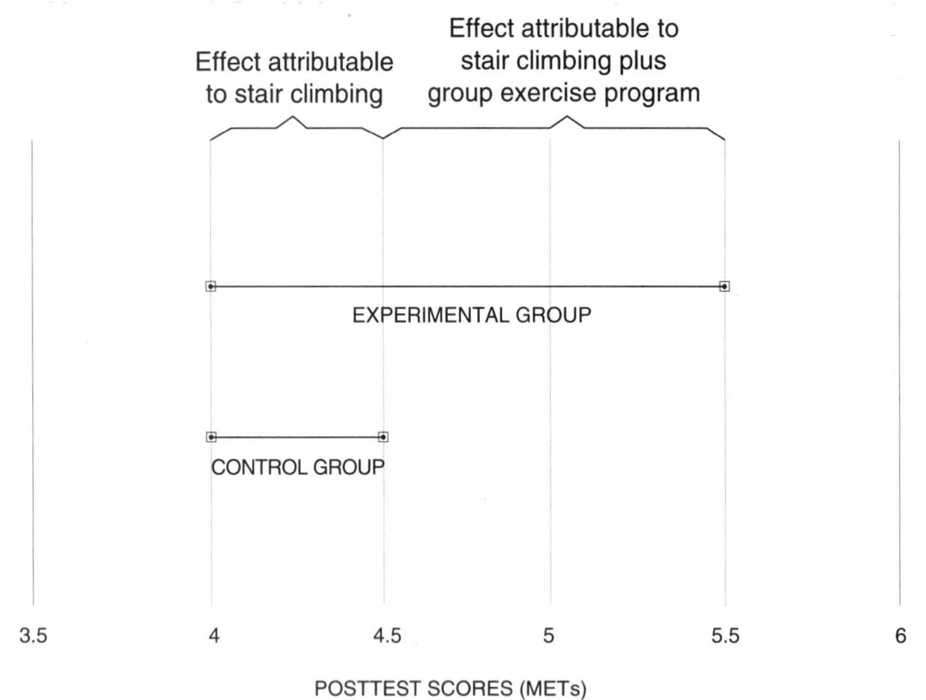

FIGURE 7–1. Separation of the effects of stair climbing from the effects of a group exercise program in a test of aerobic power. Both the control and experimental groups participated in stair climbing; only the experimental group participated in a group exercise program. Both groups had mean pretest scores of 4.0 metabolic equivalents (METs); the control group had a mean posttest score of 4.5 METs, and the experimental group had a mean posttest score of 5.5 METs. For the control group, any changes in aerobic power can be attributed to the stair climbing. For the experimental group, part of the change seen can be attributed to the stair climbing; the change above that seen in the control group can be attributed to the added effect of the group exercise program.

the researcher can minimize the chances that historical events will influence the study. If a geographical region is usually snowed in during February, a study that requires subject attendance at treatment sessions five days per week should probably be scheduled at another time of year. If testing of subjects requires a full day with half-hour rests between measurements, it might be wise to isolate subjects and researchers from radios and televisions so that news that happens to occur on the day of testing will not influence subject or researcher performance.

Use of a control group provides the researcher with some ability to separate the effects of history from the effects of the treatment. Use of a control group in this manner was illustrated by the hypothetical example of the elevator malfunction, in which the effect of stair climbing by the control group was separated from the combined effect of stair climbing and exercise group participation by the experimental group. Random assignment of subjects to groups is the best way to minimize the effects of history, because the different groups will likely be affected equally by the historical event.

In some instances, historical events that cannot be avoided may occur. In retrospective nonexperimental studies that examine differences between groups, control of history is impossible because the historical events have already occurred. If an uncontrolled historical event that may cause changes in the dependent variable does occur, it is important to collect and present information about the event. Holt and Winograd documented two historical threats to the internal validity of their findings that length of stay decreased and percentage of physical therapy referrals increased in patients seen before and after implementation of the Medicare prospective payment system. First, the percentage of patients referred to physical therapy may have been influenced by the establishment of a geriatric rehabilitation program in one of the major teaching facilities through which their resident physicians rotated. Second, length of stay may have been influenced by the introduction of a home health care program at the medical center studied. When unable to control a threat, researchers have a responsibility to present information about the threat so that readers may form an opinion about its seriousness.

Maturation

Maturation, changes within a subject due to the passage of time, is a threat to internal validity when it occurs during the course of a study and may plausibly cause changes in the dependent variable. Subjects get older, more experienced, or bored during the course of a study. Patients with neurological deficits may experience spontaneous improvement in their conditions; subjects with orthopedic injuries may become less edematous, have less pain, and be able to bear more weight with time.

As was the case with historical threats to internal validity, single-group studies do not provide a basis from which the researcher may separate the effects of maturation from the effects of treatment. Yarkony and associates used a single-group design to document the functional improvement of paraplegic patients completing an inpatient rehabilitation program.[4] Because the neurological deficit of a complete spinal cord injury is unlikely to improve after the early weeks of the injury, the maturation threat in this study was the increased experience and skill in managing their injury that the young people with paraplegia might have exhibited in the absence of a formal rehabilitation program.

Maturation effects can be controlled in several ways. The first is through use of a control group, preferably with random assignment of subjects to either the control or the experimental group. Use of the control group allows the effects of maturation alone to be observed in the control group. The treatment effects are then evaluated in terms of how much the treatment group improved in comparison with the control group.

A second way to control for the effects of maturation is to take multiple baseline measures of subjects before implementing the treatment. Suppose that you have a group of patients with ankle sprains who have persistent edema despite protected weight bearing, compression bandage wrap, elevation when possible, and use of ice packs three times daily. Documentation of baseline volume over a period of several days or weeks would provide appropriate comparison measures against which the effects of a compression/cryotherapy pump regimen could be evaluated. Figure 7–2 shows three patterns of baseline measurements: stable, irregular, and steadily progressing. Results after the intervention are interpreted in light of the baseline pattern documented before the intervention. Patients in Figure 7–2A had no change in the weeks before intervention but showed dramatic improvements after treatment. Patients in Figure 7–2B had weekly fluctuations in edema before treatment and marked improvement after treatment. Patients in Figure 7–2C showed consistent, but slow, improvement in the weeks before treatment and more rapid improvement after treatment.

Maturation effects may be seen in repeated treatment research designs. Any time patients receive more than one treatment, they may respond differently to later treatments than to earlier treatments. Performance on the dependent variable may improve for later treatments because of increased experience with the treatment, or performance may decline because of fatigue or boredom. In Brooks and associates' repeated treatment study of the torque produced by electrical stimulation of the quadriceps femoris muscle with horizontal or longitudinal electrode placement, subjects may have felt more accustomed to the electrical stimulation with time, improving performance during the second electrode placement pattern.[5] Conversely, their quadriceps femoris muscles may have fatigued during the course of the study, demonstrating decreased performance during the second electrode placement pattern. The authors randomized the order of presentation of treatments to control for maturation in this repeated treatment design.

Testing

Testing is a threat to internal validity when repeated testing itself is likely to result in changes in the dependent variable. For example, on the first day of treatment, a patient with a painful shoulder who is unfamiliar with the therapist and with the procedure for taking range-of-motion measurements may be unable to relax his shoulder girdle musculature to provide an accurate measure of his passive range of motion. Improved measurements on subsequent days may reflect familiarization with the testing procedure and more effective relaxation during testing, rather than effectiveness of the treatment.

Three basic design strategies can be used to minimize testing effects. The first is to use randomly selected experimental and control groups so that the effects of testing in the control group can be removed by comparison with the effects of testing and treatment in the experimental group. This is analogous to the removal of the effects of history and maturation through use of a control group.

The second strategy is to eliminate multiple testing through use of a posttest-only design. However, in the absence of a pretest to establish that control and experimental groups were the same at the start of the experiment, posttest-only studies must have effective random assignment of subjects to groups.

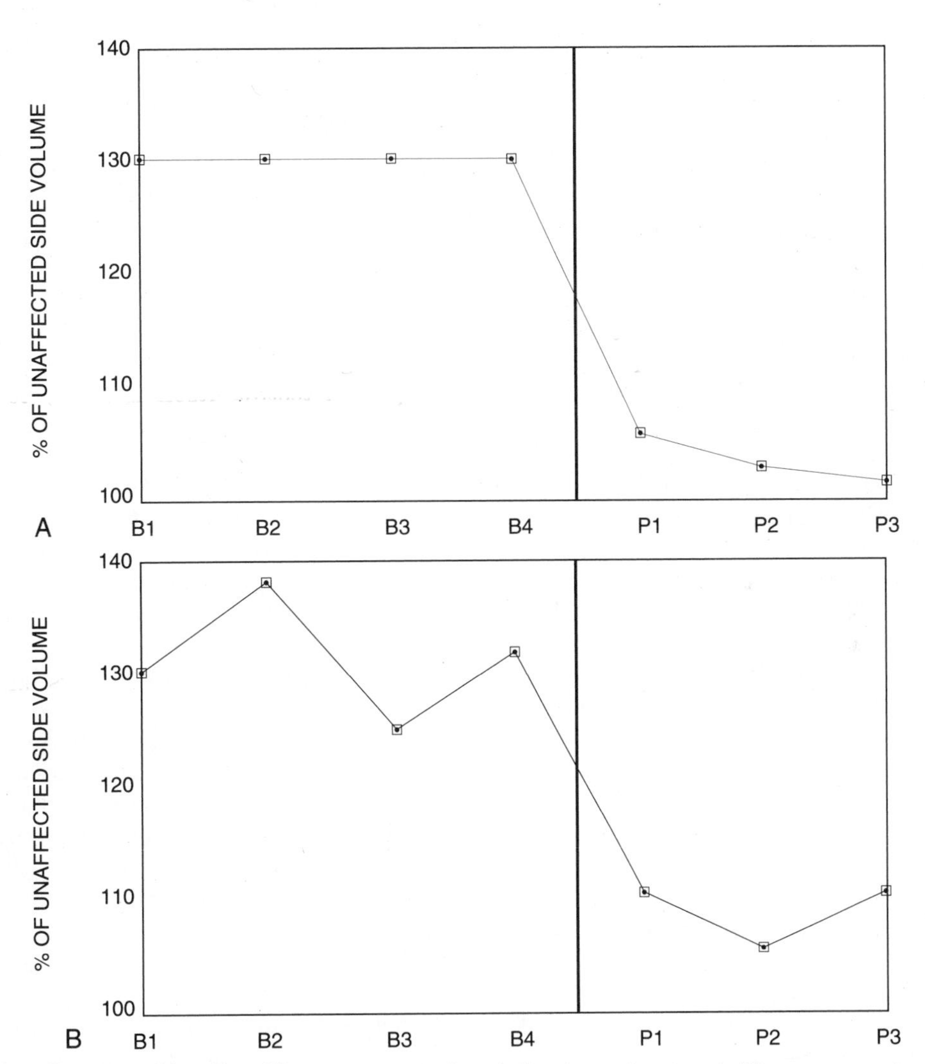

FIGURE 7–2. Patterns of baseline (B) measurements in relation to posttreatment (P) measurements. **A.** Stable baseline. **B.** Irregular baseline.

Illustration continued on following page

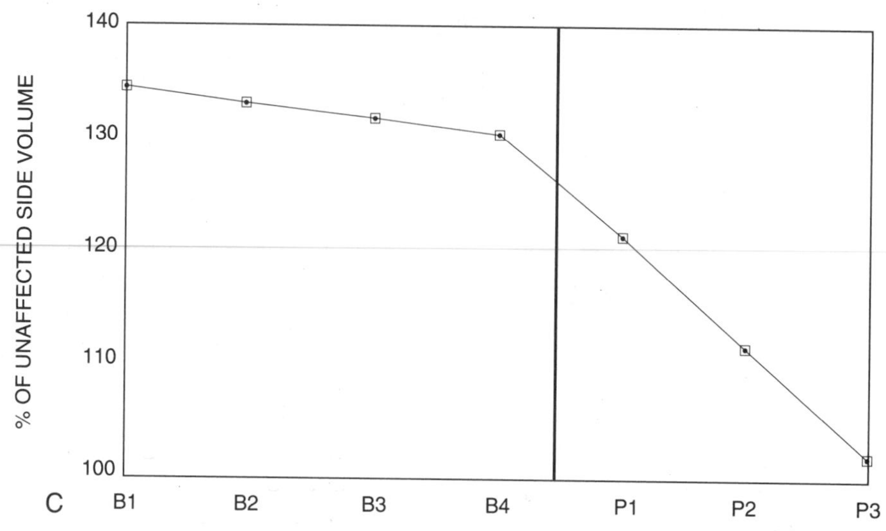

FIGURE 7–2 *Continued* **C.** Baseline with a downward trend.

The third design strategy is to conduct familiarization sessions with the testing equipment so that the effects of learning are accounted for before the independent variable is manipulated. To determine the extent of familiarization needed, the researcher should conduct a pilot study to determine how much time or how many sessions are needed before performance is stable. One drawback of multiple testing is the possibility that the familiarization process will itself constitute a "treatment." For example, if subjects familiarize themselves with an isokinetic testing regimen once a week for four weeks, they may have exercised enough during familiarization to show a training response.

Instrumentation

Instrumentation is a threat to internal validity when changes in measuring tools themselves are responsible for observed changes in the dependent variable. Many tools that record physical measurements need to be calibrated with each testing session. Calibration is a process by which the measuring tool is compared with standard measures to determine its accuracy. If inaccurate, some tools can be adjusted until they are accurate. If a tool has limited adjustability, the researcher may need to apply a mathematical correction factor to convert inaccurate raw scores into accurate transformed scores. If temperature or humidity influences measurement, this factor must be controlled, preferably through testing under constant conditions or, alternatively, through mathematical adjustment for the differences in physical environment.

Researchers themselves are measuring tools ("human instruments"). An example of the variability in the human instrument has surely been felt by almost any student: It is almost impossible for an instructor to apply exactly the same criteria to each paper in a large stack. Maybe the instructor starts out lenient but cracks down as she proceeds through the stack. Maybe the instructor who is a stickler at first adopts a more permissive attitude when the end of the stack is in sight. Maybe a middling paper is graded harshly if it follows an exemplary paper; the same paper might be graded favorably if it follows an abysmal example. A variety of observational clinical measures, such as identification of gait deviations, functional levels, or abnormal tone, may suffer from similar problems. Measurement issues in physical therapy research are addressed in detail in Chapters 10 through 12.

Statistical Regression to the Mean

Statistical regression is a threat to internal validity when subjects are selected on the basis of extreme scores on a single administration of a test. A hypothetical example illustrates the mathematical principle behind statistical regression to the mean: We have three recreational runners, each of whom has completed ten 10-km runs in an average time of 50 minutes, and a range of times from 40 to 60 minutes. The distribution in Figure 7–3A represents the race times of the three runners.

Suppose we wish to test a new training regimen designed to decrease race times to see if the regimen is equally effective with runners at different skill levels. We place runners into categories based on a single qualifying race time, have them try the training regimen for one month, and record their times at an evaluation race completed at the end of the one-month training period. At the qualifying race, we place runners into one of three speed categories based on their time in that race: Subjects in the fast group finished in less than 45 minutes, subjects in the average group finished between and including 45 and 55 minutes, and subjects in the slow group finished in greater than 55 minutes.

The times marked with a Q in Figure 7–3B show that Runner 1 performed much better than average on the day of the qualifying race (40 minutes), Runner 2 performed much worse than usual on the qualifying day (60 minutes), and Runner 3 gave an average performance (49 minutes). Runners 1 and 2 gave atypical performances on the qualifying day and in subsequent races would be expected to perform closer to their "true" running speed. Thus, even without intervention, Runner 1 would likely run the next race slower and Runner 2 would likely run the next race faster. Runner 3, who gave a typical performance, is likely to give another typical performance at the next race. In other words, the extreme scores will tend to "regress toward the mean." This regression toward the mean for the evaluation race is represented by the times marked with an E in Figure 7–3B. If we do not consider the effects of statistical regression, we might conclude that the training program has no effect on average runners, speeds up the slow runners, and slows down the fast runners.

In general, the way to control for statistical regression toward the mean is to select subjects for groups on the basis of reliable, stable measures. If the measures used to form groups are inherently variable, then subjects are best assigned to groups on the basis of a distribution of scores collected over time, rather than by a single score that might not reflect true ability.

Assignment

Assignment to groups is a threat to internal validity when groups of subjects are different from one another on some variable that is related to the dependent variable of interest. Cook and Campbell labeled this particular threat "selection."[1] The term *assignment* is more correct and differentiates between the internal validity threat related to group assignment and the external validity threat of subject selection.

Assignment threatens internal validity most often in designs in which subjects are not randomly assigned to groups or in nonexperimental designs in which study group membership cannot be manipulated by the investigator. For example, Timm used a ret-

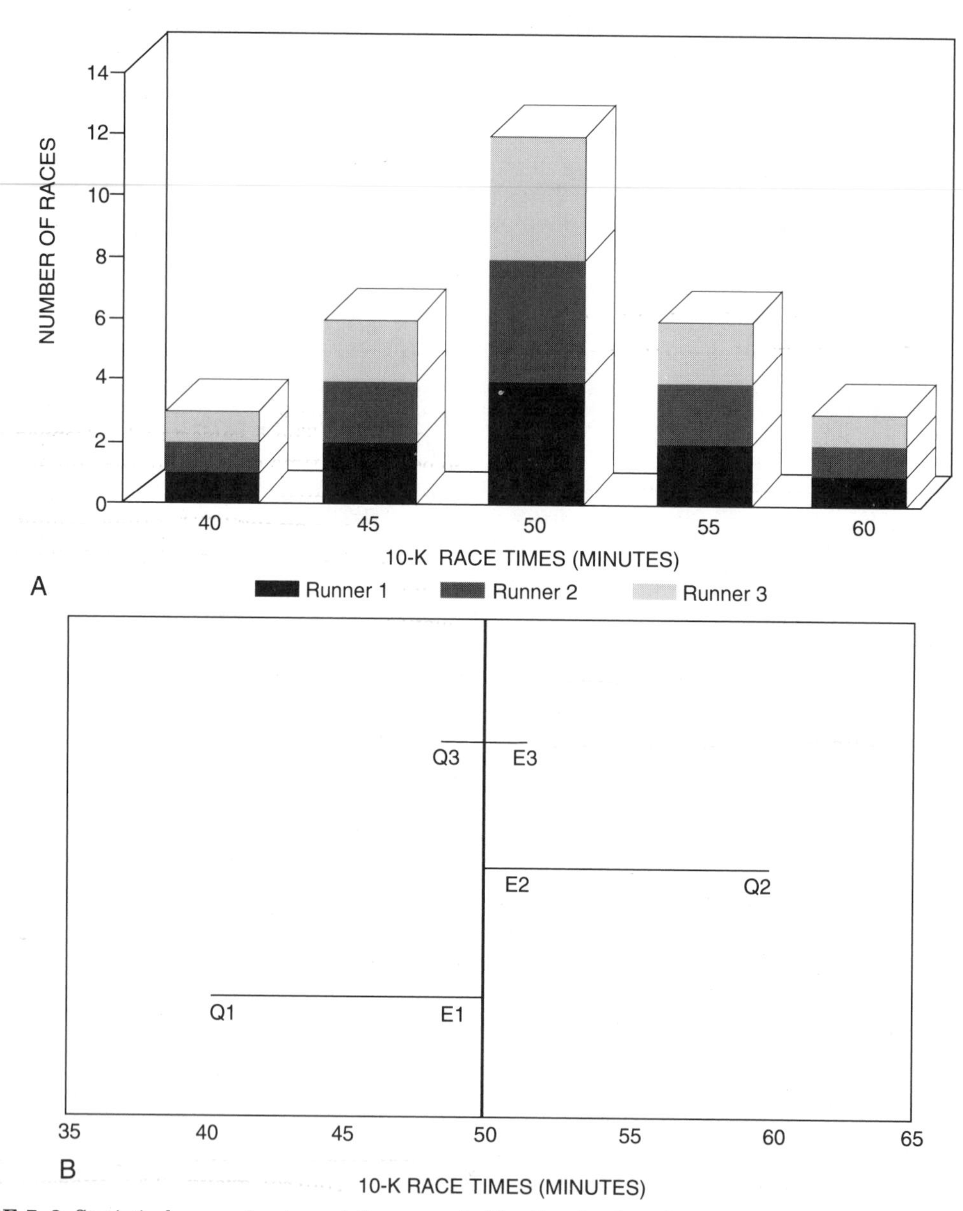

FIGURE 7–3. Statistical regression toward the mean. **A.** The distribution of race times for three runners, as shown by the different shading patterns on the bars. All three runners have an average race time of 50 minutes. **B.** The effect of statistical regression toward the mean if the runners are placed into different groups based on qualifying times at a single race. Q represents qualifying times for each runner; E represents the runners' evaluation times at a subsequent race. Runner 1 appears to have slowed from 40 to 50 minutes, Runner 2 appears to have speeded up from 60 to 50 minutes, and Runner 3 stayed approximately the same.

rospective nonexperimental design to determine the success of postoperative knee rehabilitation based on type of rehabilitation.[6] The four rehabilitation groups were as follows: no rehabilitation, home exercise, isotonic exercise, and isokinetic exercise. Because patients were placed into groups for the study based on information from medical records, there is no way to determine why individual patients underwent a particular type of rehabilitation program. Timm wisely tempered his conclusion that isokinetic exercise was the most effective method of knee rehabilitation by mentioning the possibility of assignment effects. Perhaps the superior results of the isokinetic group can be partially attributed to an assignment bias whereby motivated athletic patients were frequently placed in that group.

Control of assignment threats is most effectively accomplished through random assignment to groups within a study (see Chapter 8). When random assignment to groups is not possible, researchers may use statistical methods to "equalize" groups (see Chapter 14).

Mortality

Mortality is a threat to internal validity when subjects are lost from the different study groups at different rates or for different reasons. Despite the best efforts of the researcher to begin the study with randomly selected groups who are equivalent on all important factors, differential mortality can leave the researcher with very different groups by the end of the study. Assume that a researcher has designed a strengthening study in which one group of 50 subjects participates in a combined concentric and eccentric program of moderate intensity and another group of 50 participates in a largely eccentric program of higher intensity. Forty-five of the subjects in the moderate group complete the program, with an average increase in strength of 20%. Fifteen of the subjects in the high-intensity group complete the program, with an average increase in strength of 40%. Concluding that the high-intensity program was superior to the moderate-intensity program would ignore the differential mortality of subjects from the two groups. This problem of mortality might be written up as follows in a journal article:

> Subjects who completed the high-intensity program showed greater strength increases than did subjects who completed the moderate-intensity program. Note, however, that there was differential loss of subjects from the two groups. Ninety percent of the moderate-intensity group completed the program. The 5 subjects who dropped out did so because of time constraints that prevented regular participation in the exercise program. Only 30% of the high-intensity group completed the program. Of the 35 subjects who dropped out of the study, 5 did so because of time constraints and 30 did so because they were unable to tolerate the delayed muscle soreness associated with this exercise program. We conclude that the moderate-intensity program provides moderate strength gains and is tolerated by a majority of subjects. The high-intensity program provides impressive strength gains for the few who can tolerate the discomfort associated with the program.

An example from the literature is Amundsen and associates' study of the effect of group exercise on the aerobic power of elderly women, in which 36 women initially volunteered to participate in the exercise group.[2] Fourteen completed more than half the exercise sessions and constituted the exercise group; 15 completed less than half the exercise sessions and were not used in the data analysis; 2 could not tolerate the testing procedure; and 5 did not participate and constituted the control group. The exercise group, therefore, consisted of less than half the women who started the program. The conclusion that the exercise regimen was effective needs to be tempered by the fact that less than half of the participants completed it.

Researchers can control experimental mortality by planning to minimize possible mortality and collecting information about the lost subjects and about reasons for the loss of subjects. Researchers need to make compliance with an experimental routine as easy as possible for subjects, while maintaining the intent of the experiment. Administering treatments at a place of work or at a clinic where patients are already being treated will likely lead to higher compliance than if patients have to drive across town to participate in the study. Developing protocols that minimize discomfort are likely to lead to higher levels of retention within a study. Testing and treating on a single day will avoid the loss of subjects that inevitably accompanies a protocol that requires several days of participation.

When answering the research question requires longer term participation and its attendant loss of subjects, researchers can document the characteristics of the subjects who drop out of the study to determine if they are similar to those who remain in the study. If the dropouts have characteristics similar to those of subjects who remain in the study, and if the rate and character of dropouts are similar across study groups, then differential mortality has not occurred. Such a loss of subjects is random and affects the study groups equally.

Interactions Between Assignment and Maturation, History, or Instrumentation

Assignment effects can interact with maturation, history, or instrumentation to either obscure or exaggerate treatment effects. These interactions occur when maturation, history, or instrumentation effects act differently on treatment and control groups.

A hypothetical example of an Assignment × History interaction would be seen in Amundsen and associates' study if only one of the groups of elderly women was affected by the interruption in elevator service in the high-rise apartment.[2] If the groups used the stairs at different rates, then the study results would need to be interpreted in view of the differential effect of history on the groups. Assume that the members of the control group with the conflicting schedules went out more than the experimental group and used the stairs at least once a day to go outside to catch the bus. Members of the experimental group tended to stay home and did not use the stairs at all if the elevator was not working. In this scenario, the historical event of an elevator malfunction changed the study from a comparison of a control group versus an experimental group to a comparison of stair climbing versus group exercise. This problem might be described as follows in a journal article:

> During the course of the study, an elevator malfunction occurred that affected the control group but not the experimental group. Rather than comparing an exercising experimental group with a nonexercising control as originally planned, the comparison was between a group who participated in an eight-week group exercise program and a group who participated in a three-week stair-climbing program.

In this scenario, the hypothetical threat of an Assignment × History interaction to internal validity was uncontrollable, but explainable. Such threats can be explained only if researchers remain alert to possible threats and collect information about the extent to which subjects were affected by the threat.

An interaction between assignment and maturation occurs when different groups are maturing at different rates. If a study of the effectiveness of a rehabilitation program for patients who have had a cerebral vascular accident (CVA) used one group of patients six months after their CVA and another group two months after their CVA, the group with the more recent CVA would be expected to show greater spontaneous improvement.

An Assignment × Instrumentation interaction occurs when an instrument is more or less sensitive to change in the range at which one of the treatment groups is located. For example, assume that a researcher seeks to determine which of two methods of instruction, lecture or self study with an interactive laser video disk, results in superior student achievement in kinesiology. The students in the different instructional groups take a pretest that has a maximum score of 100 points. The group being taught by the lecture method has an average pretest score of 60; the group being taught with the laser disk technology has an average pretest score of 20. The traditional group can improve only 40 points; the video disk group can improve up to 80 points. Thus, the interaction between assignment and instrumentation exaggerates the differences in gain scores between the two groups by suppressing the gain of the group who started at 60 points. When scores "top out" and an instrument cannot register greater gains, this is termed a *ceiling effect;* when scores "bottom out" and an instrument cannot register greater declines, this is termed a *basement* or *floor effect.*

Control of interactions with assignment is accomplished through the same means that assignment, history, maturation, and instrumentation are controlled individually: random assignment to groups, careful planning, and collection of relevant information when uncontrolled threats occur. As is the case with assignment threats alone, mathematical equalization of groups can sometimes compensate for interactions between assignment and history, maturation, or instrumentation.

Diffusion or Imitation of Treatments

Diffusion of treatments is a threat to internal validity when subjects in treatment and control groups share information about their respective treatments. Assume that an experiment that evaluates the relative effectiveness of open- and closed-chain exercise in restoring quadriceps torque in patients who have undergone anterior cruciate ligament reconstruction is implemented in a single clinic. Can't you picture a member of the open-chain group and a member of the closed-chain group discussing their respective programs while icing their knees down after treatment? Perhaps the member of the open-chain group decides that stair climbing is just the thing he needs to speed his rehabilitation program along, and the member of the closed-chain group decides to buy a cuff weight and add some leg lifts to his program. If this treatment diffusion occurs, the difference between the intended treatments will be blurred.

Researchers can control treatment diffusion by minimizing contact between participants in the different groups, blinding subjects when possible, and orienting participants to the importance of sticking to the rehabilitation program to which they are assigned. Sometimes researchers will offer subjects the opportunity to participate in the alternate treatment after the study is completed if it proves to be the more effective treatment. This offer should make subjects less tempted to try the alternate treatment during the study period.

Compensatory Equalization of Treatments

Compensatory equalization of treatment is a threat to internal validity when a researcher with preconceived notions about which treatment is more desirable showers attention on subjects who are receiving the treatment the researcher perceives to be less desirable. This extra attention may alter scores on the dependent variable if the attention leads to increased compliance with treatment, increased effort during testing, or even increased self-esteem leading to a general sense of well-being.

Researchers should control compensatory equalization of treatment by avoiding topics about which they are biased or by designing studies in which their bias is controlled through researcher blinding. In addition, if a researcher has a strong sense that one treatment is more desirable than the other, he or she needs to consider whether it is ethical to contrast the two treatments in an experimental setting.

Compensatory Rivalry or Resentful Demoralization

Rivalry and demoralization are threats to internal validity when members of one group react to the perception that they are receiving a less desirable treatment than other groups. This reaction can take two forms: compensatory rivalry (a "we'll show them" attitude) and resentful demoralization (a "why bother" attitude). Compensatory rivalry tends to mask differences between control and treatment groups; resentful demoralization tends to exaggerate differences between control and experimental groups. Researchers can control rivalry and resentment by controlling the information given to subjects, blinding themselves and subjects to group membership, and having a positive attitude toward all groups.

CONSTRUCT VALIDITY

Construct validity is concerned with the meaning of variables within a study. One of the central questions related to construct validity is whether the researcher is studying a "construct as labeled" or a "construct as implemented." An example of the difference between these two constructs is illustrated by a hypothetical example wherein a researcher uses active range of motion as a dependent measure of shoulder function. The construct as labeled is "function"; the construct as implemented is "active range of motion." Some readers might consider active range of motion to be a good indicator of function, but others might consider it an incomplete indicator of function. Those who are critical of the use of active range of motion as a functional indicator are questioning the construct validity of the dependent variable.

Cook and Campbell described ten separate threats to construct validity. In this section, their list is collapsed into the four threats described below. The general strategy for controlling threats to construct validity is to develop research problems and designs through a thoughtful process that draws on the literature and theory of the discipline.

Construct Underrepresentation

Construct underrepresentation is a threat to construct validity when constructs are not fully developed within a study. In Draper's study of the effect of biofeedback on recovery of knee function after reconstruction of the anterior cruciate ligament, the independent variable construct "feedback" was not developed fully.[7] The control group received minimal feedback of any type during performance of quadriceps-setting exercises and straight leg raises; the biofeedback group received biofeedback during performance of the same exercises. As labeled, the study compared "exercise without biofeedback" with "exercise with biofeedback." On reading Draper's article, however, it becomes clear that the control group received little feedback of any kind. Perhaps, then, the comparison as implemented was actually "exercise with minimal feedback" to "exercise with biofeedback." Fuller explication of the construct of feedback would require at least a three-group study with no-feedback, verbal-feedback, and biofeedback groups.

In this same study, the general dependent measure of interest was labeled "quadriceps femoris muscle function." Muscle function was measured in two ways: (a) involved isometric quadriceps femoris muscle torque as a percentage of normal torque and (b) the number of days required to regain full knee extension. These two measures combined still probably underrepresent the construct "quadriceps femoris muscle function." A fuller representation of the construct might measure quadriceps torque at different speeds or the ability to descend stairs in a controlled manner. Some might even argue that the number of days it takes to regain full knee extension is a misrepresentation of the construct "knee extensor function" because factors other than quadriceps function, such as hamstring tightness or knee effusion, could limit the attainment of full knee extension range of motion.

Construct underrepresentation can also apply to the intensity of a construct. Kluzik and colleagues studied the effect of a neurodevelopmental treatment on reaching in children with spastic cerebral palsy.[8] They analyzed reaching motions before and after a single neurodevelopmental treatment. Although some of the individual subjects showed faster and more mature reaching patterns after the treatment, and some of the grouped data indicated significant differences after treatment, the results by no means provided unequivocal evidence of the effectiveness of the neurodevelopmental treatment. In an invited commentary accompanying publication of Kluzik and associates' article, Scholz noted the following:

> Something, albeit subtle, has resulted from the intervention. Expecting a more dramatic improvement in the reaching performance of this population following only one treatment is probably too much to ask in the first place. Future work should focus on the evaluation of long-term effects.[9(p77)]

Scholz thus recognizes that the construct has been underrepresented because it was applied only once and recommends future work with a more intense representation of the construct.

Experimenter Expectancies

Experimenter expectancy is a threat to construct validity when the subjects are able to guess the ways in which the experimenter wishes them to respond. Rosenthal, in his text on experimenter effects in behavioral research, related a classic story about experimenter expectancy, "Clever Hans."[10] Clever Hans was a horse who could provide the correct response to mathematical problems by tapping his foot the correct number of times. His owner, a mathematics teacher, did not profit from the animal's talents and did not appear to be a fraud. Hans's skills intrigued a researcher, Pfungst, who tested Hans's abilities under different controlled conditions. Pfungst found that Hans could tap out the correct answer only when his questioner was a literate individual who knew the answer to the question. He found that knowledgeable questioners unconsciously raised their eyebrows, flared their nostrils, or raised their heads as Hans was coming up to the correct number of taps. Rosenthal noted:

> Hans' amazing talents . . . serve to illustrate further the power of self-fulfilling prophecy. Hans' questioners, even skeptical ones, expected Hans to give the correct answers to their queries. Their expectation was reflected in their unwitting signal to Hans that the time had come for him to stop his tapping. The signal cued Hans to stop, and the questioner's expectation became the reason for Hans' being, once again, correct.[10(p138)]

In the story of Clever Hans, the construct as labeled was "ability to do mathematics." The construct as implemented, however, was "ability to respond to experimenter cues."

Brodzka and associates' study of long-term function of persons with bilateral below-knee amputations is an example of a study in which experimenter expectancy may have been a threat to construct validity.[11] In this study, physical therapists and occupational therapists from a rehabilitation center went to the homes of patients with bilateral below-knee amputations who had undergone post-operative rehabilitation at the center to determine their level of function in the home and community. It can be assumed that the therapists hoped to find patients who were functioning well in the face of their physical impairments. It can also be assumed that the subjects knew of the therapists' expectations. Given this, it is easy to imagine that patients might have exaggerated their abilities and that therapists might have been all too willing to believe in the exaggerated abilities. The construct as labeled was "function in the home and community"; however, the construct as implemented probably was "function in the home and community as described to a therapist who has reason to hope for high levels of function."

Researchers can control experimenter expectancy effects by limiting information given to subjects and themselves, by having different researchers who bring different expectations to the experimental setting replicate their study, and by selecting topics from which they can maintain an objective distance.

Interaction Between Different Treatments

Interaction between different treatments is a threat to construct validity when treatments other than the one of interest are administered to subjects. Snyder-Mackler and her colleagues handled this threat well in their study of the effects of helium–neon laser irradiation on skin resistance and pain in patients with trigger points.[12] Staff at one of the facilities being used as a source for subjects in this study were unwilling to discontinue the traditional physical therapy of subjects during the helium–neon laser study. The design called for two groups, laser and placebo. Because of the requirements of the one facility, the laser group consisted of six patients who received laser only and six patients who received laser plus traditional therapy. The placebo group consisted of five patients who received placebo laser and six patients who received placebo laser plus traditional therapy. Thus, the effect of group assignment to laser or placebo groups was confounded with the effects of traditional therapy. If no advantages of the laser treatment over the placebo treatment were found, would it have been because the laser was no better than a placebo or because the traditional treatment led to improvements in both groups?

To determine whether the additional treatment had an effect, Snyder-Mackler and associates analyzed three different sets of data: The entire laser group and entire placebo group were compared, the laser and placebo subgroups who did not receive additional treatment were compared, and the laser and placebo subgroups who did receive additional treatment were compared. It so happened that the threat to construct validity did not materialize in this case; the comparison between the laser and placebo groups held up regardless of whether subjects received additional treatment.

True control of interaction between different treatments is often difficult to achieve because of ethical considerations in clinical research, as demonstrated in the study cited above. However, researchers can document who receives additional treatment and can analyze data by subgroups if not all subjects are exposed to the additional treatments. If all subjects are exposed to multiple treatments, researchers need to be careful to label the treatment as it was implemented. For example, if Snyder-Mackler and colleagues had used only subjects from the facility that required the extra treatment, then the study would have been of the effects of a "combined program of helium–neon laser and traditional physical therapy" rather than simply the effect of "helium–neon laser." If only the combined treatment was given, there is no way to determine whether the laser itself would have been effective or if only the combination of traditional therapy and laser would have been effective. Even though researchers cannot always control their constructs, they should always label them accurately.

Interaction Between Testing and Treatment

Interaction between testing and treatment is a threat to construct validity when a test itself can be considered an additional treatment. As discussed in the section on testing as a threat to internal validity, controlling for the threat to internal validity made by familiarization with the test may sometimes constitute an additional treatment. In the case of isokinetic testing, repeated familiarization sessions with the equipment may constitute a training stimulus. The treatment as labeled may be "nine isokinetic training sessions"; the treatment as implemented may be "nine isokinetic training sessions and three isokinetic testing sessions."

One way to control for interaction between testing and treatment is to compare a treatment group who was pretested, a treatment group who was not pretested, a control group who was pretested, and a control group who was not pretested. This allows the researcher to compare the effects of the test and treatment combined with the effects of treatment alone, the test alone, and neither the test nor the treatment. This research plan is called a Solomon four-group design. No examples of this design were found in the physical therapy literature, presumably because of the large number of subjects that would be required to form all four groups. The posttest-only designs also control for interaction between testing and treatment by limiting testing to the end of the study.

EXTERNAL VALIDITY

External validity is concerned with the issue of to whom, in what settings, and at what times the results of research can be generalized. Cook and Campbell distinguished between generalizing *across* groups, settings, or times and generalizing *to* particular persons, settings, or times.[1] One can generalize to groups, settings, or times similar to the one studied. One can generalize across groups, settings, or times if one has studied multiple subgroups of people, settings, or times. If researchers study the effect of a proprioceptive neuromuscular facilitation technique on the biceps strength of elderly women, they can generalize their results only to elderly women. If they study the same question with a diverse group of men and women with an average age of 35 years, they can generalize their results to other diverse groups with an average age of 35. Even though the researchers have tested men and women of different age groups in the second example, they cannot generalize across age groups or sexes unless they analyze the diverse group according to subgroups. In this example, the overall group might show an increase in strength even if the elderly individuals in the group showed no change.

The question of generalizability of research results is equally applicable to descriptive research, relationship analysis, or difference analysis. Controlling the threats to external validity requires thoughtful consideration of the population to whom the results of the study can be applied, combined with practical considerations of the availability of subjects for study.

Selection

Selection is a threat to external validity when the selection process is biased in that it yields subjects who are in some manner different from the population to which the researchers hope to generalize their results. Researchers must accept that subjects who are willing to participate as research subjects may differ from the general population. As stated by Cook and Campbell, "Even when respondents belong to a target class of interest, systematic recruitment factors lead to findings that are only applicable to volunteers, exhibitionists, hypochondriacs, scientific do-gooders, those who have nothing else to do, and so forth."[1(p73)]

Amundsen and associates' study of a group exercise program for elderly women suffers from this threat to external validity.[2] First, subjects volunteered to participate in the program; presumably, this group of women differed in some way from those who did not volunteer. Maybe they had more positive attitudes toward exercise, had less to do, or were more adventuresome than those who did not volunteer. In a second self-selection process, some of the women who had originally volunteered for the study did not participate regularly. Presumably, the volunteers who participated regularly were different in some way from the volunteers who did not participate regularly. Thus, the group to which the study results can be generalized is elderly women who volunteer for and participate regularly in an exercise program. Taking a similar program and making it a mandatory part of the daily routine at a retirement center might yield disappointing results if the treatment is administered to a group who has little interest in the exercise program.

A study by Schenkman and colleagues illustrates the threat of selection to external validity in a descriptive research report.[13] The purpose of the study was to analyze whole-body movements during rising from sitting to standing. Subjects were nine women between the ages of 25 and 36. In an invited commentary accompanying the research article, VanSant expressed concern about selection by noting,

> The time is rapidly passing when we can legitimately use a sample of young adults to develop models of any movement pattern for clinical use with any group other than young adults. . . . Studies demonstrate that age differences do exist in the movement patterns used to rise from a chair.[14(p648)]

Researchers can control selection as a threat to external validity by carefully considering the target population to whom they wish to generalize results, selecting subjects accordingly, and carefully writing their research conclusions to avoid making inferences to groups or across subgroups who have not been studied.

Setting

Setting is a threat to external validity when peculiarities of the setting in which the research was conducted make it difficult to generalize the results to other settings. In a study of leg movements of preterm infants, Heriza videotaped leg movements in an effort to sample spontaneous leg movements of each infant.[15] To meet the requirements of her data analysis system, she had to stabilize the infants in some way during taping; she did so by using one hand to support the head and the other hand to maintain the trunk in a midline position. This level of interference with the child is certainly less than, for example, using a pinprick as a stimulus to begin kicking. However, the researcher and the reader still must consider the possibility that an infant's kicking behavior while he or she is supported by a human touch may differ from the infant's kicking behavior in the absence of support.

Control of threats to external validity posed by setting requires that researchers simulate as closely as possible the setting to which they hope to generalize their results. Researchers who hope their studies will have clinical applicability must try to duplicate the complexities of the clinical setting within their studies. Researchers who wish to describe subjects or settings as they exist naturally must make the research process as unobtrusive as possible.

Time

Time is a threat to external validity when the results of a study are applicable to limited time frames. For example, Draper's study of the effects of biofeedback on quadriceps muscle function is somewhat time limited.[7] The study was conducted when it was common for patients to be immobilized and remain in a non-weight-bearing condition for extended periods of time after surgery to reconstruct the anterior cruciate ligament. Restoring quadriceps function to knees treated with lengthy periods of non-weight-bearing immobilization presented a real challenge to patients and physical therapists. In this context, biofeedback may have been an effective adjunct to traditional physical therapy. In contrast, patients who undergo rehabilitation with contemporary protocols, which allow early motion and weight bearing, may never experience loss of quadriceps function that is severe enough to require biofeedback-aided exercise.

Time threats to external validity can be managed by timely presentation of research results and description of changes that make the research results less applicable in the present or future than they were when the data were collected.

RELATIONSHIP AMONG TYPES OF VALIDITY

Nineteen different threats to validity have been presented. These threats are not, however, independent entities that can be controlled one by one until the perfect research design is created. The relationship between the validity threats can be either cumulative or reciprocal.

Cumulative relationships occur when a change that influences one of the threats influences other threats in the same way. For example, researchers may initially think to use a randomly assigned control group in a study because they want to control for the effects of maturation. By controlling for maturation in this way they also control for history, assignment, testing, and so on.

Reciprocal threats occur when controlling a threat to one type of validity leads to realization of a different threat to validity. For instance, if a researcher wants to achieve the highest level of internal validity possible, he or she will standardize the experimental treatment so that there are few extraneous variables that could account for changes in the dependent measures. However, this standardization compromises external validity because the results can be applied only to settings in which the treatment would be equally well controlled.

The reciprocal relationship between validity threats is illustrated in Draper's study of biofeedback and knee rehabilitation.[7] Patients were seen for between 18 and 26 treatments. If the biofeedback group tended to come to therapy more frequently than the control group, differences between the two groups might have been related to the number of treatments rather than to the effect of biofeedback—this would be a threat to construct validity. To solve this problem, Draper could have included in her study only those patients who had completed 26 sessions. In doing so, she would have reduced external validity by narrowing the treatment setting to one in which 26 treatments were given and limiting the patients studied to those who either were very compliant or had little else to do other than attend therapy. Draper couldn't win! If she allowed patients with a greater range of treatment sessions into the study she would have limited construct validity. Conversely, if she allowed only those patients with a narrower range of treatments sessions into the study, she would have limited external validity.

SUMMARY

Threats to the believability and utility of research can be classified as threats to internal, construct, or external validity. Internal validity concerns whether the treatment caused the effect; construct validity concerns the meaning attached to concepts used within the study; and external validity concerns the persons, settings, or times to which or across which the results can be generalized. Many of the threats to validity are reciprocal because controlling one leads to problems with another.

References

1. Cook T, Campbell D. *Quasi-Experimentation: Design and Analysis Issues for Field Settings*. Chicago, Ill: Rand McNally & Co; 1979:37–94.
2. Amundsen LR, DeVahl JM, Ellingham CT. Evaluation of a group exercise program for elderly women. *Phys Ther*. 1989;69:475–483.
3. Holt P, Winograd CH. Prospective payment and the utilization of physical therapy services in the hospitalized elderly. *Am J Public Health*. 1990;80:1491–1494.
4. Yarkony GM, Roth EJ, Meyer PR, et al. Rehabilitation outcomes in patients with complete thoracic spinal cord injury. *Am J Phys Med Rehabil*. 1990;69:23–27.
5. Brooks ME, Smith EM, Currier DP. Effect of longitudinal versus transverse electrode placement on torque production by the quadriceps femoris muscle during neuromuscular electrical stimulation. *Journal of Orthopaedic and Sports Physical Therapy*. 1990;11:530–534.
6. Timm KE. Postsurgical knee rehabilitation: a five year study of four methods and 5,381 patients. *Am J Sports Med*. 1988;16:463–468.
7. Draper V. Electromyographic biofeedback and recovery of quadriceps femoris muscle function following anterior cruciate ligament reconstruction. *Phys Ther*. 1990;70:11–17.
8. Kluzik J, Fetters L, Coryell J. Quantification of control: a preliminary study of effects of neurodevelopmental treatment on reaching in children with spastic cerebral palsy. *Phys Ther*. 1990;70:65–76.
9. Scholz JP. Commentary. *Phys Ther*. 1990;70:76–78.
10. Rosenthal R. *Experimenter Effects in Behavioral Research*. Enlarged ed. New York, NY: Irvington Publishers Inc; 1976.
11. Brodzka WK, Thornhill HL, Zarapkar SE, et al. Long-term function of persons with atherosclerotic bilateral below-knee amputation living in the inner city. *Arch Phys Med Rehabil*. 1990;71:895–900.
12. Snyder-Mackler L, Barry AJ, Perkins AI, Soucek MD. Effects of helium-neon laser irradiation on skin resistance and pain in patients with trigger points in the neck or back. *Phys Ther*. 1989;69:336–341.
13. Schenkman M, Berger RA, Riley PO, et al. Whole-body movements during rising to standing from sitting. *Phys Ther*. 1990;70:638–648.
14. VanSant AF. Commentary. *Phys Ther*. 1990;70:648–649.
15. Heriza CB. Organization of leg movements in preterm infants. *Phys Ther*. 1988;68:1340–1346.

CHAPTER 8

Selection and Assignment of Subjects

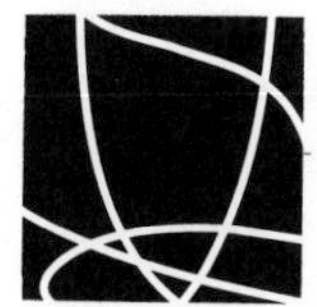

Researchers rarely have the opportunity to study all the individuals who possess the characteristics of interest within a study. Fiscal and time constraints often limit researchers' ability to study large groups of subjects. In addition, the study of very large groups may be undesirable because of the inevitable inaccuracies that result from the collection and management of large amounts of data.[1(p46)] *Sampling* is the process by which a subgroup of subjects is selected for study from a larger group of potential subjects. *Assignment* is the process by which subjects in the sample are assigned to groups within the study. This chapter acquaints readers with the major methods of selecting subjects and assigning them to groups.

SIGNIFICANCE OF SAMPLING AND ASSIGNMENT

If a group of physical therapists is interested in studying, for example, rehabilitation outcomes in patients who have undergone total knee arthroplasty (TKA), they must somehow determine which of thousands of possible subjects will be studied. The way in which subjects are identified for study, and for groups within the study, has a profound impact on the validity of the study.

Sampling methods influence the characteristics of the sample, which in turn influence the generalizability, or external validity, of a piece of research. If, for example, a sample of patients with TKA includes only subjects older than 75 years, the research results cannot be generalized to younger patient groups.

The method by which subjects are assigned to groups within the study influences the characteristics of subjects within each group, which in turn influences the internal validity of the study. Assume that we design an experiment on the effect of continuous passive range of motion (CPM) on knee range of motion after TKA. We use a posttest-only control-group design that includes one experimental group (routine rehabilitation plus CPM) and one control group (routine rehabilitation only). The threats to internal validity posed by history, maturation, testing, and assignment can all be controlled by assignment procedures that yield groups of patients with similar ages, medical problems, preoperative ambulation status, and the like.

POPULATIONS AND SAMPLES

The distinction between a population and a sample is an important one. A *population* is the total group of interest. A *sample* is a subgroup of the group of interest. *Sampling* is the procedure by which a sample of *units* or *elements* is selected from a population. In clinical research, the sampling unit may be the individual or a group of related individuals, such as graduating classes of therapists or patients treated at particular clinics.

Defining the population of interest is not a simple matter. There are generally two types of populations who are considered in research, the target population and the accessible population. The *target population* is the group to whom researchers hope to generalize their findings. The *accessible population* is the group of potential research subjects who are actually available for a given study.

Hulley and colleagues listed four types of characteristics that define populations: clinical, demographic, geographic, and temporal.[2(p18)] Clinical and demographic characteristics define the target population. The target population for our TKA study might be defined as individuals who have undergone a unilateral TKA and were at least 60 years of age at the time of the surgery. Geographic and temporal characteristics define the accessible population. The accessible population for our TKA study might consist of individuals with the aforementioned clinical and demographic characteristics who underwent surgery in one of eight Indianapolis hospitals during the five-year period from 1987 to 1991. Table 8–1 presents a hypothetical distribution of patients at the eight hospitals during this time period. This accessible population of 3,000 patients provides the basis for many of the examples in this chapter.

Once the researcher has defined the accessible population in a general way, he or she needs to develop more specific *inclusion* and *exclusion* characteristics. We already know that patients aged 60 years or older who underwent unilateral TKA at one of eight hospitals from 1987 to 1991 are included in our accessible population. Some patients who

TABLE 8–1. Hypothetical Sample of Patients Who Underwent Total Knee Arthroplasty by Hospital and Year

Hospital	1987	1988	1989	1990	1991	Total
A	22	25	28	26	24	125
B	50	55	60	40	45	250
C	48	49	52	51	50	250
D	80	78	75	71	71	375
E	72	72	77	77	77	375
F	95	107	98	97	103	500
G	100	103	95	100	102	500
H	120	130	130	122	123	625
Total	587	619	615	584	595	3,000

fit this description should, nevertheless, be excluded from participation in the study. For example, we need to decide whether to exclude patients who experienced postoperative infection, surgical revision, or rehospitalization soon after the TKA.

The decision to include or exclude subjects with certain characteristics must be made in light of the purpose of the research. If the purpose of our study is to provide a description of functional outcomes after TKA, then excluding cases with complications would artificially improve group outcomes by eliminating those likely to have a poor outcome. In contrast, if the purpose of a study is to describe the functional outcomes that can be expected after completion of a particular rehabilitation regimen, then exclusion of patients who could not complete therapy seems reasonable.

After the researcher specifies inclusion and exclusion criteria, he or she needs a sampling frame from which to select subjects. A *sampling frame* is a listing of the elements in the accessible population. In our TKA study, we would ask that someone in the medical records department in each of the eight hospitals create a sampling frame by developing a list of patients aged 60 years or older who underwent a TKA from 1987 to 1991.

Existing sampling frames are available for some populations. If we wish to study the physical therapists' opinions on physician ownership of physical therapy services, we could use either a professional association membership list or a state physical therapy licensing board list as our sampling frame. Use of an existing sampling frame necessarily defines the target population for the research. If we use the professional association membership list, we can generalize only to other professional association members; if we use the licensing board list, we can generalize to licensed physical therapists regardless of whether they belong to the professional association.

The most basic distinction between sampling methods is between *probabilistic* and *nonprobabilistic* methods. Generation of probability samples involves randomization at some point in the process; generation of nonprobability samples does not. Probability samples are preferable when the researcher hopes to generalize from an accessible population to a target population. This is because probability samples tend to have less sampling error than nonprobability samples. *Sampling error* "refers to the fact that the vagaries of chance will nearly always ensure that one sample will differ from another, even if the two samples are drawn from exactly the same target population in exactly the same random way."[1(pp 45, 46)] Probability samples tend to be less variable and better approximations of the population than nonprobability samples.

PROBABILITY SAMPLING

Four types of probability sampling are presented in this section. As required by definition, all involve randomization at some point in the sampling process. The extent of randomization, however, differs from technique to technique.

Simple Random Sampling

Simple random sampling is a procedure in which each member of the population has an equal chance of being selected for the sample, and selection of each subject is independent of selection of other subjects. Assume that we wish to draw a random sample of 300 subjects from the accessible population of 3,000 patients in Table 8–1. To literally "draw" the sample, we would write each patient's name on a slip of paper, put the 3,000 slips of paper in a rotating cage, mix the slips thoroughly, and draw out 300 of the slips. This is an example of sampling *without replacement*, because each slip of paper is not replaced in the cage after it is drawn. It is also possible to sample with replacement, in which case the selected unit is placed back in the population so that it may be drawn again. In clinical research it is not feasible to use the same person more than once for a sample, so sampling without replacement is the norm.

Drawing a sample from a cage, or even from a hat, may work fairly well when the accessible population is small. With larger populations, it becomes difficult to mix the units thoroughly. This apparently happened in the 1970 U.S. draft lottery. Capsules representing days of the year were placed in a cage for selection to determine the order in which young men would be drafted into the armed forces. Days from the later months of the year were selected considerably earlier than days from months earlier in the year. Presumably, the capsules were not mixed well, leading to a higher rate of induction among men with birthdays later in the year.[1(pp5–7)]

The preferred method for generating a simple random sample is to use random numbers that are provided in a table or generated by a computer. Table 8–2 shows a portion of the random numbers table reproduced in Appendix B.[3] Before consulting the table, the researcher numbers the units in the sampling frame. In our TKA study, the patients would be numbered from 0001 to 3000. Starting in a random place on the table, and moving in either a horizontal or vertical direction, we would include in our sample any four-digit numbers from 0001 to 3000 that we encounter. Any four-digit numbers greater than 3000 are ignored, as are duplicate numbers. The process is continued until the required number of units is selected. From within the boldface portion of Table 8–2 in Column 7, Rows 76 through 80, the following numbers, which correspond to individual subjects, would be selected for our TKA sample: 1945, 2757, and 2305.

Simple random sampling is easy to comprehend, but it is sometimes difficult to implement. If the population is large, the process of assigning a number to each population unit becomes extremely time consuming. The other probability sampling techniques are easier to implement than simple random sampling and may control sampling error as well as simple random sampling. Therefore,

TABLE 8–2. Segment of a Random Numbers Table*

	Column													
Row	***1***	***2***	***3***	***4***	***5***	***6***	***7***	***8***	***9***	***10***	***11***	***12***	***13***	***14***
71	912***27***	21199	31935	270***22***	84067	05462	352***16***	14486	29891	686***07***	41867	14951	91696	85065
72	500***01***	38140	663***21***	199***24***	72163	09538	12151	06878	919***03***	18749	344***05***	56087	82790	709***25***
73	65390	05224	72958	286***09***	814***06***	39147	25549	48542	42627	45233	572***02***	946***17***	23772	07896
74	275***04***	961***31***	83944	41575	10573	086***19***	64482	739***23***	36152	05184	94142	25299	84347	34925
75	37169	94851	39177	896***32***	00959	16487	65536	49071	39782	17095	023***30***	74301	00275	48280
76	115***08***	70225	511***11***	38351	19444	66499	7**1945**	05442	13442	78675	48081	66938	93654	59894
77	37449	30362	06694	54690	04052	531***15***	6**2757**	95348	78662	11163	81651	50245	34971	52924
78	46515	70331	85922	38329	57015	15765	9**7161**	17869	45349	61796	66345	81073	49106	79860
79	30986	81223	42416	58353	21532	30502	3**2305**	86482	05174	07901	54339	58861	748***18***	46942
80	63798	64995	46583	09765	44160	78128	8**3991**	42865	92520	83531	80377	35909	81250	54238

*Complete table appears in Appendix B.
From Beyer WH, ed. *Standard Mathematical Tables*. 27th ed. Boca Raton, Fla: CRC Press Inc; 1984.

the following three probability sampling procedures are used more frequently than simple random sampling.

Systematic Sampling

Systematic sampling is a process by which the researcher selects every *n*th person on a list. To generate a systematic sample of 300 subjects from the TKA population of 3,000, we would select every 10th person. The list of 3,000 patients might be ordered by patient number, social security number, date of surgery, or birth date. To begin the systematic sampling procedure, a random start within the list of 3,000 patients is necessary. To get a random start we can, for example, point to a number on a random numbers table, observe four digits of the license plate number on a car in the parking lot, reverse the last four digits of the accession number of a library book, or ask four different people to select numbers between zero and nine and combine them to form a starting number. There are endless ways to select the random starting number for a systematic sample. If the random starting number for a systematic sample of our TKA population is 1,786, and the sampling interval is 10, then the first four subjects selected would be the 1,786th, 1,796th, 1,806th, and 1,816th individuals on the list.

Systematic sampling is an efficient alternative to simple random sampling, and it ordinarily generates samples that are as representative of their populations as simple random sampling. The exception to this is if the ordering system used somehow introduces a systematic error into the sample. Assume that we use dates of surgery to order our TKA sample, and that for most weeks during the five-year period there were 10 surgeries performed. Because the sampling interval is 10, and there were usually 10 surgeries performed per week, systematic sampling would tend to overrepresent patients who had surgery on a certain day of the week. Table 8–3 shows an example of how patients with surgery on Monday might be overrepresented in the systematic sample; the boldface entries indicate the units chosen for the sample. If patients who have surgery on Mondays differ in some way from other patients, then a sampling bias has occurred. If certain surgeons usually perform their TKAs on Tuesday, their patients would be underrepresented in the sample. If patients who are scheduled for surgery on Monday typically have fewer medical complications than those scheduled for surgery later in the week, this will also bias the sample. It is unlikely that the assumptions made to produce this hypothetical bias would operate so systematically in real life—the number of cases per week is likely more variable than presented here, and surgeons likely perform TKAs on more than one day of the week. However, possible systematic biases such as this should be considered when one is deciding how to order the population for systematic sampling.

TABLE 8–3. Systematic Bias in a Systematic Sample

Subject	Date of Surgery	Surgeon
1786	**1–8–90 (Monday)**	**A***
1787	1–8–90 (Monday)	A
1788	1–9–90 (Tuesday)	B
1789	1–9–90 (Tuesday)	B
1790	1–10–90 (Wednesday)	C
1791	1–10–90 (Wednesday)	C
1792	1–11–90 (Thursday)	D
1793	1–11–90 (Thursday)	D
1794	1–12–90 (Friday)	E
1795	1–12–90 (Friday)	E
1796	**1–15–90 (Monday)**	**A**
1797	1–15–90 (Monday)	A

*Boldface rows indicate the patients selected for the study. If the sampling interval is 10, and approximately 10 surgeries are performed per week, patients of Surgeon A, who usually performs total knee arthroplasties on Monday, will be overrepresented in the sample.

Stratified Sampling

Stratified sampling is used when certain subgroups must be represented in adequate numbers within the sample or when it is important to preserve the proportions of subgroups in the population within the sample. In our TKA study, if we hope to make generalizations across the eight hospitals within the study, we need to be sure there are enough patients from each hospital in the sample to provide a reasonable basis for making statements about the outcomes of TKA at each hospital. On the other hand, if we want to generalize results to the "average" patient undergoing a TKA, then we need to have proportional representation of subjects from the eight hospitals.

Table 8–4 contrasts *proportional* and *nonproportional* stratified sampling. In proportional sampling, the percentage of subjects from each hospital is the same in the population and the sample (with minor deviations because subjects cannot be divided in half; compare Columns 3 and 5). However, the actual number of subjects from each hospital in the sample ranges from 12 to 62. In nonproportional sampling, the percentage of subjects from each hospital is different for the population and the sample (compare Columns 3 and 7). However, the actual number of subjects from each hospital is the same (with minor deviations because subjects cannot be divided in half).

Stratified sampling from the accessible population is implemented in several steps. First, all units in the accessible population are identified according to the stratification criteria. Second, the appropriate number of subjects is selected from each stratum. Subjects may be selected from each stratum through simple random sampling or systematic sampling. More than one stratum may be identified. For instance, we might want to ensure that each of the eight hospitals and each of the five years of the study period are equally represented in the sample. In this case, we first stratify the accessible population into eight groups by hospital, then stratify each hospital into five groups by year, and finally draw a random sample from each of the 40 Hospital × Year subgroups.

Stratified sampling is easy to accomplish if the stratifying characteristic is known for each sampling unit. In our TKA study, both the hospital and year of surgery are known for all elements in the sampling frame. In fact, those characteristics were required for placement of subjects into the accessible population. A much different situation exists, however, if we decide that it is important to ensure that certain knee replacement models

TABLE 8–4. Proportional and Nonproportional Stratified Sampling of Patients at Eight Hospitals

	Population Distribution		Proportional Sample		Nonproportional Sample	
Hospital	*N*	%	*N*	%	*N*	%
A	125	4.1	12	4.0	37	12.3
B	250	8.3	25	8.3	37	12.3
C	250	8.3	25	8.3	37	12.3
D	375	12.5	38	12.7	37	12.3
E	375	12.5	38	12.7	38	12.7
F	500	16.7	50	16.7	38	12.7
G	500	16.7	50	16.7	38	12.7
H	625	20.8	62	20.6	38	12.7
Total	3,000	100.0	300	100.0	300	100.0

are represented in the sample in adequate numbers. Stratifying according to this characteristic would require that someone read all 3,000 medical charts to determine which knee model was used for each subject. Because of the inordinate amount of time it would take to determine the knee model for each potential subject, we should consider whether simple random or systematic sampling would likely result in a good representation of each knee model.

Another difficulty with stratification is that some strata require that the researcher set classification boundaries. The strata discussed so far (hospital, year, and knee model) are discrete categories of items. Consider, though, the dilemma that would occur if we wanted to stratify on a variable such as "amount of inpatient physical therapy." If we wanted to ensure that differing levels of physical therapy are represented in the sample, we would need to decide what constitutes low, medium, and high amounts of inpatient physical therapy. Not only would we have to determine the boundaries between groups, we would also have to obtain the information on all 3,000 individuals in the accessible population. Once again, we should consider whether random or systematic sampling would likely result in an adequate distribution of the amount of physical therapy received by patients in the sample.

In summary, stratified sampling is useful when a researcher believes it is imperative to ensure that certain characteristics are represented in a sample in specified numbers. Stratifying on some variables will prove to be too costly and must therefore be left to chance. In many cases, simple random or systematic sampling will result in an adequate distribution of the variable in question.

Cluster Sampling

Cluster sampling is the use of naturally occurring groups as the sampling units. It is used when an appropriate sampling frame does not exist or when logistical constraints limit the researcher's ability to travel widely. There are often several stages to a cluster sampling procedure. For example, if we wanted to conduct a nationwide study on outcomes after TKA, we could not use simple random sampling because the entire population of patients with TKA is not enumerated—that is, a nationwide sampling frame does not exist. In addition, we do not have the funds to travel to all the states and cities that would be represented if a nationwide random sample were selected. To generate a nationwide cluster sample of patients who have undergone a TKA, therefore, we could first sample states, then cities within each selected state, then hospitals within each selected city, and then patients within each selected hospital. Sampling frames for all of these clusters exist: The 50 states are known, various references list cities and populations within each state,[4] and other references list hospitals by city and size.[5]

Each step of the cluster sampling procedure can be implemented through simple random, systematic, or stratified sampling. Assume that we have the money and time to study patients in six states. To select these six states, we might stratify according to region and then randomly select one state from each region. From each of the six states selected, we might develop a list of all cities with populations greater than 50,000 and randomly select two cities from this list. The selection could be random or could be stratified according to city size so that one larger and one smaller city within each state are selected. From each city, we might select two hospitals for study. Within each hospital, patients who underwent TKA in the appropriate time frame would be selected randomly, systematically, or according to specified strata. Figure 8–1 shows the cluster sampling procedure with all steps illustrated for one state, city, and hospital. The same

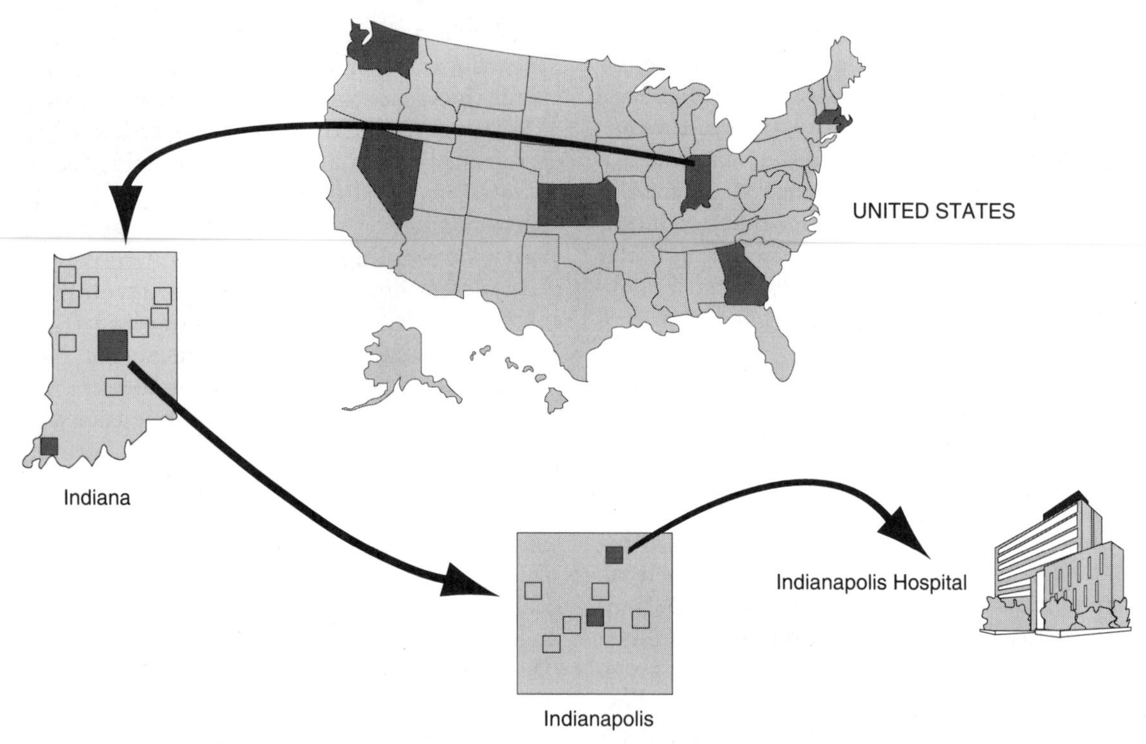

FIGURE 8–1. Partial example of cluster sampling. Six of fifty states are selected, two cities are selected in each state, and two hospitals are selected from each city. Selected units are shaded; only one state, city, and hospital is illustrated.

process would occur in the other selected states, cities, and hospitals.

Cluster sampling can save time and money compared with simple random sampling because subjects are clustered in locations. A simple random sample of patients after TKA would likely take us into 50 states and hundreds of cities. The cluster sampling procedure just described would limit the study to 12 cities in 6 states.

Cluster sampling can occur on a smaller scale as well. Assume that some researchers wish to study the effectiveness of a new electrotherapy modality on patients with chronic pain, and the accessible population consists of patients with chronic pain who seek physical therapy care in a single city. This example is well suited to cluster sampling because a sampling frame of this population does not exist. In addition, it would be difficult to train all therapists within the city to use the new modality with their patients, and there is probably a limited number of machines available for use. Cluster sampling of a few physical therapy departments or practices, and then a few therapists within each department or practice, would be efficient use of the researcher's time for both identifying appropriate patients and training therapists with the new modality.

Cluster sampling may also be necessitated by administrative constraints. Assume that researchers wish to determine the relative effectiveness of two educational approaches to third graders' developing awareness of individuals with physical disabilities: In one approach children simulate disabilities themselves, and in the other approach individuals with disabilities make presentations to the students. A superintendent is unlikely to allow the study to take place if it requires a random sampling of third graders across the school system with disruption of classrooms. Since third graders exist in clusters, it seems natural to use schools or classrooms as the sampling unit, rather than the individual pupil.

NONPROBABILITY SAMPLING

Nonprobability sampling is widely used in physical therapy research and is distinguished from probability sampling by the absence of randomization. One reason for the predominance of nonprobability sampling in physical therapy research is limited funding. Because many studies are self-funded, subject selection is confined to a single setting with a limited number of available patients, so the researcher often chooses to study the entire accessible population. There are two main forms of nonprobability sampling: convenience and purposive.

Samples of Convenience

Samples of convenience involve the use of readily available subjects. Samples of convenience that physical therapy researchers commonly use are classes of physical therapy students and patients in certain diagnostic categories at a single clinic. If we conducted our study of patients after TKA by using all patients who underwent the surgery from 1987 to 1991 at a given hospital, this would represent a sample of convenience. If patients who undergo TKA at this hospital are different in some way from the overall population of patients who have this surgery, then our study would have little generalizability beyond that facility.

The term "sample of convenience" seems to give the negative implication that the researcher has not worked hard enough at the task of sampling. In addition, we already know that probability samples tend to have less sampling error than nonprobability samples. But before you totally discount the validity of samples of convenience, it should be pointed out that the accessible populations discussed earlier in the chapter can also be viewed as large samples of convenience. An accessible population that consists of "patients post-TKA who are 60 years old or older and had the surgery at one of eight hospitals in Indianapolis from 1987 to 1991" is technically a large sample of convenience from the population of all the individuals in the world who have undergone TKA.

If an accessible population is so small that the researcher can study it in its entirety, it is generally termed a sample of convenience. If an accessible population is large enough that the researcher must select from the accessible population to obtain a representative group that is manageable for study, this is generally termed a random sample. Remember, though, that the extent to which the random sample is representative of the target population depends on the representativeness of the accessible population from which it was drawn. Figure 8–2 shows the distinctions among a target population, an accessible population, a random sample, and a sample of convenience.

Consecutive sampling is a form of convenience sampling. Consecutive samples are used in a prospective study in which the population does not exist at the beginning of the study; in other words, a sampling frame does not exist. If researchers plan a two-year study of the outcomes of TKA at a particular hospital beginning January 1, 1993, the population of interest does not begin to exist until the first patient has surgery in 1993. In a consecutive sample, all patients who meet the criteria are placed into the study as they are identified. This continues until a specified number of

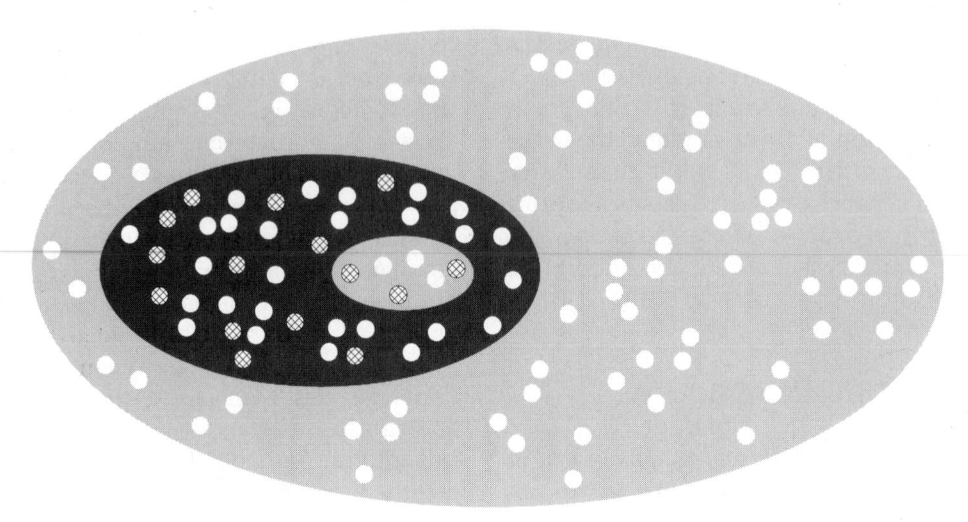

FIGURE 8–2. Distinctions among target populations, accessible populations, samples of convenience, and random samples. The white dots represent elements within the population. The large gray ellipse represents the target population. The black ellipse represents the accessible population. The small gray ellipse represents a sample of convenience. The cross-hatched dots represent a random sample from the accessible population.

patients is collected, a specified time frame has passed, or certain statistical outcomes are seen.

Purposive Sampling

Purposive sampling is used when a researcher has a specific reason for selecting particular subjects for study. Whereas convenience sampling uses whatever units are readily available, purposive sampling uses handpicked units that meet the researcher's needs. Random, convenience, and purposive samples can be distinguished if we return to the hypothetical study of different educational modes for teaching children about physical disabilities. If there are 40 elementary schools in a district and the researchers randomly select 2 of them for study, this is clearly a random sample of schools from the accessible population of a single school district. If the researchers select 2 schools in close proximity to their place of work, this constitutes a sample of convenience. If the researchers handpick 2 schools from the district that are similar in size, racial balance, and socioeconomic status of parents, this constitutes a purposive sample.

ASSIGNMENT TO GROUPS

When a study requires more than one group, the researchers need a method for assigning subjects to groups. Random assignment to groups is preferred and is appropriate even when the original selection procedure was nonrandom. Thus, many studies in the physical therapy literature use a sample of convenience combined with random assignment to groups. The goal of group assignment is to create groups that are equally representative of the entire sample. Because many statistical techniques require equal group sizes, a secondary goal of the assignment process is often to develop groups of equal size.

There are four basic ways to randomly

assign subjects to groups within a study. These methods can be illustrated by a hypothetical sample of 32 patients who have undergone TKA; age and sex are listed for each patient in Table 8–5. The sample has a mean age of 68 years and consists of 50% women and 50% men. Each of the four assignment techniques was applied to this sample; the processes are described in the following four sections, and the results are presented in Tables 8–6 to 8–9.

The design of our hypothetical study calls for four groups of patients, each undergoing a different post-TKA rehabilitation program. The four programs are variations based on two techniques for increasing range of motion (continuous passive motion [CPM] and manual stretching) and two techniques for restoring muscular function (open- and closed-chain exercise). The design is factorial, with range-of-motion technique as one independent variable and strengthening technique as the second independent variable. One group receives open-chain exercise and manual stretching, one group receives open-chain exercise and CPM, one group receives closed-chain exercise and manual stretching, and the final group receives closed-chain exercise and CPM.

Random Assignment by Individual

The first method of random assignment is to randomly assign each individual in the sample to one of the four groups. This could be done with a roll of a die, ignoring rolls of 5 and 6. When this assignment technique was applied to the hypothetical sample in Table 8–5, the open-chain/manual treatment was represented by a roll of 1, the open-chain/CPM condition by a roll of 2, the closed-chain/manual treatment by a roll of 3, and the closed-chain/CPM treatment by a roll of 4. The results of the procedure are shown in Table 8–6. Note that the group sizes range from 4 to 12 subjects.

The advantage of assignment by individual is that it is easy to do. The main disadvantage is that with a small sample size, the resulting group sizes are not likely to be equal. With a larger sample size, the probability that group sizes will be nearly equal is greater.

Random Assignment by Block

The second assignment method uses blocks of subjects to ensure equal group sizes. Say that in our sample of patients who underwent TKA, we wish to have four groups of eight subjects. To assign by block, we can use a random numbers table to select eight numbers for the first group, eight for the second group, and so on. Looking at the last two digits in each column and proceeding from left to right beginning in Column 1 of Row 71 of the random numbers table (Table 8–2), the numbers between 01 and 32 are boldface and italic, skipping any duplicates. The first

TABLE 8–5. Existing Sample Characteristics: Case Number, Sex, and Age*

1. F, 70	9. F, 62	17. M, 70	25. M, 76
2. M, 60	10. F, 78	18. F, 63	26. F, 72
3. M, 71	11. F, 68	19. M, 71	27. F, 77
4. F, 64	12. M, 81	20. F, 76	28. F, 67
5. F, 65	13. F, 69	21. F, 61	29. F, 69
6. F, 68	14. F, 60	22. M, 67	30. M, 67
7. M, 68	15. M, 66	23. M, 65	31. M, 65
8. M, 69	16. M, 66	24. M, 63	32. M, 62

*Mean age is 68 years; 50% of sample is female.

TABLE 8–6. Random Assignment by Individual

Group 1:* Open Chain/Manual	Group 2:† Open Chain/CPM**	Group 3:‡ Closed Chain/Manual	Group 4:§ Closed Chain/CPM
5. F, 65	4. F, 64	1. F, 70	6. F, 68
9. F, 62	14. F, 60	2. M, 60	7. M, 68
17. M, 70	15. M, 66	3. M, 71	8. M, 69
21. F, 61	20. F, 76	10. F, 78	14. F, 60
	24. M, 63	12. M, 81	18. F, 63
	28. F, 67	13. F, 69	19. M, 71
	30. M, 67	16. M, 66	22. M, 67
	31. M, 65		23. M, 65
	32. M, 62		25. M, 76
			26. F, 72
			27. F, 77
			29. F, 69

*n = 4, mean age = 64.5 years, women = 75.0%.
†n = 9, mean age = 65.5 years, women = 44.4%.
‡n = 7, mean age = 70.7 years, women = 42.8%.
§n = 12, mean age = 68.8 years, women = 50.0%.
**Continuous passive motion.

eight subjects who correspond to the first eight numbers constitute the first group. The next eight numbers constitute the second group, and so on. The complete results of this assignment procedure are shown in Table 8–7. Random assignment to groups by block can become time consuming with large samples.

Systematic Assignment

The process of systematic assignment is familiar to anyone who has taken a physical education class where teams were formed by "counting off." Researchers count off by using a list of the sample and systematically placing subsequent subjects into subsequent groups. Table 8–8 shows the groups generated by systematic assignment for this example. The first person was assigned to the open-chain/manual group, the second person to the open-chain/CPM group, the third person to the closed-chain/manual group, the fourth person to the closed-chain/CPM group, the fifth person to the open-chain/manual group, and so on.

Matched Assignment

In matched assignment, subjects are matched on important characteristics, and these subgroups are randomly assigned to study groups. In our sample of TKA patients, subjects were matched on both age and sex. The four youngest women in the sample were placed in a subgroup and then were randomly assigned to study groups. To randomly assign the matched subjects to groups, four different-colored poker chips, each representing a study group, were placed into a container. As shown in Table 8–9, the first chip drawn placed the youngest woman into the open-chain/manual group; the second chip drawn placed the next youngest woman into the open-chain/CPM group; and so on. The four youngest men were then placed into a subgroup and were assigned randomly to study groups. This procedure continued for the next youngest subgroups until all subjects were assigned to groups.

The matched assignment procedure is somewhat analogous to stratified sampling and has some of the same disadvantages as

TABLE 8–7. Random Assignment by Block

Group 1:* Open Chain/Manual	Group 2:† Open Chain/CPM**	Group 3:‡ Closed Chain/Manual	Group 4:§ Closed Chain/CPM
1. F, 70	2. M, 60	8. M, 69	10. F, 78
3. M, 71	4. F, 64	11. F, 68	12. M, 81
7. M, 68	5. F, 65	15. M, 66	13. F, 69
16. M, 66	6. F, 68	18. F, 63	14. F, 60
21. F, 61	9. F, 62	19. M, 71	20. F, 76
22. M, 67	17. M, 70	23. M, 65	26. F, 72
24. M, 63	25. M, 76	30. M, 67	28. F, 67
27. F, 77	31. M, 65	32. M, 62	29. F, 69

*Mean age = 67.9 years, women = 37.5%.
†Mean age = 66.3 years, women = 50.0%.
‡Mean age = 66.3 years, women = 25.0%.
§Mean age = 71.5 years, women = 87.5%.
**Continuous passive motion.

TABLE 8–8. Systematic Assignment

Group 1:* Open Chain/Manual	Group 2:† Open Chain/CPM**	Group 3:‡ Closed Chain/Manual	Group 4:§ Closed Chain/CPM
1. F, 70	2. M, 60	3. M, 71	4. F, 64
5. F, 65	6. F, 68	7. M, 68	8. M, 69
9. F, 62	10. F, 78	11. F, 68	12. M, 81
13. F, 69	14. F, 60	15. M, 66	16. M, 66
17. M, 70	18. F, 63	19. M, 71	20. F, 76
21. F, 61	22. M, 67	23. M, 65	24. M, 63
25. M, 76	26. F, 72	27. F, 77	28. F, 67
29. F, 67	30. M, 67	31. M, 65	32. M, 62

*Mean age = 67.5 years, women = 75.0%.
†Mean age = 66.9 years, women = 62.5%.
‡Mean age = 68.9 years, women = 25.0%.
§Mean age = 68.5 years, women = 37.5%.
**Continuous passive motion.

TABLE 8–9. Matched Assignment

Group 1:* Open Chain/Manual	Group 2:† Open Chain/CPM**	Group 3:‡ Closed Chain/Manual	Group 4:§ Closed Chain/CPM
14. F, 60	21. F, 61	9. F, 62	18. F, 63
31. M, 65	24. M, 63	32. M, 62	2. M, 60
28. F, 67	4. F, 64	5. F, 65	6. F, 68
15. M, 66	22. M, 67	16. M, 66	23. M, 65
1. F, 70	29. F, 69	11. F, 68	13. F, 69
30. M, 67	7. M, 68	17. M, 70	8. M, 69
10. F, 78	27. F, 77	20. F, 76	26. F, 72
3. M, 71	19. M, 71	25. M, 76	12. M, 81

*Mean age = 68.0 years, women = 50.0%.
†Mean age = 67.5 years, women = 50.0%.
‡Mean age = 68.1 years, women = 50.0%.
§Mean age = 68.4 years, women = 50.0%.
**Continuous passive motion.

stratified sampling. First, it ensures relatively equal distributions only on the variables that are matched. The possibility that other characteristics may not be evenly distributed across the groups may be forgotten in light of the homogeneity on the matched variables. In addition, the information needed for matching on some variables is difficult and expensive to obtain. If we wanted to match groups according to range of motion and knee function before surgery, we would have had to collect this data ourselves or depend on potentially unreliable retrospective data.

Consecutive Assignment

The four assignment methods presented thus far are used when an existing sample is available for assignment to groups. This is not the case when consecutive sampling is being used, for example, to identify patients as they undergo surgery or enter a health care facility. When a consecutive sample is used, then assignment to groups needs to be consecutive as well. The basic strategy used for consecutive assignment is the development of an ordered list with group assignments made in advance. As subjects enter the study they are given consecutive numbers and assigned to the group indicated for each number.

Deciding on an Assignment Method

The best assignment method will ensure that groups sizes are equal, group characteristics are similar, and group characteristics approximate the overall sample characteristics. Assignment by individuals leads to a situation where group sizes are not necessarily equal; this is more of a problem with small group studies than with large group studies. Matched assignment obviously will often lead to the least variability between groups on the matched variables, but it may not randomize other extraneous factors. In addition, it may be expensive and time consuming to collect the information on which subjects will be matched. The choice between block assignment and systematic assignment is probably arbitrary unless the researcher suspects some regularly recurring pattern in subjects. In this case, block assignment should be used. With large samples, and in the absence of a regularly recurring pattern in the subject listing, systematic assignment provides an effective and efficient way to place subjects into groups.

SAMPLE SIZE

The preceding discussion of sampling and assignment was based on one major assumption—that the researcher knows how many subjects should be in the sample and in each group. In the real world, researchers must make decisions about sample size, and these decisions have a great deal of impact on the validity of the statistical conclusions of a piece of research. A complete discussion of the determination of sample size is deferred until the statistical foundation of the text is

TABLE 8–10. Characteristics with Sample Sizes of 2

Sample 1	Sample 2	Sample 3	Sample 4
7. M, 68	27. F, 77	21. F, 61	10. F, 78
17. M, 70	11. F, 68	4. F, 64	25. F, 76

Note: In Samples 1 through 4, the mean ages are 69.0, 72.5, 62.5, and 77.0 years, respectively. The percentage of women in each sample ranges from 0.0% to 100.0%.

TABLE 8–11. Characteristics with Sample Sizes of 8

Sample 1	Sample 2	Sample 3	Sample 4
1. F, 70	1. F, 70	3. M, 71	3. M, 71
3. M, 71	6. F, 68	4. F, 64	5. F, 65
6. F, 68	7. M, 68	5. F, 65	6. F, 68
14. F, 60	17. M, 70	6. F, 68	9. F, 62
15. M, 66	22. M, 67	7. M, 68	16. M, 66
29. F, 69	25. M, 76	14. F, 60	17. M, 70
30. M, 67	27. F, 77	24. M, 63	26. F, 72
32. M, 62	30. M, 67	27. F, 77	32. M, 72

Note: In Samples 1 through 4, the mean ages are 66.6, 70.4, 67.0, and 68.3 years, respectively. The percentage of women in each sample ranges from 37.5% to 68.3%.

laid, but one general principle of sample size determination may be presented here.

This general principle is that larger samples tend to be more representative of their parent populations than smaller samples. To illustrate this principle, consider our hypothetical sample of 32 patients who underwent TKA as an accessible population from which we shall draw even smaller samples. From the population of 32 subjects, four independent samples of 2 subjects and four independent samples of 8 subjects are selected. An independent sample is drawn, recorded, and replaced into the population before the next sample is drawn.

Tables 8–10 and 8–11 show the results of the sampling, and Figure 8–3 plots the distribution of the average age of subjects in the different-sized samples. Note that average ages for the samples of eight subjects are clustered more closely around the actual population age than are the average ages for the smaller samples. This, then, is a visual demonstration of the principle that large samples tend to be more representative of their parent populations. In addition, this clustering of sample characteristics close to the population characteristics means that there is less variability from sample to sample with the larger sample sizes.

For experimental research, group sizes of 20 to 30 participants are often considered the minimum size needed to make valid generalizations to a larger population and to meet the assumptions of certain statistical tests.[6,7] For descriptive research, 10% to 20% of the population has been advanced as a minimum sample size.[7] When deciding on sample size,

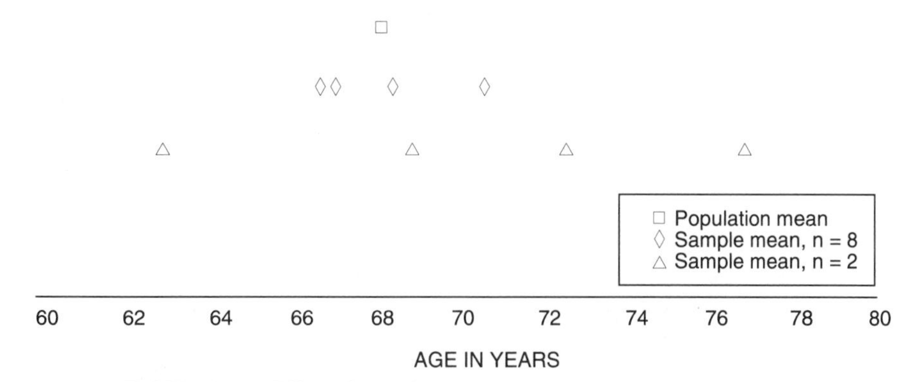

FIGURE 8–3. Effect of sample size on the stability of sample mean age.

researchers should always account for anticipated experimental mortality. If a subject's participation is required on only one day, then retention of selected subjects should be relatively high. If participation requires a commitment of a great deal of time, over a longer time period, researchers should expect that experimental mortality will be high.

Sometimes researchers are glibly advised to "get as many subjects as you can." If only 20 subjects are available, it is good advice—the researcher should try to use them all. However, if several hundred subjects are available, such advice may be inappropriate. First, recommending that sample sizes be as large as possible is ethically questionable, because this means large numbers of individuals are exposed to procedures with unknown benefits. Second, sometimes the results of research on very large groups produce statistical distinctions that are meaningless in practice, as discussed in Chapter 13.

SUMMARY

Selection and assignment of subjects influence the internal, external, and statistical conclusion validity of research. Populations are total groups of interest; samples are subgroups of populations. Probability samples use some degree of randomization to select subjects from the population. Common methods of probability sampling are simple random, systematic, stratified, and cluster sampling. Nonprobability samples do not rely on randomization. Common methods of nonprobability sampling are convenience and purposive sampling. Assignment to groups within a study can be accomplished randomly regardless of whether or not the method used to select the sample was random. Common forms of random assignment are individual, block, systematic, and matched assignment. A general principle in determining an appropriate sample size is that larger samples tend to be more representative of their parent populations than smaller samples.

References

1. Williams B. *A Sampler on Sampling*. New York, NY: John Wiley & Sons; 1978.
2. Hulley SB, Gove S, Browner WS, Cummings SR. Choosing the study subjects: specification and sampling. In Hulley SB, Cummings SR, eds. *Designing Clinical Research*. Baltimore, Md: Williams & Wilkins; 1988.
3. Beyer WH, ed. *Standard Mathematical Tables*. 27th ed. Boca Raton, Fla: CRC Press Inc; 1984.
4. *1991 Commercial Atlas and Marketing Guide*. 122nd ed. Chicago, Ill: Rand McNally & Co; 1991:321.
5. *1990 American Hospital Association Guide to the Health Care Field*. Chicago, Ill: American Hospital Association; 1990.
6. Kraemer HC, Thiemann S. *How Many Subjects? Statistical Power Analysis in Research*. Newbury Park, Calif: Sage Publications; 1987:27.
7. Gay LR. *Educational Research: Competencies for Analysis and Application*. 3rd ed. Columbus, Ohio: Merrill Publishing Co; 1987:114–115.

CHAPTER 9

Research Paradigms

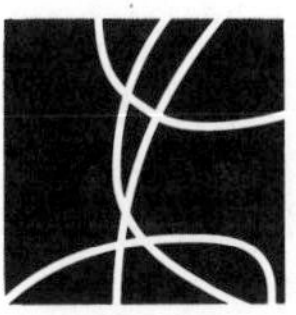

Knowledge is continually evolving. What was believed to be true yesterday may be doubted today, scorned tomorrow, and resurrected in the future. Beliefs about the methods of obtaining knowledge constitute *research paradigms*.[1(p15)] The beliefs that constitute a paradigm are often so entrenched that researchers themselves are not aware of the assumptions that undergird the research methodology they use.

The dominant research paradigm within physical therapy is the quantitative paradigm. Two competing paradigms of importance to physical therapy are the qualitative and single-system paradigms. The study of competing research paradigms in physical therapy is important for two reasons. First, research based on the competing paradigms is reported in the physical therapy literature, so consumers of the literature need to be familiar with the assumptions that undergird these paradigms. Second, competing research paradigms in any discipline emerge because the dominant paradigm is unable to answer all the important questions of the discipline. Researchers therefore need to consider research using competing paradigms not only in terms of the specific research questions it addresses, but also in terms of what the research implies about the limitations of the dominant paradigm.

In this chapter the three research paradigms used in physical therapy research are presented. First the unique qualities of each paradigm are discussed, and then the relationships among the paradigms are examined. The quantitative paradigm is discussed first. This paradigm focuses on the study of groups whose treatment is often manipulated by the investigator. Although the assumptions of this paradigm have guided much of the book thus far, in this chapter these assumptions are made explicit and the limitations of the paradigm are discussed. The qualitative paradigm is then discussed. This paradigm focuses on broad description and understanding of phenomena without direct manipulation. The final paradigm to be analyzed is the single-system paradigm, which focuses on individual responses to manipulation.

Deciding on the terminology to use for the different research paradigms is difficult. The paradigms are sometimes described in philosophical terms, sometimes in terms of components of the paradigm, and sometimes in terms of the methods that usually follow from the philosophical underpinnings of the paradigm. Table 9–1 presents the various names that have been used to identify what are being labeled in this chapter as quantitative, qualitative, and single-system paradigms.

Accurate use of the different philosophical labels requires a strong background in the history and philosophy of science, a background that most physical therapists do not have. To avoid imprecise use of the language of philosophy, the "methodological" terms are used in this text, rather than the "philosophical" terms. This choice may, however, lead to the misconception that paradigms and methods are interchangeable. They are not. A paradigm is defined by the assumptions and beliefs that guide researchers. A method is defined by the actions taken by investigators as they implement research. Adoption of a paradigm implies the use of certain methods but does not necessarily limit the researcher to those methods. Research designs, then, are specific ways of organizing methods within a study. For each paradigm, its underlying assumptions are revealed, followed by discussion of the methodological implications of the paradigm and description of specific designs associated with the paradigm.

TABLE 9–1. Terms Associated with the Three Research Paradigms

Quantitative Paradigm	Qualitative Paradigm	Single-System Paradigm
positivist	*naturalistic*	*idiographic*
received view	*phenomenological*	*N = 1*
logical positivist	*ethnographic*	*single-subject*
nomothetic	*idiographic*	
empiricist	*postpositivist*	
	new paradigm	

QUANTITATIVE PARADIGM

The quantitative paradigm is what has become known as the traditional method of science. The term *quantitative* comes from the emphasis on measurement that characterizes this paradigm. This paradigm has its roots in the 1600s with the development of Newtonian physics.[2, 3] In the early 1900s, the French philosopher Auguste Comte and a group of scientists in Vienna became proponents of related philosophical positions often labeled *positivism* or *logical positivism*.[4] This positivist philosophy is so labeled because of the central idea that one can be certain, or positive, of knowledge only if it is verifiable through measurement and observation.

Assumptions of the Quantitative Paradigm

Just as there are multiple terms for each paradigm, there are multiple views about the critical components of each paradigm. Lincoln and Guba used five basic axioms to differentiate what they refer to as positivist and naturalistic paradigms.[1(p37)] Their five axioms are presented here as the basis of the quantitative paradigm. The qualitative and single-system paradigms are developed by retaining or replacing these with alternate axioms. Table 9–2 summarizes the assumptions of the three paradigms.

Assumption 1. There is a single, objective reality. One goal of quantitative research is to determine the nature of a single, objective

TABLE 9–2. Assumptions of the Three Research Paradigms

Assumption	Paradigm		
	Quantitative	***Qualitative***	***Single-System***
Reality	Single, objective	Multiple, constructed	Single, objective
Relationship between investigator and subject	Independent	Dependent	Independent
Generalizability of findings	Desirable and possible	Situation specific	System specific
Cause-and-effect relationships	Causal	Noncausal	Causal
Values	Value free	Value bound	Value free

reality through measurement and observation of the phenomena of interest. This reliance on observation and experimentation is sometimes termed *empiricism*. A second goal of quantitative research is to predict or control this reality. After all, if researchers can empirically determine laws that regulate reality in some predictable way, then they should be able to use this knowledge to attempt to influence that reality in equally predictable ways.

Assumption 2. The investigator and subject (the object of investigation) are independent of one another. In other words, it is assumed that the investigator can be an unobtrusive observer of a reality that does not change by virtue of the fact that it is being studied. Researchers who adopt the quantitative paradigm do, however, recognize that it is sometimes difficult to achieve this independence—witness the subtle cues from investigators that led to the purported mathematical prowess of Clever Hans, the horse discussed in Chapter 7.[5] Despite the recognition of the difficulty achieving the independence of the investigator and subject, the assumption of the quantitative paradigm is that it is possible and desirable to do so.

Assumption 3. The goal of research is to develop generalizable characterizations of reality. The generalizability of a piece of research refers to its applicability to other subjects, times, and settings. The concept of generalizability leads to the classification of quantitative research as *nomothetic*, or relating to general or universal principles. Quantitative researchers recognize the limits of generalizability as threats to the external validity of their research; however, they believe that generalizability is an achievable aim and that research that fails to achieve generalizability is flawed.

Assumption 4. Cause and effect can be determined and differentiated from one another. Quantitative researchers are careful to differentiate experimental research from nonexperimental research on the basis that causal inferences can only be drawn if the researcher is able to manipulate an independent variable (the "presumed cause") in a controlled fashion while observing the effect of the manipulation on a dependent variable (the "presumed effect"). Quantitative researchers recognize that extraneous factors sometimes limit their ability to draw causal conclusions; they refer to these extraneous factors as threats to the internal validity of their research.

Assumption 5. Research is value free. The controlled, objective nature of quantitative research is assumed to eliminate the influence of the investigator's opinions and societal norms on the facts that are discovered. Inquiry is seen as the objective discovery of truths and the investigator the impartial discoverer of these truths.

Quantitative Methods

Adoption of the assumptions of the quantitative paradigm has major implications for the methods of quantitative research. In this section, five methodological issues are discussed in relation to the assumptions that underlie the quantitative paradigm: theory, selection, measurement, manipulation, and control. These issues are summarized in Table 9–3. Quotes from a single piece of quantitative research illustrate the way in which each of these methodological issues is handled within the quantitative paradigm.

Theory. The investigator performing quantitative research is expected to articulate an *a priori* theory, that is, a theory developed in advance of the research. The purpose of the research is to confirm components of the theory. This top–down notion of theory development is discussed in Chapters 2 and 4. Griffin and associates' comparison of the effectiveness of (a) high-voltage pulsed-current (HVPC), (b) intermittent pneumatic compression (IPC), and (c) placebo–HVPC treatments was an experimental study in the quantitative tradition.[6] As such, an *a priori* theoretical perspective guided the study:

> Chronic hand edema contributes to pain, decreased active motion, and further edema. . . . Identification of maximally effective methods for reducing chronic posttraumatic hand edema should result in faster recovery of hand functions. . . . High voltage pulsed current and IPC are widely used in clinical practice to reduce posttraumatic edema. . . . Controlled studies are needed to substantiate clinical reports of efficacy.[6(p279)]

The elements of this rather informal theory are that edema leads to dysfunction, that reduction of edema should enhance rehabilitation, and that there is a knowledge gap about which of two different methods of edema reduction is most effective.

Selection. Elaborate sampling and assignment procedures are expressions of the belief in the importance of generalizability:

> Chronic hand edema was defined as edema persisting for 14 to 21 days following surgery. . . . Patients were excluded if they had open wounds, severe pain, or a dystrophic component. . . . Subjects were randomly assigned to IPC, HVPC, and placebo-HVPC using a table of random digits.[6(p280)]

When quantitative researchers cannot control the nature of their subjects as well as they might like, they usually express this

TABLE 9–3. Methods of the Three Research Paradigms

Method	Paradigm		
	Quantitative	*Qualitative*	*Single-System*
Theory	*A priori*	Grounded	*A priori*
Selection and assignment	Random	Purposive	Purposive
Measurement tools	Instruments	Human	Instruments
Type of data	Numerical	Language	Numerical
Manipulation	Present	Absent	Present
Control	Maximized	Minimized	Flexible

concern as an unfortunate limitation of the research:

> The use of human subjects presents difficulties in controlled clinical studies because identical types of trauma are impossible to obtain.[6(p284)]

Measurement. The development of ever more precise measurement tools is an expression of the belief in an objective reality. Measurement deviations are viewed as errors that must be managed statistically:

> Volumetric displacements of the affected hand were recorded for 12 patients with posttraumatic hand edema, and measurements were repeated within a 10-minute period. The mean change between repeated measurements was 0.6 mL (range = −3 to 7). . . . On the basis of these findings we now consider in our facility that a reduction in hand volume must be at least 8 mL to be greater than measurement error.[6(pp282, 283)]

Measurement theory, presented in the next major section of this text, is largely based on the concept that researchers use imperfect measurement tools to estimate the "true" characteristics of a phenomenon of interest. Statistical decision making is also based on estimating true population parameters from sample statistics.

Manipulation. The manipulation that is an inherent part of experimental study is related to the quantitative paradigm assumption that researchers can determine causes and effects for changes that are observed in response to the controlled manipulation of the experimenter. Although Griffin and coworkers did not use the words *cause* and *effect* in describing their results, the causal implication was clear:

> The results of this study indicate that significant edema reduction may be obtained in some patients with chronic posttraumatic hand edema after one 30-minute treatment with IPC.[6(p284)]

Control. Control of extraneous factors is so important that this sometimes leads to construction of experimental protocols that do not resemble clinical protocols:

> Greater edema reductions might have been obtained by combining IPC or HVPC treatments with elevation of the hand, as is common in clinical practice. However, we intentionally eliminated the effect of hand elevation in order to establish the treatment effects of IPC and HVPC modalities alone.[6(p284)]

These then, are examples of five research methods—*a priori* theory development, selection for representativeness, emphasis on measurement, manipulation, and control—that flow from the underlying assumptions of the quantitative paradigm.

Quantitative Designs

The research designs presented in Chapters 5 and 6 are largely based in the quantitative paradigm. Although one of the assumptions of the quantitative paradigm is that causes and effects can be established, this does not mean that only experimental research can be conducted within the framework of the quantitative paradigm. Nonexperimental research may be as quantitative as experimental research if it is conducted in the spirit of a single objective reality, from a predetermined theoretical perspective, with a focus on identifying representative groups for study, and with the assumption that the investigator can study the subjects of interest without influencing the reality being measured.

QUALITATIVE PARADIGM

Whereas the mechanistic view of Newtonian physics provided the roots for the development of the quantitative paradigm, the relativistic view of quantum mechanics provided the roots for the development of the qualitative paradigm. Zukav contrasted the "old" Newtonian physics with the "new" quantum physics:

> The old physics assumes that there is an external world which exists apart from us. It further assumes that we can observe, measure, and speculate about the external world without changing it. . . . The new physics, quantum mechanics, tells us clearly that it is not possible to observe reality without changing it. If we observe a certain particle collision experiment, not only do we have no way of proving that the results would have been the same if we have not been watching it, all that we know indicates that it would not have been the same, because the results that we got were affected by the fact that we were looking for it.[2(pp30–31)]

Because the quantitative paradigm has proved inadequate even for the discipline of physics, a "hard" science, qualitative researchers argue that there is little justification for applying it to the "soft" sciences in which human behavior is studied.

Assumptions of the Qualitative Paradigm

The assumptions that underlie the qualitative paradigm are antithetical to the assumptions of the quantitative paradigm. Once again Lincoln and Guba's concepts, but not their terminology (they referred to the qualitative paradigm as the "naturalistic paradigm") can be used to reveal the assumptions of the qualitative paradigm. Table 9–2 provides an overview of these assumptions.

Assumption 1. The world consists of multiple constructed realities. "Multiple" means that there are always several versions of reality. "Constructed" means that participants attach meaning to events that occur within their lives and that this meaning is an inseparable component of the events themselves. Thus, reality is life as it is lived. For example, if one patient states that his therapist is cold and unfeeling, that is his reality. If another patient states that the same therapist is professional and candid, that is her reality. The notion of a single, objective reality is rejected. Researchers who adopt the qualitative paradigm believe that it is fruitless to try to determine the therapist's "actual" manner because the therapist's demeanor does not exist apart from how it is perceived by different patients.

Assumption 2. The investigator and the subject (object of investigation) are interdependent; the process of inquiry itself changes both the investigator and the subject. Whereas researchers using the quantitative paradigm seek to eliminate what they view as the undesirable interdependence of investigator and subject, researchers using the qualitative paradigm accept this interdependence as inevitable and even desirable. For example, a qualitative researcher studying the phenomenon of therapist demeanor would recognize that simply initiating such a study is likely to change the demeanor of the therapists under study.

Assumption 3. Knowledge is time and context dependent. Qualitative paradigm researchers reject the nomothetic approach and its concept of generalizability. In this sense, then, qualitative research is *idiographic*, meaning that it pertains to a particular case in a particular time and context. The goal of qualitative research is a deep understanding of the particular. Researchers who adopt the qualitative paradigm hope that this particular understanding may lead to insights about other situations, but believe that each situation is so unique that information cannot be widely applied to situations other than the one in which it was generated. Thus, qualitative researchers would recognize that different therapist demeanors are likely to be seen in different parts of the country, in different types of clinics, and with different types of patients. There would be no search for a representative demeanor that is most effective with a representative group of patients.

Assumption 4. It is impossible to distinguish causes from effects. The quantitative researchers' whole notion of cause is tied to the idea of prediction, control, and an objective reality. In contrast, researchers who adopt the qualitative paradigm believe it is more useful to describe and interpret events than to attempt to control them to establish oversimplified causes and effects. Returning to our example of therapist demeanor, a qualitative researcher would believe that it is impossible to determine whether a certain therapist demeanor caused better patient outcomes or whether certain patient outcomes caused different therapist demeanors. Because they believe causes cannot be separated from effects, qualitative researchers would focus on describing the multiple forces that shape therapist–patient interactions.

Assumption 5. Inquiry is value bound. This value ladenness is exemplified in the type of questions qualitative researchers ask, the way they define and measure constructs, and the way they interpret the results of their research. The traditional view of scientists is that they are capable of "dispassionate judgment and unbiased inquiry."[7(p109)] Frustration with the value ladenness of research has been expressed by Rubin, a prominent virologist studying acquired immune deficiency syndrome (AIDS):

> The minute someone suggests that the orthodoxy might be wrong, the establishment starts to call him crazy or a quack. One week you're a great scientist; the next week you're a jerk. Science has become the new church of America and is closing off all room for creative, productive dissent.[8(ppF1, 7)]

Rubin made this statement in response to the unwillingness of the medical community to consider that the human immunodeficiency virus (HIV) may not be the sole cause of AIDS. Thus, Rubin believes that the values of the medical research community, which is made up of researchers who have adopted the quantitative paradigm and believe themselves to be objective observers, are greatly influencing the direction of research on HIV and AIDS.

Researchers who adopt the qualitative paradigm recognize that they are unable to separate values from inquiry. They do not believe that it is productive to pretend that science is objective, particularly in light of controversies such as that cited in the example of AIDS research.

Qualitative Methods

The five assumptions of the qualitative paradigm have an enormous impact on the conduct of qualitative research. The roles of theory, selection, measurement, manipulation, and control in qualitative research are vastly different from those in quantitative research, as summarized in Table 9–3. Jensen and associates used the qualitative paradigm to structure their study of the nature of therapist–patient interactions of novice and experienced clinicians.[9] This study provides examples of the methods that follow from the beliefs of the qualitative paradigm.

Theory. Because researchers who adopt the qualitative paradigm accept the concept of multiple constructed realities, they do not begin their inquiry with a researcher-developed theoretical framework. They begin their research with an idea of what concepts or constructs may be important to understanding a certain phenomenon, but they recognize that the participants in the inquiry will define other versions of what is important. A rigid theoretical framework of the researcher would constrain the direction of the inquiry and might provide a less than full description of the phenomenon of interest:

> We call the therapeutic intervention the black box because we know so little about what happens between therapist and patient. The focus . . . was to begin to look at the black box and explore what actually happens during the time the patient is in the physical therapy clinical setting.[9(p315)]

Selection. Selection is purposive in qualitative research. This means that rather than selecting a randomized group of individuals, qualitative researchers purposely select individuals who they believe will be able to lend insight to the research problem:

> A purposive sample was used. . . . We selected therapists on the basis of experience as a practicing physical therapist. . . . At this initial level of investigation, our observations were of highly experienced and less experienced clinicians working with similar patient populations. These therapists were selected so that a variety of orthopedic outpatient settings were represented.[9(p315)]

In Jensen and associates' study, purposive sampling led to the selection of only eight therapists from four settings. Most traditional quantitative researchers would find a sample this small insufficient because (a) it would not likely be representative of a larger group and (b) small samples do not lend themselves to statistical analysis. These are not considered problems in qualitative research, because representativeness and statistical analysis are not the goals of the inquiry.

Measurement. The primary measurement tool of qualitative research is the researcher, the "human instrument." Because of the complexity of the multiple realities the qualitative researcher is seeking to describe, a reactive, thinking instrument is needed, as noted by Jensen and associates:

> We collected data through nonparticipant observation, recording of field notes, and audiotaping of each treatment session. . . . The field notes also included a rough sketch of the physical environment and a record of nonverbal activities including eye and hand contact between the therapist and the patient.[9(p316)]

The data collected in qualitative studies are usually not numerical but rather verbal and consist of feelings and perceptions rather than presumed facts. Researchers gather a great deal of descriptive data about the particular situation they are studying so that they can provide a "rich" or "thick" description of the situation. Because interpretation of the information is dependent on the time and context of the study, it is important that time and context information be well articulated.

Manipulation and Control. The qualitative researcher does not manipulate or control the research setting. Rather, the setting is manipulated in unpredictable ways by the interaction between the investigator and the subjects. The mere fact that the researcher is present or asks certain questions is bound to influence the subjects and their perception of the situation.

The natural setting is used for research. Because everything is time and context dependent, researchers who adopt the qualitative paradigm believe there is little is to be gained—and much to be lost—from creating an artificial study situation. Although Jensen and her colleagues studied their therapist–patient pairs during the course of a routine day, they would likely agree that their observation of treatment sessions changed the therapist–patient interactions in some ways. However, consider how much more the therapist–patient interactions would have been changed had they been observed in an artificial environment in which each therapist had to deal with only one patient, free from the interruptions of the telephone, other patients, and colleagues. Researchers who are guided by the quantitative paradigm would wish to create an artificial environment so that they could control these extraneous factors and focus on the interactions. Researchers, like Jensen and associates, who are guided by the qualitative paradigm view these factors as integral to therapist–patient interactions and prefer to describe them rather than control them:

> The more experienced therapists were observed to handle interruptions and tasks outside of direct treatment efficiently without disrupting the treatment session. . . . The novices we observed reacted quickly to most environmental stimuli such as intercom interruptions and patient scheduling tasks, often losing focus on direct patient care activities.[9(p320)]

Qualitative Designs

Just as the quantitative paradigm can accommodate research with the purpose of describing phenomena, analyzing relationships, or analyzing differences, so can the qualitative paradigm. Qualitative analysis of relationships and differences is done through interpretation rather than statistics. The boundaries between different types of qualitative research are less clear than the boundaries between different quantitative designs. Whereas there is relatively well-standardized terminology for the different classifications of quantitative designs (see Chapter 5), the terminology for the different types of qualitative research is far less universally accepted. Three different types of qualitative research are described here: ethnography, phenomenology, and grounded theory. Recognize that although each of the approaches serves a different purpose, there is considerable overlap between the methods used in the three approaches.

Ethnography. The purpose of ethnography is to describe a culture. Broadly, *culture* can be defined as the knowledge, beliefs, and behaviors that define a group. The group can be a societal group such as "Americans," "French-Canadians," or "Southeast Asian immigrants." The group can also be a small, specialized unit such as "burn therapists," "members of a wheelchair basketball team," or "physical therapy faculty members at a particular institution." Sometimes the terms *macroethnography* and *microethnography* are used to describe the extent of the group being described.[10(p147)] The ethnographic approach requires that the researcher, an outsider to the culture, describe the culture from the perspective of an insider. Spradley indicated that "rather than *studying people*, ethnography means *learning from people*."[11(p3)] This difference can be illustrated by contrasting the quantitative and qualitative approaches to the study of physical therapists working in a burn unit.

A quantitative approach to studying such a unit might focus on the time spent on different tasks, such as hydrotherapy; exercise; nonphysical interactions with patients; and interactions with patient families, physicians, nurses, and other therapists. The ethnographic approach would require observation and documentation of some of the same activities explored by the quantitative approach but would also focus on the emotions, feelings, and meanings of the people and activities within the unit. To do so, the ethnographer needs to request this information from the participants in the culture being studied. Questions that would be asked include, "When you say you are going to 'tank' so and so, what does this mean?", "How do you react to the death of a patient? Does this reaction differ depending on your initial impressions about a patient's chance of survival?", and "In what ways are your experiences or reactions different from those of nurses on the unit?" The qualitative researcher expresses ignorance about a culture and learns about the culture from inside "informants."

An ethnographic approach was taken to study liberal arts institutions with physical therapy programs.[12] It was assumed that the competing ideas of "liberal" and "professional" education would be evident in the interactions of various groups on campus. Data collection was accomplished through participant observation and interviews with faculty, students, and administrators. *Participant observation* is the term used to describe the process whereby a researcher enters a cultural milieu and learns about it through both observation and participation.[13] Participation can be relatively formal, such as interviews, or informal, such as dining with group members. Information from the interviews and observations is categorized and grouped into themes of meaning that characterize the culture.

Phenomenology. The purpose of the phenomenological approach to qualitative inquiry is to describe some aspect of life as it is lived by the participants.[14(p70)] The phenomenological approach is therefore somewhat narrower than the ethnographic approach. In ethnographic research, the element of interest is the culture of a group. In phenomenological research, the emphasis is on a more specific element of interest to the researcher.

The phenomenological approach was used by Peters to study the criteria that residents in long-term care facilities used to define quality care.[15] Data collection was performed through interviews with residents of the long-term care facilities. Purposive sampling was used to ensure diversity of opinion: Three different types of facilities were used, and the researcher asked contacts at the facility to identify residents whom they believed held different opinions about the quality of care at the institution. The researcher reviewed verbatim transcripts of the interviews and classified residents' responses about quality care into approximately 20 categories, which were later reduced into 10 distinct themes of quality care.

The distinction between the phenomenological and ethnographic approaches can be seen if the quality care study is recast as an ethnographic study. The purpose of the hypothetical ethnography might be to describe the culture of the long-term care facility in terms of the concept "quality care." The broader cultural approach would warrant obtaining the opinions of caregivers, residents, family, and certifying agencies such as state boards of health. Data collection would be accomplished through interviews with these groups of individuals, examination of certifying agency reports, and participant observation of the daily lives of residents of the facility. The results of this ethnography might point to the differing definitions of quality care that are held by subgroups within the facility. In contrast, Peters's phenomenological study focused on life as lived by the residents alone.

Grounded Theory. The grounded-theory approach was developed by Glaser in the 1960s.[16] The purpose of using a grounded-theory approach is to develop theories about the nature of a concept of interest. Jensen and associates' study of novice and experienced clinicians, discussed earlier as a general example of qualitative research, could be classified as grounded-theory research because one of its purposes was to "develop an initial conceptual framework"[9(p315)] about the work of physical therapists. Another example of the use of the grounded-theory approach is Scully and Shepard's study of clinical educators in physical therapy.[17] Purposive sampling was used to identify clinical educators at five diverse facilities. No *a priori* theory about the nature of clinical education or clinical educators was developed to guide the study; rather, the study results were used to generate a model of factors of importance to clinical education and clinical educators.

Data analysis in the Scully and Shepard study was performed by constant comparison.[17] The essence of the constant comparison method of data analysis is that initial data are collected, patterns of responses that indicate common underlying concepts about the culture are determined, additional data are collected, and these data are used to either confirm the initial concept organization or modify it in light of the new information.[14(pp105–113)] For example, Scully and Shepard observed that the clinical teaching situation was influenced by what they referred to as "health care institution ground rules." In their research report, they identified six health care institution factors that seemed to influence the level of supervision of students. They did not specify the actual process by which they developed these six factors, but hypothetically such a process might be as follows:

First, after observing and interviewing at one center, the researchers may classify institutional supervision norms in terms of physical structure (for example, bedside treatment implies closer supervision than treatment in the physical therapy department), patient factors (for example, the acuity of the patients' problems), and temporal factors (for example, students who have been at a facility longer may be supervised less).

Second, the researchers interview and observe at a second center, using this three-factor scheme to organize its institutional supervision factors until they identify an occurrence that cannot be classified into one of the three factors: For example, a clinical instructor becomes ill, and her student is placed suddenly into an environment with little supervision. This leads the researchers to create a fourth category within the institutional ground rules: circumstantial factors.

Third, the researchers might take this idea back to several of the therapists at the first center to see whether they recognize this fourth category, which was not observed at that clinic, as a part of the clinical education experience at their facility.

The process of data collection, concept development, and concept verification would continue until no new concepts are encountered.

Although the grounded-theory approach shares interview and observational methods with other qualitative approaches, the goal of the research is different. The goal of the ethnographic and phenomenological approaches is description of a culture or a concept as experienced by those within the culture. The goal of the grounded-theory approach is the development of a theory that is grounded in the data. The purpose of theory development is to explain phenomena and guide future inquiry.

As noted previously, the boundaries between the qualitative approaches are not clear. Some studies may not fit any of the categories; others may fit more than one of the categories. In fact, Scully and Shepard subtitled their study of clinical educators "an ethnographic study" and described the theoretical framework for their data analysis as grounded theory. Their study was classified for this chapter as grounded theory research because it clearly sought to "identify and explain"[17(p349)] some of the components of clinical education. The study does not fit this chapter's definition of ethnographic research because Scully and Shepard focused only on observation of clinical educators—they did not interview students or educators or otherwise participate in the "culture" of clinical education. Labels such as "grounded theory," "ethnography," and "phenomenology" are important because they provide a way to organize what we know about qualitative research. However, arguments about which definition is the "one true definition" tend to be counterproductive in that they violate one of the basic tenets of qualitative research—the acceptance of multiple realities. Thus, readers should use this classification of qualitative research as one way to organize information and recognize that others may use equally useful alternate classification systems.

SINGLE-SYSTEM PARADIGM

The single-system paradigm developed out of a concern that the focus of traditional group research methods was shifting away from the unit of clinical interest: the individual. Assume that a group study of the effectiveness of a particular gait training technique on gait velocity in individuals who have had an amputation is implemented in 30 individuals. If gait velocity improves for 10 patients, remains the same for 10 patients, and declines for 10 patients, then the average velocity for the group will not change very much and the group conclusion is likely to be that the treatment had no effect. This group conclusion ignores the fact that the treatment was effective for 10 patients and actually reduced velocity in 10 patients. A clinically relevant conclusion might be that the treatment has the potential to improve velocity but that clinicians should also recognize that the opposite effect is also seen in some patients. Single-system research eliminates the group conclusion and focuses on treatment effects in individuals.

Table 9–1 lists several different terms for single-system research. Ottenbacher uses the term "single system" rather than the more common "single subject" because there are some instances in which the unit of interest is group performance, rather than individual performance.[18(p45)] For example, a physical therapy administrator might wish to study departmental productivity before and after a reorganization. Because the researcher is interested not in the changes in individual therapist productivity, but in the productivity of the department as a whole, the effect of the reorganization could be studied as a single system. Because "single system" is a more inclusive term, it is used throughout this text.

Assumptions of the Single-System Paradigm

The basic assumption of the single-system paradigm is that the effectiveness of treatment depends on the subject and the setting. Single-system researchers believe that research should reflect the idiographic nature of practice by focusing on the study of individuals. Except for this focus on the individual rather than a group, the assumptions of the single-system paradigm are those of the quantitative paradigm, as shown in Table

9–2. In fact, the single-system paradigm focuses exclusively on experimental problems in which there is active manipulation of the individual under study.

The single-system paradigm is sometimes confused with the clinical case report or case study. The two are very different. The case report or case study is a description, very often a retrospective description, of a course of treatment of an individual. The case study has not been presented as a research design in this text because it does not meet the criterion of "systematic" study, as required by the definition of research adopted in Chapter 1. Single-system research, on the other hand, uses a systematic process of introduction and withdrawal of treatments to allow for controlled assessment of the effects of a treatment.

Single-System Methods

Because many assumptions are shared between the quantitative and single-system paradigms, many methods are shared as well, as shown in Table 9–3. Diamond and Ottenbacher's study of the effect of a tone-inhibiting dynamic ankle-foot orthosis (TIAFO) on stride characteristics of an adult with hemiparesis illustrates these methods in practice.[19] In this study, three walking conditions were compared: barefoot walking, a traditional plastic ankle-foot orthosis (AFO), and a TIAFO.

Theory. Single-system paradigm research generally operates from an *a priori* theoretical foundation, as demonstrated in Diamond and Ottenbacher's article:

> Based on available literature and clinical experience, we hypothesized that the TIAFO would be associated with the most normal stride.[19(p424)]

Selection. Selection of the individual for study is purposive. In Diamond and Ottenbacher's study, the subject had discontinued use of a traditional AFO but continued to have gait difficulties. Thus, the TIAFO was prescribed as an alternative to the orthosis that had not met all of his gait needs. Single-system researchers would not choose to study someone for whom they did not believe the intervention was uniquely appropriate. This is in contrast to the group approach in which, say, 30 subjects who had had cerebral vascular accidents might all be studied with the TIAFO and the traditional AFO. How likely is it that all 30 of these subjects would have problems with the traditional AFO that would require trial of the TIAFO? If, in such a study, the TIAFO was not shown to be more effective than a traditional AFO, it might be because the group needs did not warrant the use of the TIAFO. The single-system paradigm requires that the individual studied have a specific need for the treatment implemented.

Measurement. Precise measurement is an integral part of the single-system paradigm. Repeated measures taken during baseline and treatment phases are compared. Thus, measurement accuracy and reliability are critical to the ability to draw conclusions about the effects of treatment. This measurement focus is apparent in Diamond and Ottenbacher's study:

> Walking velocity (in meters per second) was measured by timing the subject with a stopwatch as he walked 11 m. Reliability of the velocity measurement was assessed by having two therapists record the time for the subject to ambulate a distance of 11 m during baseline trials.[19(p426)]

Manipulation and Control. Experimental manipulation is part of the definition of single-system research. This is illustrated in Diamond and Ottenbacher's study by their manipulation of the conditions under which the subject walked: barefoot, with an AFO, and with a TIAFO.

Finally, control of extraneous factors is important in the conduct of single-system research, as it is in quantitative research. Diamond and Ottenbacher controlled the experimental setting by randomizing the presentation of the three gait conditions and controlling the frequency of measurement sessions. Table 9–3 indicates, however, that the control in single-system paradigm research may be more flexible than it is in traditional group designs. In group designs, researchers usually attempt to control the nature of the treatment administered so that all individuals within the group receive approximately the same treatment. With the single-system designs, the treatment can be administered as it would be in the clinic. Thus the intervention can be tailored to accommodate scheduling changes, status changes, or varying patient moods.

Single-System Designs

There are four basic design variations for single-system research: A–B designs, multiple-baseline designs, alternating-treatment designs, and interaction designs.[18]

A–B Designs. In A–B designs, some pattern of initiation and removal of treatment is used to determine differences in some dependent variable on the basis of the presence or absence of the treatment. By convention, A represents baseline phases, and B represents treatment phases. An A–B design represents a baseline phase followed by a treatment phase. An A–B–A design represents a study in which a treatment phase is both preceded and followed by a baseline phase. Other variants include B–A–B and A–B–A–B designs.

Laskas and colleagues conducted a study of motor function in a child with spastic quadriplegia using an A–B–A design.[20] The dependent measures were the daily change (postactivity − preactivity) in electromyographic dorsiflexor muscle activity and the number of times the child had heel contact when assuming a standing position after activity. Seven recording sessions served as the first baseline phase (A); nine treatment and recording sessions constituted the treatment phase (B); and seven recording sessions served as the second baseline (A). Treatment consisted of 20-minute sessions of a variety of activities structured according to a neurodevelopmental treatment philosophy. During the baseline phases, the child played freely for 20 minutes. Figure 9–1 shows the results for the heel contact variable. This illustrates the typical way in which single-system results are presented. Visual analysis of this graph would lead one to conclude that the treatment phase caused a change in heel contact in standing compared with the baseline phases. Statistical analysis of single-system data is covered in Chapter 14.

Multiple-Baseline Designs. There are several variations of the multiple-baseline designs. However, they all share the same purpose, and that is to control for the effects of history. The general format for the multiple-baseline study is to conduct several single-system studies, with baselines at different times or for different durations. An example of this design is Ottenbacher and associates' study of oral sensorimotor therapy with four developmentally disabled clients.[21] The dependent measures were body weight and score on an oral–motor/feeding function scale. The baseline measurements for all clients started in the same week. However, the clients had baseline phases of two, four, six, and eight weeks, respectively.

Assume that a historical threat to internal validity occurred during the fifth week of the

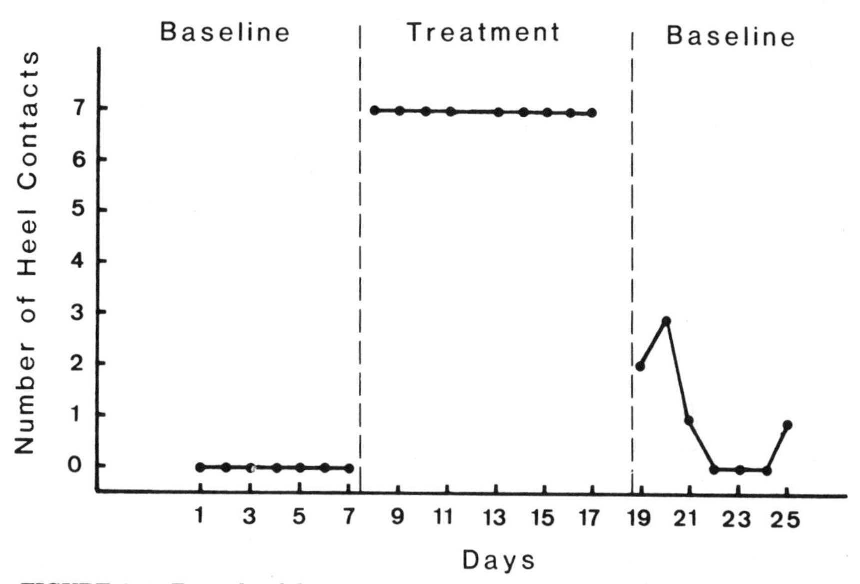

FIGURE 9–1. Example of data presentation for an A-B-A study. The study showed the frequency of heel contact in movement to standing—the number of times out of seven that the child came to a standing position with the heel contacting the floor. From Laskas CA, Mullen SL, Nelson DL, Willson-Broyles M. Enhancement of two motor functions of the lower extremity in a child with spastic quadriplegia. *Phys Ther.* 1985;65:11–16. Reprinted from *Physical Therapy* with the permission of the American Physical Therapy Association.

study. For example, if staffing improved in the fifth week of the study and remained improved during the remainder of the study, weight increases in the clients might be because of the effect of either the staff's spending more time feeding each client or the sensorimotor stimulation program. If a single case was used, it would be impossible to separate the effects of the staffing change from the effect of the sensorimotor program.

By using multiple baselines, the effect of a historical event can be analyzed. Figure 9–2 shows the hypothetical scores that assume weight increases are related to staffing and not to the effect of the sensorimotor program. The addition of the other clients allows the researcher to see that all subjects had stable baselines for the first five weeks; all subjects had increases in weight after five weeks, irrespective of the presence of the sensorimotor program; and improvement during the treatment phase seems to have been a continuation of the pattern exhibited during the baseline phase.

Alternating-Treatment Designs. Alternating-treatment designs include the use of different treatments, each administered independently of the other. In describing such designs, the letters B, C, D, E, and so on are used to represent the different treatments; A continues to represent the baseline phase or phases. This design is well suited to treatments that are expected to have short-lived effects. For example, a straightforward study of gait velocity of a patient wearing different ankle-foot orthoses might be represented by the notation A–B–A–C–A. This would mean that a baseline with no orthosis was established (A); this baseline phase was followed by gait assessments while the patient wore one orthosis, perhaps a traditional short leg

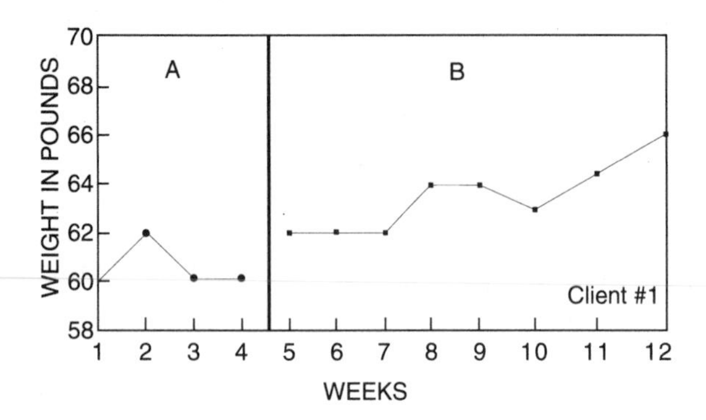

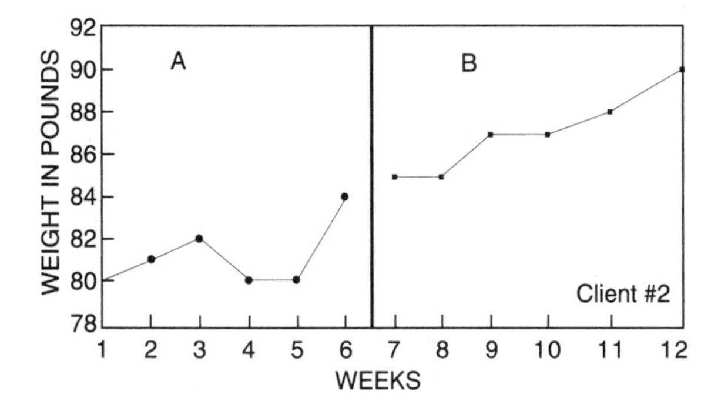

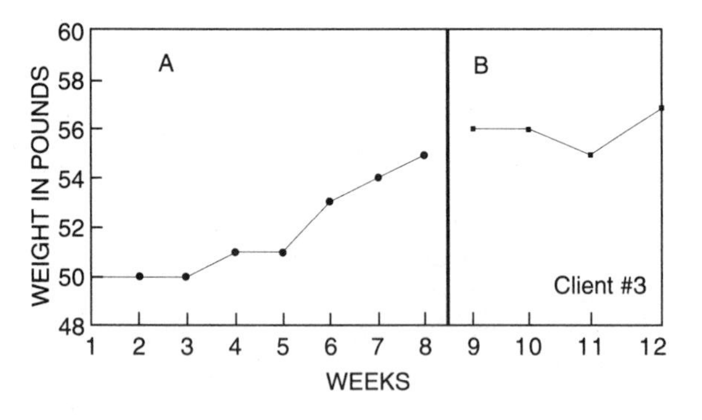

FIGURE 9–2. Example of data presentation for a multiple-baseline study. Note that all baselines (A) are stable until 5 weeks and show an increasing trend thereafter, irrespective of the intervention (B).

brace (B); this was followed by a second baseline phase (A); this was followed by gait assessment while the patient wore the second orthosis, perhaps a plastic AFO (C); and the study concluded with a final baseline phase (A). In this hypothetical case, the alternate treatments are administered in different phases of the study.

Diamond and Ottenbacher investigated this general topic in slightly more complex fashion in the study that was used earlier as a general example of single-system paradigm research.[19] Subjects walked barefoot during the baseline phase, and walked barefoot and with two different orthoses in an alternating fashion within one intervention phase. Notation for this study might be A–A, B, C–A. The commas indicate that the three conditions (A, B, and C) were alternated within a single phase. The actual sequence of measurement was as follows: (1) The first baseline phase consisted of five measurement sessions in the barefoot condition. (2) The intervention phase consisted of 12 measurement sessions, and each of the three conditions was evaluated within each session, with the order of presentation randomized within each session. (3) The second baseline phase consisted of four measurement sessions with the barefoot condition. Figure 9–3 shows the fairly consistent superiority of the TIAFO during each measurement session on the dependent measure of gait velocity. This design works particularly well when patients are experiencing overall improvements irrespective of the treatment. The alternating design lets the researcher evaluate each condition in light of the velocity that the patient exhibits on a given day. For instance, the 10th measurement session shows high velocities in all conditions and the 11th session shows a return to a more typical level for all conditions. Thus, day-to-day variability is controlled because the measure of interest is not absolute velocity, but rather the difference in velocity between conditions for a given day.

Interaction Designs. Interaction designs are used to evaluate the effect of different combinations of treatments. Assume that a comprehensive pain control program has been designed and includes the use of electroanalgesia and relaxation. Researchers might wish to differentiate the effects of these components to determine whether a single component or the combination of components is

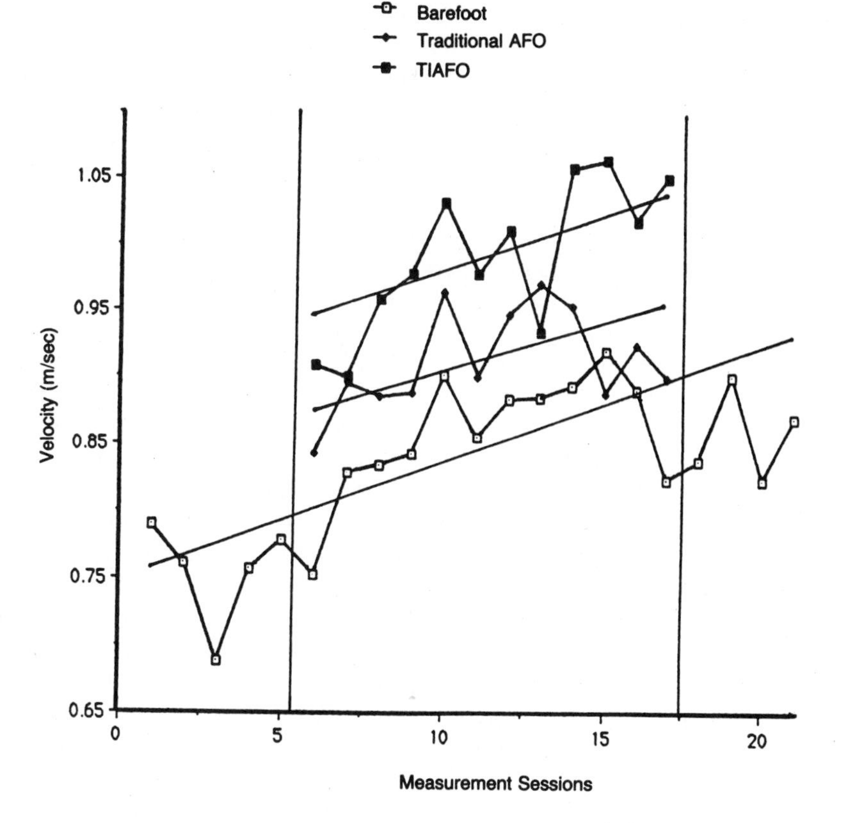

FIGURE 9–3. Example of data presentation for an alternating-treatment study. The study tested ambulation velocity in meters per second of one hemiparetic subject across three conditions (barefoot ambulation, ambulation with a prefabricated ankle–foot orthosis [AFO], and ambulation with a tone-inhibiting dynamic ankle–foot orthosis [TIAFO]) over 21 measurement sessions. From Diamond MF, Ottenbacher KJ. Effect of a tone-inhibiting dynamic ankle-foot orthosis on stride characteristics of an adult with hemiparesis. *Phys Ther.* 1990;70:423–430. Reprinted from *Physical Therapy* with the permission of the American Physical Therapy Association.

most effective. The following design could separate these effects: A–B–A–C–A–BC–A. That is, baseline phases separate an electroanalgesia phase, a relaxation phase, and a combined-treatment phase.

An example of this design is Embrey and associates' examination of the effects of neurodevelopmental treatment and orthoses on knee flexion during gait. The design of this study is A–B–A–BC–A, with neurodevelopmental treatment as the B intervention and orthoses as the C treatment. In this study, the researchers apparently were not interested in the effect of the orthoses alone; hence the absence of an isolated C treatment.

RELATIONSHIPS AMONG THE RESEARCH PARADIGMS

Some researchers believe research paradigms are mutually exclusive; if one adopts the assumptions of one paradigm, the assumptions of the others must be forsaken. Lincoln and Guba make a case for the separateness of the quantitative and qualitative paradigms:

> Postpositivism is an entirely new paradigm, *not* reconcilable with the old. . . . We are dealing with an entirely new system of ideas based on fundamentally *different*—indeed sharply contrasting—assumptions. . . . What is needed is a transformation, not an add-on. That the world is round cannot be added to the idea that the world is flat.[1(p33)]

A more moderate view is that the assumptions that underlie the different paradigms are relative, rather than absolute. Relative assumptions need not be applied to every situation; they can be applied when appropriate to a given research problem. Many authors believe that one paradigm is useful for some forms of study and other paradigms are useful for other forms of study.[13, 23, 24] This text adopts the moderate view that all forms of study have the potential to add to knowledge and understanding. The contrasting assumptions of the paradigms can be managed as we all manage many belief/action clashes on a daily basis. For example, many people believe that the world is round. However, in daily activities they act as if the world is flat by using flat maps to get from place to place and by visualizing the part of the world they are familiar with as flat. They hold one belief, but find it useful to suspend that belief in their daily activities.

Likewise, a belief in multiple constructed realities need not prevent one from studying a certain problem from the perspective of a single objective reality. A belief that it is impossible to study any phenomenon without affecting it in some way need not prevent one from attempting to minimize these effects through the design control methods discussed in Chapter 5. The potential contributions of the different research paradigms are best realized when investigators recognize the assumptions that undergird their methods and make explicit the limitations of their methods.

This moderate view also implies that paradigms can be mixed within a study to address different aspects of a research problem. For example, the study of physical therapy programs at liberal arts institutions, mentioned earlier in this chapter, combined quantitative and qualitative methods.[12] First, physical therapy students and faculty at each of 11 liberal arts institutions with physical therapy programs completed an investigator-designed questionnaire that assessed the "fit" of the physical therapy program with the institution. The assumptions that underlay the use of the questionnaire were (a) that the fit at each institution could be quantified by a single measure and (b) that fit would be problematic at some schools. This measure of fit was used to select two schools for in-depth study using qualitative methods; the school with the best fit and the one with the worst fit were selected for in-depth case study. It was believed that although a quantitative measure of fit could guide the selection of schools, a full description of the culture of each institution required qualitative study of the schools themselves. Relationships among the paradigms therefore range from lack of recognition of competing paradigms, to separation of paradigms for different purposes, to combination of paradigms within research studies. Leininger provides some useful advice to researchers struggling with which of these views to adopt:

> I hold that the researcher needs to be clear why he or she is choosing the method, the purpose of the research, and the paradigmatic views that come from each method. . . . Rather than "mix and match" for popular or peaceful coexistence reasons, thought needs to be given to the question: What are the purposes and reasons for combining or separating the . . . methods? . . . To quickly embrace one method over the other, or to combine methods *without* knowing the reasons seems highly questionable.[24(p21)]

SUMMARY

Research paradigms are the beliefs that underlie the conduct of inquiry. Currently, the dominant paradigm in physical therapy research is the quantitative paradigm, which emphasizes generalizable measurement of a single objective reality with groups of subjects whose treatment is often manipulated by the investigator. The competing qualitative paradigm emphasizes the study of multiple constructed realities through in-depth study of particular settings, with an emphasis on determining underlying meanings within a particular context. The competing single-system paradigm includes many of the beliefs of the quantitative paradigm with the important exception of the concept of generalizability; instead of studying groups, single-system studies look at changes in individuals, because the individual is the unit of interest within a discipline such as physical therapy. Some researchers believe that adoption of one paradigm precludes the use of other paradigms; other researchers believe that all three paradigms are useful when applied to appropriate questions.

References

1. Lincoln YS, Guba EG. *Naturalistic Inquiry.* Newbury Park, Calif: Sage Publications; 1985.
2. Zukav G. *The Dancing Wu Li Masters: An Overview of the New Physics.* New York, NY: Bantam Books; 1979.
3. Irby DM. Shifting paradigms of research in medical education. *Academic Medicine.* 1990;65:622–623.
4. Phillips DC. After the wake: postpositivistic educational thought. *Educational Researcher* 1983;12(5): 4–12.
5. Rosenthal R. *Experimenter Effects in Behavioral Research.* Enlarged ed. New York, NY: Irvington Publishers Inc; 1976.
6. Griffin JW, Newsome LS, Stralka SW, Wright PE. Reduction of chronic posttraumatic hand edema: a comparison of high voltage pulsed current, intermittent pneumatic compression, and placebo treatments. *Phys Ther.* 1990;70:279–286.
7. Mahoney MJ. *Scientist as Subject: The Psychological Imperative.* Cambridge, Mass: Ballinger Publishing Co; 1976.
8. Burkett, E. HIV: is it a dead end? *Indianapolis Star.* January 20, 1991:F1,7.
9. Jensen GM, Shepard KF, Hack LM. The novice versus the experienced clinician: insights into the work of the physical therapist. *Phys Ther.* 1990;70:314–323.
10. Germain C. Ethnography: the method. In: Munhall PL, Oiler CJ, eds. *Nursing Research: A Qualitative Perspective.* Norwalk, Conn: Appleton-Century-Crofts; 1986.
11. Spradley JP. *The Ethnographic Interview.* Fort Worth, Tex: Holt, Rinehart & Winston Inc; 1979.
12. Domholdt E. Physical therapy programs at liberal arts universities. *Journal of Physical Therapy Education.* 1989;3(1):20–24.

13. Jensen GM. Qualitative methods in physical therapy research: a form of disciplined inquiry. *Phys Ther.* 1989;69:492–500.
14. Oiler CJ. Phenomenology: the method. In: Munhall PL, Oiler CJ, eds. *Nursing Research: A Qualitative Perspective.* Norwalk, Conn: Appleton-Century-Crofts; 1986.
15. Peters SA. Quality care criteria defined by mobility impaired residents in long-term care facilities. Master's research project. Indianapolis, Ind: University of Indianapolis; 1990.
16. Glaser BG, Strauss AL. *The Discovery of Grounded Theory: Strategies for Qualitative Research.* Chicago, Ill: Aldine Publishing Co; 1967.
17. Scully RM, Shepard KF. Clinical teaching in physical therapy education: an ethnographic study. *Phys Ther.* 1983;63:349–358.
18. Ottenbacher KJ. *Evaluating Clinical Change: Strategies for Occupational and Physical Therapists.* Baltimore, Md: Williams & Wilkins; 1986.
19. Diamond MF, Ottenbacher KJ. Effect of a tone-inhibiting dynamic ankle-foot orthosis on stride characteristics of an adult with hemiparesis. *Phys Ther.* 1990;70:423–430.
20. Laskas CA, Mullen SL, Nelson DL, Willson-Broyles M. Enhancement of two motor functions of the lower extremity in a child with spastic quadriplegia. *Phys Ther.* 1985;65:11–16.
21. Ottenbacher K, Hicks J, Roark A, Swinea J. Oral sensorimotor therapy in the developmentally disabled: a multiple baseline study. *Am J Occup Ther.* 1983;37:541–547.
22. Embrey DG, Yates L, Mott DH. Effects of neurodevelopmental treatment and orthoses on knee flexion during gait: a single-subject design. *Phys Ther.* 1990;70:626–637.
23. Shepard KF. Qualitative and quantitative research in clinical practice. *Phys Ther.* 1987;67:1891–1894.
24. Leininger MM. Nature, rationale, and importance of qualitative research methods in nursing. In: Leininger MM, ed. *Qualitative Research Methods in Nursing.* Orlando, Fla: Grune & Stratton Inc; 1985.

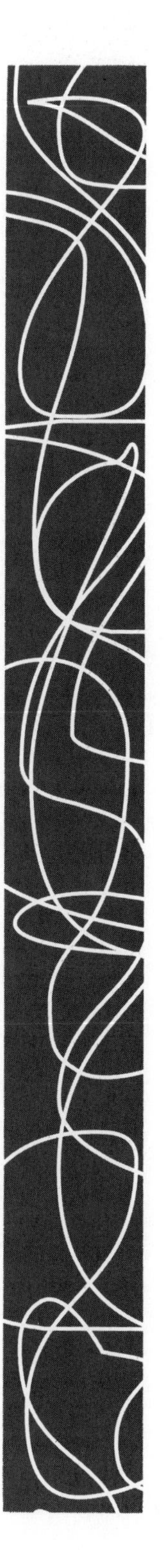

SECTION THREE

MEASUREMENT

CHAPTER 10

Measurement Theory

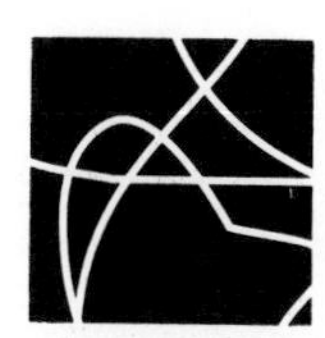

Physical therapists use measurements to help them decide what is wrong with a patient, how to treat a patient, and when to discontinue treatment. Health care insurers rely on these measurements when they make decisions about whether to reimburse the patient or physical therapist for treatment. Researchers use measurements to quantify the characteristics they study. In fact, some investigators focus the majority of their research on the evaluation of physical therapy measures. However, measurement evaluation is not reserved for these much-needed research specialists: "The user of any type of information for decision making needs to know what that information signifies and how far it can be trusted."[1] In fact, the editorial policies of *Physical Therapy* reflect a belief in this proposition by requiring that all authors document the accuracy and relevancy of the measures they use.[2]

This chapter presents a framework for understanding and evaluating the measurements used by physical therapists. It does this by presenting several definitions of measurements, discussing scales of measurement and types of variables, introducing the statistical concepts required to understand measurement theory, and discussing types of measurement reliability and validity. Chapters 11 and 12 build on this framework by presenting strategies for conducting research about measurement and a sample of the measurement tools available to physical therapists.

DEFINITIONS OF MEASUREMENT

The broadest definition of measurement is that it is "the process by which things are differentiated."[3] A narrower definition is that measurement "consists of rules for assigning numbers to objects in such a way as to represent quantities of attributes."[4] According to the first definition, classification of patients into diagnostic groups is a form of measurement; according to the second definition, it is not. This text uses the broader definition of measurement, with the addition of one qualification: Measurement is the *systematic* process by which things are differentiated. Thus, this definition emphasizes that measurement is not a random process, but one that proceeds according to rules and guidelines.

Differentiation can be accomplished with names, numerals, or numbers. For example, classifying people as underweight, normal weight, or overweight involves the assignment of names to differentiate people according to the characteristic of ideal body composition. If these groups are relabeled as Groups 1, 2, and 3 or Groups I, II, and III, then each person is assigned a numeral to represent body composition. A *numeral* is a symbol that does not necessarily have quantitative meaning;[5] it is a form of naming. Describing people not by groups but by their specific percentage of body fat (for example, 10% or 14%) would involve the assignment of a number to represent the quantity of body fat. A *number*, then, is a numeral that has been assigned quantitative meaning.

SCALES OF MEASUREMENT

Four classic scales, or levels, of measurement are presented in the literature. These scales are based on the extent to which a measure has the properties of a real-number system. A real-number system is characterized by order, distance, and origin.[6(p12)] *Order* means that higher numbers represent greater amounts of the characteristic being measured. *Distance* means that the magnitude of the differences between successive numbers is equal. *Origin* means that the number zero represents an absence of the measured quality.

Nominal Scales

Nominal scales have none of the properties of a real-number system. A nominal scale provides classification without placing any value on the categories within the classification. Because there is no order, distance, or origin to the classification, the classification can be identified by name or numeral. However, it is often better to give classifications names instead of numerals so that no quantitative difference between categories is implied. Classification of patients with cerebral palsy into quadriplegic, diplegic, and hemiplegic categories is an example of a nominal measurement. The classification itself does not rank, for example, the functional impairment of the patient—that depends on intellectual functioning, level of spasticity, and a host of other factors not implied by the classification itself.

Ordinal Scales

Ordinal scales have only one of the three properties of a real-number system: order. Thus, an ordinal scale can be used to indicate whether a person or object has more or less of a certain quality. Ordinal scales do not ensure that there are equal intervals between categories or ranks. Because the intervals on an ordinal scale are either not known or are unequal, mathematical manipulations such as addition, subtraction, multiplication, or division of ordinal numbers are not meaningful.

Many functional scales are ordinal. The amount of assistance a patient needs to ambulate is often rated as maximal, moderate, minimal, stand-by, or independent. Is the interval between maximal and moderate assistance the same as the interval between minimal and stand-by assistance? Probably not. Sometimes numerals are assigned to points on a ordinal scale, but the validity of this procedure has been questioned because the numerals are often treated as if they were quantitative numbers.[7]

Figure 10–1 illustrates the phenomenon of nonequal intervals between points on an ordinal scale of gait independence. Assume that the underlying quantity represented by the assistance categories is the proportion of the total work of ambulation that is exerted by the patient. If the patient and therapist are expending equal energy to get the patient walking, then the patient is exerting 50% of the total work of ambulation. If the patient is independent and the therapist does not need to expend any energy, then the patient is exerting 100% of the total work of ambulation. The top line of Figure 10–1 shows the assistance categories. The middle two lines show numerals that could be assigned to the assistance categories. Either set of numerals would meet the order criterion–higher numerals indicate higher levels of independence. The magnitude of the two sets of numerals varies greatly and shows the danger of thinking of ordinal numbers as real quantities. The bottom scale shows how the assistance categories might fall along a continuum of total work percentage. The categories "minimal," "stand-by," and "independent," as used by most therapists, probably fall in the top 20% of the scale. The categories "maximal" and "moderate" probably fall in the bottom 80% of the scale. Thus, the gait independence classification used by physical therapists is clearly an ordinal scale: The classification has order but does not represent equal intervals of the underlying construct that is being measured.

A second type of ordinal scale is a ranking. For a time, Martina Navratilova and Steffi Graf traded the Number 1 ranking in women's tennis between themselves. There were no other players who were even close in ability to these two. Thus, the interval between the first- and second-ranked players was very slight. The difference between the second- and third-ranked players was much larger. The intervals between ranks are usually unknown and cannot be assumed to be equal.

Interval Scales

Interval scales have the real-number system properties of order and distance, but they lack a meaningful origin. A meaningful zero point represents the absence of the measured quan-

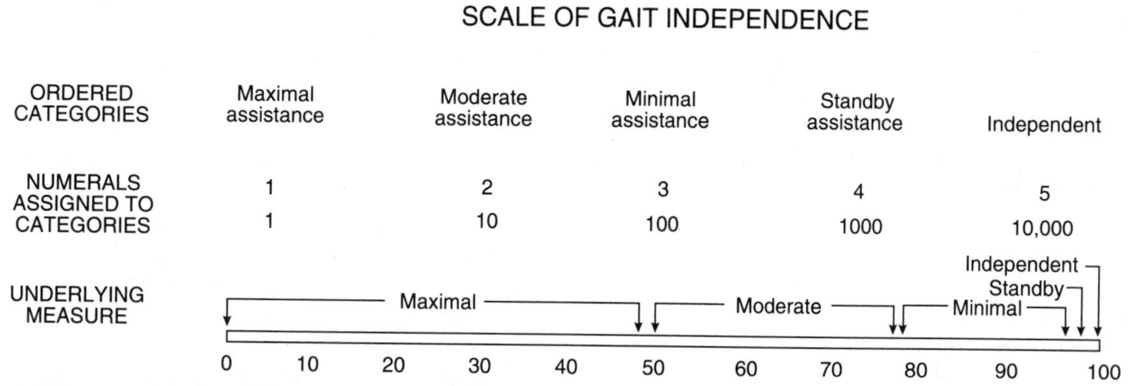

FIGURE 10–1. Level of assistance in gait as an ordinal measurement. The top row shows the assistance categories as used by many physical therapists. The bottom row shows a theoretical underlying distribution of the categories on the basis of what percentage of effort is being exerted by the patient. The middle two rows show two vastly different numbering schemes; in both schemes the numbers get larger as the amount of effort exerted by the patient increases.

tity. The Celsius and Fahrenheit temperature scales are examples of interval scales. The zero points on the two temperature scales are arbitrary: On the Fahrenheit scale it is the temperature at which salt water freezes, and on the Celsius scale it is the temperature at which fresh water freezes. Neither implies the absence of the basic property of heat—the temperature can go lower than zero on both scales. Both scales, however, have regular (but different) intervals. Because of the equal intervals, addition and subtraction are meaningful with interval scales. A 10° increase in temperature means the same thing whether the increase is from 0° to 10° or from 100° to 110°. However, multiplication and division of Fahrenheit or Celsius temperature readings are not useful because these operations assume knowledge of zero quantities. A Fahrenheit temperature of 100° is not twice as hot as a temperature of 50°; it is merely 50° hotter.

Ratio Scales

Ratio scales exhibit all three components of a real-number system: order, distance, and origin. All the arithmetic functions of addition, subtraction, multiplication, and division can be applied to ratio scales. Length, time, and weight are generally considered ratio scales because their absence is scored as zero, and the intervals between numbers are known to be equal. The Kelvin temperature scale is an example of a ratio scale because the intervals between degrees are equal and the zero point represents the absence of heat.

Determining the Scale of a Measurement

To determine the scale of a measure, the researcher must ascertain whether there is a true zero (origin), whether intervals between numbers are equal (distance), and whether there is an order to the numbers or names that constitute the measure (order). Although this sounds simple enough, there is controversy about whether some clinical measures should be considered ratio, interval, or ordinal scales.

For example, Mayhew and Rothstein do not consider isokinetic measures to be ratio measurements because some patients who can move their limbs are unable to register torque on an isokinetic dynamometer.[8(p74)] They argue that the zero point of an isokinetic measure does not represent the absence of torque and is therefore arbitrary. This controversy seems to be less about the isokinetic measures themselves than about the labels that are applied to the measurements. If one labels isokinetic measures as "torque," then Mayhew and Rothstein's concerns are valid—there are patients who can generate torque but still register zero on an isokinetic test. If, however, isokinetic measures are labeled "speed-specific torque," then the problem disappears. If a patient is unable to generate torque at the required speed, the zero measure does, in fact, represent an absence of speed-specific torque-generating capability.

The controversy about whether isokinetic devices produce interval or ratio measures is by no means the only controversy about scales of measurement. For example, does the classification of patients as underweight, normal weight, and overweight represent a nominal or ordinal scale? The numbers are placed into classes, but these classes also have an order. As another example, do scores on the Graduate Record Examination, which purports to measure aptitude for learning in graduate school, represent ordinal or interval data? Standardized tests are often treated as interval scales even though it can be argued that the underlying construct being measured is too abstract to permit assumption that intervals between scores are equal. Because the scale of measurement determines which mathematical manipulations are meaningful, controversy about measurement scales soon becomes controversy about which statistical tests are appropriate for which types of measures. These statistical controversies are discussed in Chapter 13.

TYPES OF VARIABLES

With respect to measurement, variables can be classified as continuous or discrete. A *discrete* variable is one that can assume only distinct values. Nominal scale variables are, by definition, discrete: The patients being classified must fit into a distinct category; they cannot be placed between the categories. Discrete variables that can assume only two values are called *dichotomous* variables. Examples of dichotomous variables are sex (male versus female) or disease state (present versus absent). Variables that are counts of behaviors or persons are discrete variables because fractional people or behaviors are not possible. If the measure of interest is the number of heel touches that occur in 10 standing trials, it is not possible to get a score of 7.5 on a single trial. Note, however, that it is possible to have an *average* score of 7.5 if the 10-trial sequence is repeated on four subsequent days with scores of 8, 6, 9, and 7 ($8 + 6 + 9 + 7 = 30$; $30 / 4 = 7.5$). If discrete variables can assume a fairly large range of values, have the properties of a real-number system, or are averaged across trials, then they become similar to continuous variables.

A *continuous* variable is one that theoretically can be measured to a finer and finer degree.[6(p15)] Clinicians interested in the speed of patients' ambulation might record the time it takes for patients to complete a 20-m walk. Depending on the sophistication of their measurement tools, the therapists might measure time to the nearest second or to the nearest one-thousandth of a second. If the smallest increment on a therapist's watch is the second, then measurements cannot be recorded in smaller increments even though the therapist knows that the true time required for completion of a task is not limited to whole seconds. Thus, the limits of technology dictate that continuous variables will always be measured discretely.

STATISTICAL FOUNDATIONS OF MEASUREMENT THEORY

Seven basic concepts underlie most of measurement theory: frequency distribution, mean, variance, standard deviation, normal curve, correlation coefficient, and standard error of measurement. These concepts are introduced here and expanded on in Chapter 13.

Frequency Distribution

A *frequency distribution* is nothing more than the number of times each score is represented in the data set. If a therapist measures a patient's knee flexion 10 times during one day, the following scores might be obtained: 100, 100, 90, 95, 110, 110, 95, 105, 95, 100. Table 10–1 and Figure 10–2 show two ways of presenting the frequency distribution for these 10 scores.

TABLE 10–1. Frequency Distribution of 10 Knee Flexion Measurements

Score	Frequency
90	1
95	3
100	3
105	1
110	2

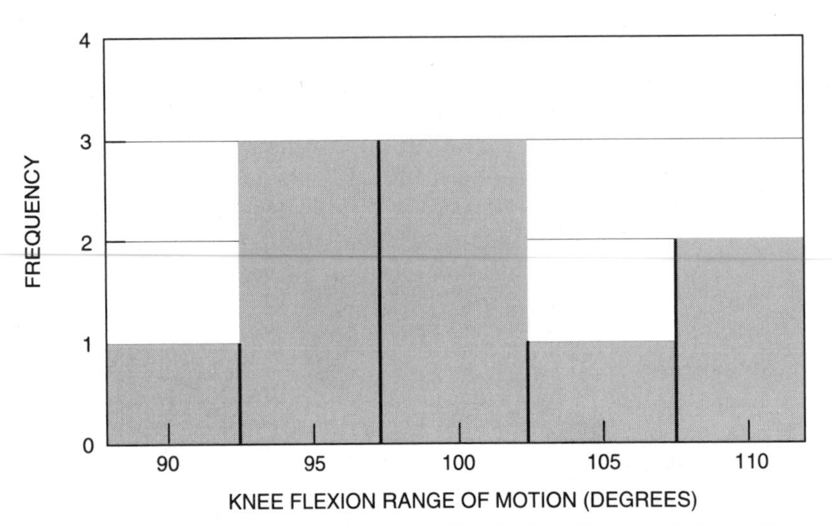

FIGURE 10–2. Histogram of the frequency distribution of hypothetical knee flexion data.

Mean

The arithmetic *mean* of a data set is the sum of the observations divided by the number of observations. Mathematical notation for the mean is

$$\overline{X} = \frac{\Sigma X}{N}$$

$\overline{X}$ is the symbol for the sample mean and is sometimes called "X-bar." Σ is the uppercase Greek letter sigma and means "the sum of." X is the symbol for each observation. N is the symbol for the number of observations. In words, the mean equals the sum of all the observations divided by the number of observations. The mean of the data set presented earlier is calculated as follows:

$$\overline{X} = \frac{(90 + 95 + 95 + 95 + 100 + 100 + 100 + 105 + 110 + 110)}{10} = 100$$

The population mean, μ, is calculated the same way, but is rarely used in practice because researchers do not have access to the entire population.

Variance

The *variance* is a measure of the variability around the mean within a data set. To calculate the variance, a researcher converts each of the raw scores in a data set to a deviation score by subtracting the mean of the data set from each raw score. In mathematical notation,

$$x = X - \overline{X}$$

The lowercase italic x is the symbol for a deviation score. The *deviation score* indicates how high or low a raw score is compared with the mean. The first two columns of Table 10–2 present the raw and deviation scores for the knee flexion data set, followed by their sums and means. Note that both the sum and the mean of the deviation scores are zero. In order to generate a nonzero index of the variability within a data set, the deviation scores must be squared. The variance is then

TABLE 10–2. Computation of the Variance in the 10 Knee Flexion Measurements

	X	x	x^2	z score
	90	−10	100	−1.59
	95	−5	25	− .79
	95	−5	25	− .79
	95	−5	25	− .79
	100	0	0	0
	100	0	0	0
	100	0	0	0
	105	+5	25	+ .79
	110	+10	100	+1.59
	110	+10	100	+1.59
Σ	1,000	0	400	
μ	100	0	40.0 = σ^2, variance	

calculated by determining the mean of the squared deviations. In mathematical notation,

$$\sigma^2 = \frac{\Sigma x^2}{N}$$

σ is the lowercase Greek sigma and when squared is the notation for the population variance. The third column in Table 10–2 shows the squared deviations from the group mean, the sum of the squared deviations, and the mean of the squared deviations. The variance is the mean of the squared deviation scores. In practice there are different symbols and slightly different formulas for the variance, depending on whether the observations represent the entire population of interest or just a sample of the population. This distinction is addressed in Chapter 13.

Although the variance is useful in many statistical procedures, it does not have a great deal of intuitive meaning because it is calculated from squared deviation scores. A measure that does have intuitive meaning is the standard deviation.

Standard Deviation

The *standard deviation* is the square root of the variance and is expressed in the units of the original measure:

$$\sigma = \sqrt{\sigma^2} = \sqrt{\Sigma x^2 / N}$$

The mathematical notations for the standard deviation and the variance make their relationship clear: The notation for the variance (σ^2) is simply the square of the notation for standard deviation (σ). The standard deviation of the knee flexion data presented in Table 10–2 is the square root of 40, or 6.3°.

Normal Curve

The distribution of groups of measurements frequently approximates a bell-shaped distribution known as the normal curve. The *normal curve* is a symmetrical frequency distribution that can be defined in terms of the mean and standard deviation of a set of data. Any raw score within the distribution can be converted into a *z score*, which indicates how many standard deviations the raw score is above or below the mean. A *z* score is calculated by subtracting the mean from the raw score, creating a deviation score, and then dividing the deviation score by the standard deviation:

$$z = \frac{x}{\sigma}$$

The fourth column of Table 10–2 shows each raw score as a *z* score. Raw scores were transformed into *z* scores by dividing each of the deviation scores (x) by the standard deviation of 6.3°. The *z* score tells us, for example, that a measurement of 90° is 1.59 standard deviations below the mean.

In a normal distribution, 68.27% of the scores fall within 1 standard deviation above or below the mean; 95.44% of the scores fall within 2 standard deviations above or below the mean; and 99.74% of the scores fall within 3 standard deviations above or below the mean. Figure 10–3 shows a diagram of the normal curve, with the percentages of scores that are found within each standard deviation. Figure 10–4A shows the normal curve that corresponds to the knee flexion data set. The mean is 100°, and the standard deviation is 6.3°. Figure 10–4B shows that if the knee flexion scores are normally distributed, we could expect about 98% of our measurements to exceed the score of 87.4°. Figure 10–4C shows that we could expect about 68% of our measures to fall between 93.7° and 106.3°. Predicting the probability of obtaining certain ranges of scores is one of the most basic of statistical functions.

Correlation Coefficient

A *correlation coefficient* is a statistical summary of the degree of relationship that exists between two or more measures.[9] The relationship can be between either different variables (such as strength and range of motion) or repeated measures of the same variables (such as range-of-motion measures of the same patient taken by three different therapists). There are many different types of correlation coefficients; the computational distinctions between them are discussed in Chapter 15.

A correlation coefficient of 0.0 means that there is no relationship between the variables; a correlation coefficient of 1.0 indicates that there is a perfect relationship between the variables. Values in between these two

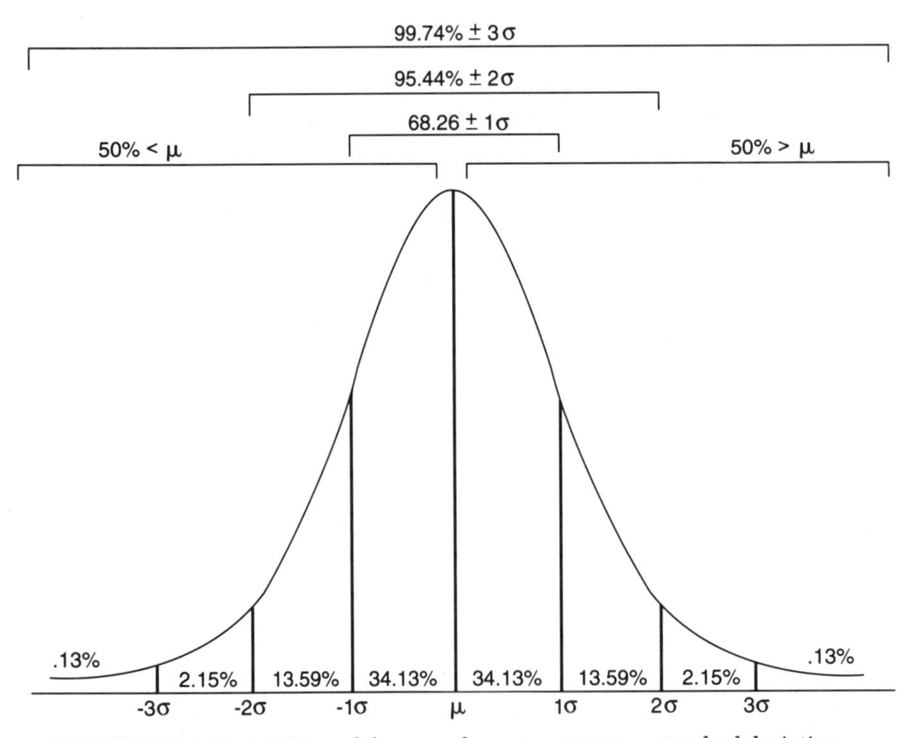

FIGURE 10–3. Probabilities of the normal curve. μ, mean; σ, standard deviation.

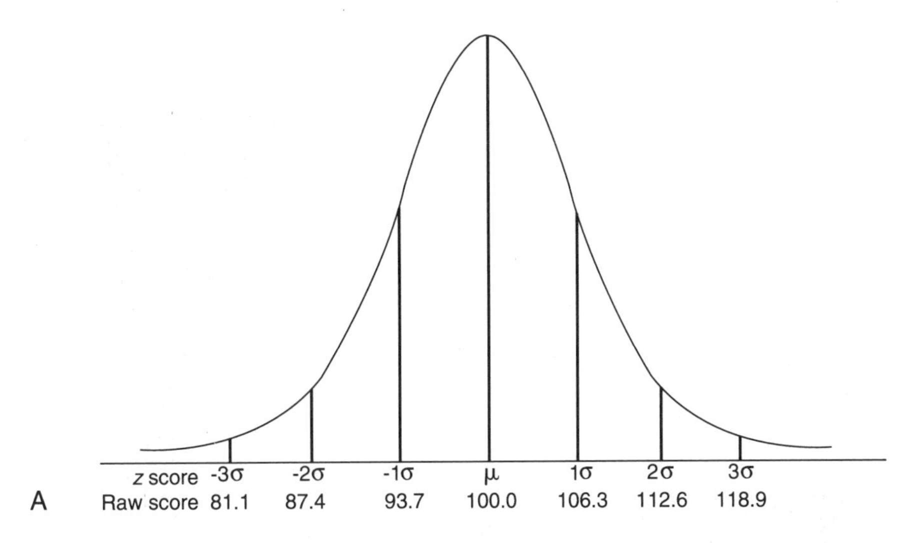

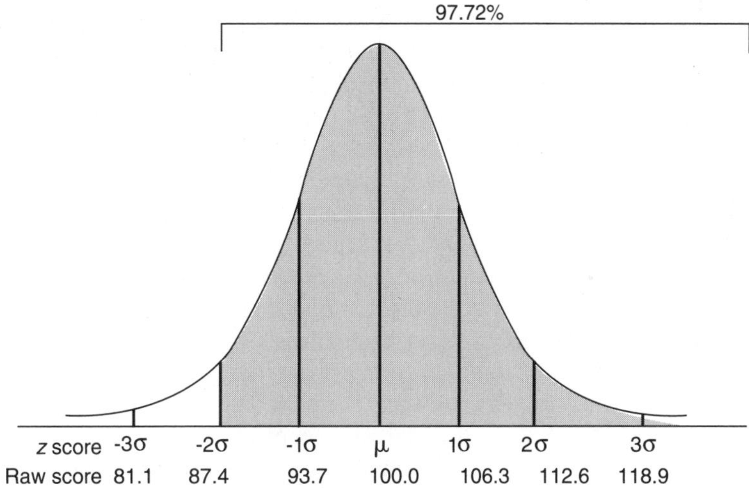

FIGURE 10–4. Probabilities of the normal curve applied to hypothetical range-of-motion data with a mean of 100 and a standard deviation of 6.3. **A.** The range-of-motion values that correspond to 1, 2, and 3 standard deviations above and below the mean. **B.** The probability of obtaining a score greater than 87.4° (the shaded area) is 97.72%. **C.** The probability of obtaining a score between 93.7° and 106.3° (the shaded area) is 68.26%. μ, mean; σ, standard deviation.

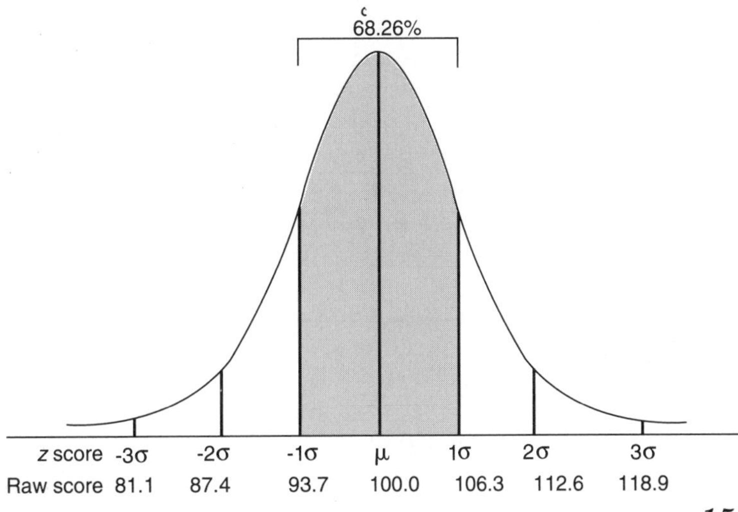

extremes indicate intermediate levels of relationship. Some correlation coefficients can also have values from 0.0 to −1.0. A negative correlation indicates an inverse relationship between variables (that is, as the values for one variable become larger, the values for the other become smaller). In this text, r is used as a general symbol for a correlation coefficient. The specific notation for each type of coefficient is introduced when needed.

Standard Error of Measurement

In addition to knowing the relationship between repeated measurements, the researcher may wish to know how much a score is likely to vary with repeated measurements of the same subject. To determine the amount of measurement error, a researcher can take many repeated measures of the same subject and calculate the standard deviation of the scores; this standard deviation is known as the *standard error of measurement* (SEM). In practice, it is difficult to determine the standard error of measurement directly. Consider the effect of measuring knee flexion up to 100 times in a patient with limited knee motion to determine the standard error of measurement. The patient's knee flexion might improve during the course of testing by virtue of the exercise associated with taking so many measurements. Conversely, the patient's knee flexion might be reduced as the knee became progressively more painful. In any event, taking so many repeated measurements would likely result in a confounding of measurement error with actual treatment effects.

Because of the difficulty in directly determining the standard error of measurement, it is often estimated as follows:[10(p62)]

$$\text{SEM} = \sigma\sqrt{1 - r}$$

Assume that a researcher takes two knee flexion measurements on each of 10 patients. If the standard deviation of the measures is 5° and the correlation between the two measures is .80, then the estimated SEM is 2.2°.

$$\text{SEM} = 5\sqrt{1 - .80} = 5\sqrt{.20} = 5(.44) = 2.2$$

The SEM is a standard deviation of measurement errors, and measurement errors are assumed to be normally distributed. Thus, by combining our knowledge of the probabilities of the normal curve with this value for the SEM, we can conclude that approximately 68% of the time, a repeated measurement of knee flexion would be within 1 standard deviation of the mean or ± 2.2° of the original measurement. Approximately 96% of the time, a repeated measurement of knee flexion would be within 2 standard deviations of the mean or ± 4.4° of the original measurement.

MEASUREMENT FRAMEWORKS

There are two basic frameworks in which measurement is conducted and evaluated: norm referenced and criterion referenced. *Norm-referenced* measures are those used to judge individual performance in relation to group norms. The statistical concepts of the mean and standard deviation are integral to norm-referenced measures. An example of a norm-referenced measure of importance to physical therapists practicing in the United States is the physical therapy licensing examination. The examination is administered and scored nationally, and each state determines the level of proficiency it requires of licensees. The level of proficiency is expressed as a standard deviation from the mean; most states license individuals who receive a score that is 1.5 standard deviations below the mean or higher for a particular administration of the test.[11] If one administration of the 200-item test results in a mean of 150 and a standard deviation of 10, a state with a 1.5

standard deviation requirement would license therapists who received a score of 135 or higher on that administration of the test ($\overline{X}$ − 1.5[σ] = 150 − 1.5[10] = 135). If a second test administration resulted in a mean of 145 and a standard deviation of 12, the same state would license therapists who scored 127 or higher on the second test (145 − 1.5[12] = 127). Thus, therapists are not held to an absolute standard of performance; they are evaluated with respect to the norms of the group with whom they took the examination and the difficulty of the particular test taken.

Many clinical measurements are norm referenced. Blood pressure and pulse rates are evaluated against a range of normal values, muscular performance can be compared with average performance for age- and sex-matched groups, and a patient's function after a stroke may be compared with that of patients with comparable lesions.

A *criterion-referenced* measure is one in which each individual's performance is evaluated with respect to some absolute level of achievement. When a teacher establishes 75% as the minimum passing score in a course, this is a criterion-referenced measurement. If all students exceed the 75% criterion, all pass. If only 25% exceed the criterion, only 25% pass. Therapists use a criterion-referenced framework when they set specific performance criteria that patients have to meet in order to resume athletic competition or take an assistive device home.

MEASUREMENT RELIABILITY

Reliability is the "degree to which test scores are free from errors of measurement."[12(p19)] Other terms that are similar to reliability are *accuracy*, *stability*, and *consistency*. This section of the chapter introduces reliability theories, components, and measures.

Two Theories of Reliability

Two basic measurement theories—classical measurement theory and generalizability theory—provide somewhat different views of reliability. Classical measurement theory rests on the assumption that every measurement, or obtained score, consists of a true component and an error component. In addition, each person has a single true score on the measurement of interest. Because we can never know the true score for any measure, the relationship between repeated measurements is used to estimate measurement errors. A measurement is said to be reliable if the error component is small, thus allowing consistent estimation of the true quantity of interest. With classical measurement theory, all variability within a person's score is viewed as measurement error.[13]

Classical theories of reliability have been extended into what is known as generalizability theory. Generalizability theory recognizes that there are different sources of variability for any measure. Measurements are studied in ways that permit the researcher to divide the measurement error into sources of variability, or *facets*, of interest to the researcher.

To understand the differences between these two approaches, consider the measurement of forward head position with a device that provides a measurement in centimeters. Classical measurement theory assumes that every person has a true value for forward head position and that variations in a person's scores are measurement errors about the true score. In contrast, generalizability theory recognizes that differences in scores may be related to any number of different facets. Facets of interest to a given researcher for this example might be the subject's level of relaxation, his or her level of comfort with the particular examiner taking the measurement, the skill of the examiner, and the accuracy of the device used to measure forward head position. The generalizability approach seems to have a great deal of promise for the study of measurements in physical therapy because it acknowledges and provides a way to quantify the many sources of variability that physical therapists see in their patients from day to day.

Components of Reliability

Several components of reliability are examined frequently: instrument, intrarater, interrater, and intrasubject reliability. Although it is often difficult to completely separate these components from one another, readers of the literature need to be able to conceptualize the different components so that they can determine which components or combinations of components are being studied.

Instrument Reliability. The reliability of the instrument itself may be assessed. There are three broad categories of physical therapy measurements: biophysiological, self-report, and observational. Different instruments are used to take the different types of measurements, and the appropriate approach for determining an instrument's reliability depends on which type of instrument it is.

Biophysiological measurements are obtained through the use of mechanical or electrical tools such as the dynamometer, goniometer, spirometer, scale, and electromyograph. The reliability of these instruments is assessed by taking repeated measurements across the range of values expected to be found in actual use of the device. Assessment of scores on two or more administrations of a test is often called *test–retest reliability*. For example, Stratford and colleagues determined the test–retest reliability of a hand-held dynamometer by repeated application of known loads from 10 to 60 kg.[14] If the output of a device is in analog format (that is, the tester determines the value by examining a scale on the device), then it is impossible to separate the reliability of the device from the examiner's ability to read the scale accurately. If the device output is in digital format, separation of device reliability from examiner reliability is easier because the digital reading leaves little room for examiner interpretation.

Self-report measurements are obtained through the use of instruments that require subjects to give their own account of the phenomenon under study. Written surveys, standardized tests, pain scales, and interviews are examples of self-report measures. Forms of reliability for self-report tests include test–retest reliability, in which subjects take the same test on two or more occasions; parallel-form reliability, in which similar forms of a test are each administered once; split-half reliability, in which portions of a test are compared with each other; and internal consistency, in which responses to individuals items are evaluated. The reader is referred to standard texts on educational or psychological measurement for a fuller description of assessment of the reliability of written tests.[1, 3, 15]

Observational measurements require only a human instrument with systematic knowledge of what to observe. The examiner may be an unobtrusive observer or may play a more active role. The knowledge may be in the examiner's head, or the examiner may use a check-list, such as the Movement Assessment of Infants (MAI).[16] The MAI is an example of a tool that uses both active and passive observation: Some of the categories in the MAI require observation of movement without intervention; however, the tone assessment portion of the examination requires hands-on manipulation of the infant.

Manual muscle testing and placement of patients into gait independence categories are additional examples of physical therapy measures that require only a human instrument with the knowledge of what to observe. The reliability of observational scales with multiple items can be examined for internal consistency in much the same manner as are written tests. Because the tester is the instrument, determining the reliability of observational measures is linked to determining intrarater and interrater reliability, described below.

Intrarater Reliability. A strict definition of *intrarater reliability* is "the consistency with which one rater assigns scores to a single set of responses on two occasions."[17(p141)] If a researcher is using videotape analysis to determine step length, he or she can view the same videotape on two different dates. Because the behavior being assessed both times is identical, any variability in scores is, in fact, related to measurement errors of the researcher. For most of the measurements we take in physical therapy, however, we do not have the ability to exactly reproduce the movement of interest, as a videotape would. If a therapist wishes to assess intrarater reliability of knee extension performance as measured by a hand-held dynamometer, the patient will have to perform the movement two or more times. In doing so, any variability in the force measurements can be attributed to either the examiner's measurement error or the subject's inconsistent performance. It is often difficult to separate the two.

Interrater Reliability. A strict definition of *interrater reliability* holds that it is the "consistency of performance among different raters or judges in assigning scores to the same objects or responses. . . [It] is determined when two or more raters judge the performance of one group of subjects at the same point in time."[17(p140)] If two therapists simultaneously observe and rate an infant's spontaneous movements as part of a developmental assessment, the comparison between their scores would be a pure measure of interrater reliability because they observed the exact same episode of movement. If they observed the child at two different times, however, it would be impossible to separate the variability attributable to differences in the examiners from the variability attributable to actual differences in the child's behavior from time to time.

A variation of intertester reliability, triangulation, is used to document the consistency of the results of qualitative research. *Triangulation* consists of comparing responses across several different sources,[18] which in effect become different raters of the phenomenon of interest. The reader is referred to the literature on qualitative research for a further discussion of reliability issues in qualitative research.[18, 19]

Intrasubject Reliability. The final component of reliability is associated with actual changes in subject performance from time to time. Some measurements in physical therapy may appear to be unreliable simply because the phenomenon being measured is inherently variable. It may be unreasonable to think, for example, that single measurements of spasticity could be reproducible because spasticity is such a changing phenomenon. Unless one has a perfectly reliable instrument and a perfectly reliable examiner, it is impossible to derive a pure measure of subject variability. Thus, most test–retest reliability calculations reflect some combination of instrument errors, tester errors, and true subject variability. Chapter 11 presents research designs for evaluating the different reliability components or combinations of components.

Quantification of Reliability

Reliability is quantified in two ways, as either relative or absolute reliability. *Relative reliability* examines the relationship between two or more sets of repeated measures; *absolute reliability* examines the variability of the scores from measurement to measurement.[10]

Relative Reliability. *Relative reliability* is based on the idea that if a measurement is reliable, individual measurements within a group will maintain their position within the group on repeated measurement. For example, people who score near the top of a distribution on a first measure would be expected to stay near the top of the distribution even if their actual scores changed from time to time. Relative reliability is measured with some form of a correlation coefficient, which, as mentioned earlier in this chapter, indicates the degree of association between repeated measurements of the variable of interest. Different correlation coefficients are used with different types of data, as shown in Table 10–3.[20–22] The mathematical basis of the correlation coefficients and the rationale for choosing a particular coefficient are discussed in greater detail in Chapter 15.

We know that a correlation coefficient of 1.0 indicates a perfect association between repeated measures. How much less than 1.0 can a correlation be if it is to be considered reliable? This question is not easily answered. Currier cites two different sources in which adjectives were used to describe ranges of correlation coefficients (for example, .80 to 1.0 was described as "very reliable" and .69 and below was said to constitute "poor reliability").[23] There are problems with using adjectives to describe ranges of correlation coefficients. First, there are many different formulas for correlation coefficients, and these different formulas may result in vastly different coefficients for the same data.[24] Second, there is not universal agreement about the appropriateness of the different formulas.[25, 26]

TABLE 10–3. Correlation Coefficients

Name of Coefficient	Type of Data Required	No. of Repeated Measures Compared
Pearson product–moment correlation	Continuous	Two
Intraclass correlation	Continuous	Two or more
Spearman rank order correlation	Ranked	Two
Kendall's tau	Ranked	Two
Cohen's kappa	Nominal	Usually two; can be modified to accommodate more than two

Third, the value of a correlation coefficient is greatly affected by the range of scores used to calculate the coefficient. Correlation coefficients evaluate the consistency of an individual's position within a group; if the group as a whole shows little variability on the measure of interest, there is little mathematical basis for determining relative positions and the correlation between the repeated measurements will be low. Thus, other things being equal, the interrater reliability correlation coefficient calculated on a group of patients with knee flexion range-of-motion values between 70° and 90° would be lower than one calculated with a broader range of values, say, between 30° and 90°.

Fourth, most of the correlation coefficients are not very good at detecting systematic errors. A systematic error is one that is predictable. For example, assume that on a first measurement of limb girth a researcher used one tape measure and on a second measurement used a different tape measure that was missing the first centimeter. There would be a systematic measurement error of 1 cm on the second measure. However, if each subject's position within the group were maintained, the correlation coefficients would remain high despite the absolute difference.

Because of these four problems with correlation coefficients, a rigid criterion for acceptable reliability is inappropriate. In addition, the component of reliability being studied affects the interpretation of the correlation coefficient. For example, one would ordinarily expect there to be less variability in scores recorded on a single day than in scores recorded over a longer time period. Similarly, intrarater reliability coefficients are generally higher than interrater reliability coefficients. Finally, if a researcher is deciding which of two measurement tools to use and has found that one has an intrarater reliability of .99 and the other an intrarater reliability of .80, then .80 seems unacceptable. On the other hand, if a highly abstract concept is being measured and a researcher is deciding between two instruments with intratester reliability coefficients of .45 and .60, then .60 may become acceptable.

Because of the limitations of determining relative reliability with correlation coefficients, researchers should often supplement relative information with absolute information.

Absolute Reliability. *Absolute reliability* indicates the extent to which a score varies on repeated measurement. The statistic used to measure absolute reliability is the SEM, described earlier in the chapter.

Unfortunately, many researchers who report measurement studies in the physical therapy literature specify only the relative reliability of the measurement and not the absolute reliability.[27] For a physical therapist to make meaningful statements about whether a patient or subject's condition has changed, the therapist must know how much variability in the scores could be expected solely because of measurement errors. This is illustrated in Diamond and associates' study of the reliability of diabetic foot evaluation.[28] The interrater reliability coefficients for selected foot biomechanical measurements ranged from .58 to .89. The SEM of these same measurements ranged from 1° to 4°, but the smaller SEMs were not always associated with the higher correlation coefficients! For example, the interrater reliability coefficient for tibial varum was .66 and the SEM was 1°. This indicates that approximately 96% of the time, the true value for tibial varum would be expected to fall within ±2° of the observed measurement (observed score ±2 SEMs). Conversely, a higher correlation coefficient (.89) was associated with interrater reliability for calcaneal inversion, but this measurement had an SEM of 3°. In this instance, we would expect that approximately 96% of the time the true value for calcaneal inversion would be within ±6° of the observed measurement.

Thus in Diamond and associates' study, the correlation coefficient and the SEM provided contradictory information: The correlation coefficients implied that measurement of calcaneal inversion was more reliable than tibial varum, but the SEM results implied the opposite. Because correlation coefficients and SEMs provide different and often contradictory views of reliability, it is important that researchers document both. Documenting both may prohibit straightforward interpretation of the results of a measurement study, but uncertainty based on complete information is preferable to a false sense of certainty based on incomplete information.

MEASUREMENT VALIDITY

Measurement validity is the "appropriateness, meaningfulness, and usefulness of the specific inferences made from test scores."[12(p9)] Reliability is a necessary, but not sufficient, condition for validity. An unreliable measure is also an invalid measurement, because measurements with a great deal of error have little meaning or utility. A reliable measure is valid only if, in addition to being repeatable, it provides meaningful information.

Earlier we defined *research validity* as the extent to which the conclusions of research are believable and useful. Note that although the two types of validity relate to different areas—measurement and research design, respectively—they are similar in that they both relate to the *utility* of findings and not to the findings themselves. Thus, measurement validity is not a quality associated with a particular instrument or test, but rather is a quality associated with the way in which test results are applied.

For example, active range-of-motion measurements may provide a valid indication of muscle performance in patients with full passive range of motion. The same active range-of-motion measures do not provide valid information about muscle performance in patients with significantly restricted passive motion. In these patients, the measure is not a meaningful indicator of muscle performance but rather an indicator of some combination of joint mobility and muscle performance.

Measurement validity is often subdivided into several categories. Construct, content, and criterion validity are discussed below.

Construct Validity

Construct validity is the validity of the abstract constructs that underlie measures. For example, strength is a construct that is poorly delineated in the physical therapy literature. When physical therapists speak of strength, they may mean many different things. Strength may be conceptualized as the ability to move a body part against gravity, the ability to generate speed-specific torque, the ability to lift a certain weight a certain number of times in a certain time period, or the ability to accomplish some functional task. In fact, Mayhew and Rothstein believe that the construct strength is so poorly delineated that the term *muscle performance* should be used instead.[8(p58)] Manual muscle tests, isokinetic tests, work performance tests, and functional tests may all be valid measures of a particular conceptualization of strength or muscle performance.

To maximize construct validity, physical therapy researchers must first be very clear about the constructs they wish to measure. If strength is an important construct within a study, is it best conceptualized as functional strength, static strength, eccentric strength, or some other aspect of this extremely broad construct? Once the underlying construct of interest is clarified, it must be operationalized to make it measurable. An *operational definition* is a specific description of the way in which a construct is presented or measured within a study. For example, Ellison and associates studied patterns of hip rotation motions in healthy subjects and patients with low back pain.[29] They provided operational definitions of healthy subjects (university students and staff who had no low back or hip pain that prevented them from working or attending school in the past year), patients with low back pain (patients at one clinic who were undergoing treatment for back pain at the time of the study), hip rotation measurements (a detailed description of measurements taken in the prone position), and a range-of-motion pattern classification (a detailed description of rules for placing each subject into one of four groups).

Although developing operational definitions is necessary for construct validity, it does not *guarantee* construct validity. One might argue that in Ellison and associates' study, the patient group was defined too broadly or that hip rotation measures should have been taken in the sitting position. Supplying readers with the operational definitions used in a study allows them to form their own opinion of the validity of the measurements.

Content Validity

Content validity is the extent to which a measure is a complete representation of the concept of interest. Content validity is more often a concern with self-report or observational tools than with biophysiological ones. When students come away from a test saying, "Can you believe how many questions there were on . . . ?", they are talking about the content validity of the test, because they are questioning whether the emphasis on the exam was an accurate representation of the course content.

A rehabilitation instrument that may have questionable content validity is the Katz Index of Activities of Daily Living, a standardized tool used to document the functional abilities of individuals with disabilities.[30] It covers dressing, walking, bathing, feeding, transferring, and toileting. It does not, however, include grooming, wheelchair activities, stair climbing, or bed mobility—activities that are often included on other functional scales. If these omitted activities are important indicators of activities of daily living, the content validity of the Katz index is low. When a researcher is designing a questionnaire or a functional scale, he or she should have its content validity evaluated by knowledgeable peers before it is used. The input of peers may lead to the addition of items, the deletion of irrelevant or redundant items, or reassessment of the emphasis given to particular topics.

Criterion Validity

Criterion validity is the extent to which one measure is systematically related to other measures or outcomes. Whereas relative reliability compares repeated administrations of the *same* measurement, criterion validity compares administration of *different* measures. The mathematical basis for determining the degree of association between two different measures is similar to that for determining the association between repeated administrations of the same measurement. Therefore the correlation coefficients used to determine relative reliability are often used to measure criterion validity as well. The epidemiological concepts of specificity and sensitivity, described in Chapter 6, are also often useful for determining criterion validity. Criterion validity can be subdivided into concurrent and predictive validity on the basis of the timing of the different measures.

Concurrent validity is at issue when one is comparing a measuring tool with a measurement standard. The two tests are performed closely in time to maximize the chances of measuring the same phenomenon. Stratford and associates' comparison of isokinetic torque curve patterns and arthroscopic diagnosis of tears in the anterior cruciate ligament (ACL) is an example of a study of concurrent validity.[31] A particular pattern of torque curves was thought to be indicative of ACL tears. The measurement standard for determining the presence of an ACL tear is examination of the ligament through an arthroscope. The concurrent validity of the torque curve tracings was determined by calculation of the sensitivity and specificity of the torque curve pattern compared with the arthroscopic results. The degree of association between the two measures was low, indicating that torque tracings are not valid indicators of ACL tears.

Predictive validity relates to whether a test done at one point in time is predictive of future status. Harris and associates studied the predictive validity of the MAI, described earlier in this chapter.[32] They compared the risk scores of four-month-old infants with pediatrician assessments of their motor development at two years. More than 80% of the children who showed cerebral palsy at two years had been identified as at risk by the MAI when they were four months old. However, there was also a 44% rate of false-positive tests, in which children rated normal at two years had had an abnormal MAI at 4 months. Thus, the MAI showed good sensitivity (it identified as abnormal a high percentage of children eventually determined to have cerebral palsy) but low specificity (it also identified as abnormal a high percentage of children who were apparently normal at two years of age). Determining the predictive validity of a screening measure such as the MAI is an essential, although obviously time-consuming, process. The premise of many screening tests is that they allow early identification of some phenomenon that is not usually apparent until some later date. The usefulness of such measures cannot be determined unless their predictive validity is known.

SUMMARY

Measurement is a systematic process by which things are differentiated. Measurements can be identified by scale (nominal, ordinal, interval, or ratio), type (discrete or continuous), and framework (norm referenced or criterion referenced). Statistical concepts of importance to measurement theory include the frequency distribution, mean, variance, standard deviation, normal curve, correlation, and SEM. Reliability is the extent to which a measure is free from error. The components of reliability include instrument, tester, and subject variability. Relative measures of reliability are correlation coefficients; the absolute measure of reliability is the SEM. Validity is the meaningfulness and utility of an application of a measurement. The components of validity include construct, content, and criterion validity.

References

1. Thorndike RL, Hagen EP. *Measurement and Evaluation in Psychology and Education.* 4th ed. New York, NY: John Wiley & Sons; 1977:21.
2. Journal editorial policies. *Phys Ther.* 1991;70:86.
3. Hopkins KD, Stanley JC. *Educational and Psychological Measurement and Evaluation.* 6th ed. Englewood Cliffs, NJ: Prentice-Hall Inc; 1981:3.
4. Nunnally JC. *Psychometric Theory.* 2nd ed. New York, NY: McGraw-Hill; 1978:3.
5. Kerlinger FN. *Foundations of Behavioral Research.* 3rd ed. Fort Worth, Tex: Holt, Rinehart & Winston Inc; 1986:392.
6. Safrit MJ. An overview of measurement. In: Safrit MJ, Wood TM, eds. *Measurement Concepts in Physical Education and Exercise Science.* Champaign, Ill: Human Kinetics Books; 1989.
7. Merbitz C, Morris J, Grip JC. Ordinal scales and foundations of misinference. *Arch Phys Med Rehabil.* 1989;70:308–312.
8. Mayhew TP, Rothstein JM. Measurement of muscle performance with instruments. In: Rothstein JM, ed. *Measurement in Physical Therapy.* New York, NY: Churchill Livingstone; 1985.
9. Glass GV, Hopkins KD. *Statistical Methods in Education and Psychology.* 2nd ed. Englewood Cliffs, NJ: Prentice-Hall Inc; 1984:79.
10. Baumgartner TA. Norm-referenced measurement: reliability. In: Safrit MJ, Wood TM, eds. *Measurement Concepts in Physical Education and Exercise Science.* Champaign, Ill: Human Kinetics Books; 1989.
11. American Physical Therapy Association. *1992 State Licensure Guide.* Alexandria, Va: American Physical Therapy Association; 1992.
12. American Educational Research Association, American Psychological Association, and National Committee on Measurement in Education. *Standards for Educational and Psychological Testing.* Washington, DC: American Psychological Association; 1985.
13. Morrow JR. Generalizability theory. In: Safrit MJ, Wood TM, eds. *Measurement Concepts in Physical Education and Exercise Science.* Champaign, Ill: Human Kinetics Books; 1989:74.
14. Stratford PW, Norman GR, McIntosh JM. Generalizability of grip strength measurements in patients with tennis elbow. *Phys Ther.* 1989;69:276–281.
15. Cronbach LJ. *Essentials of Psychological Testing.* 5th ed. New York, NY: Harper & Row; 1990.
16. Harris SR, Haley SM, Tada WL, Swanson MW. Reliability of observational measures of the Movement Assessment of Infants. *Phys Ther.* 1989; 64:471–477.
17. Waltz CF, Strickland OL, Lenz ER. *Measurement in Nursing Research.* Philadelphia, Pa: FA Davis Co; 1984.
18. Lincoln YS, Guba EG. *Naturalistic Inquiry.* Newbury Park, Calif: Sage Publications; 1985.
19. LeCompte MD, Goetz JP. Problems of reliability and validity in ethnographic research. *Review of Educational Research.* 1982;52:31–60.
20. Cohen J. A coefficient of agreement for nominal scales. *Educational and Psychological Measurement.* 1960;20:37–46.
21. Haley SM, Osberg JS. Kappa coefficient calculation using multiple ratings per subject: a special communication. *Phys Ther.* 1989;69:970–974.
22. Bartko JJ. The intraclass correlation coefficient as a measure of reliability. *Psychological Reports.* 1966;19:3–11.

23. Currier DP. *Elements of Research in Physical Therapy*. 3rd ed. Baltimore, Md: Williams & Wilkins; 1990:167.
24. Shrout PE, Fleiss JL. Intraclass correlations: uses in assessing rater reliability. *Psychological Bulletin*. 1979;86:420–428.
25. Bartko JJ, Carpenter WT. On the methods and theory of reliability. *J Nerv Ment Dis*. 1976;163:307–317.
26. Hart DL. Commentary. *Phys Ther*. 1989;69:102–103.
27. Stratford P. Reliability: consistency or differentiating among subjects? *Phys Ther*. 1989;69:299–300.
28. Diamond JE, Mueller MJ, Delitto A, Sinacore DR. Reliability of a diabetic foot evaluation. *Phys Ther*. 1989;69:797–802.
29. Ellison JB, Rose SJ, Sahrmann SA. Patterns of hip rotation range of motion: a comparison between healthy subjects and patients with low back pain. *Phys Ther*. 1990;70:537–541.
30. Gresham GE, Phillips TF, Labi MLC. ADL status in stroke: relative merits of three standard indexes. *Arch Phys Med Rehabil*. 1980;61:355–358.
31. Stratford P, Agostino V, Armstrong B, Stewart T, Weininger S. Diagnostic value of knee extension torque tracings in suspected anterior cruciate ligament tears. *Phys Ther*. 1987;67:1533–1536.
32. Harris SR, Swanson MW, Andrews MS, Sells CJ, Robinson NM, Bennett FC, Chandler LS. Predictive validity of the "Movement Assessment of Infants." *Developmental and Behavioral Pediatrics*. 1984; 5:336–342.

CHAPTER 11

Methodological Research

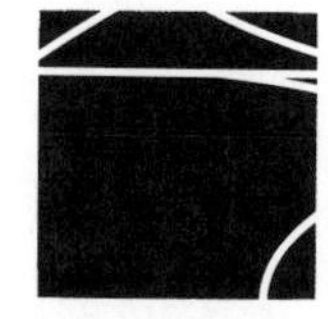

The goals of methodological research are to document and improve the reliability and validity of clinical and research measurements. Because measurement is an integral part of clinical and research documentation, research that examines physical therapy measurements is important to the profession. In addition to the importance of measurement as a topic in its own right, documentation of the reliability and validity of the measures used within a study is a necessary component of all research. This chapter provides a framework for the design of methodological research. Reliability designs are presented first, followed by validity designs.

RELIABILITY DESIGNS

The reliability of a measurement is influenced by many factors, including (1) the sources of variability studied, (2) the subjects selected, and (3) the range of scores exhibited by the sample. Each of these factors is illustrated in this chapter by a hypothetical example of measurement of joint range of motion. The hypothetical example is supplemented by relevant examples from the literature. After these three general factors are discussed, two specialized types of reliability studies are considered: reliability optimization and reliability documentation within nonmethodological research.

Sources of Variability to Be Studied

Differences found in repeated measurements of the same characteristic can be attributed to instrument, intrarater, interrater, and intrasubject components. Within each of these components there are many additional sources of variability. When designing reliability studies, researchers must clearly delineate which of the reliability components they wish to study and which sources of variability they wish to study within each component. To assist with this task, it is helpful to list the four reliability components and all possible sources of variation for each component. Table 11–1 shows potential sources of variability in passive range-of-motion scores as measured with a universal goniometer. There are two steps in delineating the sources of variability to be studied: (1) determining which reliability components to study and (2) determining the level of standardization of the measurement protocol.

Determining the Reliability Components

Once the sources of variability within the measurement are delineated, the researcher must determine which of the components will be the focus of his or her methodological study. As is the case with all research design, the investigator designing methodological research must identify a problem that needs to be studied. Is there a knowledge deficit about the interinstrument reliability of goniometers of different sizes or designs? Is it important to establish the degree of variation that can be expected in a particular measurement made by a single therapist? What is the magnitude of differences that could be expected if several therapists take measurements on the same person? Is subject performance consistent across days or weeks?

Each of these questions relates to one of the four components of reliability: instrument, intrarater, interrater, and intrasubject. However, in many methodological studies, more than one of the reliability components are examined. For example, Morrow and his colleagues studied interinstrument, intratester, and intertester reliability in a single study of a particular method of determining body composition through skinfold measurements.[1] Three testers (intertester reliability) performed three measurement trials (intratester reliability) with each of three different skinfold calipers (interinstrument reliability) on all subjects.

TABLE 11–1. Sources of Variability in Passive Range-of-Motion Measurements with a Universal Goniometer

Sources of Variability
INSTRUMENT
Loose axis (slips during measurement)
Tight axis (too difficult to move precisely)
Interinstrument differences
INTRARATER
Variations in subject positioning
Inconsistent identification of landmarks
Variable end-range pressure
Inconsistent stabilization
Reading errors
INTERRATER
Variations in subject positioning
Inconsistent identification of landmarks
Variable end-range pressure
Inconsistent stabilization
Differing ability to gain subjects' trust
Different end-digit preference
Reading errors
INTRASUBJECT
Varying levels of pain
Differing tolerance to end-range pressure
Mood changes
Differing activities prior to measurement
Biological variation

Determining the Level of Standardization

The second step in identifying the sources of variability to study is to determine the degree of standardization in the measurement protocol. The degree of standardization is the number of sources of variability within a reliability component that are controlled.

Consider three different reasons to study intertester reliability of goniometric measurements. The purpose of one study might be to determine interrater reliability of goniometric measurements as they occur in the clinic, without any standardization of technique between therapists. The purpose of a second study might be to determine the upper limits of interrater reliability with a highly standardized protocol. The purpose of a third study might be to determine interrater reliability with a level of standardization that would be feasible for most clinics to achieve.

The preceding three purpose statements correspond to three general approaches to reliability that are seen in literature: nonstandardized, highly standardized, and partially standardized. The three approaches differ in the extent to which the sources of variability are controlled within each of the reliability components under study. For intertester reliability in the measurement of passive motion with a goniometer, Table 11–1 lists seven possible sources of variability: positioning, landmark identification, end-range pressure, stabilization, patient trust in the therapist, end-digit preference (some therapists always round measurements to the nearest 5°, others round to even numbers only, and others do not round off at all), and reading errors. Let's consider how nonstandardized, highly standardized, and partially standardized studies would be applied to these sources of variability to determine intertester reliability of goniometric measurement.

Nonstandardized Approach. A completely nonstandardized approach would control none of these sources of variability and would establish the lower limit for the reliability component studied. The basic design of a nonstandardized study of intertester reliability would be to have each therapist take measurements privately so as not to influence the technique of the other therapists within the study.

The number of therapists used within the study and the number of times each patient is measured would be determined by the research setting and the nature of the measurement. Hibner studied intertester reliability of goniometric measurements of the shoulder joint in patients with shoulder dysfunction.[2] The clinic at which the study was conducted had a total of four physical therapists and physical therapist assistants who took goniometric measurements. Because of the small number of personnel involved, it was relatively easy for all four therapists or assistants to take one measurement on each subject within the study. Furthermore, it was believed that patients could tolerate four repeated measures.

Contrast the clinical situation in Hibner's study with that of Watkins and associates' study of the reliability of goniometric measures of knee range of motion.[3] The clinic in Watkins and associates' study had 14 therapists who could participate in the study. Because it was not reasonable to expect that all 14 therapists could be available to measure each patient or that patients could tolerate that many repeated measures in a single sitting, each patient was measured by only two different, randomly selected, therapists.

Highly Standardized Approach. In contrast to a nonstandardized approach, a highly standardized approach would control many of the possible sources of variability to determine the upper limits of the reliability of the component. Whereas a nonstandardized approach seeks to document the reliability of measurements as they commonly occur, a highly standardized approach seeks to document reliability in an ideal situation. A highly standardized approach to taking measurements may be a useful way of separating measurement error from subject variability.

In a highly standardized study of intertester goniometric reliability, positioning, stabilization, landmarks, end-range pressure, and end-digit preference would all be controlled. Positioning for shoulder internal rotation, for example, could be controlled by having all therapists take the measurements with the patient supine on the same firm plinth. Stabilization could be controlled by strapping the patient's chest to prevent substitution of scapular or trunk movements. To control inconsistent identification of landmarks, landmarks could be marked on the subjects and left in place while all therapists take their measurements. End-range pressure could be standardized by having an assistant provide a predetermined force as documented by a hand-held dynamometer. Finally, end-digit preference could be controlled by instructing therapists to report the measurement to the nearest degree. The experimental protocol for such a study might be that one therapist positions each patient and three other therapists each take a measurement in rapid succession. Such a protocol would establish the upper limits of intertester reliability and would eliminate the effects of subject variation because the subject would not be moved between measurements.

Mayerson and Milano used a highly standardized approach to study goniometric measurement reliability.[4] A healthy subject was positioned in 22 consistent extremity joint positions; two therapists each took two measurements at each position. The protocol eliminated variability due to subject positioning, stabilization, end-range pressure, and changes in subject motion. Thus, the protocol provided a test of the reliability of goniometer placement and reading. They found that both intertester and intratester differences could confidently be expected to fall within 4° of each other in a highly standardized measurement protocol.

Partially Standardized Approach. The third approach to determining the sources of variability to be studied within an investigation of reliability is the partially standardized approach. As indicated by its name, this approach falls between the extremes of the nonstandardized and highly standardized approaches by standardizing a few sources of variability while leaving others nonstandardized. The sources of variability that are standardized often reflect the realities of the clinic. The hypothetical highly standardized study of internal rotation range of motion described above is probably unrealistic for routine clinical use: An assistant is not always available to position the patient, and landmarks are likely to be washed off between treatment sessions. A partially standardized measurement protocol might therefore standardize positioning and stabilization but allow landmark determination and end-range pressure to vary among therapists. The experimental protocol for a partially standardized study requires educating the examiners in the standardized methods to be employed in the study.

Youdas and colleagues used a partially standardized approach to study the reliability of cervical range-of-motion measurements taken by visual estimation, with a universal goniometer, and with a cervical range of motion instrument.[5] Therapists were trained in the use of a standardized protocol for positioning of the subjects; placement of the measuring devices and a warm-up protocol for subjects were also standardized.

The appropriate level of standardization for reliability studies is debated in the rehabilitation literature. Some researchers argue for the use of nonstandardized approaches applicable to clinical settings;[6] others argue for the use of highly and partially standardized approaches to isolate which aspects of measurements are unreliable.[4,7] It seems reasonable to accept that each approach is useful for specific purposes. Nonstandardized studies describe reliability as it is; highly standardized studies present idealized reliability estimates and examine the impact of limited sources of variability on reliability; partially standardized studies describe reliability with moderate levels of standardization that should be achievable in clinical settings.

Subject Selection

As is the case with all types of research, subject selection in reliability studies influences the external validity of the study; the study results can be generalized only to the types of subjects studied. Therefore, the reliability of an instrument should be determined using the individuals on whom the instrument will be used in practice. If the measure is a clinical one, it is best to determine its reliability on patients who would ordinarily require this measurement as part of their care. Watkins and associates did just this in their study of the reliability of knee range-of-motion measurements.[3] In fact, they even divided their patients into diagnostic categories to determine whether the measurements were more reliable for patients with certain types of knee dysfunction. The inappropriate use of normal subjects to establish the reliability of clinical measures may inflate reliability estimates because normal subjects may be easier to measure than patients. Pain, obliteration of landmarks because of deformity, or difficulty following directions because of neurological impairment may make it difficult to take measurements in patients.

If a researcher ultimately wishes to determine norms for certain characteristics, it is appropriate to determine the reliability of the measurements using normal subjects. If the measurement in question is part of a screening tool, such as a flexibility test that might be administered at a fitness fair, then a broad sampling of the individuals likely to be screened should be used to establish the reliability of the measurement.

Range of Scores

The reliability of a measure should be determined over the range of scores expected for that measure. There are two reasons for this. First, as discussed in Chapter 10, a restricted range of scores will lead to low reliability coefficients even in the presence of small absolute differences in repeated measurements. The use of normal subjects often restricts the range of scores within a study.

Second, reliability may vary at different places in the range of scores because of difficulties unique to taking measurements at particular points in the range. For example, Lohman and coworkers examined the reliability of body composition determination with skinfold measurements in female college basketball players, a group expected to be close to ideal body fat.[8] The authors were careful to note that their findings could not be generalized to groups with higher percentages of body fat, because larger measurement errors may be encountered with thicker skinfolds.

Optimization Designs

In many instances, researchers have found less than satisfactory reliability for physical therapy measures, particularly as they are implemented in the clinic.[9–11] Such research is useful because it may lead to a healthy skepticism about the measurements we use. In and of itself, however, *documenting* the reliability of a clinical measure does nothing to *improve* its reliability. Improving the reliability of physical therapy measures requires that researchers study ways to optimize reliability. There are two basic designs for optimization research: standardization and mean designs.

Standardization Designs. The standardization designs compare the reliabilities of measurements taken under different sets of conditions. For example, suppose that the result of a nonstandardized reliability study was that the SEM for passive internal range of motion was 10°. Furthermore, the result of a highly standardized, but clinically unfeasible, study was that the SEM was 1°. A standardization study might be developed with a goal of determining what level of standardization is needed to achieve an SEM of 3°. To do so, a researcher might determine reliability with standardized positioning. If, despite the positioning change, the SEM is still too large, both position and upper chest stabilization might be standardized. The level of standardization would be increased until the reliability goal was met. A reverse sequence could also be implemented by starting with a highly standardized procedure and eliminating standardization procedures that are not feasible in the clinic.

Hibner used a standardization design to try to improve the reliability of shoulder range-of-motion measurements taken in a single clinic.[2] He started with a nonstandardized procedure and found large SEMs for all six motions studied. The optimization procedure Hibner used was to make positioning among therapists consistent. This improved the SEM for several measures. A next step to further improve the reliability of the measurements might focus on identification of landmarks and goniometer placement or on stabilization of the trunk to prevent substitution.

Mean Designs. The mean designs compare the reliabilities of single measurements and also compare the reliabilities of measurements averaged across several trials. This design is particularly appropriate for measures that are difficult to standardize for clinical use or for characteristics that are expected to show a great deal of natural variation. Stratford and colleagues studied the reliability of grip strength measurements in patients with tennis elbow.[12] Three measurements of grip strength were taken for each patient on each of two days. With such a design the researcher can determine the reliability between two single measures (for example, the first and second trials on one day), between two averages of two measures (for example, the average of the first two trials on one day and the average of the first two trials on the second day), and between two averages of three measures (the average of the three trials on the first day and the average of three trials on the second day). Mathematical extension of the reliability formulas can predict the reliability that would be found with additional measurements on additional days. Such information allows clinicians to make knowledgeable decisions about the test protocols they establish.

Measurement Reliability in Nonmethodological Studies

Useful research studies must be based on measurements that are reliable. Measurement reliability in nonmethodological studies should often be addressed at two times during the study: during the design phase and during the implementation phase.

In the design phase, the researcher must determine which of several possible instruments to choose, which of several possible measurement protocols to follow, and which of several raters to use. Studies of interinstrument, interrater, or intrarater reliability components may be needed to make these decisions.

When conducting a pilot reliability study, the researcher needs to simulate the research conditions as closely as possible. The same types of subjects, settings, time pressures, and the like should be employed. The results of a pilot reliability study conducted after clinic hours, when therapists and subjects have much time and few distractions, may differ from those of the actual study if the actual study takes place during clinic hours, when time is short and distractions abound.

Reliability measures should also be taken during implementation of a study. Several authors have found a decline in reliability from that seen during a training phase to that occurring during the experimental phase.[13,14] In addition, reliability studies conducted during a short time frame before a study may not adequately reflect the subject variability that might be seen during the longer time frame of the actual study. Researchers can establish reliability during the course of a study by taking repeated measures of all subjects, using pretest and posttest scores of a control group as the reliability indicator, or taking repeated measures of selected subjects at random. Which strategy is adopted depends on factors such as the expense of the measures, the risks of repeated measurements to subjects, and the number of subjects in the study.

VALIDITY DESIGNS

As discussed previously, the validity of a measurement is the extent to which a particular use of the measurement is meaningful. Measures are validated through argument about and research into the soundness of the interpretations made from them. To make sound interpretations, a researcher must first be confident that the measurements are reproducible, or reliable. Recall that although reliability is necessary for validity, it does not validate the meaning behind the measure. This section of the chapter presents several designs for research to determine the construct, content, and criterion validity of measurements.

Construct Validation

Constructs are artificial frameworks that are not directly observable. Strength, function, proprioception, and pain are constructs used frequently in physical therapy. Because the constructs themselves are not directly observable, there are no absolute standards against which measurements can be compared to determine if they are valid indicators of the constructs. Consider, for example, all the different measures that physical therapists use to represent the construct of strength: manual muscle testing, the number of times that a particular weight can be lifted, hand-held dynamometers, and a multitude of isokinetic tests. All are appropriate for some purposes, but none is a definitive measure of strength.

In the absence of a clear-cut standard, persuasive argument becomes one means by which the construct validity of measurements is established.[15] A researcher who wishes to assess strength gains following a particular program of exercise must be prepared to defend the appropriateness of the measurements he or she used for the type of exercise program studied. Such considerations include whether the measure should test concentric or eccentric contractions, whether the test should be isometric or should sample strength throughout the range of motion, and whether the test should be conducted in an open or closed kinetic chain position.

A second way in which construct validity is established is through examination of the convergence and divergence of measures thought to represent similar and different constructs, respectively. Provost and associates compared two assessment tools designed to identify sensorimotor problems in preschool children.[16] One scale, the Peabody Developmental Motor Scale, consists of two scales: one for gross and one for fine motor scores. Each scale is further divided into skill categories. The other scale, the Miller Assessment for Preschoolers, consists of three major areas: sensory and motor ability, cognitive abilities, and combined abilities.

The gross motor scales of the Peabody and Miller assessments both measure basic body movement abilities that underlie the construct gross motor skill. Although there is no absolute standard of gross motor skill against which these scales can be compared, if the two scales are highly correlated, this provides evidence that the scales are measuring the same thing. Persuasive argument may then be used to establish whether what is being measured is the construct of gross motor skill.

The fact that there are separate scales for gross and fine motor scores indicates that the test developers believe that the two types of motor skills represent separate constructs. If fine and gross motor skill are really different, one would expect to find a low association between the gross and fine motor scales on the same instrument or between instruments. Construct validity is best supported when the scores on items thought to represent the same construct are highly associated (convergence) and when scores on items that are theoretically different have a low association (divergence).

Content Validation

Content validation involves documenting that a test provides an adequate sampling of the behavior or knowledge that it is measuring. To determine the content validity of a measure, a researcher compares the items in the test against the actual practice of interest. There are four basic issues a researcher must consider when determining content validity: the sample on whom the measure is validated, the content's completeness, the content's relevance, and the content's emphasis. As an example, consider the content validity of the Blue MACS, an assessment tool used widely to evaluate students on clinical rotations in physical therapy.[17] The Blue MACS consists of detailed descriptions of physical therapist behaviors that should be components of more than 40 clinical activities. If the Blue MACS has content validity, then it should accurately represent the demands that clinical practice places on physical therapists.

To determine content validity, a researcher needs to determine an appropriate group on whom the content can be validated. To determine the content validity of the Blue MACS, should a random sampling of physical therapists be selected for observation of their practice? Should therapists with less than two years of experience constitute the sample? Should students on clinical rotations be studied? If the Blue MACS is viewed as a tool that determines readiness for entry-level physical therapy practice, then the group of new therapists may be the most appropriate group on whom the content should be validated. If the Blue MACS is viewed as a tool that assesses performance on clinical rotations, then the student group may be the appropriate group on whom the tool should be validated.

Once the subject group has been identified, test content can be compared with actual practice. If the validity were perfect, all activities of the observed therapists would be represented in the Blue MACS, and all items in the Blue MACS would be demonstrated in actual practice. In addition, more emphasis would be placed on items that are frequently performed in actual practice and less emphasis would be placed on infrequently performed items.

Criterion Validation

The criterion validation of a measure is determined by comparing it with an accepted standard of measurement. The major considerations in designing a criterion validation study are selecting the criterion, timing the administration of the tests, and selecting a sample for testing.

Three different criteria against which a test is compared are found in the literature. The first criterion is essentially instrumentation accuracy. The accuracy of the measurement provided by an instrument is determined by comparing the reading on the device with a standard measure. Examples in the literature include loading a dynamometer with known weights to determine whether the device output is accurate and comparing the angular measurements of a goniometer with known angles.[3, 12] Complex instruments have specific standardization procedures that allow the investigator to check the instrument against known standards and either make adjustments until the device readings accurately reflect the standard or develop equations that can be used to correct for inaccuracies.[18]

The second criterion is a concurrent one. A concurrent criterion is applied at the same time the test in question is validated. Burdett and colleagues determined the validity of four instruments for measuring lumbar spine and pelvic positions by comparing the external measures with the criteria of angles drawn from radiographs taken in the same position.[19]

The third criterion is predictive. A measure has predictive validity if the result of its administration at one point in time is highly associated with future status. There are three difficulties in doing predictive studies: determining the criterion itself, determining the timing of administration of the criterion, and maintaining a good sample of subjects measured on both occasions. Harris and associates studied the predictive validity of the Movement Assessment of Infants (MAI) by comparing children's scores on the MAI at four months of age with an assessment of their motor development at one to two years.[20] Note that the criterion used was a motor criterion. If the MAI predicts both cognitive and motor development, then using only a motor criterion may underestimate the predictive validity of the MAI.

The importance of timing is also illustrated in the MAI validity study. By assessing motor development at one to two years, Harris and associates were testing relatively gross motor abilities. If status at Age 5 were assessed, perhaps fine motor deficits would begin to show themselves in problems with handwriting and drawing. If status at Age 12 were assessed, subtle coordination problems may show up as the child begins to participate in sports activities.

The third difficulty with predictive validity studies is the sample available for study. Because these studies extend over time, there may be differential loss of subjects. For example, in Harris and associates' study, only 80% of the children with four-month MAI scores also had one- or two-year motor assessment scores.[20] It is possible that the majority of the children who were not followed-up were normal. Differential loss of normal subjects would likely result in inflated validity estimates.

SUMMARY

Methodological research is conducted to document and improve measuring tools by assessing their reliability and validity. The major components of reliability are instrument, intrarater, interrater, and intrasubject reliability. Reliability research can be classified according to whether the measurement protocol used is nonstandardized, partially standardized, or highly standardized. Subjects should be selected on the basis of whether they would likely be assessed with the tool in clinical situations; in addition, subjects who demonstrate a wide range of scores should be selected. Construct validity is determined through logical argument and assessment of the convergence of similar tests and divergence of different tests. Content validity is determined by assessing the completeness, relevancy, and emphasis of the items within a test. Criterion validity is determined by comparing one measure with an accepted standard of measurement.

References

1. Morrow JR Jr, Fridye T, Monaghen SD. Generalizability of the AAHPERD health related skinfold test.

Research Quarterly for Exercise and Sport. 1986;57:187–195.

2. Hibner RJ. Standardization of goniometry of the shoulder in the clinic. Master's research project. Indianapolis, Ind: University of Indianapolis; 1990.
3. Watkins MA, Riddle DL, Lamb RL, Personius WJ. Reliability of goniometric measurements and visual estimates of knee range of motion obtained in a clinical setting. *Phys Ther.* 1991;71:90–96.
4. Mayerson NH, Milano RA. Goniometric reliability in physical medicine. *Arch Phys Med Rehabil.* 1984;65:92–94.
5. Youdas JW, Carey JR, Garrett TR. Reliability of measurements of cervical spine range of motion—comparison of three methods. *Phys Ther.* 1991;71:98–104.
6. Riddle DL. Commentary. *Phys Ther.* 1991;71:105–106.
7. Youdas JW, Carey JR, Garrett TR. Author response. *Phys Ther.* 1991;71:106.
8. Lohman TG, Pollock ML, Slaughter MH, Brandon LJ, Boileau RA. Methodological factors and the prediction of body fat in female athletes. *Med Sci Sport Exerc.* 1984;16:92–96.
9. Riddle DL, Rothstein JM, Lamb RL. Goniometric reliability in a clinical setting: shoulder measurements. *Phys Ther.* 1987;67:668–673.
10. Elveru RA, Rothstein JM, Lamb RL. Goniometric reliability in a clinical setting: subtalar and ankle joint measurements. *Phys Ther.* 1988;68:672–677.
11. Potter NA, Rothstein JM. Intertester reliability for selected clinical tests of the sacroiliac joint. *Phys Ther.* 1985;65:1671–1675.
12. Stratford PW, Norman GR, McIntosh JM. Generalizability of grip strength measurements in patients with tennis elbow. *Phys Ther.* 1989;69:277–281.
13. Mitchell SK. Interobserver agreement, reliability, and generalizability of data collected in observational studies. *Psychol Bull.* 1979;86:376–390.
14. Taplin PS, Reid JB. Effects of instructional set and experiment influence on observer reliability. *Child Dev.* 1973;44:547–554.
15. Cronbach LJ. *Essentials of Psychological Testing.* New York, NY: Harper & Row; 1990:185.
16. Provost B, Harris MB, Ross K, Michnal D. A comparison of scores on two preschool assessment tools: implications for theory and practice. *Physical and Occupational Therapy in Pediatrics.* 1988;8:35–51.
17. The Texas Consortium for Physical Therapy Clinical Education Inc. *The Blue MACS: Mastery and Assessment of Clinical Skills.* 4th ed. Berryville, Va: Forum Medicum Inc; 1989.
18. Geddes LA, Baker LE. *Principles of Applied Biomedical Instrumentation.* 3rd ed. New York, NY: John Wiley & Sons; 1989:8–9.
19. Burdett RG, Brown KE, Fall MP. Reliability and validity of four instruments for measuring lumbar spine and pelvic positions. *Phys Ther.* 1986;66:677–684.
20. Harris SR, Swanson MW, Andrews MS, Sells CJ, Robinson NM, Bennett FC, Chandler LS. Predictive validity of the "Movement Assessment of Infants." *Developmental and Behavioral Pediatrics.* 1984; 5:336–342.

CHAPTER 12

Measurement Tools for Physical Therapy Research

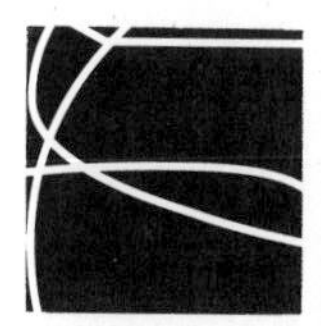

After defining a research problem, the researcher must confront the question of how to measure the constructs of interest within a study. Physical therapy researchers have a wide range of instruments from which to choose. These instruments include devices or procedures used in the clinic, instruments designed primarily for research use, observational methods that require only the skills of the researcher, and self-report instruments that require written or oral responses from subjects.

To assist physical therapists in evaluating the vast array of measurement tools available to them, the American Physical Therapy Association (APTA) has published *Standards for Tests and Measurements in Physical Therapy Practice.*[1] This document provides a framework from which test developers, researchers, teachers, and test users can evaluate the measures they use. An additional document published by the APTA is called the *Resource and Buyer's Guide,* and it provides information about the suppliers of many of the measurement tools that are discussed in this chapter.[2]

This chapter introduces the wide range of measuring tools that are reported in the physical therapy literature. As mentioned in Chapters 10 and 11, the reliability of a measure depends on the way in which data are collected, and validity depends on the use to which a measurement is put rather than on the measurement itself. Therefore, in this chapter no judgments are made about the relative merits of the measurement tools presented. Instead, references that discuss the reliability, validity, and use of the various tools in physical therapy research are cited. These references provide a foundation of information on which readers can base their decision on whether to use a particular measure in their own study. The chapter is organized around 12 major constructs that physical therapists measure: muscle performance; joint motion; physiological function; pain; functional status; biomechanics; anthropometrics; postural control; sensation; developmental status; behavior; and self-report measures of personal characteristics, opinions, and attitudes. A variety of measures are described for each construct.

MEASURING MUSCLE PERFORMANCE

The term "muscle performance," suggested by Mayhew and Rothstein,[3(p58)] describes the very broad spectrum of qualities related to the function of the muscular system. Four different aspects of muscle performance are discussed in this section: force generation, electrical activity, muscle tone, and microscopic composition.

Force Generation

Physical therapists are often interested in the force-generating capacity of muscles: How much pressure can a subject exert? How much weight can a subject lift? How many times can a subject complete a movement? All of these questions relate either to the force generated by a muscle or to extensions of the concept of force, such as torque, work, and power. Measurements of muscular force or its extensions range from simple measures that rely on the examiner's judgment to complex instruments which cost thousands of dollars. Six types of measures are discussed below: manual muscle testing, hand-held dynamometry, weights, cable tensiometers and strain gauges, hand dynamometers, and isokinetic dynamometers.

Manual Muscle Testing. Manual muscle testing procedures are familiar to all physical therapists. Manual muscle tests do not require equipment and rely instead on therapist judgments about a subject's ability to move against gravity or against a force exerted by the examiner. In 1985, Lamb reviewed the literature on manual muscle testing and concluded that the reliability and validity of the major approaches to manual muscle testing had not been well established.[4] Since his review, at least two studies have evaluated the reliability of manual muscle testing as it is used in contemporary practice. In one study high levels of intratester reliability were found for several muscle groups that were selected because of their ease of testing;[5] in the other study relatively low intertester reliability was found for nonstandardized testing of two muscles thought to be difficult to test.[6] A major limitation of manual muscle testing as a research tool is its ordinal nature; that is, the intervals between the various grades are not established.

Hand-Held Dynamometry. Hand-held dynamometry is an instrumented extension of manual muscle testing (Figure 12–1). However, rather than relying on the physical therapist's judgment of the external load the patient is able to withstand, hand-held dynamometers provide quantitative output of the force exerted against the instrument. The test–retest reliability of hand-held dynamometry has been determined to be relatively high for patients with brain damage,[7, 8] healthy children and children with muscular dystrophy,[9] and patients with chronic orthopedic disorders.[5] Good interrater reliability has been shown with a group of patients with diverse neurological diagnoses.[10] Bohannon used hand-held dynamometry to assess the influence of head–neck position on elbow flexion in patients who had had a stroke.[11]

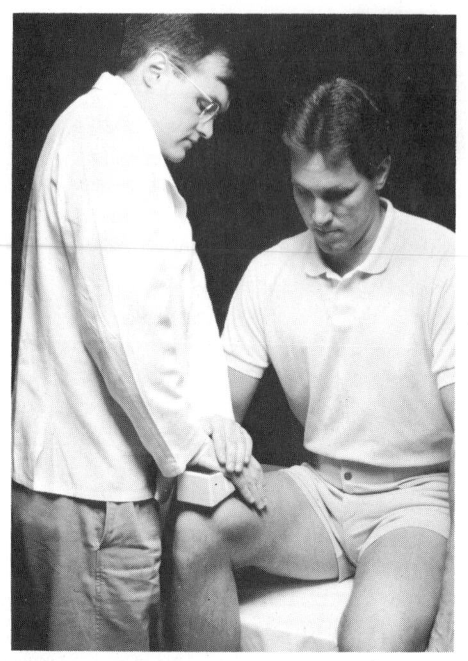

FIGURE 12–1. Hand-held dynamometer. Photo courtesy of Lafayette Instruments, 3700 Sagamore Parkway North, Lafayette, IN 47903.

Weights. The use of weights to document muscle performance was popularized by DeLorme in the 1940s.[12] Muscle performance is quantified by determining the maximum amount of weight that a subject is able to move through either a single repetition (one-repetition maximum) or 10 repetitions (10-repetition maximum). Weiss and associates used a one-repetition maximum as their measure of strength in a study of heavy resistance training of triceps surae muscles.[13]

Cable Tensiometers and Strain Gauges. Cable tensiometers and strain gauges are mechanical and electrical versions of basically the same tool. In both, there is a device that is fixed on one end and secured to the subject's limb at the other end. When the subject exerts force against the device, quantitative output is obtained. With the cable tensiometer, a meter located along the cable measures the tension on the cable. The strain gauge measures changes in the electrical resistance of the materials that are placed under stress. Mayhew and Rothstein[3(pp 68, 69)] note the following limitations to strength testing with cable tensiometers: Few clinicians are exposed to the device, tensiometers are not available in most clinical settings, fixation equipment is needed for accurate testing, and two testers are often needed to meet the positioning requirements of the test. Many of the same limitations apply to the strain gauges.

Pelletier and associates used a cable tensiometer to document strength changes in a single-system experimental design to determine the effect of isometric exercise in an individual with hemophilia.[14] Vaughan used a strain gauge to measure muscle strength in a study of the effect of immobilization on several muscle performance characteristics.[15]

Hand Dynamometers. Several different types of dynamometers are designed to measure grip or pinch strength (Figure 12–2). Fess has reviewed the literature on the reliability and validity of hand dynamometry.[16] Mathiowetz and associates documented normative data for grip and pinch strength in adults.[17] Jansen and Minerbo used both grip and pinch gauges in a nonexperimental research study of immobilization protocols after flexor tendon surgery.[18]

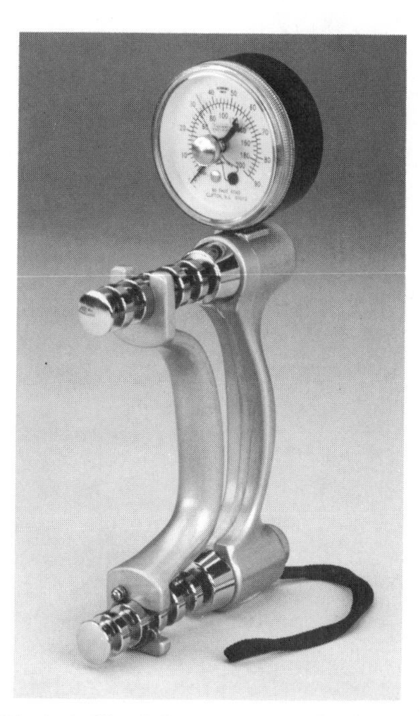

FIGURE 12–2. Hand dynamometer. Photo courtesy of Lafayette Instruments, 3700 Sagamore Parkway North, Lafayette, IN 47903.

Isokinetic Dynamometers. Pioneered in the 1960s, isokinetic devices allow exercise and muscle testing to be conducted under constant velocity throughout the range of motion (Figure 12–3). Clinicians now have a choice of several different commonly available brands of isokinetic dynamometers.[19] In addition, specialized isokinetic dynamometers have been developed for testing trunk musculature. In a modification of the isokinetic concept, devices have been developed that permit "isoinertial" testing and exercise against constant resistance throughout the range of motion.[20]

The dynamometers are interfaced with computers that provide many different measures of muscle performance, such as peak torque, torque:body weight ratios, endurance factors, and torque measurements at certain ranges of motion. In addition, all of these measures can be taken at different speeds. Some of the machines allow testing of eccentric as well as concentric muscle contractions. A researcher should use caution when comparing measurements taken with different brands of machines, because the measurements from different dynamometers are not interchangeable.[21, 22]

Despite the sophistication of these instruments, the validity of some of the commonly used isokinetic measures has been questioned. For example, a commonly used measure is the peak torque:body weight ratio. This ratio is calculated in an attempt to standardize peak torque values to permit comparison among individuals of different sizes. However, the correlation between peak torque and body weight has been found to be low, making the usefulness of the ratio questionable.[23] In

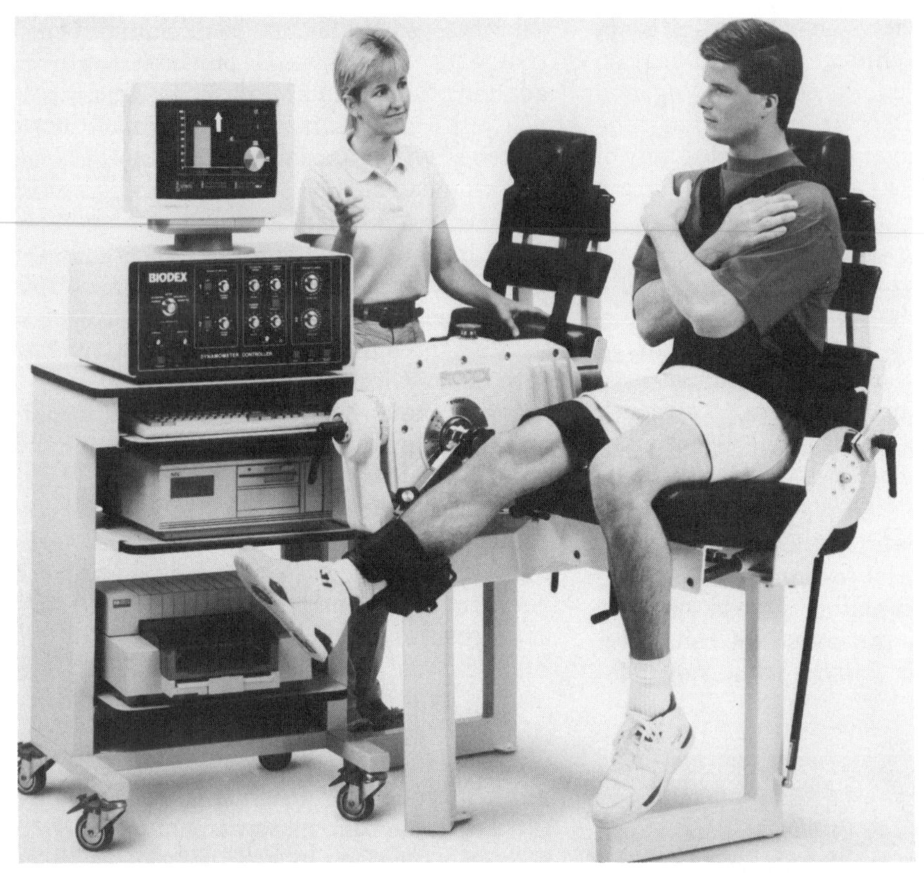

FIGURE 12–3. Isokinetic dynamometer. Photo courtesy of Biodex Corporation, PO Box 703, Shirley, NY 11967.

addition, there are measurement issues related to correcting torque measurements for gravity, damping the signal, and calibrating the machines. Rothstein and associates and Winter and associates have reviewed some of the major issues involved with isokinetic testing.[19, 24]

Electrical Activity

A second aspect of muscle performance is the electrical activity of the muscle, as documented by electromyography (EMG). EMG has been used as a diagnostic tool, a biofeedback tool, and a tool for kinesiological and biomechanical research. Five characteristics of the EMG potential have been noted: duration, frequency, amplitude, characteristics of the wave form, and characteristics of the sound generated.[25] EMG potentials can be detected by both surface electrodes and fine wire electrodes. Surface electrodes pick up more activity from large muscle masses; fine wire electrodes are inserted into the muscle through a hollow needle and allow the study of smaller, deeper muscles (Figure 12–4).[26]

A major concern in the interpretation of EMG results is the extent to which the EMG signal is indicative of muscle force-generating capacity. Muscular length and the type of contraction influence the relationship be-

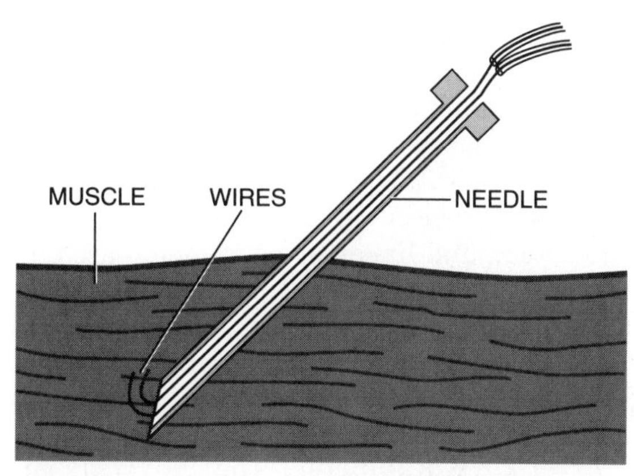

FIGURE 12–4. Bipolar fine wire electromyographic electrode. Redrawn from Snyder-Mackler L, Robinson AJ. *Clinical Electrophysiology, Electrotherapy, and Electrophysiologic Testing*. Baltimore, MD: Williams & Wilkins; 1989:37.

tween EMG activity and muscular force.[27] Guidelines for human EMG research have been developed and published by the Society for Psychophysiological Research.[28]

Two recently reported studies illustrate the different uses of EMG in research. In a study of postural adjustments during balance testing, Duncan and colleagues used surface EMG to determine the timing and sequence of activation of various muscle groups during postural responses.[29] Hanten and Schulthies used fine wire electrodes to study the EMG activity of the vastus medialis oblique and vastus lateralis muscles during performance of two different exercises.[30]

Muscle Tone

Muscle tone is yet another aspect of muscle performance that interests physical therapists. A general definition of muscle tone is the "responsiveness of muscles to passive elongation or stretch."[31(p139)] A clinical manifestation of abnormal muscle tone is a disorder in the timing of different muscular actions when movement is attempted. It is difficult to measure muscle tone because it is a fluctuating phenomenon. In addition, muscle tone may change with touch and movement. Despite these difficulties, muscle tone has been quantified by description of responses to elongation and by measurement of EMG activity, range of motion, and force.

One of the simplest measures of muscle tone is the Ashworth scale of spasticity. This ordinal scale requires that the examiner judge resistance to movement according to descriptions of five or six grades of spasticity. Bohannon and Smith found their modification of the Ashworth scale to have good interrater reliability.[32] Another ordinal scale of muscle tone is the 0 to 4+ scale used to quantify the deep tendon reflexes.[33]

Range-of-motion measurements have also been used to indicate spasticity. Worley and colleagues used two different range-of-motion measures to quantify spasticity: the resting position of the joint and the position at which resistance to passive movement was encountered.[34]

An additional use of range-of-motion measures for documentation of spasticity is the pendulum test. In this test, the spasticity of the quadriceps femoris muscles is indicated by the pattern of movement after the lower leg is dropped from a position of full knee extension with the subject in a supine position and the lower legs dangling from the supporting surface. A limb with no spasticity swings rapidly to the resting position of 90° of knee flexion. The slightly spastic leg "catches" earlier in the range of motion, and the highly spastic leg may not move at all from the extended position. The points in the range of motion at which catches or oscillations occur have been documented with an electrogoniometer attached to the limb and with a goniometer incorporated within an isokinetic dynamometer.[35–37] Bajd and associates used a pendulum test to document spasticity changes in patients with spinal cord injury following electrical stimulation.[38]

EMG has also been used to document tone or spasticity.[39] Patterns of muscle activation may indicate changes in muscle tone, and the magnitude of muscular activity may be used to determine whether a spasticity-reducing treatment is effective. Wolf and colleagues and Dickstein and colleagues have used EMG data to document muscle activation changes with various treatments.[40, 41]

Microscopic Composition

The fourth aspect of muscle performance studied by physical therapists is the microscopic composition of muscles. Biochemical and histochemical analysis of muscle tissue can determine the proportion of different fiber types within muscle units, the organization of motor units within a muscle, the motor units that have been fatigued by a given maneuver, and the extent of muscular degeneration or regeneration. Brown used histochemical analysis to determine the effects of resistance exercise on skeletal muscles in rats and the effect of short-wave diathermy on skeletal muscle injury in rabbits.[42, 43] Sinacore and colleagues used histochemical and biochemical analysis to study the order of activation of muscle fibers during electrical muscle stimulation in a human subject.[44]

MEASURING JOINT MOTION AND POSITION

Along with the measurement of muscle performance, the measurement of joint range of motion and position is one of the most frequently used evaluative procedures in physical therapy. These measurements can be classified into three broad categories: extrinsic joint movements, intrinsic movements within a joint, and joint or body segment position. Miller has reviewed many issues in the measurement of joint motion.[45]

Extrinsic Joint Motions

Many different clinical and research tools are available for the documentation of extrinsic joint motions. The universal goniometer, gravity-referenced goniometers, electrogoniometers, and linear measurements are discussed in this section. Gajdosik and Bohannon have reviewed the literature on measurement of the extrinsic range of motion of the joints of the extremities.[46]

Universal Goniometer. The universal goniometer is the most familiar clinical tool for measuring joint range of motion. Several authors have provided guidelines for using the goniometer.[47, 48] Many authors have documented the reliability of measurements taken with the universal goniometer.[49–51] The universal goniometer is used to measure both isolated joint movements and the combined movement of several segments, such as the cervical or lumbar spine and hips.

When evaluating passive range of motion, the examiner exerts a force against one of the limbs involved in the motion. Thus, the amount of force the examiner uses becomes a variable that may affect the reliability and validity of the range-of-motion measure. A measurement technique using a universal goniometer to measure range of motion and a dynamometer to standardize the force exerted for passive range-of-motion measurements has been termed *torque range of motion.*[52]

Gravity-Referenced Goniometers. Gravity-referenced goniometers have some mechanism by which the measurement is referenced to either the horizontal or vertical. Some use the concept of a carpenter's level, and others use the principle of a plumb bob. The term *inclinometer* is sometimes used for gravity-referenced goniometers because they measure the degree of inclination from the vertical (Figure 12–5). Merritt and associates

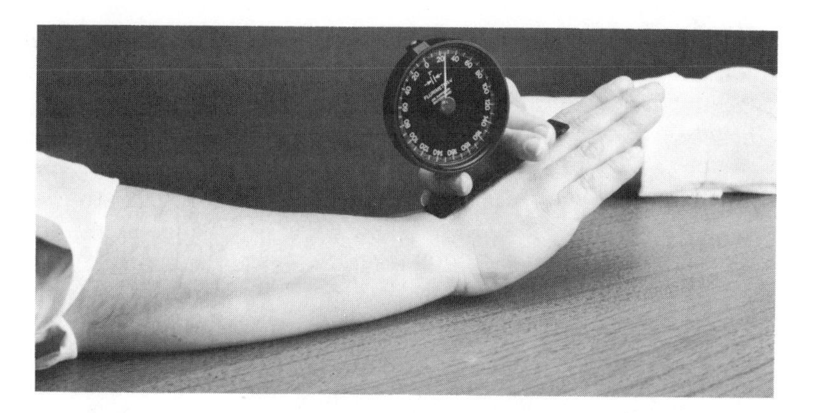

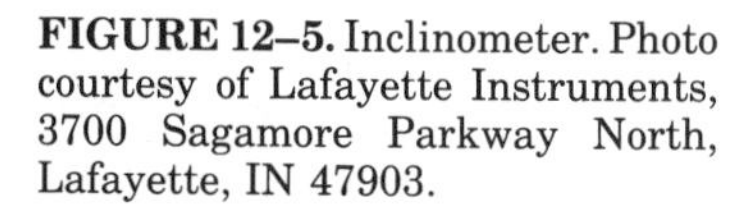
FIGURE 12–5. Inclinometer. Photo courtesy of Lafayette Instruments, 3700 Sagamore Parkway North, Lafayette, IN 47903.

and Burdett and colleagues have described the use of inclinometers to measure trunk flexibility.[53, 54] Specialized goniometers have been designed for the measurement of cervical spine motions (Figure 12–6). In addition to gravity referencing, these goniometers permit stabilization of the device on the head. Youdas documented the reliability of one of the specialized cervical measurement devices.[55]

Electrogoniometers. Electrogoniometers detect differences in electrical potential that occur when the positions of the arms of the instrument change in relation to each other.

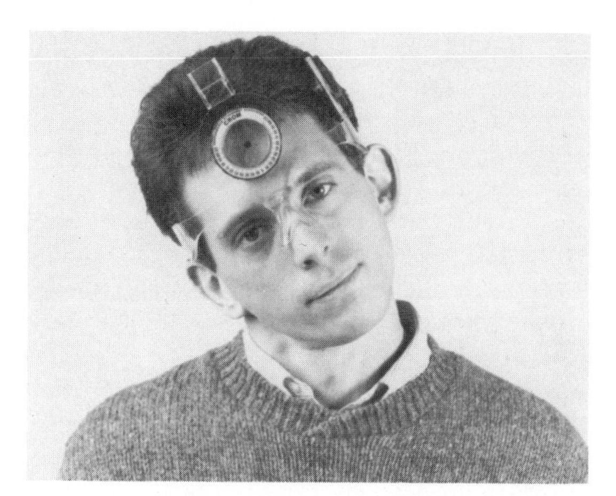
FIGURE 12–6. Cervical range-of-motion instrument. Photo courtesy of Performance Attainment Associates, 958 Lydia Drive, Roseville, MN 55113.

The electrogoniometer must be secured to the individual's body segment in such a way that (a) the axis of the goniometer corresponds to the axis of the joint being measured and (b) the axis and arms do not slip. Electrogoniometers may be planar (two dimensional) or triaxial (three dimensional).[56] Condon and Hutton used an electrogoniometer to collect the range-of-motion data needed for their study of dorsiflexion range of motion during four stretching procedures.[57]

Linear Measurements. The angles of some isolated or combined joint movements are so difficult to measure that a variety of linear measurement techniques have been developed. Temporomandibular joint opening is often documented by measuring the distance between the upper and lower incisors. Greater distance represents greater motion of the joint. Anterior and lateral protrusions of the jaw may also be measured by the distance between the incisors after each maneuver.[48(pp132–134)] Trunk motion may be documented by the distance between the fingertips and the floor at the extremes of the range of motion or skin distraction measures that document changes in the distance between two skin markers when a patient moves from the resting position to the extreme of range of motion.[53, 54] Batti'e and colleagues used a skin distraction measure to document lumbar flexion in their study of lumbar flexibility in adults.[58] Fingertip-to-palm distance, finger abduction distance, and thumb abduction distance from the palm are frequently measured linearly.[59]

Intrinsic Joint Motions

The extent of intrinsic joint motion is frequently the judgment of the clinician, with the motion generally described as hypomobile, normal, or hypermobile. McClure and associates have studied the intertester reliability of such clinical judgments with regard to medial knee ligament integrity.[60] Measurement of anterior–posterior knee instability has become more objective with the introduction of knee arthrometers (Figure 12–7).[61, 62]

Joint Position and Posture

Measurement of joint position and posture is related to measurement of joint motion. However, rather than the movement of a body part, the resting position of a segment or the resting relationship between body segments is documented. Goniometers can be used to document resting positions, although there must be a relevant reference point with which the resting position can be compared. Cervical spine posture has been documented by measuring the linear distance between the most anterior portion of the cervical curvature and the most posterior portion of the thoracic curve.[63] Lumbar spine position has been documented by using a flexible ruler to match the position of the spine and then using trigonometric calculations to generate an angular measurement.[64] Link and colleagues used a flexible ruler to measure subjects' lumbar position while they were standing and sitting in two styles of chairs.[65]

MEASURING PHYSIOLOGICAL FUNCTION

Physical therapists often use exercise or relaxation techniques that can be expected to produce changes in cardiovascular, pulmo-

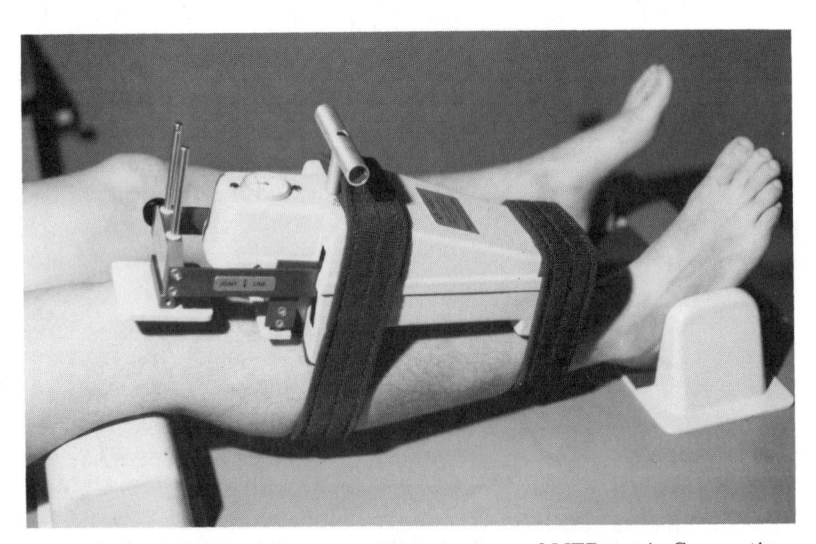

FIGURE 12–7. Knee arthrometer. Photo courtesy of MEDmetric Corporation, 7542 Trade Street, San Diego, CA 92121.

nary, or autonomic nervous system functions. Kispert, Sinacore and Ehsani, and Protas have all reviewed the literature related to cardiopulmonary measurements.[66–68]

Cardiovascular Measures

Heart Rate. Heart rate may be determined by palpation; by commercial heart rate monitors that attach to a subject's earlobe, finger, wrist, or chest; or by electrocardiographic equipment. Electrocardiographic measurement is considered the standard against which other measures of heart rate are evaluated. Sedlock and associates found a high degree of accuracy of self-determination of pulse rate after exercise in their comparison of heart rate determined through palpation of radial and carotid pulses with heart rate obtained with an electrocardiograph.[69] Araujo and associates documented the accuracy of five different heart rate monitors when subjects were at rest.[70]

Heart rate is sensitive to many factors, such as patients' activity prior to measurement, the time of day, the temperature of the room, patients' anxiety about the procedure, patients' food and drink consumption, and patients' emotional state. Researchers need to carefully control these factors, regardless of which method of measurement they choose.

Blood Pressure. Blood pressure may be determined directly with invasive measurement of pressures within arteries, or it may be determined indirectly through auscultation by an examiner or the use of an automated blood pressure device. The American Heart Association has provided guidelines for the measurement of blood pressure with sphygmomanometers.[71] Several researchers have compared measurements taken with different blood pressure monitoring equipment.[72–74]

Like heart rate, blood pressure is a labile phenomenon that may differ within an individual on the basis of the individual's emotional state, physical activity, and food and drink consumption. No matter which instrumentation a researcher uses to measure blood pressure, he or she must carefully control extraneous factors that may alter blood pressure.

Fitness. Maximum oxygen consumption (max VO_2) is the standard against which other measures of fitness are compared. Max VO_2 is measured by analyzing the exhaled gases of a person who exercises in graded increments until oxygen consumption levels off or begins to decrease.[75] Such measures may be obtained manually through systems that collect expired gases or automatically by systems that analyze expired gases continuously (Figure 12–8).[76] Nelson and colleagues used automated oxygen consumption measurement in a study of changes in fitness during training.[77] Gussoni and associates used manual oxygen consumption measurement in a study of the energy cost of walking with hip joint impairment.[78]

In addition to *direct* measurements of oxygen consumption, numerous tests *estimate* oxygen consumption by determining the distance a subject can run or walk in a specified period of time or the heart rate a subject achieves during a submaximal bout of bicycling, walking or jogging on a treadmill, or ascending and descending a step.[75, 79] Amundsen and associates used a step test to estimate the fitness of elderly women before and after an exercise program.[80]

Blood Flow. Because several physical therapy techniques are purported to work by increasing local blood flow, physical therapy researchers may have an interest in measuring the blood flow to an area before and after a given treatment. Doppler flowmeters provide a noninvasive way of determining blood flow. The hand-held Doppler device contains transmitting and receiving ultrasound

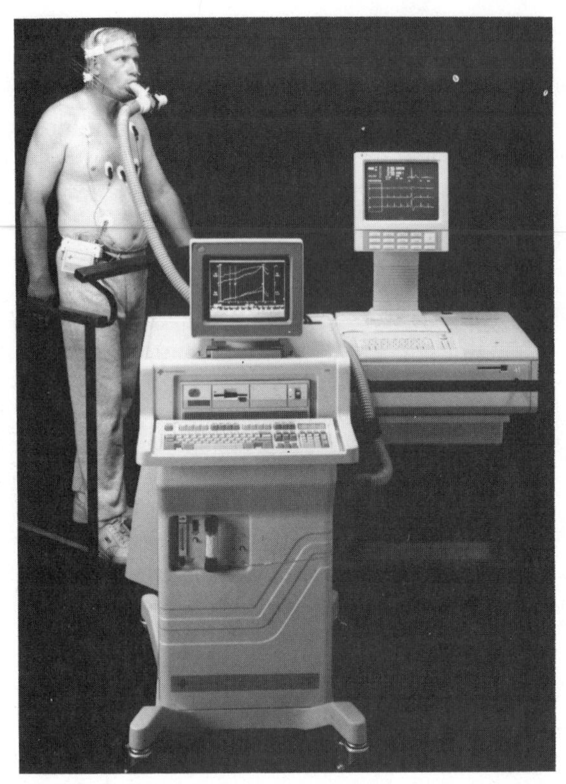

FIGURE 12–8. Automatic gas analysis system for evaluating maximum oxygen consumption. Photo courtesy of Sensormedics, 22705 Savi Ranch Parkway, Yorba Linda, CA 92687.

crystals that are placed over the vessel in which blood flow is being measured. The blood flow pattern can be printed on a chart recorder, providing both quantitative measures of flow and qualitative interpretations based on the shape of the curve.[81, 82] Walker and associates used a Doppler flowmeter to study the effect of high-voltage pulsed electrical stimulation on blood flow.[83] Skin temperature changes have also been used as an indirect measure of blood flow.[84]

Pulmonary Measures

The measures of pulmonary function can be grossly divided into those that assess the mechanics of breathing and those that assess physiological function. One of each type of test is described below.

Forced Expiratory Volume. Forced expiratory volume (FEV) is measured to assess a person's ability to move air out of the lungs. A spirometer measures the volume of air expired after a maximal inspiration (Figure 12–9). FEV_1 is a variant of FEV that documents the proportion of air that is expelled in the first second of a forced exhalation. Protas has reviewed reliability issues in pulmonary function testing.[68] Cerny used FEV, FEV_1, and related measures to document pulmonary function in children with cystic fibrosis.[85]

Oxygen Saturation. Noninvasive oximeters can be used to measure the level of oxygen saturation in the blood. Because oxygen saturation is related to arterial oxygenation, oximetry provides a useful measure of physiological function. Cerny used an ear oxime-

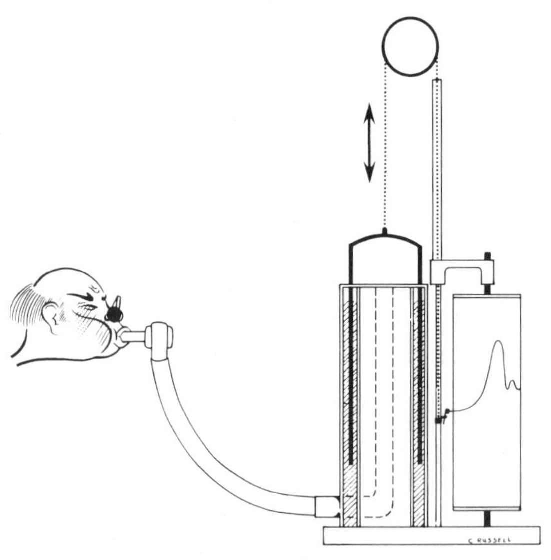

FIGURE 12–9. Spirometer. From Shaffer TH, Wolfson MR, Gault JH. Respiratory physiology. In: Irwin S, Tecklin JS, eds. *Cardiopulmonary Physical Therapy*. St. Louis, Mo: CV Mosby Co; 1985:176.

ter that clips to the earlobe to measure saturation in children with cystic fibrosis.[85] Kelly and colleagues used a pulse oximeter attached to the foot to determine saturation levels in preterm infants.[86]

Autonomic Function

Physical therapists are often interested in whether the goal of relaxation has been achieved. However, few investigators have effectively quantified changes in autonomic function that should indicate relaxation. Measures that have been used include heart rate,[84, 87, 88] blood pressure,[84] galvanic skin response,[84] skin temperature,[84] and respiratory sinus arrhythmia.[87, 88] Galvanic skin response is related to sweat gland activity, which in turn is related to autonomic arousal.[89] Respiratory sinus arrhythmia—the rhythmic increase in heart rate associated with inspiration and the decrease associated with expiration—is thought to be an indication of vagal, or parasympathetic, tone.[87]

MEASURING PAIN

Pain is an abstract construct that a researcher can never directly observe. Quantification of pain usually takes one of three forms: use of descriptive words, assignment of numbers to indicate intensity, or documentation of tolerance to experimentally induced pain.

Using Descriptive Words

The most frequently cited tool that uses descriptive words to document pain is the McGill pain questionnaire.[90] Although the questionnaire consists of four parts, the second part is the most commonly quantified. It asks patients to indicate which of up to 20 words in 20 different categories best describes their pain. Longobardi and colleagues used the McGill pain questionnaire to study pain reduction caused by transcutaneous electrical nerve stimulation in patients with distal extremity pain.[91]

Assigning Numbers to Pain Intensity

Researchers may use a visual analog scale (VAS) to quantify the nature of pain. The typical VAS is a 10-cm line with words such as "worst pain I ever felt" and "no pain" at the ends of the line. The subject marks the line at the point that represents his or her pain perception.[92] The investigator then measures the distance from the end of the line that represents no pain to the subject's mark. Price and colleagues have examined the reliability and validity of the VAS for both chronic and experimental pain.[93] Longobardi and colleagues used a VAS to supplement the information they obtained with the McGill pain questionnaire in patients with distal extremity pain.[91]

Another instrument, the Pain Disability Index, quantifies not the pain itself, but the level of disability resulting from the pain. Tait and associates have described this index and its use with patients in pain.[94]

Experimentally Induced Pain

Pain has been induced experimentally by electrical stimulation, thermal stimulation, or induction of extremity ischemia through use of a tourniquet.[95] Noling and colleagues used electrical stimulation to induce pain in their study of the effect of auricular transcutaneous electrical nerve stimulation on pain threshold at the wrist. The electrical stimulation was increased in small increments until the subject identified the sensation as painful. The researchers evaluated the effectiveness of the treatment by determining changes in the amount of current tolerated before and after the treatment.[96]

MEASURING FUNCTIONAL STATUS

Restoration of physical function is the ultimate goal of physical therapy. Despite this, physical therapists seem to document physical impairments such as range-of-motion limitation or muscle performance deficits far more frequently than they document functional status. Assessment of functional status takes two main forms: assessment of activities of daily living and assessment of task-specific function.

Tests of Activities of Daily Living

The state of the art in functional status assessment has been reviewed by Jette and by Guccione and associates.[97, 98] They compared several measures that assess activities of daily living (ADL). Others have reviewed the reliability, validity, and ordinal scaling of functional status assessments.[99–102] One of the most frequently reported ADL assessments is the Barthel Index. The Barthel Index evaluates subjects' performance of 10 functional tasks according to the level of independence shown in each task. Scores on each task are added together to generate a single numerical score for physical function. Yarkony and colleagues used a modification of the Barthel Index as the dependent measure in their study of rehabilitation outcomes in patients with thoracic spinal cord injury.[103]

Task-Specific Functional Assessment

Physical therapists are often interested in a patient's ability to return to his or her previous employment setting. Assessing the ability to return to previous work depends on whether the patient can perform tasks that are specific to the work environment. Baxter-Petralia and associates have reviewed the major tools used to evaluate the physical capacity of the hand and upper extremity.[104] Physical therapists working in occupational rehabilitation may also use more global assessments of functional capacity that determine the patient's ability to lift, push, pull, or carry certain amounts of weight; assess the patient's tolerance for standing, sitting, and walking; determine the pace at which the patient can work; and assess the patient's safety during various work-related maneuvers.[105, 106] Physical therapists who work with athletes may find sport skill tests useful for the study of athletic function.[107]

MEASURING MOVEMENT USING BIOMECHANICAL ANALYSIS

Biomechanical analysis of movement is highly technical and can be divided into kinematics (the study of movement) and kinetics (the study of the forces that underlie movement). Winter's classic text on biomechanics provides basic information about the various biomechanical procedures.[56]

Kinematics

A major kinematic measurement technique is the filming of subjects in motion. Motion picture cameras (cinematography) can shoot at fast speeds to capture very fast motions. Video techniques sample at a slower number of frames per second and can be used for slower motions. Before a subject is filmed, body landmarks are marked with tape or lights that are easily visualized on the film. The coordinates of the landmarks are determined by a process called *digitizing*. Cinematographic digitizing is accomplished by projecting each frame of the film onto a digitizing pad and identifying the landmarks with an electronic pointer that determines the coordinates for each point. An interface with a computer allows relatively efficient calculation of angles between body segments from the marked coordinates. Video digitizing is accomplished by displaying each of the video frames on a monitor and using a computer mouse to identify the points of interest; the coordinates are stored in a computer. Optoelectric systems use light-emitting diodes as landmarks and require no hand digitizing (Figure 12–10).[108, 109]

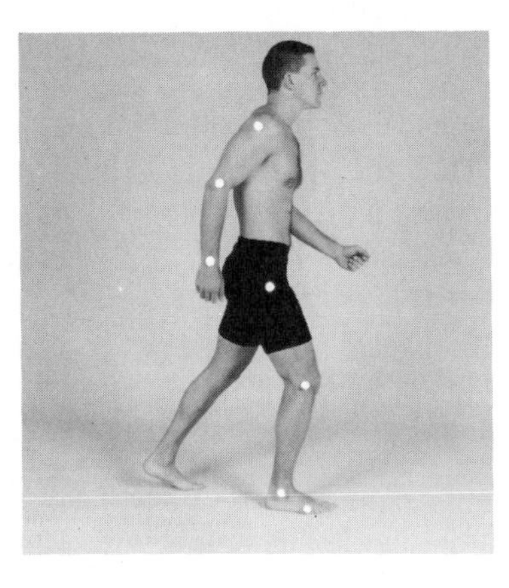

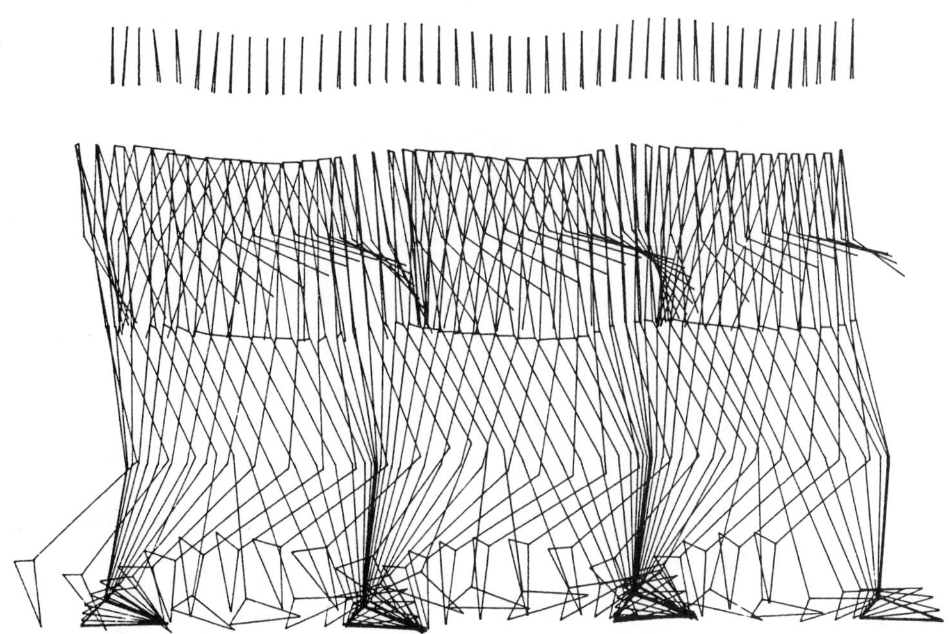

FIGURE 12–10. Video motion measurement system. **A**. Light-emitting diodes affixed to subject. **B**. Stick figures generated from video of subject with diodes. Courtesy of Peak Performance Technologies, Suite 601, 7388 South Revere Parkway, Englewood, CO 80112.

Blanke and Hageman used high-speed (100 frames per second) cinematography and digitizing to compare the gait characteristics of young and elderly men.[110] Heriza used videotaping (60 frames per second) and digitizing to study leg movements in preterm infants.[111] Kluzik and colleagues used an optoelectrical video system to analyze reaching movements in children with cerebral palsy.[112]

In addition to filming, kinematic studies may use electrogoniometers (see Extrinsic Joint Motions) and accelerometers to measure motion. Accelerometers attach to a limb segment and measure the acceleration of that segment. Like electrogoniometers, accelerometers may be uniaxial or triaxial.[108, 109]

Less technical approaches to kinematic studies of gait are footprint analysis,[113, 114] use of a floor grid,[115] and direct measurement of angles from projected video images.[114]

Kinetics

Kinetics is the study of the forces that underlie movements. One tool of kinetic analysis is EMG, which is used to study patterns of muscular activation during movement, as discussed earlier in the chapter (see Electrical Activity). A second major kinetic measurement tool is the force platform. The force platform is typically used in gait studies to determine ground reaction forces.[116] Schuit and colleagues used a force platform to analyze the effect of heel lifts on ground reaction force patterns in subjects with leg-length discrepancies.[117] Integration of film, EMG, and force platform data can provide a very complex description of the kinetics of movement throughout a range of motion.[109, 116]

MEASURING SIZES AND PROPORTIONS OF BODY PARTS (ANTHROPOMETRIC MEASURES)

Anthropometric measures document the size and proportions of segments of the human body. Major items assessed include segmental length, surface area, girth, volume, and body composition.

Segmental Length

Standardized procedures for determining segmental length, such as forearm or leg length, have been described by Lohman and associates.[118] Accurate measurement of segmental lengths requires an anthropometric caliper set and a narrow metal tape measure.

Surface Area

The most common reason that physical therapists measure surface area is to document the size of wounds. Bohannon and Pfaller describe three methods of quantifying the size of wound through the use of transparent wound tracings: superimposing the tracing on graph paper; weighing a cutout of the tracing; and using a planimeter, which calculates surface area directly.[119] Kloth and Feedar superimposed wound tracings on graph paper to document wound size in their study of the effectiveness of a high-voltage current on wound healing.[120]

Girth

Girth is determined by measuring the circumference of a body segment at reproducible levels. For example, calf girth might be measured at the level of the tibial tubercle and at 5, 10, 15, and 20 cm distal to the tibial tubercle. Lohman recommends the use of a metal tape to prevent stretching and deformation of the tape itself, which may occur with fabric or plastic tapes.[118] Controlled-tension tapes may also be used. Controlled-tension tapes have a spring on one end that allows the examiner to pull the tape to a consistent pressure at each measurement (Figure 12–11). This reduces the variability that occurs when an examiner uses different amounts of tension on the tape on different measuring occasions or when different examiners use different amounts of tension. A controlled-tension tape was used by Weiss and colleagues to document circumference changes in response to heavy resistance exercise of the triceps surae muscles.[13]

Girth has sometimes been used to document muscle hypertrophy after an exercise program. Use of girth in this fashion must be assessed carefully because an increase in girth caused by an increase in muscle size may be attenuated by a decrease in body fat that may accompany initiation of an exercise program.[121]

Volume

Volumeters collect and measure water displaced by immersing a limb to a certain point (Figure 12–12). Waylett-Rendall and Seibly documented the accuracy of a commercially available volumeter.[122] Griffin and associates used a volumeter to document volume changes after intermittent compression or electrical stimulation in patients with chronic hand edema.[123]

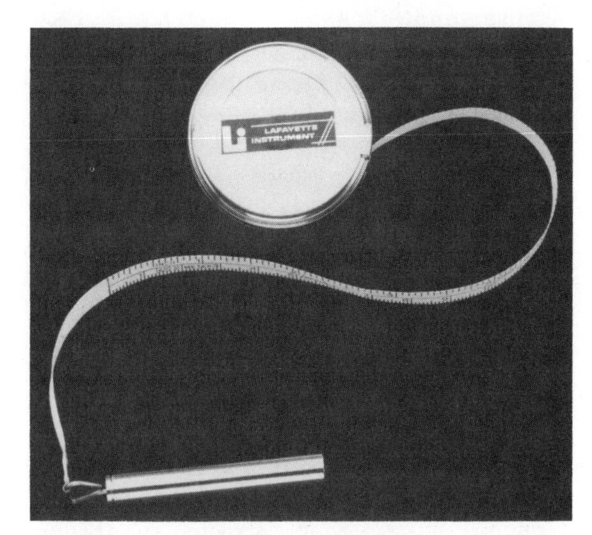

FIGURE 12–11. Controlled tension tape measure. Photo courtesy of Lafayette Instruments, 3700 Sagamore Parkway North, Lafayette, IN 47903.

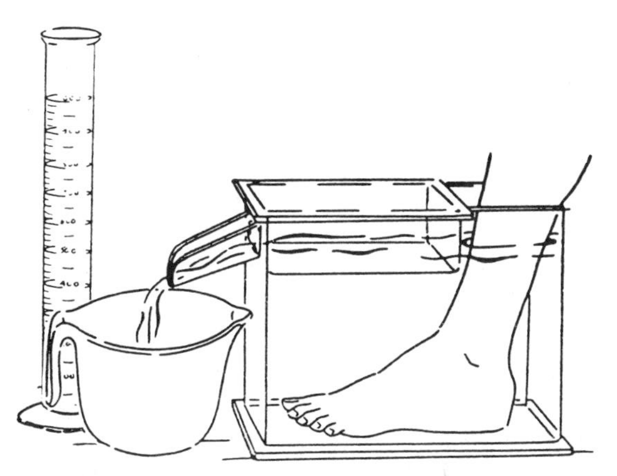

FIGURE 12–12. Foot volumeter. Courtesy of Volumeters Unlimited, 1307 Sandra Way, Redlands, CA 92374.

Body Composition

The proportion of lean body mass to fat is often of interest to physical therapists. The proportion may be calculated for the whole body or for a particular body segment. Subcutaneous fat thickness has been determined with skinfold calipers,[124] ultrasound,[125] magnetic resonance imaging,[125] and computerized axial tomography.[121] Measurements of subcutaneous fat thickness are often used as variables in equations calculated to predict body density or percentage of body fat.[124, 126] Researchers must be sure that the equations they are using were developed for use with a population similar to the one they are studying.

Measures of body density that do not depend on measurement of subcutaneous fat thickness are hydrostatic weighing and body impedance analysis. Hydrostatic weighing requires that the subject be able to tolerate complete immersion in either a specially designed tank or a Hubbard tank that has been modified to include a scale.[127] Body impedance analysis is easier to accomplish because it requires only that electrodes be placed in a few limb locations.[128]

MEASURING POSTURAL CONTROL

Postural control has been defined as the ability to maintain equilibrium in a gravitational field.[129] Measurement of postural control has traditionally been divided into measurement of static balance and measurement of dynamic balance. Berg has recently reviewed the literature on the measurement of balance.[130]

Static Balance

In tests of static balance, subjects either do not move or do not have their balance challenged in any way. Researchers often measure static balance with the subject under different sensory conditions to differentiate sensorimotor impairments from neuromuscular or musculoskeletal dysfunction.

Some of the most frequently cited measures of static balance are variations on the Romberg test. Differences in body sway are observed with subjects' eyes open and closed as they stand with their feet together, in a heel-to-toe position, or on one leg.[131] The length of time that subjects can maintain these positions is often determined. Bohannon and colleagues studied the timed static balance tests and determined normative values for individuals in each decade from 20 to 70 years of age.[132]

Shumway-Cook and Horak have developed a series of balance tests that vary sensory input to a greater extent than simply having the subjects open or close their eyes.[133] Three visual conditions are included: eyes open, eyes closed, and inaccurate visual input. Two different supporting surfaces are included: firm and compliant. Each visual condition is combined with each surface condition, yielding a total of six trials under different sensory conditions.

Documentation of sway in standing has also been used to quantify postural control. Fernie and Holliday used a system in which a belt was hooked to a patient, and cables from the belt ran to potentiometers that were stimulated when the patient swayed.[134] Speed of sway and the amplitude of movement were both used as indicators of balance ability in normal subjects and amputees. Sway can also be documented with a force platform. Dettman and colleagues used a force platform to quantify postural stability in patients with hemiplegia.[135]

Dynamic Balance

In tests of dynamic balance, patients either move or have their balance challenged in some way. A relatively simple dynamic measure is the Postural Stress Test developed by Wolfson and colleagues.[136] In this test, a belt is attached to a patient, and weights of different proportions of body weight are dropped to cause a predictable displacement force to the subject. The subject's reaction to the force is graded according to the number of trials in which his or her balance response was effective, as well as the strategy the subject used to maintain balance. Chandler and colleagues found that the Postural Stress Test differentiated between elderly subjects who fell and young and elderly subjects who did not fall.[137]

Other means of providing postural displacements are moveable platforms and "visual" pushes that modify the visual environment to cause an inappropriate postural response that is then corrected by the patient.[138, 139]

Another type of dynamic balance test is a

performance test. Mathias and colleagues developed what they called the "Get-up and Go" test, in which patients perform a sequence of maneuvers including rising from a chair, walking, turning, and sitting down.[140] Berg and colleagues are in the process of developing and validating a functional measure of balance that includes some of the same components as the "Get-up and Go" test.[141]

MEASURING SENSATION

Sensation is a complex phenomenon mediated by a diverse set of mechano-, thermo-, nocio-, chemo-, and electroreceptors.[142] There are numerous clinical tests of specific components of the sensory system. Two of the most easily quantified tests of cutaneous sensation are two-point discrimination and monofilament sensibility.

Two-point discrimination determines the minimum distance between two points that is detectable by a patient. Nolan provides procedures for two-point discrimination testing and normative data for two-point discrimination in different parts of the body for young adult men and women.[143–146]

The ability to detect different calibers of monofilaments provides another objective view of sensation.[147] The ends of different monofilaments are pressed into the surface of the skin until they bend. The patient is asked to indicate when he or she perceives a sensation. Subjects with better cutaneous sensation are able to detect smaller monofilaments than those with impaired sensation. Mueller and colleagues used a monofilament test to determine whether there were sensation differences between diabetic patients with and without foot ulcers and a nondiabetic control group.[148]

MEASURING DEVELOPMENT

Many different standardized tools are used to assess children's developmental status. Campbell reviewed many of the tools and noted that they test nine different theoretical aspects of motor development: speed, static body balance, dynamic body balance, coordination, strength, visual–motor tracking, response speed to a visual stimulus, visual–motor control of the hand, and upper extremity speed and precision in manipulation.[149] Tests used frequently include the Bayley Scales of Infant Development,[150] the Peabody Developmental Motor Scales,[150] and the Movement Assessment of Infants.[151] Harris used both the Bayley and Peabody scales to determine the effect of neurodevelopmental treatment on children with Down's syndrome.[152]

Several references provide broad-based information about various developmental tests. Stengel and colleagues' chapter in *Pediatric Neurologic Physical Therapy* provides a detailed overview of developmental testing from the perspective of physical therapists.[153] *Tests and Measurements in Child Development* and *Mental Measurements Yearbook* are comprehensive references that include test descriptions, information about obtaining the tests, and reviews of literature related to the tests.[154, 155]

MEASURING BEHAVIOR

Sometimes one is interested in whether treatment has affected some behavior that has either been absent or inconsistently demonstrated in the past. A general approach to quantifying behavior is behavior sampling. The subject is observed at different times or in different situations to determine the presence or absence or the frequency with which a particular behavior occurs within the given time frame.[156] In a directed behavioral analysis, the client is asked to perform skills during the observation. Hulme and associates used directed behavioral analysis to determine whether adaptive seating devices influenced the sitting, head control, and reaching and grasping activities of adolescents with multiple handicaps.[157] In undirected behavioral analysis, researchers observe and document behavior unobtrusively rather than requesting performance of a certain skill. Horowitz and Sharby used an undirected approach to study the development of prone extension postures in healthy infants.[158]

MEASURING PERSONAL CHARACTERISTICS, OPINIONS, AND ATTITUDES (SELF-REPORT MEASURES)

Self-report measures are the foundation of *survey research.* The basic assumption of survey research is that meaningful information can be obtained by asking the parties of interest what they know, what they believe, and how they behave. This section of the chapter considers the types of information that can be gleaned by self-report measures, the methods of collecting that information, the types of items that can be used to collect the desired information, and the use of existing self-report instruments.

Types of Self-Report Information

The scope of information that can be obtained through self-report instruments is vast. Concrete facts, knowledge, and behavior can be documented, as can abstract opinions and personal characteristics. The physical therapy literature contains examples of each of the five types of survey information just mentioned. Holcomb and associates conducted a primarily factual study about the scholarly productivity of physical therapy faculty members.[159] Uili and colleagues studied physicians' knowledge of physical therapy procedures.[160] Glazer-Waldman and associates studied the health behaviors of physical therapists.[161] Durant and associates studied the patients' opinions about direct access to physical therapy services.[162] Rezler and French studied the personality types and learning preferences of several groups of students in the allied health professions.[163]

Data Collection Methods

There are three classic methods of collecting survey data: personal interviews, telephone interviews, and written questionnaires. Although written questionnaires can be administered in person, the most common method is to administer them through the mail. Each of the three methods has its advantages and disadvantages, as indicated in Table 12–1. Procedural guidelines for developing questions, conducting interviews, and administering questionnaires are offered in Chapter 19.

One specialized questionnaire approach, the *Delphi technique*, uses several rounds of questionnaires that compensate for some of the limitations of administration of a single questionnaire. The Delphi technique was designed as a consensus-generating technique that eliminates the interpersonal factors that influence group decisions made in traditional meetings. These factors include the undue influence of a dominant personality and the willingness of less vocal members to acquiesce for the sake of achieving consensus.[164]

In a Delphi study, respondents complete and return a first-round questionnaire. A group of experts evaluate the first-round responses and compile results; the results are returned to the respondents for review and comment (the second round). The experts review the second-round responses and compile results; again, the results are sent back to the respondents for a third round. This iterative sequence is repeated until the responses from a round are consistent with the responses of the previous round. Miles-Tapping and colleagues used a Delphi approach to

TABLE 12–1. Advantages and Disadvantages of Interviews and Questionnaires

Characteristic	Method: Personal Interview	Telephone Interview	Mailed Questionnaire
Time	Very time consuming	Time consuming	Efficient
Cost	Personnel to do interviews, travel	Personnel to do interviews, long-distance telephone	Clerical personnel, printing and mailing
Geographic distribution of respondents	Greatly limited unless well funded	Somewhat limited unless well funded	Least limited because mailing is less expensive than travel
Depth of response	Can be extensive	Somewhat limited	Limited
Anonymity	Difficult to achieve	Difficult to achieve	Easily achieved
Literacy of respondents	Can sample those unable to read/write	Can sample those unable to read/write	Respondents must be able to read and write
Ability to clarify questions	Possible	Possible	Impossible
Scheduling	Must coordinate researcher's and respondents' schedules	Must coordinate researcher's and respondents' schedules	Completed at respondents' convenience

determine Canadian physical therapists' priorities for clinical research.[165]

Types of Interview and Questionnaire Items

Although the format of interview and questionnaire items is limited only by the creativity of the researcher, several standard item formats exist. The broadest distinction among item types is open- versus closed-format items. The closed-format items are divided further into multiple-choice, Likert-type, semantic differential, and Q-sort items.

Open-Format Items

Open-format items permit a flexible response. Interviews frequently include open-format items, and it is these open-format items that allow for the greater breadth of response that is listed as an advantage of using the interview in survey research. Suppose that a researcher is interested in identifying the sources of job satisfaction and dissatisfaction for hospital-based physical therapists. An open-format interview question might be, "What about your job is satisfying to you?" Respondents would be free to structure their responses as desired. Some might emphasize aspects of patient care, others might focus on working with a respected leader within the department, others might discuss the quality of interactions among coworkers, and others might list several different satisfying aspects of their work.

Questionnaires may also include open-format items, although the depth of response depends on the respondents' ability to communicate in writing and their willingness to provide an in-depth answer in the absence of an interviewer who can prompt them and provide encouragement during the course of their response.

The major difficulty with open-format items is their analysis. The researcher must sift and categorize the responses into a relatively small number of manageable categories. The literature on the qualitative research paradigm provides guidelines for the classification of responses from open-format items.[166, 167] The categorization of responses from open-format items is sometimes used as the basis for writing the fixed alternatives needed for closed-format items.

Closed-Format Items

Closed-format items restrict the range of possible responses. Mailed questionnaires often include a high proportion of closed-format responses. In addition, highly structured interviews may use closed-format responses. In such a case, the interview becomes an orally administered questionnaire, and the breadth of response characteristic of the interview format is lost. Four types of closed-format items are common: multiple-choice, Likert-type, semantic differential, and Q-sort items.

Multiple-Choice Items. Multiple-choice items can be used to measure knowledge, behavior, opinions, or personal characteristics. Some researchers design closed-format items that allow some flexibility of response by including "other" as a possible response and permitting respondents to write in a response of their choice.[168] In a study comparing public opinion responses to open- and closed-format items, few respondents took advantage of the "other" category in closed-format items.[169]

In a variation of the multiple-choice item, a vignette may be used as the stem of the item. A vignette is a short story or scenario that sets a scene. Kvitek and associates used vignettes to determine the goals that physical therapists would set for two different patients with amputations.[170] Each patient's age, level of amputation, occupation, and marital status were described in the vignettes. Vignettes permit researchers to evaluate responses to a complex circumstance that may better approximate clinical settings than traditional multiple-choice items.

Likert-Type Items. Likert-type items, named for their originator, are used to assess the strength of response to a declarative statement. The most typical set of responses includes "strongly agree," "agree," "undecided," "disagree," and "strongly disagree." Many others are available, a few of which are "very important" to "very unimportant," "strongly encourage" to "strongly discourage," and "definitely yes" to "definitely no."[171(p55)] Likert-type items were included in the Maslach Burnout Inventory used by Deckard and Present to study the impact of role stress on the emotional and physical well-being of physical therapists.[172]

Semantic Differential Items. Semantic differential items are based on the work of Osgood and colleagues in the 1950s.[173] Semantic differential items consist of adjective pairs that represent different ends of a continuum. The respondent indicates the place on the continuum that best represents the item or person being described. If semantic differential items were used to study physical therapists' opinions about their department, word pairs such as "cohesive–fragmented," "invigorating–dull," and "organized–disorganized" might be used to elicit their opinions. Semantic differential items were used by Streed and Stoecker to assess the levels of stereotyping in physical therapy and occupational therapy students.[174]

Q-Sort Items. A Q-sort is a method of forced-choice ranking of many alternatives.[175] It could be used to study job satisfaction in physical therapists. To do so, the researcher would generate a set of, say, 50 items about the job that might be important to physical therapists. Example items might be "chance to rotate among services," "weekends off," and "availability of physical therapist assistants." Each item would be written on a single card. Each therapist in the study would be asked to sort the cards into categories based on a preset distribution. For example, for our 50-card sort there might be five categories with the following forced distribution: exceedingly important (4 cards), very important (10 cards), moderately important (22 cards), minimally important (10 cards), and of negligible importance (4 cards). This distribution would force therapists to differentiate among a set of job satisfaction items by identifying the very few that are most important as well as the very few that are least important. Responses could be quantified by assigning numerals to each category (exceedingly important = 5; of negligible importance = 1) and adding the scores for each item across therapists. Items with the highest scores would be those that were consistently placed in the more important categories.

Freihofer and Felton used Q-sort methodology to determine that family members of dying patients valued the following nursing behaviors most highly: keeping patients pain free, promoting their physical comfort, and maintaining good grooming.[176]

Existing Self-Report Instruments

Researchers who wish to study behaviors and attitudes have a wide range of existing instruments available to them. Several of the studies cited in the section above used existing instruments: the Myers-Briggs Type Indicator,[163] the Maslach Burnout Inventory,[172] the Health Team Stereotyping Scale,[174] and the Health Risk Appraisal.[161] Existing instruments that are commercially available and frequently cited in the literature can be identified from references such as *Mental Measurements Yearbook* and *Tests in Print*.[155, 177] The text *Instruments for Clinical Nursing Research* includes descriptions of existing measures for constructs such as quality of life, coping, hope, self-care, and body image.[178] An instrument that was developed for a single study can often be obtained by writing the researcher. Even if an instrument has been used only once before, there is a base of information about the tool on which subsequent research can build. Thus, researchers are encouraged to seek out existing self-report tools that meet their needs before they develop their own.

SUMMARY

A vast array of measurement tools are available to physical therapists. Tools for the measurement of 12 major constructs within physical therapy have been widely reported: muscle performance; joint motion; physiological function; pain; functional status; biomechanics; anthropometrics; postural control; sensation; developmental status; behavior; and personal characteristics and attitudes. Physical therapy clinicians must critically evaluate the measures they use to document patient status, readers of the literature need to critically examine the measurement tools described in research reports, and researchers must critically evaluate their measurement options to determine which tool is most appropriate for the study at hand.

References

1. *Standards for Tests and Measurements in Physical Therapy Practice*. Alexandria, Va: American Physical Therapy Association; 1990.
2. *Resource and Buyer's Guide*. Alexandria, Va: American Physical Therapy Association; 1992.
3. Mayhew TP, Rothstein JM. Measurement of muscle performance with instruments. In: Rothstein JM, ed. *Measurement in Physical Therapy*. New York, NY: Churchill Livingstone; 1985:57–102.
4. Lamb RL. Manual muscle testing. In: Rothstein JM, ed. *Measurement in Physical Therapy*. New York, NY: Churchill Livingstone; 1985:47–55.
5. Wadsworth CT, Krishnan R, Sear M, Harrold J, Nielsen DH. Intrarater reliability of manual muscle testing and hand-held dynametric muscle testing. *Phys Ther*. 1987;67:1342–1347.
6. Frese E, Brown M, Norton BJ. Clinical reliability of manual muscle testing: middle trapezius and gluteus medius muscles. *Phys Ther*. 1987;67:1072–1076.
7. Bohannon RW. Test-retest reliability of hand-held dynamometry during a single session of strength assessment. *Phys Ther*. 1986;66:206–209.
8. Riddle DL, Finucane SD, Rothstein JM, Walker ML. Intrasession and intersession reliability of

hand-held dynamometer measurements taken on brain-damaged patients. *Phys Ther.* 1989;69:182–189.

9. Stuberg WA, Metcalf WK. Reliability of quantitative muscle testing in healthy children and in children with Duchenne muscular dystrophy using a hand-held dynamometer. *Phys Ther.* 1988; 68:977–982.
10. Bohannon RW, Andrews AW. Interrater reliability of hand-held dynamometry. *Phys Ther.* 1987; 67:931–933.
11. Bohannon RW, Andrews AW. Influence of head-neck rotation on static elbow flexion force of paretic side in patients with hemiparesis. *Phys Ther.* 1989;69:135–137.
12. Spielholz NI. Scientific bases of exercise programs. In Basmajian JV, Wolf SL, eds. *Therapeutic Exercise.* 5th ed. Baltimore, Md: Williams & Wilkins; 1990:58.
13. Weiss LW, Clark FC, Howard DG. Effects of heavy-resistance triceps surae muscle training on strength and muscularity of men and women. *Phys Ther.* 1988;68:208–213.
14. Pelletier JR, Findley TW, Gemma SA. Isometric exercise for an individual with hemophilic arthropathy. *Phys Ther.* 1987;67:1359–1364.
15. Vaughan VG. Effects of upper limb immobilization on isometric muscle strength, movement time, and triphasic electromyographic characteristics. *Phys Ther.* 1989;69:119–129.
16. Fess EE. Documentation: essential elements of an upper extremity assessment battery. In: Hunter JM, Schneider LH, Macklin EJ, Callahan AD, eds. *Rehabilitation of the Hand: Surgery and Therapy.* 3rd ed. St. Louis, Mo: CV Mosby Co; 1990:53–81.
17. Mathiowetz V, Kashman N, Volland G, Weber K, Dowe M, Rogers S. Grip and pinch strength: normative data for adults. *Arch Phys Med Rehabil.* 1985;66:69–74.
18. Jansen CWS, Minerbo G. A comparison between early dynamically controlled mobilization and immobilization after flexor tendon repair in zone 2 of the hand: preliminary results. *Journal of Hand Therapy.* 1990;3:20–25.
19. Rothstein JM, Lamb RL, Mayhew TP. Clinical uses of isokinetic measurements: critical issues. *Phys Ther.* 1987;67:1840–1844.
20. Parnianpour M, Li F, Nordin M, Kahanovitz N. A database of isoinertial trunk strength tests against three resistance levels in sagittal, frontal, and transverse planes in normal male subjects. *Spine.* 1989;14:409–411.
21. Francis K, Hoobler T. Comparison of peak torque values of the knee flexor and extensor muscle groups using the Cybex II and Lido 2.0 isokinetic dynamometers. *Journal of Orthopaedic and Sports Physical Therapy.* 1987;8:481–483.
22. Thompson MC, Shingleton LG, Kegerreis ST. Comparison of values generated during testing of the knee using the Cybex II Plus and Biodex Model B-2000 isokinetic dynamometers. *Journal of Orthopaedic and Sports Physical Therapy.* 1989;11:108–115.
23. Brown M, Kohrt WM, Delitto A. Peak torque to body weight ratios in older adults: a re-examination. *Physiotherapy Canada.* 1991;43:7–11.
24. Winter DA, Wells RP, Orr GW. Errors in the use of isokinetic dynamometers. *Eur J Appl Physiol.* 1981;46:397–408.
25. Echternach JL. Measurement issues in nerve conduction velocity and electromyographic testing. In: Rothstein JM, ed. *Measurement in Physical Therapy.* New York, NY: Churchill Livingstone; 1985:281–304.
26. Soderberg GL, Cook TM. Electromyography in biomechanics. *Phys Ther.* 1984;64:1813–1820.
27. Portney L. Electromyography and nerve conduction velocity tests. In: O'Sullivan SB, Schmitz TJ, eds. *Physical Rehabilitation: Assessment and Treatment.* 2nd ed. Philadelphia, Pa: FA Davis Co; 1988:159–194.
28. Fridlund AJ, Cacioppo JT. Guidelines for human electromyographic research. *Psychophysiology.* 1986;23:567–589.
29. Duncan PW, Studenski S, Chandler J, Bloomfeld R, LaPointe LK. Electromyographic analysis of postural adjustments in two methods of balance testing. *Phys Ther.* 1990;70:88–96.
30. Hanten WP, Schulthies SS. Exercise effect on electromyographic activity of the vastus medialis oblique and vastus lateralis muscles. *Phys Ther.* 1990;70:561–565.
31. O'Sullivan SB. Motor control assessment. In: O'Sullivan SB, Schmitz TJ, eds. *Physical Rehabilitation: Assessment and Treatment.* 2nd ed. Philadelphia, Pa: FA Davis Co; 1988:135–158.
32. Bohannon RW, Smith MB. Interrater reliability of a modified Ashworth scale of muscle spasticity. *Phys Ther.* 1987;67:206–207.
33. Minor MAD, Minor SD. *Patient Evaluation Methods for the Health Professional.* Reston, Va: Reston Publishing Co Inc; 1987:181.
34. Worley JS, Bennett W, Miller G, Miller M, Walter B, Harmon C. Reliability of three clinical measures of muscle tone in the shoulders and wrists of post-stroke patients. *Am J Occup Ther.* 1991;45:50–58.
35. Bajd T, Vodovnik L. Pendulum testing of spasticity. *J Biomed Eng.* 1984;6:9–16.
36. Bohannon RW, Larkin PA. Cybex II isokinetic dynamometer for the documentation of spasticity. *Phys Ther.* 1985;65:46–47.
37. Bohannon RW. Variability and reliability of the pendulum test for spasticity using a Cybex II isokinetic dynamometer. *Phys Ther.* 1987;67:659–661.
38. Bajd T, Gregoric M, Vodovnik L, Benko H. Electrical stimulation in treating spasticity resulting from spinal cord injury. *Arch Phys Med Rehabil.* 1985;66:515–517.
39. Corcos DM. Strategies underlying the control of disordered movement. *Phys Ther.* 1991;71:25–38.
40. Wolf SL, LeCraw DE, Barton LA. Comparison of motor copy and targeted biofeedback training techniques for restitution of upper extremity function among patients with neurologic disorders. *Phys Ther.* 1989;69:719–735.

41. Dickstein R, Pillar T, Shina N, Hocherman S. Electromyographic responses of distal ankle musculature of standing hemiplegic patients to continuous anterior-posterior perturbations during imposed weight transfer over the affected leg. *Phys Ther.* 1989;69:484–491.
42. Brown M. Resistance exercise effects on aging skeletal muscle in rats. *Phys Ther.* 1989;69:46–53.
43. Brown M, Baker RD. Effect of pulsed short wave diathermy on skeletal muscle injury in rabbits. *Phys Ther.* 1987;67:208–214.
44. Sinacore DR, Delitto A, King DS, Rose SJ. Type II fiber activation with electrical stimulation: a preliminary report. *Phys Ther.* 1990;70:416–422.
45. Miller PJ. Assessment of joint motion. In: Rothstein JM, ed. *Measurement in Physical Therapy.* New York, NY: Churchill Livingstone; 1985:103–136.
46. Gajdosik RL, Bohannon RW. Clinical measurement of range of motion: review of goniometry emphasizing reliability and validity. *Phys Ther.* 1987;67:1867–1872.
47. American Academy of Orthopaedic Surgeons. *Joint Motion: Method of Measuring and Recording.* Chicago, Ill: American Academy of Orthopaedic Surgeons; 1965.
48. Norkin CC, White DJ. *Measurement of Joint Motion: A Guide to Goniometry.* Philadelphia, Pa: FA Davis Co; 1985.
49. Boone DC, Azen SP, Lin CM, Spence C, Baron C, Lee L. Reliability of goniometric measurements. *Phys Ther.* 1978;58:1355–1360.
50. Rothstein JM, Miller PJ, Roettger RF. Goniometric reliability in a clinical setting: elbow and knee measurements. *Phys Ther.* 1983;63:1611–1615.
51. Mayerson NH, Milano RA. Goniometric reliability in physical medicine. *Arch Phys Med Rehabil.* 1984;65:92–94.
52. Breger-Lee D, Bell-Krotoski J, Brandsma JW. Torque range of motion in the hand clinic. *Journal of Hand Therapy.* 1990;1:7–13.
53. Merritt JL, McLean TJ, Erickson RP, Offord KP. Measurement of trunk flexibility in normal subjects: reproducibility of three clinical methods. *Mayo Clin Proc.* 1986;61:192–197.
54. Burdett RG, Brown KE, Fall MP. Reliability and validity of four instruments for measuring lumbar spine and pelvic positions. *Phys Ther.* 1986;66:677–684.
55. Youdas JW, Carey JR, Garrett TR. Reliability of measurement of cervical spine range of motion—comparison of three methods. *Phys Ther.* 1991;71:98–104.
56. Winter DA. *Biomechanics and Motor Control of Human Movement.* 2nd ed. New York, NY: John Wiley & Sons; 1990.
57. Condon SM, Hutton RS. Soleus muscle electromyographic activity and ankle dorsiflexion range of motion during four stretching procedures. *Phys Ther.* 1987;67:24–30.
58. Batti'e MC, Bigos SJ, Sheehy A, Wortley MD. Spinal flexibility and individual factors that influence it. *Phys Ther.* 1987;67:653–658.
59. Cambridge CA. Range-of-motion measurement of the hand. In: Hunter JM, Schneider LH, Macklin EJ, Callahan AD, eds. *Rehabilitation of the Hand: Surgery and Therapy.* 3rd ed. St. Louis, Mo: CV Mosby Co; 1990:82–92.
60. McClure PW, Rothstein JM, Riddle DL. Intertester reliability of clinical judgments of medial knee ligament integrity. *Phys Ther.* 1989;69:268–275.
61. Wroble RR, Van Ginkel LA, Grood ES, Noyes FR, Shaffer BL. Repeatability of the KT–1000 arthrometer in a normal population. *Am J Sports Med.* 1990;18:396–399.
62. Neuschwander DC, Drez D, Pains RM, Young JC. Comparison of anterior laxity measurements in anterior cruciate deficient knees with two instrumented testing devices. *Orthopedics.* 1990;13:299–302.
63. Klasen P. The intratester and intertester reliability of the posture gauge. Master's research project. Indianapolis, Ind: University of Indianapolis; 1990.
64. Lovell FW, Rothstein JM, Personius WJ. Reliability of clinical measurements of lumbar lordosis taken with a flexible ruler. *Phys Ther.* 1989;69:96–102.
65. Link CS, Nicholson GG, Shaddeau SA, Birch R, Gossman MR. Lumbar curvature in standing and sitting in two types of chairs: relationship of hamstring and hip flexor muscle length. *Phys Ther.* 1990;70:611–618.
66. Kispert CP. Clinical measurements to assess cardiopulmonary function. *Phys Ther.* 1987;67:1886–1890.
67. Sinacore DR, Ehsani AA. Measurements of cardiovascular function. In: Rothstein JM, ed. *Measurement in Physical Therapy.* New York, NY: Churchill Livingstone; 1985:225–280.
68. Protas EJ. Pulmonary function testing. In: Rothstein JM, ed. *Measurement in Physical Therapy.* New York, NY: Churchill Livingstone; 1985:229–254.
69. Sedlock DA, Knowlton RG, Fitzgerald PI, Tahamont MV, Schneider DA. Accuracy of subject-palpated carotid pulse after exercise. *The Physician and Sportsmedicine.* 1983;11(4):106–116.
70. Araujo J, Born DG, Thomas TR. An evaluation of five portable heart monitors. Abstract. *Med Sci Sports Exerc.* 1981;13:124.
71. Kirkendall WM, Feinleib M, Freis ED, Mark AI. Recommendations for human blood pressure determination by sphygmomanometers. *Hypertension.* 1981;3:510A–519A.
72. Barker WF, Hediger ML, Katz SH, Bowers EJ. Concurrent validity studies of blood pressure instrumentation: the Philadelphia blood pressure project. *Hypertension.* 1984;6:85–91.
73. O'Brien E, Fitzgerald D, O'Malley K. Blood pressure measurement: current practice and future trends. *Br Med J.* 1985;290:729–733.
74. Lightfoot JT, Tankersley C, Rowe SA, Freed AN, Fortney SM. Automated blood pressure measurements during exercise. *Med Sci Sports Exerc.* 1989;21:698–707.

75. McArdle WD, Katch FI, Katch VL. *Exercise Physiology: Energy, Nutrition, and Human Performance.* 3rd ed. Philadelphia, Pa: Lea & Febiger; 1991:212–213.
76. Wasserman K, Hansen JE, Sue DY, Whipp BJ. *Principles of Exercise Testing and Interpretation.* Philadelphia, Pa: Lea & Febiger; 1987:242–244.
77. Nelson AG, Arnall DA, Loy SF, Silvester LJ, Conlee RK. Consequences of combining strength and endurance training regimens. *Phys Ther.* 1990; 70:287–294.
78. Gussoni M, Margonato V, Ventura R, Veicsteinas A. Energy cost of walking with hip joint impairment. *Phys Ther.* 1990;70:295–301.
79. American College of Sports Medicine. *Guidelines for Exercise Testing and Prescription.* 4th ed. Philadelphia, Pa: Lea & Febiger; 1991:39–43.
80. Amundsen LR, DeVahl JM, Ellingham CT. Evaluation of a group exercise program for elderly women. *Phys Ther.* 1989;69:475–483.
81. Fronek A, Coel M, Bernstein EF. Quantitative ultrasonographic studies of lower extremity flow velocities in health and disease. *Circulation.* 1976;53:957–960.
82. Hurley JJ, Hershey FB, Auer AI, Binnington HB. Noninvasive evaluation of peripheral arterial status: the physiologic approach. In: Levin ME, O'Neal LW, eds. *The Diabetic Foot.* St. Louis, Mo: CV Mosby Co; 1983:120–132.
83. Walker DC, Currier DP, Threlkeld AJ. Effects of high voltage pulsed electrical stimulation on blood flow. *Phys Ther.* 1988;68:481–485.
84. Reed BV, Held JM. Effects of sequential connective tissue massage on autonomic nervous system of middle-aged and elderly adults. *Phys Ther.* 1988;68:1231–1234.
85. Cerny FJ. Relative effects of bronchial drainage and exercise for in-hospital care of patients with cystic fibrosis. *Phys Ther.* 1989;69:633–639.
86. Kelly MK, Palisano RJ, Wolfson MR. Effects of a developmental physical therapy program on oxygen saturation and heart rate in preterm infants. *Phys Ther.* 1989;69:467–474.
87. Cottingham JT, Porges SW, Lyon T. Effects of soft tissue mobilization (Rolfing pelvic lift) on parasympathetic tone in two age groups. *Phys Ther.* 1988;68:352–356.
88. Cottingham JT, Porges SW, Richmond K. Shifts in pelvic inclination angle and parasympathetic tone produced by Rolfing soft tissue manipulation. *Phys Ther.* 1988;68:1364–1370.
89. Marcer D. *Biofeedback and Related Therapies in Clinical Practice.* Rockville, Md: Aspen Publishers Inc; 1986:14.
90. Melzack R. The McGill pain questionnaire: major properties and scoring methods. *Pain.* 1975;1:277–299.
91. Longobardi AG, Clelland JA, Knowles CJ, Jackson JR. Effects of auricular transcutaneous electrical nerve stimulation on distal extremity pain: a pilot study. *Phys Ther.* 1989;69:10–17.
92. Bowsher D. Acute and chronic pain and assessment. In: Wells RE, Ramption V, Bowsher D, eds. *Pain Management in Physical Therapy.* Norwalk, Conn: Appleton & Lange; 1988.
93. Price DD, McGrath PA, Rafii A, Buckingham B. The validation of visual analogue scales as ratio scale measures for chronic and experimental pain. *Pain.* 1983;17:45–56.
94. Tait RC, Pollard A, Margolis RB, Duckro PN, Krause SJ. The Pain Disability Index: psychometric and validity data. *Arch Phys Med Rehabil.* 1987;68:438–441.
95. Echternach JL. Evaluation of pain in the clinical environment. In: Echternach JL, ed. *Pain.* New York, NY: Churchill Livingstone; 1987.
96. Noling LB, Clelland JA, Jackson JR, Knowles CJ. Effect of transcutaneous electrical nerve stimulation at auricular points on experimental cutaneous pain threshold. *Phys Ther.* 1988;68:328–332.
97. Jette AM. State of the art in functional status assessment. In: Rothstein JM, ed. *Measurement in Physical Therapy.* New York, NY: Churchill Livingstone; 1985.
98. Guccione AA, Cullen KE, O'Sullivan SB. Functional assessment. In: O'Sullivan SB, Schmitz TJ, eds. *Physical Rehabilitation: Assessment and Treatment.* 2nd ed. Philadelphia, Pa: FA Davis Co; 1988.
99. Merbitz C, Morris J, Grip JC. Ordinal scales and foundations of misinference. *Arch Phys Med Rehabil.* 1989;70:308–312.
100. Keith RA. Functional assessment measures in medical rehabilitation: current status. *Arch Phys Med Rehabil.* 1984;65:74–78.
101. Sheikh K. Disability scales: assessment of reliability. *Arch Phys Med Rehabil.* 1986;67:245–249.
102. Kaufert JM. Functional ability indices: measurement problems in assessing their validity. *Arch Phys Med Rehabil.* 1983;64:260–267.
103. Yarkony GM, Roth EJ, Meyer PR, Lovell LL, Heinemann AW. Rehabilitation outcomes in patients with complete thoracic spinal cord injury. *Am J Phys Med Rehabil.* 1990;69:23–27.
104. Baxter-Petralia PL, Bruening LA, Blackmore SM, McEntee PM. Physical capacity evaluation. In: Hunter JM, Schneider LH, Macklin EJ, Callahan AD, eds. *Rehabilitation of the Hand: Surgery and Therapy.* 3rd ed. St. Louis, Mo: CV Mosby Co; 1990.
105. Isernhagen SJ. Functional capacity evaluation. In: Isernhagen SJ, ed. *Work Injury: Management and Prevention.* Rockville, Md: Aspen Publishers Inc; 1988.
106. Key GL. Industrial physical therapy: an introduction. In: Gould JA. *Orthopaedic and Sports Physical Therapy.* 2nd ed. St. Louis, Mo: CV Mosby Co; 1990.
107. Bosco JS, Gustafson WF. *Measurement and Evaluation in Physical Education, Fitness, and Sports.* Englewood Cliffs, NJ: Prentice-Hall; 1983:227–272.
108. Robertson G, Sprigings E. Kinematics. In: Dainty DA, Norman RW, eds. *Standardized Biomechanical Testing in Sport.* Champaign, Ill: Human Kinetics Publishers Inc; 1987.
109. Dainty D, Gagnon M, Lagasse P, Norman R, Robertson G, Sprigings E. Recommended procedures.

In: Dainty DA, Norman RW, eds. *Standardized Biomechanical Testing in Sport.* Champaign, Ill: Human Kinetics Publishers Inc; 1987.
110. Blanke DJ, Hageman PA. Comparison of gait of young men and elderly men. *Phys Ther.* 1989; 69:144–148.
111. Heriza CB. Organization of leg movements in preterm infants. *Phys Ther.* 1988;68:1340–1346.
112. Kluzik J, Fetters L, Coryell J. Quantification of control: a preliminary study of effects of neurodevelopmental treatment on reaching in children with spastic cerebral palsy. *Phys Ther.* 1990;70:65–76.
113. Rose-Jacobs R. Development of gait at slow, free, and fast speeds in 3- and 5-year-old children. *Phys Ther.* 1983;63:1251–1259.
114. Burdett RG, Borello-France D, Blatchly C, Potter C. Gait comparison of subjects with hemiplegia walking unbraced, with ankle-foot orthosis, and with air-stirrup brace. *Phys Ther.* 1988;68:1197–1203.
115. Robinson JL, Smidt GL. Quantitative gait evaluation in the clinic. *Phys Ther.* 1981;61:351–353.
116. Gagnon M, Robertson G, Norman R. Kinetics. In: Dainty DA, Norman RW, eds. *Standardized Biomechanical Testing in Sport.* Champaign, Ill: Human Kinetics Publishers Inc; 1987.
117. Schuit D, Adrian M, Pidcoe P. Effect of heel lifts on ground reaction force patterns in subjects with structural leg-length discrepancies. *Phys Ther.* 1989;69:663–670.
118. Lohman TG, Roche AF, Martorell R, eds. *Anthropometric Standardization Reference Manual.* Champaign, Ill: Human Kinetics Publishers Inc; 1988.
119. Bohannon RW, Pfaller BA. Documentation of wound surface area from tracings of wound perimeters. *Phys Ther.* 1983;63:1622–1624.
120. Kloth LC, Feedar JA. Acceleration of wound healing with high voltage, monophasic, pulsed current. *Phys Ther.* 1988;68:503–508.
121. Cureton KJ, Collins MA, Hill DW, McElhannon FM. Muscle hypertrophy in men and women. *Med Sci Sports Exerc.* 1988;20:338–344.
122. Waylett-Rendall J, Seibly DS. A study of the accuracy of a commercially available volumeter. *Journal of Hand Therapy.* 1991;4:10–13.
123. Griffin JW, Newsome LS, Stralka SW, Wright PE. Reduction of chronic posttraumatic hand edema: a comparison of high voltage pulsed current, intermittent pneumatic compression, and placebo treatments. *Phys Ther.* 1990;70:279–286.
124. Jackson AS, Pollack ML. Practical assessment of body composition. *The Physician and Sportsmedicine.* 1985;13(5):76–90.
125. Hayes PA, Sowood PJ, Belyavin A, Cohen JB, Smith FW. Subcutaneous fat thickness measured by magnetic resonance imaging, ultrasound, and calipers. *Med Sci Sports Exerc.* 1988;20:303–309.
126. Oppliger RA, Spray JA. Skinfold measurement variability in body density prediction. *Research Quarterly for Exercise and Sport.* 1987;58:178–183.
127. Williams D, Anderson T, Currier D. Underwater weighing using the Hubbard tank vs the standard tank. *Phys Ther.* 1984;64:658–664.
128. Caton JR, Mole PA, Adams WC, Heustis DS. Body composition analysis by bioelectrical impedance: effect of skin temperature. *Med Sci Sports Exerc.* 1988;20:489–491.
129. Horak FB. Clinical measurement of postural control in adults. *Phys Ther.* 1987;67:1881–1885.
130. Berg K. Balance and its measure in the elderly: a review. *Physiotherapy Canada.* 1989;41:240–246.
131. Briggs RC, Gossman MR, Birch R, Drews JE, Shaddeau SA. Balance performance among noninstitutionalized elderly women. *Phys Ther.* 1989;69:748–756.
132. Bohannon RW, Larkin PA, Cook AC, Gear J, Singer J. Decrease in timed balance test scores with aging. *Phys Ther.* 1984;64:1067–1070.
133. Shumway-Cook A, Horak FB. Assessing the influence of sensory interaction on balance. *Phys Ther.* 1986;66:1548–1550.
134. Fernie GR, Holliday PJ. Postural sway in amputees and normal subjects. *J Bone Joint Surg.* 1978;60-A:895–898.
135. Dettman MA, Linder MT, Sepic SB. Relationships among walking performance, postural stability, and functional assessments of the hemiplegic patient. *Am J Phys Med.* 1987;66:77–90.
136. Wolfson LI, Whipple R, Amerman P, Kleinberg A. Stressing the postural response: a quantitative method for testing balance. *J Am Geriatr Soc.* 1986;34:845–850.
137. Chandler JM, Duncan PW, Studenski SA. Balance performance on the postural stress test: comparison of young adults, healthy elderly, and fallers. *Phys Ther.* 1990;70:410–415.
138. Badke MB, Duncan PW. Patterns of rapid motor responses during postural adjustment when standing in healthy subjects and hemiplegic patients. *Phys Ther.* 1983;63:13–20.
139. Ring C, Matthews R, Nayak USL, Isaacs B. Visual push: a sensitive measure of dynamic balance in man. *Arch Phys Med Rehabil.* 1988;69:256–260.
140. Mathias S, Nayak USL, Isaacs B. Balance in elderly patients: the "get-up and go" tests. *Arch Phys Med Rehabil.* 1986;67:387–389.
141. Berg K, Wood-Dauphinee S, Williams JI, Gayton D. Measuring balance in the elderly: preliminary development of an instrument. *Physiotherapy Canada.* 1989;41:304–311.
142. Schmitz TJ. Sensory assessment. In: O'Sullivan SB, Schmitz TJ, eds. *Physical Rehabilitation: Assessment and Treatment.* 2nd ed. Philadelphia, Pa: FA Davis Co; 1988.
143. Nolan MF. Clinical assessment of cutaneous sensory function. *Clinical Management in Physical Therapy.* 1984;4(2):26–29.
144. Nolan MF. Two-point discrimination assessment in the upper limb in young adult men and women. *Phys Ther.* 1982;62:965–969.
145. Nolan MF. Limits of two-point discrimination ability in the lower limb in young adult men and women. *Phys Ther.* 1983;63:1424–1428.

146. Nolan MF. Quantitative measure of cutaneous sensation: two-point discrimination values for the face and trunk. *Phys Ther.* 1985;65:181–185.
147. Holewski JJ, Graf PM. Aesthesiometry: quantification of cutaneous pressure sensation in diabetic peripheral neuropathy. *J Rehabil Res Dev.* 1988;25:1–10.
148. Mueller MJ, Diamond JE, Delitto A, Sinacore DR. Insensitivity, limited joint mobility, and plantar ulcers in patients with diabetes mellitus. *Phys Ther.* 1989;69:453–462.
149. Campbell SK. Assessment of the child with CNS dysfunction. In: Rothstein JM, ed. *Measurement in Physical Therapy.* New York, NY: Churchill Livingstone; 1985:207–228.
150. Harris SR, Heriza CB. Measuring infant movement: clinical and technological assessment techniques. *Phys Ther.* 1987;67:1877–1880.
151. Washington KA, Harris SR. Mental and motor performance of low-birthweight infants with normal developmental outcomes. *Pediatric Physical Therapy.* 1989;1:159–165.
152. Harris SR. Effects of neurodevelopmental therapy on motor performance of infants with Down's syndrome. *Dev Med Child Neurol.* 1981;23:477–483.
153. Stengel TJ, Attermeier SM, Bly L, Heriza CB. Evaluation of sensorimotor dysfunction. In: Campbell SK, ed. *Pediatric Neurologic Physical Therapy.* New York, NY: Churchill Livingstone; 1984.
154. Johnson OG. *Tests and Measurements in Child Development: Handbook II: Volume I.* San Francisco, Calif: Jossey-Bass Publishers; 1976.
155. Conoley JC, Kramer JJ, eds. *The Tenth Mental Measurements Yearbook.* Lincoln, Neb: Buros Institute of Mental Measurements of the University of Nebraska-Lincoln; 1989.
156. Shaugnessy JJ, Zechmeister EB. *Research Methods of Psychology.* 2nd ed. New York, NY: McGraw-Hill Publishing Co; 1990:59–61.
157. Hulme JB, Gallacher K, Walsh J, Niesen S, Waldron D. Behavioral and postural changes observed with use of adaptive seating by clients with multiple handicaps. *Phys Ther.* 1987;67:1060–1067.
158. Horowitz L, Sharby N. Development of prone extension postures in healthy infants. *Phys Ther.* 1988;68:32–36.
159. Holcomb JD, Selker LG, Roush RE. Scholarly productivity: a regional study of physical therapy faculty in schools of allied health. *Phys Ther.* 1990;70:118–124.
160. Uili RM, Shepard KF, Savinar E. Physician knowledge and utilization of physical therapy procedures. *Phys Ther.* 1984;64:1523–1530.
161. Glazer-Waldman HR, Hart JP, LeVeau BF. Health beliefs and health behaviors of physical therapists. *Phys Ther.* 1989;69:204–210.
162. Durant TL, Lord LJ, Domholdt E. Outpatient views on direct access to physical therapy in Indiana. *Phys Ther.* 1989;69:850–857.
163. Rezler A, French R. Personality types and learning preferences of students in six allied health professions. *J Allied Health.* 1975;4:20–25.
164. Goodman CM. The Delphi technique: a critique. *J Adv Nurs.* 1987;12:729–734.
165. Miles-Tapping C, Dyck A, Brunham S, Simpson E, Barber L. Canadian therapists' priorities for clinical research: a Delphi study. *Phys Ther.* 1990;70:448–454.
166. Lincoln YS, Guba EG. *Naturalistic Inquiry.* Newbury Park, Calif: Sage Publications; 1985:332–356.
167. Spradley JP. *The Ethnographic Interview.* Fort Worth, Tex: Holt, Rinehart & Winston Inc; 1979;173–203.
168. Michels E. *Using and Understanding Surveys: An Introductory Manual.* Alexandria, Va: American Physical Therapy Association; 1985.
169. Schuman H, Scott J. Problems in the use of survey questions to measure public opinion. *Science.* 1987;236:957–959.
170. Kvitek SDB, Shaver BJ, Blood H, Shepard KF. Age bias: physical therapists and older patients. *J Gerontol.* 1986;41:706–709.
171. Orlich DL. *Designing Sensible Surveys.* Pleasantville, NY: Redgrave Publishing Co; 1978.
172. Deckard GJ, Present RM. Impact of role stress on physical therapists' emotional and physical well-being. *Phys Ther.* 1989;69:713–718.
173. Osgood CE, Suci GJ, Tannenbaum PH. *The Measurement of Meaning.* Urbana, Ill: University of Illinois Press; 1957.
174. Streed CP, Stoecker JL. Stereotyping between physical therapy students and occupational therapy students. *Phys Ther.* 1991;71:16–24.
175. Stephenson W. *The Study of Behavior: Q Technique and Its Methodology.* Chicago, Ill: University of Chicago Press; 1975.
176. Freihofer P, Felton G. Nursing behaviors in bereavement: an exploratory study. *Nurs Res.* 1976;25:332–337.
177. Mitchell JV Jr, ed. *Tests in Print III.* Lincoln, Neb: University of Nebraska Press; 1983.
178. Frank-Stromberg M. *Instruments for Clinical Nursing Research.* Norwalk, Conn: Appleton & Lange; 1988.

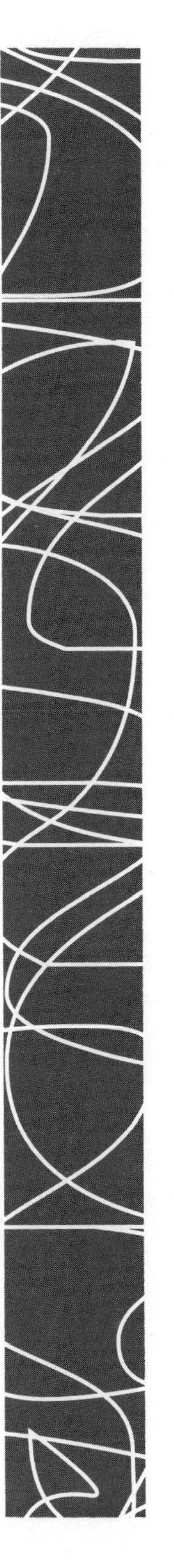

SECTION FOUR

DATA ANALYSIS

CHAPTER 13

Statistical Reasoning

Data Set
Frequency Distribution
Central Tendency
Mean
Median
Mode
Variability
Range
Variance
Standard deviation
Normal Distribution
z score
Percentages of the normal distribution
Sampling Distribution
Confidence intervals of the sampling distribution
Significant Difference
Null hypothesis
Alpha level
Probability determinants
Errors
Power
Statistical Conclusion Validity
Low power
Clinical insignificance
Error rate problems
Violated assumptions

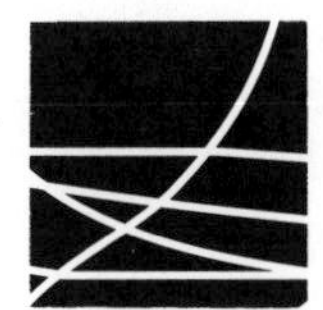

Statistics has a bad name. Consider this tongue-in-cheek sampling from the irreverent *Journal of Irreproducible Results*:

> We all know that you can prove anything with statistics. So I recently proved that nobody likes statistics, except for a few professors. If you don't believe that, just ask the person on the street. I did. The first person I saw referred to the subject as "sadistics." The second person, an old gentleman along the Mississippi River, muttered something about "liars, damned liars, and statisticians."[1(p13)]

Although quips about statistics are amusing, the discipline of statistics should not be confused with the conclusions that researchers draw from statistical analyses. Statistics is a discipline in which mathematics and probability are applied in ways that allow researchers to make sense of their data. Although there are many different statistical tests and procedures—too many to include even in textbooks devoted solely to statistics—there are remarkably few central concepts that underlie all of the tests.

In this chapter, the central concepts of statistics are introduced. Readers should be prepared to read this chapter, and Chapters 14 and 15, which cover particular statistical tests, very slowly. Careful reading, examination of the tables and figures, and independent calculation of the examples in this chapter should provide a strong basis for understanding not only the following chapters but, more important, the data analysis and results portions of research articles in the physical therapy literature.

The chapter begins by presenting a data set that is used for all of the statistical examples in this and the following two chapters. Next, the concepts of frequency distribution, central tendency, variability, and normal distribution, which were introduced in Chapter 10, are reviewed and expanded. Then the new concepts of sampling distribution, significant difference, and power are explained. Finally, the concepts are integrated by a discussion of statistical conclusion validity.

DATA SET

Achieving a conceptual understanding of statistical reasoning is greatly enhanced by performing simple computational examples. Thus, a small hypothetical data set has been developed for use throughout this and the following two chapters. Our data set consists of 30 hypothetical patients, 10 at each of three clinics, who have undergone rehabilitation for a total knee arthroplasty. Eighteen pieces of information are available for each patient:

- Case number
- Clinic attended
- Sex
- Age
- Three-week knee flexion range of motion (ROM)
- Six-week knee flexion ROM
- Six-month knee flexion ROM
- Six-month knee extensor torque
- Six-month knee flexor torque
- Six-month gait velocity
- Four six-month activities of daily living (ADL) indexes
- Four six-month deformity indexes.

The ADL and deformity indexes were adapted for the purposes of this data set from a knee-rating system used at Brigham and Women's Hospital in Boston.[2] Table 13–1 provides an outline of the data set, indicating abbreviations for each variable, the unit of measurement when appropriate, and the meaning of any numerical coding. Table 13–2 presents the actual data set.

FREQUENCY DISTRIBUTION

A *frequency distribution* is a tally of the number of times each score is represented in a data set. There are four ways of presenting a frequency distribution: frequency distribution with percentages, grouped frequency distribution with percentages, frequency histogram, and stem-and-leaf plot.

Frequency Distribution with Percentages. Table 13–3 shows a frequency distribution with percentages for the variable three-week ROM. The first column lists the scores that were obtained. The second column, absolute frequency, lists the number of times that each score was obtained. For example, two subjects had three-week ROM values of 67°. The third column, relative frequency, lists the percentage of subjects who received each score. This is calculated by dividing the number of subjects with that score by the total number of subjects. From this column we find that the four subjects who had scores of 81 represent 13.3% of the sample [(4/30) × 100 = 13.3%]. The fourth column, cumulative frequency, is formed by adding the relative frequencies of the scores up to and including the one in which you are interested. For example, you might be interested in the percentage of patients who had ROM scores of less than 50° three weeks postoperatively. From the cumulative frequency column you find that 26.7% of the sample had ROM values of 49° or less.

A variation of this basic display is needed if there are missing values in the sample. Suppose that Patients 3 through 5 missed their three-week evaluation appointments. Table 13–4 presents a revised frequency distribution that accounts for these three missing pieces of data. Note that another column, adjusted frequency, has been added. The adjusted frequency is calculated by dividing the number of observations for each score by the number of valid scores for each variable,

TABLE 13–1. Data Set Specifications for Patients Who Underwent Rehabilitation After Total Knee Arthroplasty

Variable Code	Variable Name	Variable Values
CASE	Case number	01–30
CN	Clinic number	1 = Community Hospital 2 = Memorial Hospital 3 = Religious Hospital
SEX	Patient sex	0 = male 1 = female
AGE	Patient age	In years at last birthday
W3R	Three-week range of motion (ROM) at each clinic	To nearest degree
W6R	Six-week ROM	To nearest degree
M6R	Six-month ROM	To nearest degree
E	Six-month extension torque	To nearest Newton • meter (N•m)
F	Six-month flexion torque	To nearest N•m
V	Gait velocity	To nearest cm/sec
DFC	Deformity: flexion contracture	1 = >15° 2 = 6–15° 3 = 0–5°
DVV	Deformity: varus/valgus angulation in stance	1 = >10° valgus 2 = >5° varus or 6–10° valgus 3 = 5° varus to 5° valgus
DML	Deformity: mediolateral stability	1 = marked instability 2 = moderate instability 3 = stable
DAP	Deformity: anteroposterior stability with knee at 90° flexion	1 = marked instability 2 = moderate instability 3 = stable
ADW	Activities of daily living (ADLs): distance walked	5 = unlimited 4 = 4–6 blocks 3 = 2–3 blocks 2 = indoors only 1 = transfers only
AAD	ADL: assistive device	5 = none 4 = cane outside 3 = cane full-time 2 = two canes or crutches 1 = walker or unable
ASC	ADL: stair climbing	5 = reciprocal, no rail 4 = reciprocal, with rail 3 = one at a time, with or without rail 2 = one at a time, with rail and assistive device 1 = unable to climb stairs
ARC	ADL: rising from a chair	5 = no arm assistance 4 = single arm assistance 3 = difficult with two arm assistance 2 = needs assistance of another 1 = unable to rise

TABLE 13–2. Data Set for Patients Who Underwent Rehabilitation After Total Knee Arthroplasty

Case	CN	Sex	Age	W3R	W6R	M6R	E	F	V	DFC	DVV	DML	DAP	ADW	AAD	ASC	ARC
01	1	1	50	95	90	100	170	100	165	2	1	2	1	5	5	5	5
02	1	0	87	32	46	85	100	60	100	2	2	1	1	3	4	4	2
03	1	0	66	67	78	100	130	70	130	1	1	2	2	4	5	5	4
04	1	0	46	92	85	105	175	95	170	2	2	1	2	5	5	5	5
05	1	0	53	87	85	105	157	86	150	1	2	2	2	5	4	5	5
06	1	0	76	58	50	95	88	52	135	2	1	2	2	4	4	4	4
07	1	1	43	92	95	110	120	75	153	1	1	1	1	5	5	5	5
08	1	1	46	88	90	100	130	90	145	2	3	3	2	4	5	5	5
09	1	1	43	84	80	95	132	92	147	1	1	1	2	5	5	5	4
10	1	1	48	81	90	105	156	98	145	2	2	3	2	5	5	4	5
11	2	0	92	34	63	90	87	53	95	3	2	2	2	3	3	3	3
12	2	0	65	56	71	90	160	95	150	2	3	2	2	4	4	5	5
13	2	0	76	45	63	78	92	60	120	1	2	1	2	4	3	3	4
14	2	0	92	27	35	65	85	49	85	3	3	3	3	2	1	1	2
15	2	1	68	76	70	95	170	102	165	2	3	2	2	4	3	5	5
16	2	1	79	49	56	98	81	37	93	2	2	2	1	3	2	3	2
17	2	1	85	47	58	84	87	46	70	3	2	2	2	2	1	2	2
18	2	1	82	50	60	80	93	63	94	1	1	2	2	3	2	2	2
19	2	0	81	40	40	83	96	58	101	2	2	2	2	3	2	1	2
20	2	1	90	67	70	95	103	63	103	1	1	3	2	2	2	2	3
21	3	0	66	32	67	105	180	105	180	1	2	1	1	5	5	5	5
22	3	0	72	50	67	105	150	85	150	2	3	3	2	5	4	4	4
23	3	0	68	60	65	95	154	89	156	2	3	3	2	4	4	4	4
24	3	0	77	84	80	105	141	83	146	2	2	2	1	3	3	4	3
25	3	0	60	81	85	100	168	93	178	3	3	3	2	4	5	5	5
26	3	1	75	81	94	110	146	84	135	2	1	3	3	5	5	5	5
27	3	1	73	84	90	100	120	74	134	2	2	2	3	4	4	4	4
28	3	1	72	81	95	103	110	68	120	2	1	2	3	4	5	3	4
29	3	1	72	82	90	104	116	74	126	3	2	3	1	4	3	4	3
30	3	1	63	91	95	106	137	86	131	2	1	3	3	4	5	5	5

Note: All variables are identified in Table 13–1.

rather than by the number of subjects. In this case, there are 27 valid scores. The relative frequency of a ROM score of 81° is now 14.8% [(4/27) × 100 = 14.8%]. The cumulative frequency is the sum of the adjusted frequencies. If many data points are missing, it is often misleading to present the frequencies as percentages of the total sample; use of adjusted frequencies corrects the problem.

Grouped Frequency Distribution with Percentages. The grouped frequency distribution is another way frequency information is commonly presented. When there are many individual scores in a distribution, the characteristics of the distribution may be grasped more easily if scores are placed into groups. Table 13–5 presents a grouped frequency distribution for the three-week ROM values. From this grouped distribution it is readily apparent that the group with the highest frequency is that with scores from 80° to 89°.

A disadvantage of the grouped frequency distribution is that information is lost. Table 13–5 indicates that there are three subjects whose scores range from 30° to 39°. But what does this mean? This could mean all three patients had scores of 39, three patients had scores of 30, or the three had a variety of scores within this range.

Frequency Histogram. Another way to

TABLE 13–3. Frequency Distribution of Three-Week Range of Motion Values

Score (degrees)	Absolute Frequency	Relative Frequency (%)	Cumulative Frequency (%)
27	1	3.3	3.3
32	2	6.7	10.0
34	1	3.3	13.3
40	1	3.3	16.7
45	1	3.3	20.0
47	1	3.3	23.3
49	1	3.3	26.7
50	2	6.7	33.4
56	1	3.3	36.7
58	1	3.3	40.0
60	1	3.3	43.3
67	2	6.7	50.0
76	1	3.3	53.3
81	4	13.3	66.6
82	1	3.3	70.0
84	3	10.0	80.0
87	1	3.3	83.3
88	1	3.3	86.6
91	1	3.3	90.0
92	2	6.7	96.7
95	1	3.3	100.0
Total	30	100.0	

TABLE 13–4. Frequency Distribution of Three-Week Range of Motion Scores, Modified for Missing Values

Score (degrees)	Absolute Frequency	Relative Frequency (%)	Adjusted Frequency (%)	Cumulative Frequency (%)
27	1	3.3	3.7	3.7
32	2	6.7	7.4	11.1
34	1	3.3	3.7	14.8
40	1	3.3	3.7	18.5
45	1	3.3	3.7	22.2
47	1	3.3	3.7	25.9
49	1	3.3	3.7	29.6
50	2	6.7	7.4	37.0
56	1	3.3	3.7	40.7
58	1	3.3	3.7	44.4
60	1	3.3	3.7	48.1
67	1	3.3	3.7	51.8
76	1	3.3	3.7	55.5
81	4	13.3	14.8	70.3
82	1	3.3	3.7	74.3
84	3	10.0	11.1	85.1
88	1	3.3	3.7	88.8
91	1	3.3	3.7	92.5
92	1	3.3	3.7	96.2
95	1	3.3	3.7	100.0
Missing	3	10.0	Missing	
Total	30	100.0	100.0	

TABLE 13–5. Grouped Frequency Distribution for Three-Week Range of Motion Values

Scores (degrees)	Frequency	Relative Frequency (%)	Cumulative Frequency (%)
20–29	1	3.3	3.3
30–39	3	10.0	13.3
40–49	4	13.3	26.7
50–59	4	13.3	40.0
60–69	3	10.0	50.0
70–79	1	3.3	53.3
80–89	10	33.3	86.7
90–99	4	13.3	100.0
Total	30	100.0	

present a grouped frequency distribution is a histogram. A histogram presents each grouped frequency as a bar on a graph. The height of each bar represents the frequency of observations in the group. Figure 13–1 shows a histogram of the three-week ROM data. Like the grouped frequency distribution from which the histogram is generated, information is lost because one does not know how the scores are distributed within each group.

Stem-and-Leaf Plot. A final way of presenting frequency data is the stem-and-leaf plot. This plot presents data concisely, without losing information in the grouping process. Each individual score is divided into a "stem" and a "leaf," as shown in Table 13–6. In this instance the stem is the digit representing the multiple of 10 (20, 30, 40, etc.), and the leaf is the digit representing the multiple of 1 (1, 2, 3, 4, etc.). The row with the stem of 5 has leaves of 0, 0, 6, 8. The stems and leaves together represent the four scores of 50, 50, 56, and 58. The stem-and-leaf plot, like the histogram, provides a good visual picture of the frequency distribution.

CENTRAL TENDENCY

Researchers often wish to collapse a set of data into a single score that represents the whole set. In other words, the researcher is interested in the central tendency of the data. The three commonly used measures of central

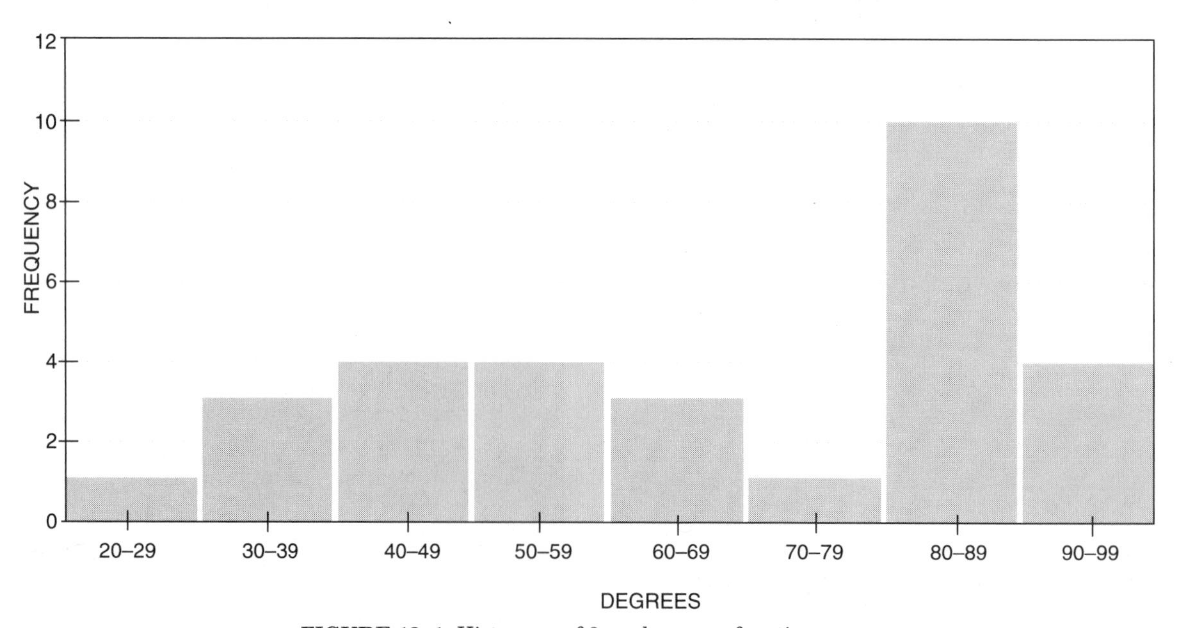

FIGURE 13–1. Histogram of 3-week range of motion scores.

TABLE 13–6. Stem-and-Leaf Plot of Three-Week Range of Motion Frequency Distribution

Stem	Leaf	Total
2	7	1
3	2 2 4	3
4	0 5 7 9	4
5	0 0 6 8	4
6	0 7 7	3
7	6	1
8	1 1 1 1 2 4 4 4 7 8	10
9	1 2 2 5	4
Total		30

tendency are the mean, the median, and the mode. If a distribution is perfectly symmetrical, then the mean, median, and mode are all identical. If the distribution is asymmetrical, they differ.

Mean

The arithmetic *mean* of a data set is the sum of the observations divided by the number of observations. Recall from Chapter 10 that mathematical notation for the mean is as follows:

$$\overline{X} = \frac{\Sigma X}{N}$$

In words, this equation says the mean is the sum of all the observations divided by the number of observations. The mean of the three-week ROM scores for Clinic 1 is 77.6° [(95 + 32 + 67 + 92 + 87 + 58 + 92 + 88 + 84 + 81)/10 = 77.6]. The mean is a versatile measure of central tendency because it uses information from all the scores in the distribution. However, extreme values can distort the mean. In this example, 7 of the 10 scores are greater than 80°, but the very low score of 32° pulls the mean down to 77.6°.

Median

The *median* is the "middle" score of a distribution, or the score above which half of the distribution lies. To calculate the median, a researcher must first rank the scores. When the distribution has an odd number of scores, the middle score is easy to locate: (N + 1)/2 = the middle ranked score. Thus, in a sample of 987 scores, the 494th ranked score is the median. When the number of scores in a distribution is even, as in our example, the median is calculated by finding the mean of the two middle scores: [N/2] and [(N/2) + 1]. In a sample with 988 scores, the median is the mean of the 494th and 495th ranked scores. Table 13–7 presents the frequency distribution for the 10 three-week measurements we are considering. The median, as shown, is 85.5°. The median is a useful measure of central tendency when the distribution contains a few extreme values that distort the mean. The disadvantage of the median is that it does not include information from all of the scores in the distribution.

Mode

The *mode* is the score that occurs most frequently in a distribution. If there are two modes, the distribution is termed *bimodal*. Our example of three-week ROM scores has a mode of 92, as shown in Table 13–7. The mode is often used to describe nominal data, which have neither the property of order nor the property of distance and therefore cannot provide a median and mean.

VARIABILITY

The variability of a data set is the amount of spread in the data. Two different groups might have the same mean score, yet have very different characteristics. For example, a

TABLE 13–7. Median and Mode Calculations for Three-Week Range of Motion Values for Clinic 1

Score (degrees)	Absolute Frequency	Cumulative (%)	Median[a]	Mode[b]
32	1	10.0		
58	1	20.0		
67	1	30.0		
81	1	40.0		
84	1	50.0		
			85.5	
87	1	60.0		
88	1	70.0		
92	2	90.0		92
95	1	100.0		

[a]Median is the "middle" score. When there is an even number of scores, the two middle scores are averaged. In this example, the median is (84 + 87) / 2 = 85.5.
[b]Mode is the score that occurs most frequently.

sample of female college athletes might have the same mean weight as a sample of female nonathletes at the school. However, the athletes would be expected to have a relatively narrow range of weights, whereas the nonathletes would be expected to range in weight from the very underweight to the very overweight. The three measures of variability are range, variance, and standard deviation.

Range

The *range* is the difference between the highest and lowest values in the distribution. In the group of 10 patients from Clinic 1, the range is 63° (95 − 32 = 63). Although the range is technically a single score, it is often reported by presenting both the high and low scores so that readers will understand not only the range but also the magnitude of the scores in the distribution.

Variance

The *variance* is a measure of variability that, like the mean, requires that every score in the distribution be used in its calculation. Although the calculation of the variance was presented in Chapter 10, it is reviewed here with our three-week ROM data from Clinic 1. To calculate the variance, we convert each of the raw scores in the data set to a *deviation score* by subtracting the mean of the data set from each raw score. In mathematical notation,

$$x = X - \overline{X}$$

Recall from Chapter 10 that the lowercase, italic x is the symbol for a deviation score. The deviation score indicates how high or low a raw score is compared with the mean. The first two columns of Table 13–8 present the raw and deviation scores for the knee flexion data set and, below them, their sums and means. Note that both the sum and the mean of the deviation scores are zero. To generate a nonzero index of the variability within a data set, we must square the deviation scores. We can then calculate the *population variance* by determining the mean of the squared deviations. In mathematical notation,

$$\sigma^2 = \frac{\Sigma x^2}{N}$$

TABLE 13–8. Computation of the Variance, *z* Scores, and Probabilities for Three-Week Range of Motion Scores at Clinic 1

	X	x	x^2	*z* score	*p*
	32	−45.6	2,079.36	−2.30	.011
	58	−19.6	384.16	− .99	.161
	67	−10.6	112.36	− .53	.298
	81	3.4	11.56	.17	.433
	84	6.4	40.96	.32	.374
	87	9.4	88.36	.47	.319
	88	10.4	108.16	.52	.302
	92	14.4	207.36	.73	.233
	92	14.4	207.36	.73	.233
	95	17.4	302.76	.88	.189
Σ =	776	0	3,542.40		
$\bar{X}$ =	77.6	0	354.24	= population variance (σ^2)	
			18.82	= population standard deviation (σ)	
$s^2 = \frac{\Sigma x^2}{N - 1}$			393.60	= sample variance (s^2)	
			19.84	= sample standard deviation (s)	

We know from Chapter 10 that σ is the lowercase Greek sigma and when squared is the notation for the variance. The third column in Table 13–8 shows the squared deviations from the group mean and, below them, their sum and mean. The population variance is used when all of the members of a population are known. In practice this rarely occurs, so the *sample variance* is used to *estimate* the population variance. The sample variance is calculated by dividing the sum of the squared deviations by N − 1, as follows:

$$s^2 = \frac{\Sigma x^2}{N - 1}$$

The symbol for the sample variance is s^2. In our example, the sample variance is calculated by dividing 3,542.40 (the sum of the squared deviations) by 9 (N − 1), as shown in Table 13–8.

The rationale for dividing the sum of the squared deviations by N − 1 rests on the concept of *degrees of freedom*. Although an abstract concept, degrees of freedom can be understood in a general sense through the use of an illustration. In a sample of 10 values with a known mean, 9 of the values are "free" to fluctuate, as long as the investigator has control over the final value. We know that for our sample of 10 observations with a mean of 77.6°, the sum of those 10 observations adds up to 776. If we wanted to generate another sample with a mean of 77.6°, we could select 9 numbers randomly as long as we could manipulate the 10th value. If 9 randomly selected numbers happen to each have a value of 100, then they add to a total of 900. The sample can still have a mean value of 77.6° if the 10th value is manipulated to be −124 (900 − 124 = 776; 776/10 = 77.6). This phenomenon is termed degrees of freedom, or the number of items that are free to fluctuate. Thus, for the mean, there are always N − 1 degrees of freedom. Statisticians have found that using the degrees of freedom for the mean as the denominator of the sample variance formula leads to an unbiased estimation of the population variance. The degrees of freedom concept is used in the computation of many different statistical tests.

Standard Deviation

As just defined, the population variance is the mean of the squared deviations from the mean, and the sample variance is the sum of the squared deviations from the mean, divided by the degrees of freedom for the mean. Although the variance is useful in many statistical procedures, it does not have a great deal of intuitive meaning because it is calculated from squared deviation scores. A measure that has such meaning is the *standard deviation*. The standard deviation is the square root of the variance and is expressed in the units of the original measure. The population standard deviation is the square root of the population variance; the sample standard deviation is the square root of the sample variance:

$$s = \sqrt{s^2}$$

The mathematical notations for the sample standard deviation and the sample variance make their relationship clear: The notation for the variance *(s^2)* is simply the square of the notation for standard deviation *(s)*. In practice, the entire population is not usually measured, so the sample standard deviation is used as an estimate of the population standard deviation. The sample standard deviation of the knee flexion data presented in Table 13–8 is the square root of 393.60, or 19.84°.

Taken together, the measures of central tendency and variability are referred to as descriptive measures. When these measures are used to describe a population, they are known as *parameters;* when they are used to describe a sample, they are known as *statistics*. Because researchers can rarely measure all the subjects within a population, they use sample statistics such as the mean and standard deviation as estimates of the corresponding population parameters.

NORMAL DISTRIBUTION

The normal distribution is central to many of the statistical tests that are presented in subsequent chapters. Groups of measurements frequently approximate a bell-shaped distribution known as the normal curve. The *normal curve* is a symmetrical frequency distribution that can be defined in terms of the mean and standard deviation of a set of data.

z Score

Any score within a distribution can be standardized with respect to the mean and standard deviation of the data. That is, each score can be expressed in terms of how many standard deviations it is above or below the mean. The result of such a standardization procedure is called a z score. A z score is calculated by dividing the deviation score ($x = X - \overline{X}$) by the standard deviation:

$$z = \frac{x}{s}$$

When a normally distributed set of data is converted to z scores, the distribution of the z scores is known as the *standard normal distribution*. The standard normal distribution has a mean of zero and a standard deviation of 1.0. The fourth column of Table 13–8 shows our 10 raw three-week ROM scores as z scores. This was done by dividing each of the deviation scores *(x)* by the standard deviation *(s)* of 19.84°. The z score tells us, for example, that a measurement of 32° is 2.30 standard deviations below the mean.

Percentages of the Normal Distribution

In a normal distribution the percentage of scores that fall within a certain range of scores is known. Approximately 68% of scores fall within 1 standard deviation above or below the mean. Approximately 96% of the scores fall within 2 standard deviations of the mean, and almost 100% of the scores fall within 3 standard deviations of the mean. Figure 13–2 shows a diagram of the normal curve, with the exact percentages of scores that are found within each standard deviation.

Figure 13–3A shows the normal curve that

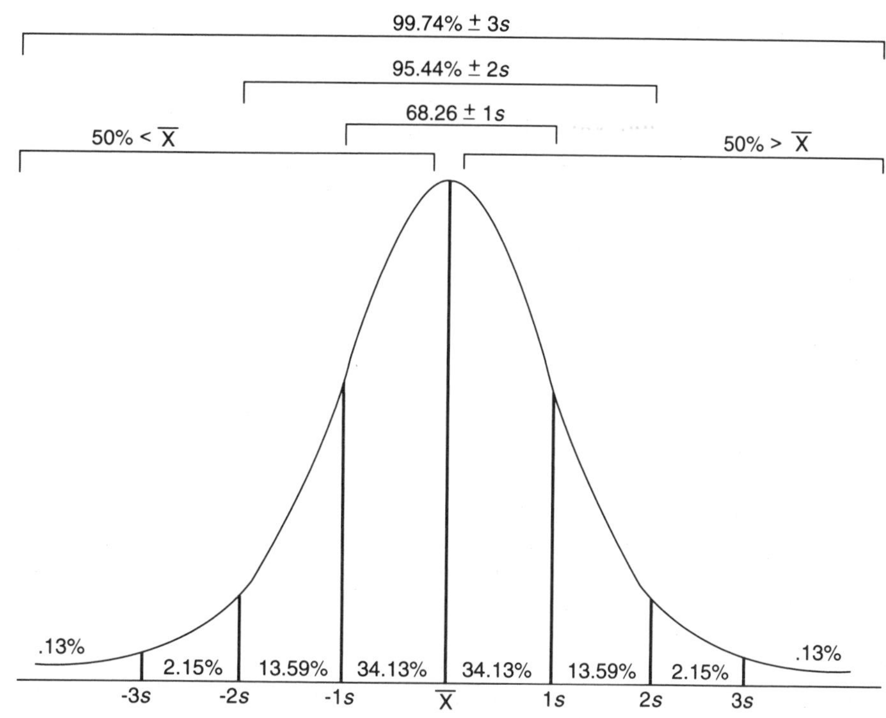

FIGURE 13–2. Percentages of the normal distribution. $\overline{X}$, mean; *s*, standard deviation.

corresponds to our three-week ROM data for Clinic 1. The sample mean is 77.6°, and the sample standard deviation is 19.84°. The x axis is labeled with both *z* scores and the raw scores that correspond to 1, 2, and 3 standard deviations above and below the mean. Figure 13–3B shows that if the knee flexion scores are normally distributed, we would estimate that 98% of our measurements would exceed the score of 37.92°; Figure 13–3C shows that we could expect 68% of our measurements to fall between 57.76° and 97.44°. Predicting the probability of obtaining certain ranges of scores is basic to most of the statistical testing presented in Chapter 14.

We know from the preceding paragraphs the approximate probability of obtaining scores within 1, 2, and 3 standard deviations of the mean. A table of *z* scores can provide exact probabilities of achieving scores at any level within the distribution. Earlier we calculated that 32° of ROM at three weeks postoperatively was 2.30 standard deviations below the mean for patients at Clinic 1. Without a table, we know only that the probability of obtaining scores outside the second standard deviation is approximately 2%. Consulting a *z* table tells us the exact probability of obtaining scores that are less than or equal to 2.30 standard deviations below the mean. Appendix C provides a *z* table.

To identify the *z* score of 2.30 in Appendix C, look in the far lefthand column for the stem 2.3, and then read across the uppermost row to the leaf .00. The intersection of the row and column gives a value of .011 or, if stated as a percentage, 1.1%. The picture of the normal curve above the table shows that the proportion indicated is either at the upper or lower tail of the curve, depending on whether the *z* score is positive or negative. Because the curve is symmetrical, there is no

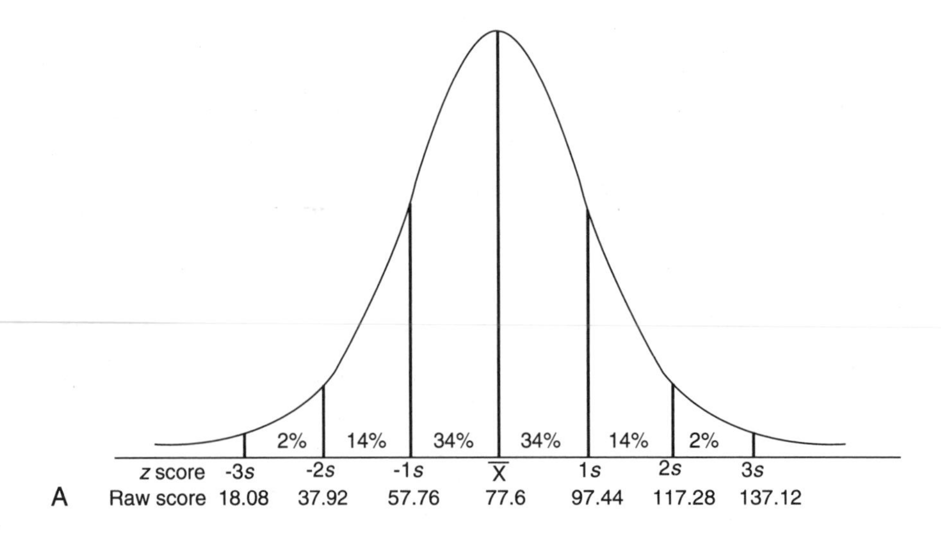

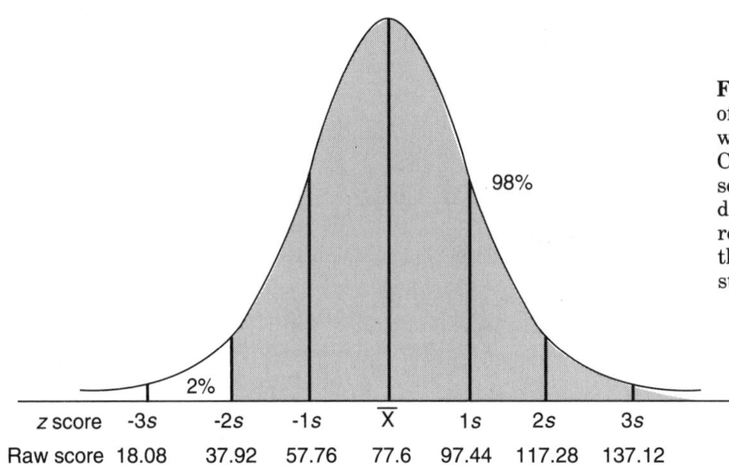

FIGURE 13–3. A. Percentages of the normal distribution for 3-week range-of-motion scores at Clinic 1. **B.** Shaded area represents approximately 98% of the distribution. **C.** Shaded area represents approximately 68% of the distribution. $\overline{X}$, mean; *s*, standard deviation.

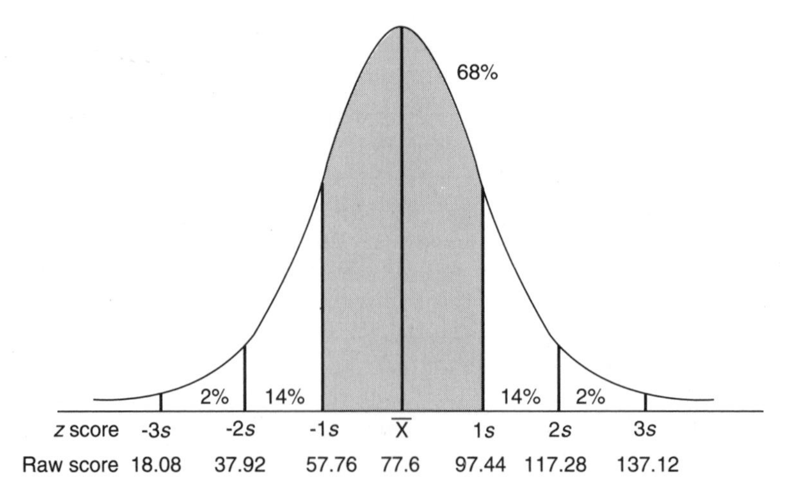

need for separate tables of positive and negative z scores; researchers simply need to know that the probabilities associated with positive z scores lie in the upper portion of the curve and the probabilities associated with negative z scores lie in the lower portion of the curve. The final column of Table 13–8 gives the probabilities associated with each z score. Readers may wish to use the z table in Appendix C to confirm that they understand how these probabilities were obtained.

SAMPLING DISTRIBUTION

To understand statistical testing, it is extremely important to understand sampling distributions. The sampling distribution is a specific type of normal distribution. Imagine that you had access to the entire population of individuals who had total knee arthroplasties in a given year. If we drew a random sample of 10 individuals from this large population and examined their three-week ROM values, we might get a sample with a mean of 77.6°, as in the example from Clinic 1. If we drew another random sample of 10 individuals, we might get a mean of 98.2°. If we drew another random sample, we might get a mean of 59.1°. Assume that we drew 10 samples and obtained means of 77.6°, 98.2°, 59.1°, 84.5°, 78.9°, 45.6°, 89.5°, 64.3°, 68.7°, and 75.4°. Using each of these mean scores to represent each sample, we can calculate both a mean of the sample means (74.18°) and a standard deviation of the sample means (15.37°).

TABLE 13–9. Computation of the Mean, Sample Variance (s^2), and Sample Standard Deviation (s) for the Sampling Distribution of Three-Week Range of Motion Scores

	X	x	x^2
	98.2	24.02	576.96
	89.5	15.32	234.70
	84.5	10.32	106.50
	78.9	4.72	22.28
	77.6	3.42	11.70
	75.4	1.22	1.48
	68.7	−5.48	30.03
	64.3	−9.88	97.61
	59.1	−15.08	227.41
	45.6	−28.58	816.82
Σ =	741.8	0	2,125.49
$\bar{X}$ =	74.18	0	

$s^2 = \frac{\Sigma x^2}{N - 1} = 236.16$

$s = 15.37$

Table 13–9 shows the calculations that provide this mean and standard deviation. The calculations are the same as those presented in Table 13–8; the only difference is that each score in the distribution in Table 13–9 represents a group rather than an individual, as in Table 13–8. The distribution of the means of several samples drawn from the same population is called a *sampling distribution*. The mean of the sampling distribution is assumed to be the mean of the population. The standard deviation of the sampling distribution is called the *standard error of the mean*, or the SEM. Note that SEM is also the abbreviation for the standard error of measurement (see Chapter 10). When this abbreviation is used, it should be made clear whether it refers to the standard error of the mean or the standard error of measurement. The term "error" does not refer to a mistake made by the researcher. Rather, "error" denotes the inevitable differences that are found between a population and the samples that are drawn from the population.

The SEM varies with sample size. When we draw sample sizes of 10, the presence of just one extremely low or high value alters the mean greatly. For example, assume that we have 9 scores of 75° and one score of 115°; the mean is 79°—4° away from the modal score of 75°. Do the same to a sample of 100 with 99 scores of 75° and one score of 115°. The mean in this case is 75.4°—less than half a degree higher than the majority of scores.

Thus, the means of large samples are more stable than means of small samples because they are less influenced by extreme scores. This stability is reflected in the magnitude of the SEM: The SEM of a sample distribution generated from a large sample is small; the SEM of a sampling distribution generated from a small sample is large.

Researchers often do not have the time or resources to draw repeated samples from a population to determine the SEM of the resulting sampling distribution. Therefore, the SEM is usually estimated from a single sample drawn for study. As just noted, the sample size greatly affects the variability of mean scores, so the SEM estimation formula takes sample size into account:

$$\text{SEM} = \frac{s}{\sqrt{N}}$$

The estimate of the SEM is found by dividing the sample standard deviation *(s)* by the square root of the number in the sample. This estimated SEM, or one of several mathematical variations, is used in the calculation of many of the statistical tests discussed in Chapter 14. For our single sample with a mean of 77.6°, a standard deviation of 19.84°, and a sample size of 10, the estimated SEM is 6.27° ($19.84/\sqrt{10} = 6.27$).

Confidence Intervals of the Sampling Distribution

Because the sampling distribution is a normal distribution, we can find the probability of obtaining a sample with a certain range of mean scores by consulting a *z* table. The procedure is the same as discussed earlier, except that the scores now represent sample means rather than individual scores. Earlier we started with a particular *z* score and determined the probability of obtaining scores that either equaled or exceeded the selected score. We can also use the *z* table in reverse by specifying a particular probability in which we are interested and determining the *z* score that corresponds to that probability. This reverse process is used to determine *confidence intervals* (CIs) about the mean.

Recall that the sample mean of three-week ROM scores at Clinic 1 is 77.6°, the standard deviation is 19.84°, and the SEM is 6.27°. We recognize that the obtained sample mean is only an estimate of the population mean because of the phenomenon of sampling error. We can use the probabilities of the sampling distribution to identify a range of mean scores that is likely to include the true population mean. If we take the mean score (77.6) and subtract and add one SEM ($77.6 - 6.27 = 71.33$; $77.6 + 6.27 = 82.87$), we get a range of means from 71.33° to 82.87°. From our knowledge of the probabilities of the normal distribution we know that approximately 68% of the scores in a distribution fall within the first standard deviation from the mean. Thus, there is an approximately 68% chance that the true population mean lies somewhere between 71.33° and 82.87°. This is known as the 68% CI.

In practice, researchers usually report a 90%, 95%, or 99% CI. To generate these intervals, we need to determine what *z* scores correspond to them. For the 90% CI, 10% is excluded—5% (.05) in the upper tail of the distribution and 5% in the lower tail of the distribution. For the 95% and 99% CIs, the percentages excluded in each tail are 2.5% (.025) and .5% (.005), respectively. Refer to the *z* table in Appendix C to confirm that the *z* scores that correspond to .05 and .025 are 1.645 and 1.960, respectively. The *z* table included in this text was selected for its simplicity and conciseness. However, this simplicity is at the expense of some precision in the very low probability ranges. Thus, we cannot determine from this table the exact *z* score that corresponds to .005. From a more complete table printed elsewhere the value is found to be 2.576.[3(p380)] Thus, the desired CI of the mean is determined by adding and subtracting the appropriate number of SEMs to and from the mean. In mathematical notation,

$$90\%\ CI = \overline{X} \pm 1.645\ (SEM)$$
$$95\%\ CI = \overline{X} \pm 1.960\ (SEM)$$
$$99\%\ CI = \overline{X} \pm 2.576\ (SEM)$$

Inserting the values of 77.6° ($\overline{X}$) and 6.27° (SEM), we find the following:

90% CI = 67.3° to 87.9°
95% CI = 65.3° to 89.9°
99% CI = 61.4° to 93.7°

We are 90% confident that the true population mean is somewhere between 67.3° and 87.9°; we are 99% confident that it lies somewhere between 61.4° and 93.7°. The computations given here are for the simplest calculation of a CI for the population mean. CIs can also be calculated for population proportions, for the difference between population proportions, and for the difference between population means.[3(pp69–103)]

SIGNIFICANT DIFFERENCE

Researchers often wish to do more than describe their data. They wish to determine whether there are differences between groups who have been exposed to different treatments. The branch of statistics that is used to determine whether, among other things, there are significant differences between groups is known as *inferential statistics*. The theoretical basis of inferential statistics is that population parameters can be inferred from sample statistics. The determination of whether two sample means are significantly different from one another is actually a determination of the likelihood that the two sample means are drawn from populations with the same means. The sampling distribution of the mean is used as the basis for making these inferential statements—it is the link between the observed samples and the theorized population.

When we compare two groups who have received different experimental treatments, we almost always find that there is some difference between the means of the two groups. For example, assume that we wish to determine the effect of continuous passive motion on three-week ROM in our patients who have had total knee arthroplasty. Assume that the patients at Clinic 1 received continuous passive motion postoperatively and that the patients at Clinic 3 did not. The mean three-week ROM score for Clinic 1 is 77.6°; for Clinic 3, it is 72.6°. This is a difference of 5.0°. We wonder whether this difference is a true difference between the two groups or chance variation due to sampling error.

If it is highly likely that the difference was due to sampling error, then we conclude that there is *no significant difference* between the two group means. In other words, if sampling errors are a likely explanation for the difference between the means of the groups, then it is likely that the two groups were drawn from populations with the same means. Conversely, if it is highly unlikely that the difference between the groups was the result of sampling errors, then we conclude that there is a *significant difference* between the groups. If sampling error is not a likely explanation for differences between the groups, then it is likely that the two groups come from populations with different means. To determine whether the difference between groups is significant, we test a null hypothesis at a particular alpha level, as described next.

Null Hypothesis

The seemingly convoluted language needed to describe the meaning of a statistically significant difference derives from the fact that the statistical hypothesis that is tested is the hypothesis of "no difference." This hypothesis is referred to as the *null hypothesis*, or H_0. The formal null hypothesis for determining whether there are different mean three-week ROM scores between Clinics 1 and 3 is as follows:

$$H_0: \mu_1 = \mu_3$$

Thus, the null hypothesis is that the population mean for Clinic 1 is equal to the population mean for Clinic 3. For now we will assume that the alternative hypothesis, or H_1, is that the population mean of Clinic 1 is greater than the population mean of Clinic 3:

$$H_1: \mu_1 > \mu_3$$

Other alternative hypotheses are possible and are addressed later with specific statistical tests. In statistical testing, we determine the probability that the null hypothesis is true. If the probability is sufficiently low, we conclude that the null hypothesis is false, accept the alternative hypothesis, and conclude that there are significant differences between the groups. If the probability that the null hypothesis is true is high, we conclude that the null hypothesis is true, accept the null hypothesis, and conclude that there are no significant differences between the groups.

Alpha Level

Before conducting a statistical analysis of differences, researchers must determine how much of a probability of drawing an incorrect conclusion they are willing to tolerate. To use null hypothesis terminology, how low is the "sufficiently low" probability needed to detect a significant difference? The conventional level of chance that is tolerated is 5%, or .05. This is referred to as the *alpha (α) level*. If a difference in means is significant at the .05 level, this means that 5% of differences of this magnitude would have been the result of chance fluctuations caused by sampling errors. That is, 95% of the time the difference would represent a true difference and 5% of the time the difference would represent sampling error. Occasionally the more stringent level of .01 is used, as is the more permissive level of .10.

There are two twists that occur with alpha levels as they are reported in research. The first is the distinction between the alpha level and the obtained probability; the second is inflation and correction of the alpha level during performance of multiple statistical tests.

The distinction between the alpha level and the obtained probability (p) level is the distinction between what the researcher is willing to accept as chance and what the actual results are. The alpha level is specified before the data analysis is conducted; the probability level is a product of the data analysis. Researchers may set the alpha level at .05, meaning that they are willing to accept a 5% chance that significant findings may actually be the result of sampling error. In studies in which significant differences are found, the actual probability that a given result will occur by chance may be much less than the alpha level set by the researcher.

Assume that the result of a statistical test comparing two group means is that the probability that the difference will occur by chance is .001. This means that in only 1 of 1,000 instances would a difference of this magnitude likely be the result of sampling error. Now that computers are available to calculate statistics, such precise probability levels are often reported. Because the obtained probability level of .001 is less than the preset alpha level of .05, the researcher concludes that there is a significant difference between the groups. Does the reporting of the obtained probability level of .001 somehow indicate that the researcher changed the alpha level during the course of the data analysis? No. The reporting of a specific probability level simply indicates to the reader the extent to which the obtained probability was lower or higher than the alpha set by the researcher.

The second twist that is given to an alpha level in a study is called *alpha level inflation.* This occurs when researchers conduct many statistical tests within a given study. Using an alpha level of 5%, we know that the probability that differences occurred by chance is 5% for each test. If we conduct many tests, the overall probability of obtaining chance significant differences increases. This increase is alpha level inflation. When researchers conduct multiple tests, they may correct for alpha level inflation by using a more stringent alpha level for each individual test. They may obtain a more stringent alpha by using, for example, the *Bonferroni adjustment.* This adjustment divides the total alpha level for the experiment, called the experiment-wise alpha, by the number of statistical tests conducted to determine a test-wise alpha level.[3(p128)] For example, a researcher may set the experiment-wise alpha at .05 and conduct 10 tests, each with a test-wise alpha level of .005 (.05/10 = .005). Some researchers consider this adjustment too stringent and compensate by setting a higher experiment-wise alpha level. For example, if a researcher sets the experiment-wise alpha at .15 and conducts 7 tests, the adjusted test-wise alpha level would be .0214.

An example of the use of the Bonferroni adjustment is found in Moncur's study of physical therapist competencies in rheumatology.[4] To compensate for using each piece of data in 7 different analyses, she divided her alpha level of .05 by 7 to arrive at a test-wise alpha level of .007.

Statistical analysis requires that the researcher set an alpha level. If the statistical test results in an obtained probability that is less than the predetermined alpha level, the result is deemed statistically significant. Whether a result is statistically significant or not often depends on the way in which the researcher sets the alpha level. Thus, tests of statistical significance do not provide absolute conclusions about the meaning of data. Rather, these tests provide the researcher with information about the probability that the obtained results occurred by chance. The researcher then draws statistical conclusions about whether a statistically significant difference exists. Researchers and readers then need to interpret the statistical conclusions in light of their knowledge of the subject being studied.

Probability Determinants

Three pieces of information are essential to the determination of statistical probabilities: effect size, or differences *between* groups; variability, or differences *within* a group; and sample size. In this section, the effect of each of these determinants is illustrated conceptually, without determination of actual probabilities. Actual probabilities are determined in subsequent chapters when specific statistical tests are discussed.

Between-Groups Variability. To illustrate the influence of the size of the difference between two groups, let us compare the differences in mean three-week ROM scores between Clinics 1 through 3. Clinic 1 has a mean of 77.6°, Clinic 2 a mean of 49.1°, and Clinic 3 a mean of 72.6°. If within-group variability and sample size are held constant, then a larger between-groups difference is associated with a smaller probability that the difference occurred by chance. Thus, there is a relatively low probability that the large 28.5° difference in the three-week ROM means for Clinics 1 and 2 occurred by chance.

Conversely, there is a relatively high probability that the smaller 5.0° difference in the three-week ROM means for Clinics 1 and 3 did occur by chance.

Within-Group Variability. The second piece of information used to determine the probability that a difference is a true difference is the variability within a group. If between-groups variability and sample size are held constant, the differences between groups with lower within-group variability have a lower probability of occurring by chance than differences between groups with high within-group variability. Assume that we have two groups of 100 with means of 72.6° and 77.6°. If the groups have high within-group variability—say, standard deviations of 30.0°—curves representing their sampling distributions would look like those drawn in Figure 13–4A. The sampling distributions, which each have an SEM of 3 ($30/\sqrt{100} = 3$), overlap a great deal.

Because of the overlap in sampling distributions, there is a high probability that the two samples came from populations that have the same mean. Because this probability is high, we conclude that the difference in means occurred by chance; that is, the difference between the means of the two groups is not significant.

Contrast Parts A and B in Figure 13–4. Part B illustrates the same between-groups difference, 5.0°. However, the within-group variability has been reduced sharply. In this example, each group standard deviation is set at 10.0°, meaning that the SEM is 1° ($10/\sqrt{100} = 1$). With a SEM of only 1°, the two curves overlap very little. Because they do not overlap very much, there is a low probability that the samples could have been drawn from populations with the same mean. Because this probability is low, we can conclude that the difference in means did not occur by chance; that is, the difference between the means of the two groups is a significant one. Even small differences between groups can be statistically significant if the within-group variability is sufficiently low.

Sample Size. The third piece of information used to determine the probability that a difference is a true difference is the sample size. We already know that the mean of a large sample is more stable than a mean of a small sample. Assume that we have two groups of 100, each with a standard deviation of 10.0°, and a mean difference between the groups of 5.0°. Because of the large sample sizes, we are confident that the mean values are stable indicators of the means of the populations from which the samples are drawn. The estimated SEM for each group's sampling distribution is 1.0° ($10/\sqrt{100} = 1$); Figure 13–5A shows the minimal overlap between the two sampling distributions. This minimal overlap leads us to conclude that it is unlikely that the differences between the two groups are due to chance; in other words, there is a significant difference between the groups.

Now assume that we have two groups of 10 subjects each. The mean difference between the groups is the same as the previous example (5.0°), as is the standard deviation of each group (10.0°). Because we know that sample sizes of only 10 are sensitive to extreme values, we know that the mean of a sample of 10 is considerably less stable than a mean from a sample of 100. This is reflected in the calculation of the estimated SEM. With a standard deviation of 10° and a sample size of 10, the SEM becomes 3.16° ($10/\sqrt{10} = 3.16$). Figure 13–5B shows the curves that correspond to the sampling distributions of our smaller samples. The curves overlap considerably, leading us to conclude that the samples might well have been drawn from populations with the same mean; that is, there is no significant difference between the means of the two groups. Thus, if the sample size is large enough, even small between-

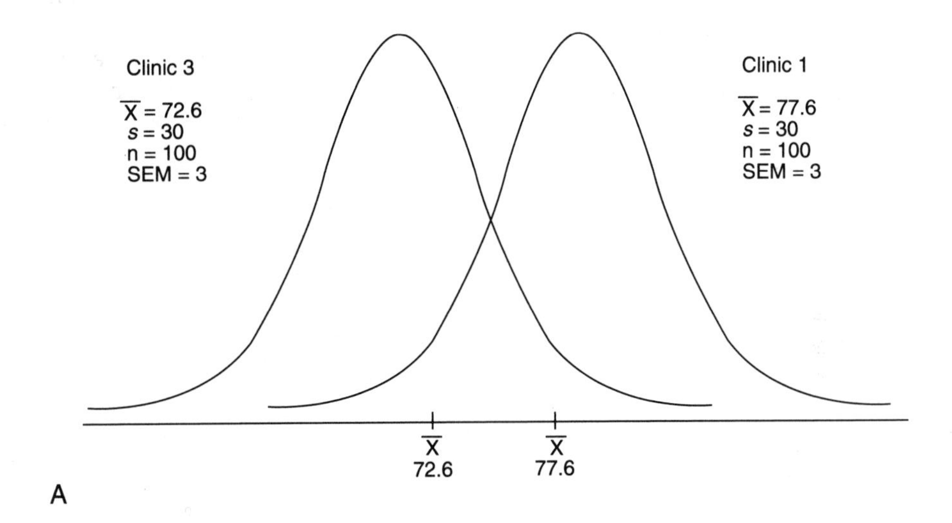

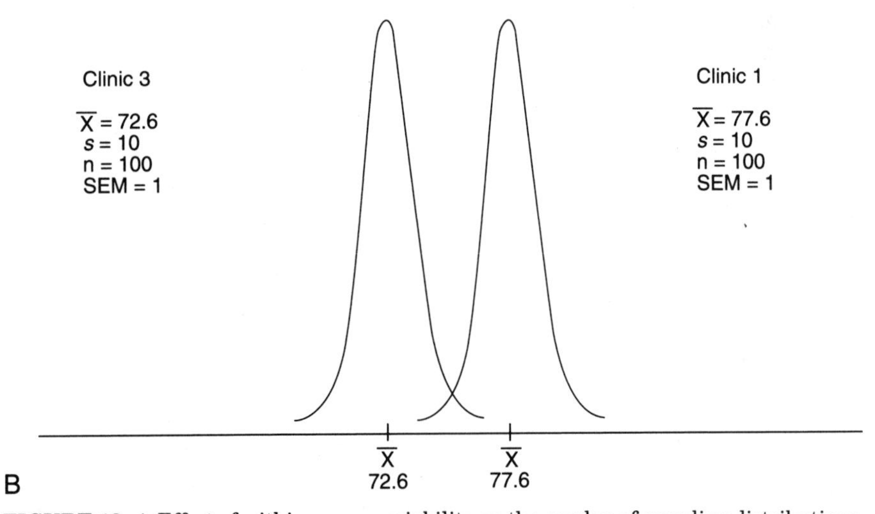

FIGURE 13–4. Effect of within-group variability on the overlap of sampling distributions. **A.** High variability leads to overlap of sampling distributions. **B.** Low variability leads to minimal overlap of sampling distributions. $\overline{X}$, mean; *s*, standard deviation; n, number of subjects; SEM, standard error of the mean.

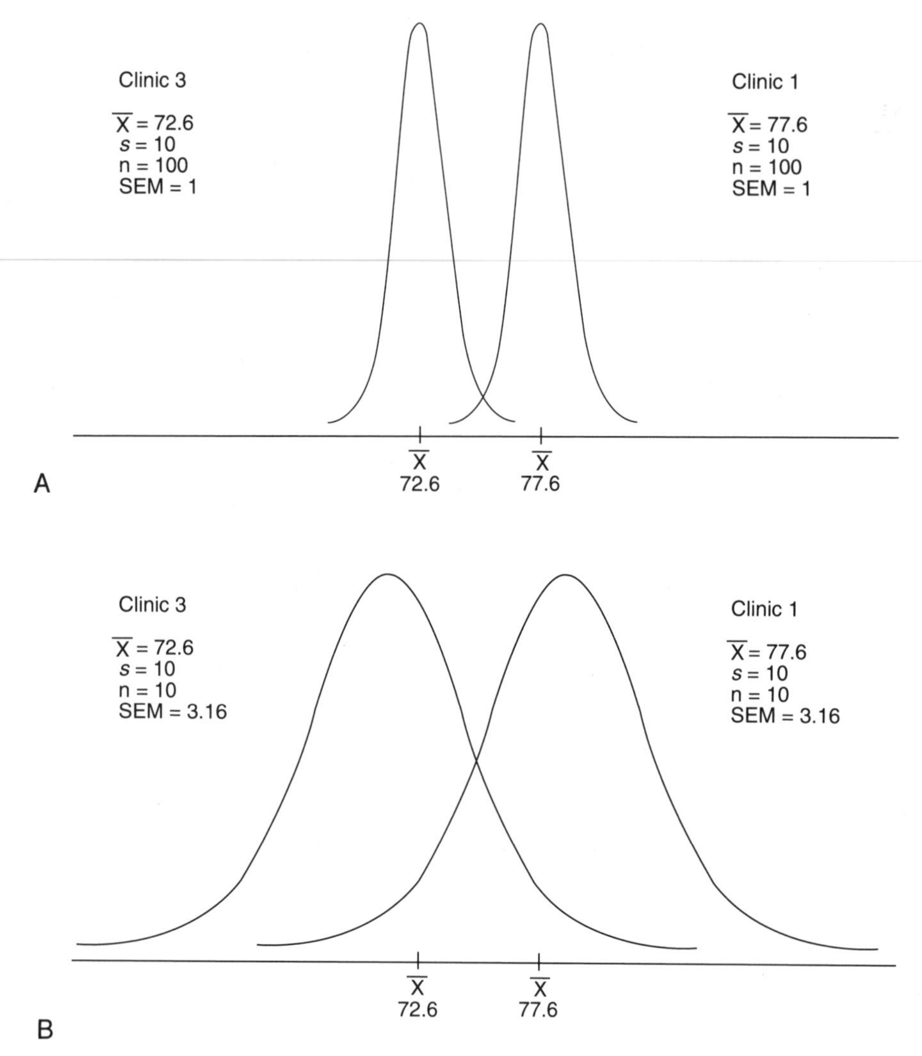

FIGURE 13–5. Effect of sample size on the overlap of sampling distributions. **A.** Large sample size leads to low overlap. **B.** Small sample size leads to extensive overlap. $\overline{X}$, mean; *s*, standard deviation; n, number of subjects; SEM, standard error of the mean.

groups differences may be statistically significant and, conversely, if the sample size is too small, even large between-groups differences may not be statistically significant.

ERRORS

Because researchers determine statistical differences by making probability statements, there is always the possibility that the statistical conclusion has been reached in error. Unfortunately, researchers never know when an error has been made, they only know the probability of making that error. There are two types of statistical errors, labeled simply Type I and Type II. Figure 13–6 shows the difference between them. The columns represent the two possible states of reality: there

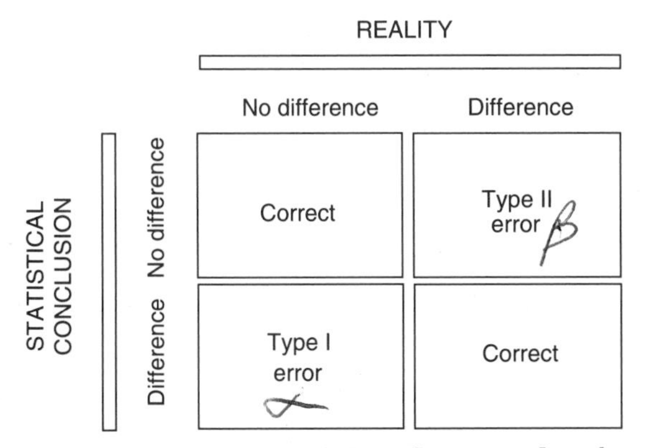

FIGURE 13–6. Type I and Type II errors reflect the relationship between statistical conclusions and reality.

is or is not a difference between groups. The rows represent the two statistical conclusions that can be drawn: there is or is not a difference between groups. The intersection of the columns and rows creates four different combinations of statistical conclusions and reality. If the statistical conclusion is that there is no difference between groups and there is in fact no difference, then we have made a correct statistical conclusion. If the statistical conclusion is that there is a difference between groups and this is in fact the case, then we have also come to a correct statistical conclusion.

However, if the statistical conclusion is that there is a difference between groups when in fact there is no difference, then we have come to an erroneous statistical conclusion. This error is called a Type I error. The probability of making a Type I error is alpha. Recall that researchers set alpha according to the amount of chance they are willing to tolerate. An alpha level of .05 means that the researcher is willing to accept a 5% chance that significant results occurred by chance. Thus, alpha is the probability that significant results will be found when in fact no significant difference exists. Researchers never know when they have committed a Type I error; they only know the probability that one occurred. If researchers wish to decrease the probability of making a Type I error, they simply reduce alpha.

A Type II error occurs when the statistical conclusion is that there is no difference between the groups when in reality there is a difference. The probability of making a Type II error is beta. Beta is related to alpha but is not as easily obtained. Figure 13–7 shows the relationship between alpha and beta.

For this example we assume samples of 25 with standard deviations of 10°, giving us an SEM of 2.0° ($10/\sqrt{25} = 2$). We also assume that Clinic 3, with a mean of 72.6°, is the standard against which Clinic 1, with a mean of 77.6°, is being compared. Our null hypothesis is that $\mu_1 = \mu_3$. Our alternative hypothesis is that $\mu_1 > \mu_3$. In words, we wish to determine whether the mean of Clinic 1 is significantly greater than the mean of Clinic 3. Alpha is set at 5% in Part A of Figure 13–7.

To determine beta, we first must determine the point on the Clinic 3 curve above which only 5% of the distribution lies. From the *z* table we find that .05 corresponds to a *z* score of 1.645. A *z* score of 1.645 corresponds in this case to a raw score of 75.9° [through algebraic rearrangement, $\overline{X} + (z)(SEM) = X$; $72.6 + (1.645)(2) = 75.9$]. Thus, if Clinic 1's mean is greater than 75.9° (1.645 SEM above Clinic 3's mean), it would be considered significantly different from Clinic 3's mean of 72.6° at the 5% level. The dark shading at the upper tail of Clinic 3's sampling distribution corresponds to the alpha level of 5% and is the probability of making a Type I error. This darkly shaded area is sometimes referred to as the *rejection region* because the null hypothesis of no difference between groups would be rejected if a group mean within this area were obtained. Any group mean less than 75.9° degrees would not be identified as statistically different from the group mean of 72.6°.

The entire part of the curve below the rejection region (including the parts that are

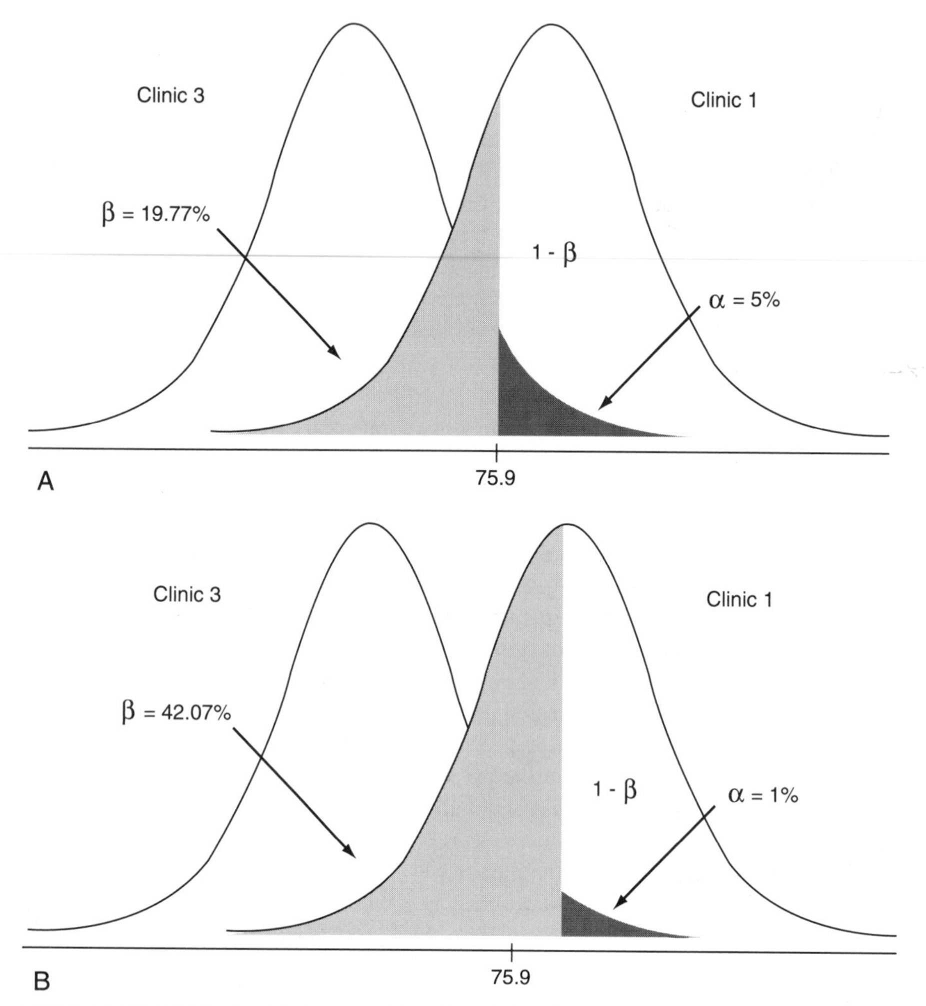

FIGURE 13–7. Relationship between Type I and Type II errors. **A.** α (probability of making a Type I error) is 5% and β (probability of making a Type II error) is 19.77%. **B.** α is 1% and β is 42.07%.

lightly shaded) is termed the *acceptance region* because the null hypothesis of no difference between groups would be accepted if a group mean within this area were obtained.

Shift your attention now to the lightly shaded lower tail of the sampling distribution of Clinic 1. Using the *z* table, we can determine the probability of obtaining sample means less than 75.9°, if the population mean was actually 77.6°. To do so, we convert 75.9 to a *z* score in relation to 77.6: $z = (X - \overline{X})/SEM$; $(75.9 - 77.6)/2 = -.85$. Using the *z* table, we find that 19.77% of Clinic 1's sampling distribution will fall below a *z* score of −.85. This percentage is the probability of making a Type II error. If Clinic 1, in reality, has a mean that is significantly greater than Clinic 3's mean, we would fail to detect this difference almost 20% of the time because of the overlap in the sampling distributions. Almost 20% of Clinic 1's sampling distribution falls within the acceptance region of Clinic 3's sampling distribution.

There is an inverse relationship between

the probability of making Type I and II errors. When the probability of one increases, the probability of the other decreases. Figure 13–7B shows that, for this example, when the probability of making a Type I error is decreased to 1%, the Type II error increases to 43%. Thus, in setting the alpha level for an experiment, the researcher must find a balance between the likelihood of detecting chance differences (Type I error—alpha) and the likelihood of ignoring important differences (Type II error—beta).

POWER

The *power* of a test is the likelihood that it will detect a difference when one exists. Recall that beta was the probability of ignoring an important difference when one existed. The probability of detecting a true difference, or power, is therefore $1 - \beta$, as shown in the Clinic 1 curves in Figure 13–7. Recall that the size of the between-groups difference, the size of the sample, and the variability within the sample are the factors that determine whether significant differences between groups are detected. When the sampling distributions of the groups have minimal overlap, the power of a test is high. Factors that contribute to nonoverlapping sampling distributions are large between-groups differences, small within-group differences, and large sample sizes.

Ottenbacher and Barrett have shown that power is often lacking in rehabilitation research.[5] This is because between-groups differences are often small, sample sizes are usually small, and within-group variability is often large. This lack of statistical power in our literature may mean that promising treatment approaches are not pursued because research has failed to show a significant advantage to the approaches. The power of a given statistical test can be determined by consulting published power tables.[6, 7]

Researchers may increase a test's statistical power in three ways. First, they can maximize between-groups differences by carefully controlling extraneous variables and making sure they apply experimental techniques consistently. Note, however, that rigid controls may reduce a study's external validity by making the conditions under which it was conducted very different from the clinical situation to which the researcher wishes to generalize the results.

Second, researchers can reduce within-group variability by studying homogeneous groups of subjects or by using subjects as their own controls in repeated measures designs. Note that these strategies also may reduce external validity by narrowing the group of patients to whom the results can be generalized.

Third, researchers can increase sample size. Increasing sample size does not have the negative impact on external validity that the other two solutions have. However, the increased cost of research with more subjects is an obvious disadvantage to this strategy.

Published power tables can also be used to determine what sample size is needed to achieve a particular power rating. The variables needed to determine sample size requirements are

- Desired power (Ottenbacher and Barrett recommend a power level of .80[5])
- The alpha level that will be used in the research
- An estimate of the size of the between-groups difference that would be considered clinically meaningful
- An estimate of the within-group variability expected.

A researcher can obtain these values from previous research or from a pilot study. In some instances it is difficult to determine sample size because there is no previous information on which to base one's estimates.

STATISTICAL CONCLUSION VALIDITY

Readers have previously been introduced to the research design concepts of internal, external, and construct validity. The final type of design validity that a researcher must consider when evaluating a research report is statistical conclusion validity. Four threats to statistical conclusion validity, modified from Cook and Campbell, are presented in this section.[8]

Low Power

When statistically insignificant results are reported, readers must ask whether the nonsignificant result is a true indication of no difference or the result of a Type II error. Researchers who give power estimates provide their readers with the probability that their analysis could detect differences and, in doing so, provide information readers need to make a decision about the potential usefulness of further study in the area.

Whether or not a power analysis is provided, readers should examine nonsignificant results to determine whether any of the nonsignificant changes were in the desired direction or of a clinically important magnitude. If the nonsignificant differences seem clinically useful and the probability of making a Type II error seems high (sample size was small, the within-group variability was large, or an analysis showed less than 80% power), then readers should be cautious about dismissing the results altogether. Studies with promising nonsignificant results should be replicated with more powerful designs.

An example of a study with low power is Palmer and associates' report of the effects of two different types of exercise programs in patients with Parkinson's disease.[9] Seven patients participated in each exercise program. No significant changes were found in measures of rigidity, although some showed nonsignificant changes in the desired direction. A power analysis of this study reveals that it had, at most, a 50% power level.[5] Because the probability of making a Type II error was so high, the nonsignificant findings should not necessarily be taken to mean that exercise was not useful for these patients. A logical next step in investigating the effects of exercise for patients with Parkinson's disease is to replicate this study with a more powerful design.

Clinical Insignificance

If the power of a test is sufficiently great, it may detect differences that are so small that they are clinically insignificant. This occurs when samples are large and groups homogeneous. Just as readers need to examine the between-groups differences of statistically insignificant results to determine whether there is promise in the results, they must also examine statistically significant between-groups differences to determine whether they are clinically meaningful.

Error Rate Problems

Inflation of alpha when multiple tests are conducted within a study is referred to as an error rate problem because the probability of making a Type I error rises with each additional test. As discussed earlier, some researchers compensate for multiple tests by dividing an experiment-wise alpha among the tests to be conducted. Although division of alpha controls the experiment-wise alpha, it also dramatically reduces the power of each test. Readers must determine whether they believe that researchers who have conducted multiple tests have struck a reasonable balance between controlling alpha and limiting the power of their statistical analyses.

A study of balance function in elderly people illustrates alpha level inflation.[10] In this study, three groups were tested: nonfallers, recent fallers, and remote fallers. Five different measures of balance function were obtained on each of two types of supporting surfaces for each of two types of displacement stimuli. The combination of all these factors produced 20 measures for each subject. In the data analysis nonfallers were compared with recent fallers, recent fallers were compared with remote fallers, and nonfallers were compared with remote fallers on each of the 20 measures. This yielded a total of 60 different tests of statistical significance. With this many tests, the overall probability that a Type I error was committed was far higher than the .05 level set for each analysis. Statistical techniques that would have permitted comparison of more than two groups or more than one dependent variable simultaneously could have been used to prevent this alpha level inflation; these techniques are presented in Chapter 14.

Violated Assumptions

Each of the statistical tests that are presented in Chapters 14 and 15 is based on certain assumptions that should be met for the test to be valid. These assumptions are that the observations were made independently of one another, that subjects were randomly sampled, that the data were normally distributed, and that the variance of the data was approximately equal across groups. These assumptions, and the consequences of violating them, are discussed in detail in Chapters 14 and 15.

SUMMARY

All statistical analyses are based on a relatively small set of central concepts. Descriptive statistics are based on the concepts of central tendency (mean, median, or mode) and variability (range, variance, and standard deviation) within a data set. The distribution of many variables forms a bell-shaped curve known as the normal distribution. The percentage of scores that fall within a certain range of the normal distribution is known and can be used to predict the likelihood of obtaining certain scores. The sampling distribution is a special normal distribution that consists of a theoretical distribution of sample means.

Inferential statistical tests use sampling distributions to determine the likelihood that different samples came from populations with the same characteristics. A significant difference between groups indicates that the probability that the samples came from populations with the same characteristics is lower than a predetermined level, alpha, that is set by the researcher. There is always a probability that one of two statistical errors will be made: A Type I error occurs when a significant difference is found when in fact there is no difference; a Type II error occurs when a difference actually exists but is not identified by the test. The power of a test is the probability that it will detect a true difference. The validity of statistical conclusions is threatened by low power, clinically insignificant results, alpha level inflation with multiple tests, and violation of statistical assumptions.

References

1. Chottiner S. Statistics: toward a kinder, gentler subject. *Journal of Irreproducible Results.* 1990; 35(6):13–15.
2. Ewald FC, Jacobs MA, Miegel RE, Walker PS, Poss R, Sledge CB. Kinematic total knee replacement. *J Bone Joint Surg.* 1984;66-A:1032–1040.
3. Shott S. *Statistics for Health Professionals.* Philadelphia, Pa: WB Saunders Co; 1990.
4. Moncur C. Perception of physical therapy competencies in rheumatology: physical therapists versus rheumatologists. *Phys Ther.* 1987;67:331–339.
5. Ottenbacher KJ, Barrett KA. Statistical conclusion

validity of rehabilitation research: a quantitative analysis. *Am J Phys Med Rehabil.* 1990;69:102–107.
6. Kraemer HC, Thiemann S. *How Many Subjects? Statistical Power Analysis in Research.* Newbury Park, Calif: Sage Publications; 1987.
7. Cohen J. *Statistical Power Analysis for the Behavioral Sciences.* 2nd ed. Hillsdale, NJ: Lawrence Erlbaum Associates; 1988.
8. Cook TD, Campbell DT. *Quasi-experimentation: Design and Analysis Issues for Field Settings.* Chicago, Ill: Rand McNally College Publishing Co; 1979:37–94.
9. Palmer SS, Mortimer JA, Webster DD, Bistevins R, Dickinson GL. Exercise therapy for Parkinson's disease. *Arch Phys Med Rehabil.* 1986;67:741–745.
10. Ring C, Nayak USL, Isaacs B. Balance function in elderly people who have and who have not fallen. *Arch Phys Med Rehabil.* 1988;69:261–264.

↑ BG (b/t group)
↓ WG (w/in group)
↑ SS (sample sizes)

CHAPTER 14

Statistical Analysis of Differences

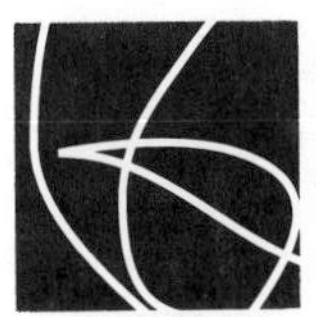

Researchers use statistical tests when they wish to determine whether a significant difference exists between two or more sets of numbers. In this chapter, the general statistical concepts presented in Chapter 13 are applied to the specific statistical tests of differences commonly reported in the physical therapy literature. The distributions most commonly used in statistical testing are presented first, followed by the general assumptions that underlie statistical tests of differences. The sequence of steps common to all statistical tests of differences is then outlined. Finally, the specific tests of differences are presented. Each is illustrated with an example from the hypothetical knee arthroplasty data set presented in Chapter 13 as well as an example from the literature.

DISTRIBUTIONS FOR ANALYSIS OF DIFFERENCES

In Chapter 13 the rationale behind statistical testing is developed in terms of the standard normal distribution and its z scores. Use of this distribution assumes that the population standard deviation is known. Because the population standard deviation is usually *not* known, we cannot ordinarily use the standard normal distribution and its z scores to draw statistical conclusions from samples. Therefore, researchers conduct most statistical tests using distributions that resemble the normal distribution but are altered somewhat to account for the errors that are made when population parameters are estimated. The three most common distributions used for statistical tests are the t, F, and chi-square (χ^2) distributions, pictured in Figure 14–1. Just as we determined the probability of obtaining certain z scores based on the standard normal distribution, we can determine

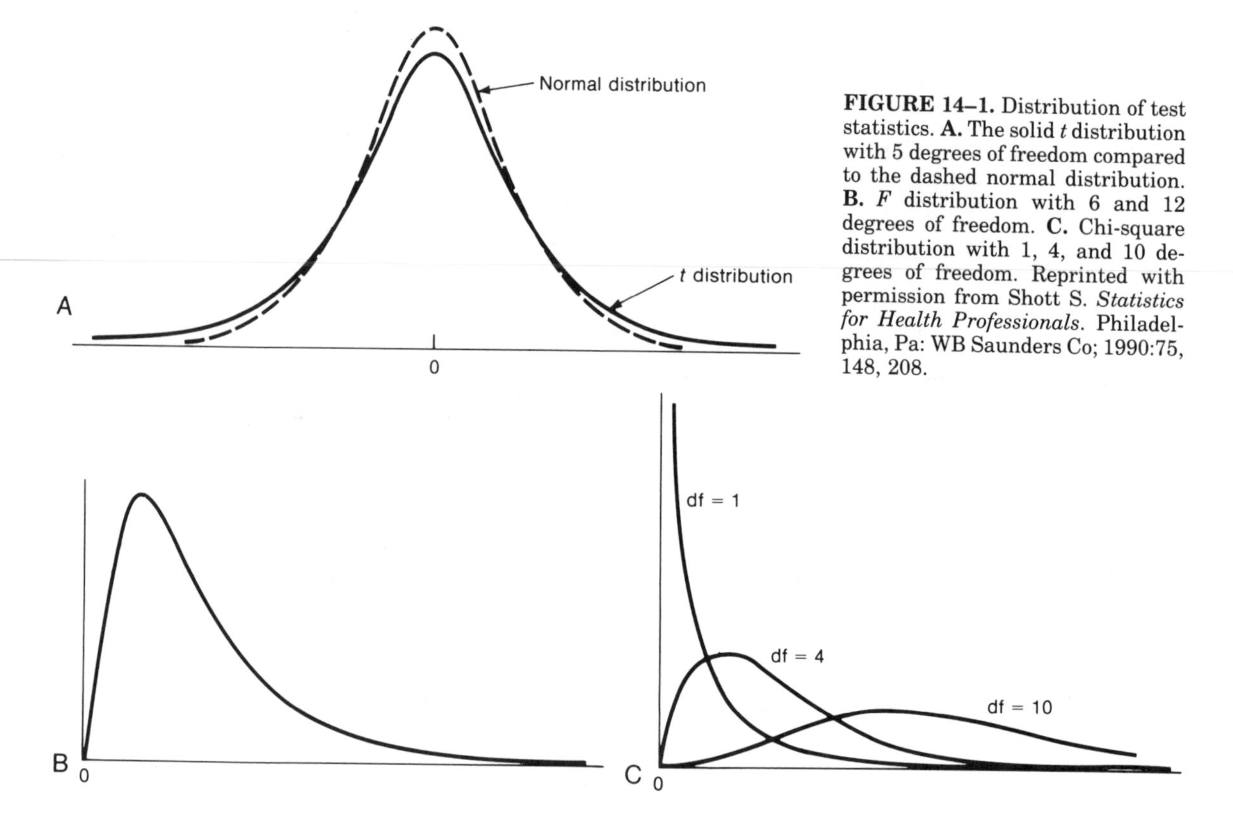

FIGURE 14–1. Distribution of test statistics. **A.** The solid *t* distribution with 5 degrees of freedom compared to the dashed normal distribution. **B.** *F* distribution with 6 and 12 degrees of freedom. **C.** Chi-square distribution with 1, 4, and 10 degrees of freedom. Reprinted with permission from Shott S. *Statistics for Health Professionals.* Philadelphia, Pa: WB Saunders Co; 1990:75, 148, 208.

the probability of obtaining certain *t, F,* and chi-square statistics based on their respective distributions.

***t* Distribution.** The *t* distribution is a symmetrical distribution that is essentially a "flattened" *z* distribution (Figure 14–1A). Compared with the *z* distribution, a greater proportion of the *t* distribution is located in the tails and a lesser proportion in the center of the distribution. The *z* distribution is spread to form the *t* distribution to account for the errors that are introduced when population parameters are estimated from sample statistics. The shape of a *t* distribution varies with its degrees of freedom, which is based on sample size. Because estimation of population parameters is more accurate with larger samples, *t* distributions become more and more similar to *z* distributions as sample size and degrees of freedom increase.

***F* Distribution.** The *F* distribution is a distribution of squared *t* statistics (Figure 14–1B). It is asymmetrical and, because it is generated from squared scores, consists only of positive values. The actual shape of a particular *F* distribution depends on two different degrees of freedom—one associated with the number of groups being compared and one associated with the sample size.

Chi-Square Distribution. The chi-square distribution is a distribution of squared *z* scores (Figure 14–1C). As is the case with the *t* and *F* distributions, the shape of the chi-square distribution varies with its degrees of freedom.

ASSUMPTIONS OF TESTS OF DIFFERENCES

Statistical tests of differences are either parametric or nonparametric. Parametric tests are based on specific assumptions about the distribution of populations. They use sample statistics such as the mean, standard deviation, and variance to estimate differences between population parameters. The two major classes of parametric tests are *t* tests and analyses of variance (ANOVAs).

Nonparametric tests are not based on specific assumptions about the distribution of populations. They use rank or frequency information to draw conclusions about differences between populations.[1, 2] Parametric tests are usually assumed to be more powerful than nonparametric tests and are often preferred to nonparametric tests.[3(p229)] However, parametric tests cannot always be used because the assumptions on which they are based are more stringent than the assumptions for nonparametric tests.

Parametric Assumptions

Three parametric assumptions are commonly accepted: independence or dependence of samples, random selection, and homogeneity of variance. A fourth assumption is controversial and relates to the measurement level of the data.

Independence or Dependence of Samples. The first basic assumption that must be met for parametric testing concerns whether the different sets of numbers being compared are independent or dependent. Sets are independent when values in one set tell nothing about values in another set. When two or more groups consist of different, unrelated individuals, the observations made about the samples are independent. For example, the three-week range of motion (ROM) scores for patients in Clinics 1 through 3 in our hypothetical knee arthroplasty study are independent of one another. Knowing the three-week ROM values for patients at Clinic 1 provides us with no information about three-week ROM values at Clinic 2 or Clinic 3.

When the sets of numbers consist of repeated measures on the same individuals, they are said to be dependent. The three-week, six-week, and six-month ROM scores for patients across the three clinics are dependent measures. A patient's six-week score is expected to be related to the three-week score. Repeated measures taken on the same individual are not the only type of dependent measures, however. If we compare male and female characteristics by using brother–sister pairs, we have dependent samples. If we study pairs or trios of individuals matched for factors such as income, education, age, height, and weight, then we also have dependent samples.

Different statistical tests are used with independent versus dependent samples, and the assumption of either independence or dependence must not be violated. The researcher must select the correct test according to whether the samples are independent or dependent.

Random Selection from Normally Distributed Populations. The second basic assumption of parametric testing is that the subjects are randomly selected from normally distributed populations. However, this assumption may be violated as long as the data sets used in the analysis are relatively normally distributed. Even when the data sets are not normally distributed, statistical researchers have shown that the various statistical tests are *robust,* meaning that they usually still provide an appropriate level of rejection of the null hypothesis. The extent to which a data set is normally distributed may be tested; however, the details are beyond the scope of this text.[4(p68)]

When data are extremely nonnormal, one data analysis strategy is to convert, or *transform,* the data mathematically so that they become normally distributed. Squaring, taking the square root of, or calculating a logarithm of raw data are common transformations. Parametric tests can then be conducted on the transformed scores. A second strategy for dealing with nonnormality is to use nonparametric tests, which do not require normally distributed data.

Homogeneity of Variance. The third basic assumption of parametric testing is that the population variances of the groups being tested are equal, or *homogeneous*. When the sample sizes of the groups being tested are equal, the homogeneity-of-variance assumption can usually be violated without significant alteration of probability levels.

Homogeneity of variance may be tested statistically.[4(p264)] If homogeneity of variance is tested and the variances of the groups are found to differ significantly, then nonparametric tests must be used.

Measurement-Level Assumption. The final, and most controversial, assumption for parametric testing concerns the measurement level of the data. As noted earlier, one distinction between parametric and nonparametric tests is that the two types of tests are used with different types of data. Nonparametric tests require rankings or frequencies—nominal and ranked ordinal data meet this need, and interval and ratio data can be converted into ranks or grouped into categories to meet this need. Parametric tests require data from which means and variances can be calculated—interval and ratio data clearly meet this need; nominal data clearly do not. The controversy, then, surrounds the use of parametric statistics with ordinal measurements.

Contemporary references indicate that the traditional belief that parametric tests can be conducted only with interval or ratio data is not valid.[5, 6(p24)] Although ordinal-scaled variables do not have the property of equal intervals between numerals, the distribution of ordinal data is often approximately normal. As long as the data themselves meet the parametric assumptions, regardless of the origin of the numbers, then parametric tests can be conducted. As is the case with all statistical tests of differences, the researcher must interpret parametric statistical conclusions that are based on ordinal data in light of their clinical or practical implications.

For example, a common type of ordinal measurement used by physical therapists is a scale of the amount of assistance a patient needs to accomplish various functional tasks. The categories maximal, moderate, minimal, standby, and no assistance could be coded numerically from 1 to 5, with 5 representing no assistance. Assume that four different groups have mean scores of 1.0, 2.0, 4.0, and 5.0 and that these group means have been found to be significantly different from one another. If the researchers believe that the "real" interval between maximal and moderate assistance is greater than the interval between standby and no assistance, they might interpret the difference between the groups with means of 1.0 and 2.0 to be more clinically important than the difference between the groups with means of 4.0 and 5.0. It is reasonable to conduct parametric tests with ordinal data as long as interpretation of the tests accounts for the nature of the ordinal scale.

Nonparametric Assumptions

Because the nonparametric tests are not derived from means, standard deviations, and variances, the parametric assumptions of normality and homogeneity of variance do not apply. Each nonparametric test is, however, based on the assumption that data are from either independent or dependent samples. As is the case with the parametric tests, the independence or dependence assumption must not be violated.

STEPS IN THE STATISTICAL TESTING OF DIFFERENCES

The statistical testing of differences can be summarized in 10 basic steps, regardless of the particular test used. A general assumption of these steps is that researchers intend to perform parametric tests and perform nonparametric tests only if the assumptions for parametric testing are not met. The steps are as follows:

1. State the null and alternative hypotheses in parametric terms.
2. Decide on an alpha level for the test.
3. Determine whether the samples are independent or dependent.
4. Determine whether parametric assumptions are met. Revise hypotheses if nonparametric tests are chosen.
5. Determine the appropriate statistical test, given the above information.
6. Calculate the test statistic.
7. Determine the degrees of freedom for the test statistic.
8. Determine the probability of obtaining the calculated test statistic, taking into account the degrees of freedom. Computer statistical packages generate the precise probability of obtaining a given test statistic for the given degrees of freedom. If a computer package is not available, then statistical tables are used to determine critical values of the test statistic. The critical value is the value of the test statistic above which the specified proportion of the distribution lies. If the alpha level is .05, then 5% of the distribution of the test statistic lies above the critical value.
9. Compare the probability obtained in Step 8 with the alpha level established in Step 2. If the obtained probability is less than the alpha level, the test has identified a statistically significant difference; that is, the null hypothesis is rejected. If the obtained probability is equal to or greater than the alpha level, the test has failed to identify a statistically significant difference; that is, the null hypothesis is not rejected. If statistical tables are used rather than computer probabilities, the obtained test statistic is compared with the critical value of the test statistic. If the obtained value exceeds the critical value, the test has identified a statistically significant difference. If the obtained value is less than or equal to the critical value, the test has failed to identify a statistically significant difference.
10. Evaluate the statistical conclusions in light of clinical knowledge. If the result is statistically significant but the differences between groups seem clinically insignificant, this discrepancy should be discussed. If the result is statistically insignificant but the differences between groups appear clinically important, a power analysis should be conducted and discussed in light of the discrepancy between the statistical and clinical conclusions.

Table 14–1 lists these steps and specifies differences in the procedure based on whether a computer or a calculator and statistical tables are used to conduct the analysis. The remainder of this chapter illustrates how these 10 steps are implemented for several different statistical tests of differences.

TABLE 14–1. Ten Steps in the Statistical Testing of Differences

Step	Computation Method: *Computer Package*	Computation Method: *Calculator and Tables*
1	State hypotheses.	State hypotheses.
2	Determine alpha level.	Determine alpha level.
3	Determine whether samples are independent or dependent.	Determine whether samples are independent or dependent.
4	Run frequency and descriptive programs to determine whether parametric assumptions are met.	Plot frequencies and calculate descriptive statistics to determine whether parametric assumptions are met.
5	Determine appropriate test.	Determine appropriate test.
6	Use appropriate programs to calculate test statistic.	Use appropriate formulas to calculate test statistic.
7	Program calculates the degrees of freedom.	Calculate the degrees of freedom.
8	Program calculates the probability of obtaining the test statistic given the degrees of freedom.	Determine the critical value of the test statistic given the degrees of freedom and predetermined alpha level.
9	Compare the obtained probability with the alpha level to draw statistical conclusion.	Compare the obtained test statistic with the critical value of the test statistic to draw statistical conclusion.
10	Evaluate the statistical conclusions in light of clinical knowledge.	Evaluate the statistical conclusions in light of clinical knowledge.

STATISTICAL ANALYSIS OF DIFFERENCES

The hypothetical total knee arthroplasty data set is used in the rest of this chapter to illustrate 15 different statistical tests of differences. All analyses were conducted with the Statistical Package for the Social Sciences (SPSS).[7] Formulas and computations are included with the first few examples to illustrate how the test statistics are calculated. However, the purpose of this chapter is to enable readers to understand the results of tests, not to perform statistical analyses. Researchers who wish to analyze small data sets by hand can refer to any number of good research and statistical references for the formulas and tables needed to do so.[3,4,8,9]

The 15 tests presented in this chapter are organized by the type of difference being analyzed, rather than by statistical technique. For most of the differences, both a parametric and a nonparametric test are given. Although the number of tests may seem daunting, there are actually only a few basic tests that are varied according to the number of groups being compared, whether the samples are independent or dependent, the nature of the data, whether parametric assumptions are met, and the number of variables being compared simultaneously. Table 14–2 presents an overview of the tests presented in this chapter. This is not an exhaustive list of statistical tests of differences, but it provides the reader with background in more than 80% of the tests of differences that are reported in the physical therapy and rehabilitation literature.[10,11]

Differences Between Two Independent Groups

Assume that Clinics 1 and 2 have different postoperative activity protocols for their patients who have had total knee arthroplasty. We wonder whether there are differences in three-week ROM results between patients at

TABLE 14–2. Statistical Tests for Analyzing Differences

Design	Independent Samples		Dependent Samples	
	Parametric	*Nonparametric*	*Parametric*	*Nonparametric*
Two samples, 1 independent variable (IV), 1 dependent variable (DV)	Independent *t* test	Mann-Whitney	Paired-*t* test	Wilcoxon signed rank (ranks) McNemar (frequencies)
Two or more samples, 1 IV, 1 DV	One-way analysis of variance (ANOVA)	Kruskal-Wallis ANOVA (ranks) Chi-square (frequencies)	Repeated measures ANOVA	Friedman's ANOVA (ranks)
Two or more samples, >1 IV, 1 DV	Two-way ANOVA		Two-factor repeated measures ANOVA	
Two or more samples, 1 IV, >1 DV	Multivariate ANOVA			
Two or more samples, intervening variable	Analysis of covariance			
Single system				Celeration line approaches

Clinic 1 and Clinic 2. The null and alternative hypotheses we intend to test are as follows:

$$H_0: \mu_1 = \mu_2$$

$$H_1: \mu_1 \neq \mu_2$$

We set alpha at 5% and determine that we have independent samples because different, unrelated patients make up the samples from the two clinics. Now we have to determine whether our data meet the assumptions for parametric testing. Table 14–3 shows the descriptive statistics and stem-and-leaf plots for the three-week ROM data for the two groups. The variances, although not identical, are at least of similar magnitude. The ratio of the larger variance to the smaller variance is 1.85, which is less than the 2.0 maximum recommended for meeting the homogeneity-of-variance assumption for the independent *t* test.[3(p117)] The plot for Clinic 1 is negatively *skewed;* that is, it has a long tail of lower numbers. The plot for Clinic 2 looks fairly symmetrical. Under these conditions some researchers would proceed with a parametric test, and others would use a nonparametric test because of the nonnormal shape of the Clinic 1 data. The parametric test of differences between two independent sample means is the independent *t* test; the nonparametric test is either the Mann-Whitney test or the Wilcoxon rank sum test.

Independent t *Test*

Like most test statistics, the test statistic for the independent *t* test is the ratio of the differences between the groups to the differences within the groups. The pooled formula

TABLE 14–3. Independent *t* Test

Clinic	1	2
Data	3 2	2 7
	5 8	3 4
	6 7	4 0 5 7 9
	8 1 4 7 8	5 0 6
	9 2 2 5	6 7
		7 6
Mean	$\overline{X}_1 = 77.6$	$\overline{X}_2 = 49.1$
Variance	$s_1^2 = 393.62$	$s_1^2 = 212.58$
Standard deviation	$s_1 = 19.84$	$s_2 = 14.58$

$$t = \frac{\overline{X}_1 - \overline{X}_2}{\left(\sqrt{\frac{(n_1 - 1)s_1^2 + (n_2 - 1)\,s_2^2}{n_1 + n_2 - 2}}\right)\left(\sqrt{\frac{1}{n_1} + \frac{1}{n_2}}\right)} = \frac{28.5}{(17.4)\,(.447)} = 3.66$$

for the independent t is presented at the bottom of Table 14–3. The numerator is simply the difference between the two sample means. The denominator is a form of a standard error of the mean created by pooling the standard deviations of the samples and dividing by the square root of the pooled sample sizes. When the t formula is solved by inserting the values from our example, a value of 3.66 is obtained. A separate variance formula is available for use if the difference between the two group variances is too great to permit pooling.[3(p119)] The computer-generated two-tailed probability of obtaining a t statistic of 3.66 with 18 degrees of freedom ($n_1 + n_2 - 2$) is .002. Because .002 is less than the predetermined alpha level of .05, we reject the null hypothesis. We conclude that the mean three-week ROM scores of the populations from whom the Clinic 1 and Clinic 2 patients are drawn are significantly different from one another. The difference between the means of the two groups is 28.5°. Because this difference seems clinically important, our statistical and clinical conclusions concur.

In determining our statistical conclusions in the paragraph above, a two-tailed probability was used. The t test is one of only a few statistical tests that require the researcher to differentiate between directional and nondirectional hypotheses before conducting the test. The alternative hypothesis given at the beginning of this section, $\mu_1 \neq \mu_2$, is *nondirectional,* meaning that we are open to the possibility that Clinic 1's mean ROM is either greater than *or* less than Clinic 2's mean ROM. If Clinic 1's mean is greater than Clinic 2's mean, as in our example, the t statistic would be positive. If, however, Clinic 2's mean is greater than Clinic 1's mean, the value of t would be negative. Because our research hypothesis allows for either a positive or a negative t, the probability that t will be greater than $+3.66$ *and* the probability that t will be less than -3.66 must both be accounted for. The two-tailed probability of .002 is the sum of the probability that t will exceed $+3.66$ and the probability that t will be less than -3.66.

A *directional hypothesis* is used occasionally as the alternative to the null hypothesis. A directional hypothesis specifies which of the means is expected to be greater than the other. Use of a directional hypothesis is justified only if there is existing evidence of the direction of the effect or when only one outcome is of interest to the researcher. Researchers who use a directional hypothesis are interested in only one tail of the t distribution. Because the two-tailed probability is the sum of the probabilities in the upper and lower tails of the distribution, the one-tailed probability is determined by dividing the two-tailed probability in half. Thus, for our example, the two-tailed probability of .002 becomes a one-tailed probability of .001.

In this example both the one- and two-tailed probabilities are so low that both lead to the same statistical conclusion. Imagine, though, if the two-tailed probability for a test were .06. If we set alpha at .05 and conduct a two-tailed test, there is no significant difference between groups. However, if we conduct a one-tailed test we divide the two-tailed probability in half to get a one-tailed probability of .03. This is less than our alpha level of .05; thus with the one-tailed test we conclude that there is a significant difference between groups. As can be seen, the one-tailed test is more powerful than the two-tailed test. Researchers should not be tempted to abuse this power by conducting one-tailed tests unless they have an appropriate rationale for doing so.

Independent t tests are often used to analyze pretest–posttest designs when there are only two groups and two measurements on each subject. One strategy is to perform an independent t test on the pretest data; if there is no significant difference between groups at pretest, then an independent t test is run on the posttest data to determine whether there was a significant treatment effect. A second strategy is to create gain scores by subtracting the pretest value from the posttest value for each subject. An independent t test is then run on the gain scores to determine whether one group had a significantly greater change than the other. Egger and Miller provide a useful description of different options for analyzing pretest–posttest designs, along with guidelines for making decisions among the options.[12]

An independent t test would typically be summarized in a journal article as follows:

DATA ANALYSIS

An independent t test was used to determine whether there was a significant difference between mean three-week range of motion (ROM) values at Clinics 1 and 2. A two-tailed test was conducted with alpha set at .05.

RESULTS

The mean three-week ROM at Clinic 1 was 28.5° greater than at Clinic 2; this difference was statistically significant (Table 1).

Mann-Whitney or Wilcoxon Rank Sum Test

These two equivalent tests are the nonparametric alternatives to the independent t test. If the assumptions for the independent t test are violated, researchers may choose to analyze their data with one of these tests. When nonparametric tests are employed, the hypotheses need to be stated in more general terms than the hypotheses for parametric tests.

H_0: The populations from which the Clinic 1 and Clinic 2 samples are drawn are identical.

H_1: One population tends to produce larger observations than the other population.[3(p238)]

To perform the Mann-Whitney test, a researcher ranks the scores from the two groups, irrespective of original group membership. Table 14–4 shows the ranking of three-week ROM scores for Clinics 1 and 2.

Table 1. Three-Week Range of Motion Difference Between Clinics.

Clinic	N	$\bar{X}$	s	t	p
1	10	77.6°	19.84°	3.66	.002
2	10	49.1°	14.58°		

TABLE 14–4. Mann-Whitney or Wilcoxon Rank Sum Test

	Clinic 1	Clinic 2
	Score (Rank)	*Score (Rank)*
	32 (2)	27 (1)
	58 (10)	34 (3)
	67 (11.5)	40 (4)
	81 (14)	45 (5)
	84 (15)	47 (6)
	87 (16)	49 (7)
	88 (17)	50 (8)
	92 (18.5)	56 (9)
	92 (18.5)	67 (11.5)
	95 (20)	76 (13)
Rank sum	(142.5)	(67.5)

When a number occurs more than once, its ranking is the mean of the multiple ranks it occupies. For example, the two 67s are the 11th and 12th ranked scores in this distribution, so each receives a rank of 11.5. The next-ranked number, 76, receives the rank of 13. The sum of the Clinic 1 ranks is 142.5; the sum of the Clinic 2 ranks is 67.5.

To understand the logic behind the Mann-Whitney, imagine that our two clinics have vastly different scores that do not overlap at all. The Clinic 2 ranks would be 1 through 10, which add up to 55; the Clinic 1 ranks would be 11 through 20, which add up to 155. Now suppose the opposite case, in which the scores are very similar. The Clinic 2 scores might get all the odd ranks, which add up to 100; the Clinic 1 scores might get all the even ranks, which add up to 110. When the two samples are similar, their rank sums will be similar. When the samples differ greatly, the rank sums will be very different. The rank sums (67.5 and 142.5) of our two samples of patients with total knee arthroplasty fall between the two extremes of (a) 55 and 155 and (b) 100 and 110. To come to a statistical conclusion, we need to determine the probability of obtaining the rank sums of 67.5 and 142.5 if in fact the populations from which the samples are drawn are identical. To do so, we transform the higher rank sum into a z score and calculate the probability of obtaining the z score.

An alternative form of the Mann-Whitney test uses a U statistic, which is converted into a z score. In this example, the computer-generated z score is 2.84 and the associated two-tailed probability is .0046. We conclude from this that there is a significant difference between the scores from Clinic 1 and the scores from Clinic 2. Given the 28.5° difference in the means and the 37.5° difference in the medians between the clinics, this difference seems clinically important. Once again, our statistical and clinical conclusions concur.

The results of a Mann-Whitney test might be written up as follows in a journal article:

DATA ANALYSIS

Because the distribution of Clinic 1's range of motion (ROM) scores was nonnormal, we chose to analyze differences between the two groups with a nonparametric Mann–Whitney test. The 5% significance level was used for hypothesis testing.

RESULTS

A significant difference between the three–week ROM scores for the two groups was found. Table 1 shows descriptive measures and rank sums for both groups.

Table 1. Three–Week Range of Motion Difference Between Clinics.

Clinic	Median	$\bar{X}$	s	Rank Sum[a]
1	85.5°	77.6°	19.84°	142.5
2	48.0°	49.1°	14.58°	67.5

[a]Significant at $p < .05$.

Literature Examples

Draper used an independent t test to determine whether the number of days required to achieve full knee ROM after anterior cruciate ligament reconstruction was significantly different between groups who did and did not receive electromyographic biofeedback during quadriceps femoris muscle exercise.[13] Griffin and colleagues used Mann-Whitney tests to determine whether there were different rates of healing of pressure ulcers between a group who received high-voltage pulsed current and a group who received a placebo treatment.[14]

Differences Between Two or More Independent Groups

If Clinics 1 through 3 all have different postoperative protocols for their patients who have undergone total knee arthroplasty, we might wonder whether there are significant differences in mean three-week ROM scores among the three clinics. To test this question statistically, we develop the following hypotheses:

H_0: $\mu_1 = \mu_2 = \mu_3$

H_1: At least one of the population means is different from another population mean.

We shall set alpha at .05 for the analysis. The samples are independent because they consist of different, unrelated subjects. The descriptive measures and stem-and-leaf plots for all three clinics are presented in Table 14–5. The scores for both Clinics 1 and 3 appear to be nonnormal; the variances are similar. If we believe that the parametric assumptions have been met, we test the differences with a one-way ANOVA. If we do not believe that the parametric assumptions have been met, the comparable nonparametric test is the Kruskal-Wallis test. A chi-square test of association can be used to test differences between groups when the dependent variable consists of nominal-level data.

One-Way ANOVA

ANOVA techniques partition the variability in a sample into between-groups and within-group variability. A ratio is created with between-groups variability as the numerator and within-group variability as the denominator. This ratio is an F statistic, which is distributed as shown in Figure 14–1B, dis-

TABLE 14–5. Frequencies and Descriptive Statistics for Three-Week Range of Motion at Clinics 1 Through 3

Clinic	1	2	3
Data		2 7	
	3 2	3 4	3 2
	4	4 0579	4
	5 8	5 06	5 0
	6 7	6 7	6 0
	7	7 6	7
	8 1478		8 111244
	9 225		9 1
$\overline{X}$	77.6	49.1	72.6
s^2	393.62	212.58	357.38
s	19.84	14.58	18.90

cussed earlier. Because the F distribution is a squared t distribution, F cannot be negative. This means that all the extreme values for F are in the upper tail of the distribution, eliminating the need to differentiate between one- and two-tailed tests. The ANOVA is a very versatile statistical technique, and many different variations of it are available. All of the ANOVA techniques are based on partitioning variability to create an F ratio that is evaluated against the probabilities of the F distribution.

The ANOVA required in our example is known as a *one-way ANOVA*. "One-way" refers to the fact that only one independent variable is examined. In this case, the independent variable is clinic, and it has three levels—Clinic 1, Clinic 2, and Clinic 3. Table 14–6 shows the calculations needed to determine the F statistic. Although time consuming, the calculations presented here are not difficult. To compute the F statistic, we must first know the individual group means as well as the grand mean. The *grand mean* is the

TABLE 14–6. One-Way Analysis of Variance Calculations of Sum of Squares Total (SST), Within Group (SSW), and Between Groups (SSB)

Clinic No.	Raw Score	Deviation from Grand Mean	Deviation²	Deviation from Group Mean	Deviation²
1	32	−34.4	1,183.36	−45.6	2,079.36
1	58	−8.4	70.56	−19.6	384.16
1	67	.6	.36	−10.6	112.36
1	81	14.6	213.16	3.4	11.56
1	84	17.6	309.76	6.4	40.96
1	87	20.6	424.36	9.4	88.36
1	88	21.6	466.56	10.4	108.16
1	92	25.6	655.36	14.4	207.36
1	92	25.6	655.36	14.4	207.36
1	95	28.6	817.96	17.4	302.76
2	27	−39.4	1,552.36	−22.1	488.41
2	34	−32.4	1,049.76	−15.1	228.01
2	40	−26.4	696.96	−9.1	82.81
2	45	−21.4	457.96	−4.1	16.81
2	47	−19.4	376.36	−2.1	4.41
2	49	−17.4	302.76	−.1	.01
2	50	−16.4	268.96	.9	.81
2	56	−10.4	108.16	6.9	47.61
2	67	.6	.36	17.9	320.41
2	76	9.6	92.16	26.9	723.61
3	32	−34.4	1,183.36	−40.6	1,648.36
3	50	−16.4	268.96	−22.6	510.76
3	60	−6.4	40.96	−12.6	158.76
3	81	14.6	213.16	8.4	70.56
3	81	14.6	213.16	8.4	70.56
3	81	14.6	213.16	8.4	70.56
3	82	15.6	243.36	9.4	88.36
3	84	17.6	309.76	11.4	129.96
3	84	17.6	309.76	11.4	129.96
3	91	24.6	605.16	18.4	338.56
Σ			13,303.40 (SST)		8,671.70 (SSW)

$$SSB = (77.6 - 66.4)^2 (10) + (49.1 - 66.4)^2 (10) + (72.6 - 66.4)^2 (10) = 4{,}631.7$$

Note: Clinic 1 mean = 77.6°, Clinic 2 mean = 49.1°, and Clinic 3 mean = 72.6°.

mean of all of the scores across the groups; for our three samples the grand mean is 66.4°.

The total variability within the data set is determined by calculating the sum of the squared deviations of each individual score from the grand mean. This is called the *total sum of squares* (SST). The SST calculation is shown in the fourth column of Table 14–6. The second column shows the raw scores; the third column, the deviation of each raw score from the grand mean; and the fourth column, the squared deviations. The sum of these squared deviations across all 30 subjects is the SST.

The within-group variability is determined by calculating the sum of the squared deviations of the individual scores from the group mean. This is known as the *within-group sum of squares* (SSW). The second column of Table 14–6 shows the raw scores; the fifth column, the deviations of each raw score from its group mean; and the final column, the squared deviations. The sum of all of the 30 squared deviation scores in the fifth column is the SSW.

The between-groups variability is determined by calculating the sum of the squared deviations of the group means from the grand mean, with each deviation weighted according to sample size. This is known as the *between-groups sum of squares* (SSB) and is shown at the bottom of Table 14–6.

The SST is the sum of the SSB and the SSW. Conceptually, then, the total variability in the sample is partitioned into variability attributable to differences between the groups and variability attributable to differences within each group.

The next step in calculating the F statistic is to divide the SSB and SSW by appropriate degrees of freedom to obtain the mean square between groups (MSB) and the mean square within group (MSW), respectively. The degrees of freedom for the SSB is the number of groups minus 1; the degrees of freedom for the SSW is the total number of subjects minus the number of groups. The F statistic is the MSB divided by the MSW. Thus, for our example, the MSB is 2,315.85:

$$\text{MSB} = \text{SSB} / (\text{groups} - 1) = 4{,}631.7 / 2 = 2{,}315.85$$

The MSW is 321.17:

$$\text{MSW} = \text{SSW} / (\text{N} - \text{groups}) = 8{,}671.7 / 27 = 321.17$$

The F statistic is 7.21:

$$F = \frac{\text{MSB}}{\text{MSW}} = \frac{2{,}315.85}{321.17} = 7.21$$

Large F values indicate that the differences between the groups are large compared with the differences within groups. Small F values indicate that the differences between groups are small compared with the differences within groups. The computer-generated probability for our F of 7.21 with 2 and 27 degrees of freedom is .0031. Because this is less than our predetermined alpha level of .05, we can conclude that there is at least one significant difference among the three means that were compared.

If a one-way ANOVA does not identify a significant difference among means, then the statistical analysis is complete. If, as in our example, a significant difference is identified, the researcher must complete one more step. Our overall, or *omnibus*, F test tells us that there is a difference among the means. It does not tell us whether Clinic 1 is different from Clinic 2, whether Clinic 2 is different from Clinic 3, or whether Clinic 1 is different from Clinic 3. To determine the sources of the differences identified by the omnibus F, we must make multiple comparisons between pairs of means.

Conceptually, conducting multiple-comparison tests is similar to conducting t tests between each pair of means, but with a correction to prevent inflation of the alpha level. A comparison of two means is called a *con-*

trast. Common multiple-comparison procedures, in order of decreasing power, are

- planned orthogonal contrasts
- Newman-Keuls test
- Tukey test
- Bonferroni test
- Scheffé test.[4(p386)]

The more powerful tests identify smaller differences between means as significant. Various assumptions must be met for the different multiple-comparison procedures to be valid.

Using a Newman-Keuls procedure on our example, the mean ROM scores for Clinic 1 (77.6°) and Clinic 3 (72.6°) were not found to be significantly different, and the mean ROM score for Clinic 2 (49.1°) was found to differ significantly from the mean ROM scores for both Clinics 1 and 3. From a clinical viewpoint, it seems reasonable to conclude that the 5° difference between Clinics 1 and 3 is not important but the difference of more than 20° between Clinic 2 and Clinics 1 and 3 is.

There are two additional twists to the multiple-comparison procedure: (a) whether the contrasts are planned or post hoc and (b) whether the multiple-comparison results are consistent with the omnibus test.

In *planned contrasts,* the researcher specifies which contrasts are of interest before the statistical test is conducted. If, for some reason, the researcher is not interested in differences between Clinics 2 and 3, then only two comparisons need to be made: Clinic 1 versus Clinic 3 and Clinic 1 versus Clinic 2.

If planned contrasts are not specified in advance, all possible multiple comparisons should be conducted as post hoc tests. As more multiple comparisons are conducted, each contrast becomes more conservative to control for alpha inflation.

Occasionally, the omnibus F test identifies a significant difference among the means, but the multiple-comparison procedure fails to locate any significant contrasts. One response to these conflicting results is to believe the multiple-comparison results and conclude that despite the significant F there is no significant difference among the means. Another response is to believe the F-test results and use progressively less conservative multiple-comparison procedures until the significant difference between means is located. A one-way ANOVA might be reported in the literature as follows:

DATA ANALYSIS

One-way analysis of variance (ANOVA) was used to determine whether there were significant three-week range of motion (ROM) differences among the three clinics. Alpha was set at .05; Newman-Keuls post hoc comparisons were conducted.

RESULTS

Tables 1 and 2 show the descriptive statistics and ANOVA summary for the tests of differences between the three-week ROM means at the three clinics. The omnibus test identified a significant difference among the means. The post hoc analysis showed that the differences of greater than 20° between Clinic 2 and both Clinics 1 and 3 was significant, but that the 5° difference between Clinics 1 and 3 was not.

Table 1. Three-Week Range of Motion at Clinics 1, 2, and 3.

Clinic	N	$\bar{X}$	s
1	10	77.6°	19.8°
2	10	49.1°	14.6°
3	10	72.6°	18.9°

Table 2. Summary of Analysis of Variance for Three-Week Range of Motion at Clinics 1, 2, and 3.

Source	Sum of Squares	Degrees of Freedom	Mean Square	F
Between groups	4,631.7	2	2,315.8	7.21[a]
Within group	8,671.7	27	321.2	
Total	13,303.4	29		

[a]p = .0031.

Kruskal-Wallis Test

The Kruskal-Wallis test is the nonparametric equivalent of the one-way ANOVA. If the assumptions of the parametric test are not met, the nonparametric test should be performed. The hypotheses for the nonparametric test must be stated in more general terms than the hypotheses for the parametric test:

H_0: The three samples come from populations that are identical.

H_1: At least one of the populations tends to produce larger observations than another population.[3(p241)]

To conduct the Kruskal-Wallis test, a researcher ranks the scores, irrespective of group membership. The ranks for each group are then summed and plugged into a formula to generate a Kruskal-Wallis (KW) statistic. The distribution of the KW statistic approximates a chi-square distribution. The computer-generated value of the KW statistic for our example is 11.10; the respective probability is .0039. Because .0039 is less than the alpha level of .05 that we set before conducting the test, we conclude that there is a significant difference somewhere among the groups.

An appropriate multiple-comparison procedure to use when a Kruskal-Wallis test is significant is the Mann-Whitney test with a Bonferroni adjustment of alpha. We have three comparisons to make, and each is tested at an alpha of .017. The probabilities associated with the three Mann-Whitney tests are as follows: For Clinic 1 compared with Clinic 2, p = .0046; for Clinic 1 compared with Clinic 3, p = .2237; and for Clinic 2 compared with Clinic 3, p = .0072. Thus, the multiple comparisons tell us that there is no significant difference between Clinics 1 and 3 and that Clinic 2 is significantly different from both Clinics 1 and 3. In this example the nonparametric conclusions are the same as the parametric conclusions. The results of a Kruskal-Wallis test might be reported in a journal article as follows:

DATA ANALYSIS

Three-week range of motion differences among the three clinics were studied with a Kruskal-Wallis (KW) analysis of variance with an alpha level of .05. A nonparametric test was used because the data at Clinics 1 and 3 were not normally distributed. Post hoc comparisons were made with three Mann-Whitney tests. The Bonferroni adjustment was used to set alpha at .017 (.05 / 3 = .017) for each post hoc comparison to compensate for the alpha level inflation that occurs with multiple tests.

RESULTS

A significant difference among the three-week range of motion scores at the three clinics was found (KW = 11.10, p = .0039). Clinics 1 and 3, with medians of 85.5° and 81.0°, respectively, were not significantly different from one another (p = .2237). Both were significantly different from Clinic 2, which had a median of 48.0° degrees (for Clinic 1 versus 2, p = .0046; for Clinic 2 versus 3, p = .0072).

Chi-Square Test of Association

Assume that we still wish to determine whether there are differences in the three-week ROM scores of the three clinics. However, let us further assume that previous research has shown that the ultimate functional outcome after total knee arthroplasty depends on having regained at least 90° of knee flexion by three weeks postsurgery. If such evidence existed, we might no longer be interested in the absolute three-week ROM scores at our three clinics. We might instead be interested in the proportion of patients who achieve 90° of knee flexion three weeks postoperatively. Our hypotheses would be as follows:

H_0: There is no association between the clinic and ROM category proportions.

H_1: There is an association between the clinic and ROM category proportions.

Table 14–7 presents the data in the contingency table format needed to calculate chi-square. A *contingency table* is simply an array of data organized into a column variable and a row variable. In this table, clinic is the row variable and consists of three levels. ROM category is the column variable and consists of two levels. Calculation of the chi-square statistic is based on differences between observed frequencies and frequencies that would be expected if the null hypothesis were true.

TABLE 14–7. Chi-Square (χ^2) Test of Association

	Three-Week Knee Flexion Range of Motion Category	
Clinic No.	*<90°*	*≥90°*
1	7 (8.67)	3 (1.33)
2	10 (8.67)	0 (1.33)
3	9 (8.67)	1 (1.33)
Total	26	4

$$\chi^2 = \Sigma \frac{(O - E)^2}{E} = (.32) + (.20) + (.01) + (2.10) + (1.33) + (.08) = 4.04^a$$

Note: Values are actual frequencies. Expected frequencies are in parentheses.
[a] p = .1327.

To determine the observed frequencies, we need to examine the raw data and place each subject in the appropriate ROM category. To determine the expected frequencies, we need to determine the distribution of scores if the proportion in each ROM category were equal across the clinics. In our example, 26 of the 30 subjects overall have ROM scores less than 90°. If these patients were equally distributed among the clinics, each clinic would be expected to have 8.7 (26 / 3 = 8.7) patients with ROM less than 90°. There are 4 subjects with ROM greater than or equal to 90°. If these 4 subjects were equally distributed among clinics, each clinic would be expected to have 1.3 (4 / 3 = 1.3) subjects with ROM greater than or equal to 90°. In this example, the expected frequencies are easy to calculate because there is an equal number of patients in each group. If there are unequal numbers, the expected frequencies are proportionate to the numbers in each group.

An alternative test, the *chi-square test of goodness of fit,* compares the observed frequencies with the hypothesized expected frequencies. For example, if we knew of previous research results that indicated that 80% of patients with total knee arthroplasty achieved 90° of motion by three weeks postoperatively, then we might test each of our clinic proportions against this hypothesized proportion.

In the chi-square statistic, the squared deviation of each expected cell frequency from the observed frequency is divided by the expected frequency for that cell; this is done for every cell, and the values are added together, as shown at the bottom of Table 14–7. If the dependent variable consists of only two categories, then a variation of chi-square called *Fisher's exact test* is sometimes used. If the expected frequencies are below five in a number of the cells of the table, the chi-square statistic is sometimes modified with *Yates' correction.*[4(p288)]

Table 14–7 shows the chi-square calculation for our example. The chi-square of 4.04, with 2 degrees of freedom (the number of columns − 1 × number of rows − 1), is associated with a probability of .1327. Because this probability is higher than the .05 we set as our alpha level, we conclude that there is no significant difference in the proportions of patients in the two ROM categories across the three clinics.

Note that the statistical conclusions of the chi-square analysis differ from those of the ANOVA and Kruskal-Wallis test. The ANOVA, which used all the original values of the data for the analysis, detected a difference among groups. The Kruskal-Wallis test, based on a ranking of the original data, also detected a difference. The chi-square test of association, however, using only nominal data, which eliminated much of the information in the original data set, failed to detect a difference among the groups.

In general, if ratio or interval data exist, it is not wise to convert them to a lower measurement level unless there is a strong theoretical rationale for doing so. Given the hypothetical rationale that was used to set up this chi-square example, we would conclude that patients at all three clinics are likely to have equally poor functional outcomes because of the low proportion of patients at any of the clinics who achieved 90° of motion by three weeks postoperatively. Chi-square results might be written up in a journal article as follows:

DATA ANALYSIS

Patients at each clinic were placed into one of two three-week range of motion (ROM) categories. The limited-progress category included those with less than 90° of flexion; the normal-progress category included those with ROM greater than or equal to 90°. The chi-square test of association (alpha = .05) was used to determine whether patients in the two categories were equally distributed across the three clinics.

RESULTS

Chi-square analysis showed no significant difference in the distribution of three-week ROM categories across the clinics (Table 1).

Table 1. Frequency and Percentage of Three-Week Range of Motion Categories Across Clinics.[a]

	<90°		≥90°	
Clinic	*Frequency*	*%*	*Frequency*	*%*
1	7	70.0	3	30.0
2	10	100.0	0	0.0
3	9	90.0	1	10.0

[a] $\chi^2_2 = 4.04$, $p = .133$.*

*Subscript 2 is the degrees of freedom for the chi-square statistic. Throughout this chapter, degrees of freedom is presented as a subscript when statistic values are presented mathematically.

Literature Examples

A one-way ANOVA was used to analyze differences between a treatment and a control group in Weiss's study of the effects of heavy-resistance exercise on triceps surae muscularity.[15] This example shows that although an ANOVA can analyze differences between many groups simultaneously, it is equally appropriate when only two groups are being compared.

Moncur used the Kruskal-Wallis test to analyze differences in the perceptions of physical therapy clinical educators, physical therapists with identified interests in arthritis, and rheumatologists of the importance of various physical therapy competencies in treating arthritic patients.[16] Post hoc multiple comparisons were made with the Mann-Whitney test.

Mayer and colleagues used the chi-square test of association to determine whether there were significant differences in the rate of returning to work in patients who had completed a functional restoration program versus patients who had dropped out of the program and patients who had not entered a program.[17]

Differences Between Two Dependent Samples

Suppose that we are interested in whether there is a change in ROM from three weeks postoperatively to six weeks postoperatively for patients across all three of our clinics. The hypotheses we test are as follows:

$$H_0: \mu_{\text{3-week ROM}} = \mu_{\text{6-week ROM}}$$

$$H_1: \mu_{\text{3-week ROM}} \neq \mu_{\text{6-week ROM}}$$

We shall set the alpha level at .05. In this example, the two measures are dependent—they are repeated measures taken on the same individuals. When determining whether the data are suitable for parametric testing, remember that the relevant data are the differences between the pairs, rather than the raw data. Table 14–8 presents the distributions of the differences for the entire sample. The differences were calculated by subtracting the three-week ROM values from the six-week ROM values given in Table 13–2. A positive difference therefore indicates an improvement in ROM over the three-week time span. The distribution of difference scores is asymmetrical, with a greater proportion of scores in the lower end of the range. The parametric test of differences for two dependent samples is the paired-*t* test. The corresponding nonparametric test is the Wilcoxon signed rank test. The test of differences between two dependent samples for nominal data is the McNemar test.

Paired-t Test

To calculate the paired-*t* test, we first determine the difference between each pair of measurements. The mean difference and standard deviation of the differences are cal-

TABLE 14–8. Difference Between Six-Week and Three-Week Range of Motion Scores Across Clinics

Stem	Leaves
−0	8 7 6 5 4 4 2
0	0 2 3 3 4 4 5 6 7 8 8 9
1	0 1 1 3 4 4 5 7 8
2	9
3	5

Mean of the differences: 7.0°
Standard deviation of the differences: 10.03°

$$t = \frac{\overline{X}_d}{\frac{S_d}{\sqrt{n}}} = \frac{7.0}{\frac{10.03}{\sqrt{30}}} = 3.82$$

culated, and then the mean is compared with a mean difference of zero. The mean of our example differences is 7.0°; the standard deviation of the differences is 10.03°. We calculate the t statistic for paired samples by dividing the mean difference by the standard error of the mean differences, as shown at the bottom of Table 14–8. The probability associated with the t statistic of 3.82 with 29 degrees of freedom (number of pairs − 1) is .001. Because .001 is less than the alpha level of .05, we conclude that there is a significant difference between three-week and six-week ROM scores. Clinically, an average 7.0° difference in motion over three weeks seems modest for this population, particularly considering that few patients are even close to achieving the maximal mechanical ROM of their new knee joints. Therefore, the statistical conclusion must be tempered with a statement about the relatively small size of the difference. Paired-t test results might be reported in a journal article as follows:

DATA ANALYSIS

The difference between six-week and three-week range of motion (ROM) values was analyzed with a paired-t test. A two-tailed test with alpha at .05 was conducted.

RESULTS

The difference between the six-week and three-week ROM scores ranged from −8° to +35°, with a mean of 7.0° and a standard deviation 10.03°. A positive difference indicates an improvement in ROM score from Week 3 to Week 6. Twenty-two subjects improved in the three-week time span; eight either did not change or experienced a decrease in ROM. The difference in motion was statistically significant, $t_{29} = 3.82$, $p = .001$.

DISCUSSION

Although the difference in ROM between the three-week and six-week measurements was statistically significant, the clinical importance of an average 7.0° change over three weeks must be questioned, particularly because so few subjects were close to the mechanical flexion limits of their prostheses. Because we had anticipated much larger changes, we conclude that the postoperative progress of these subjects, although statistically significant, is limited.

Wilcoxon Signed Rank Test

The Wilcoxon signed rank test is the nonparametric version of the paired-t test. The nonparametric hypotheses relate to the median:

H_0: The difference between the population medians is equal to zero.

H_1: The difference between the population medians is not equal to zero.

To conduct the Wilcoxon signed rank test, we calculate the difference between each pair of numbers. We rank the nonzero differences according to their absolute value and then separate them into the ranks associated with positive and negative differences. If there is no difference from one time to the next, then the sum of the positive ranks should be approximately equal to the sum of the negative ranks. Table 14–9 shows the sums of the positive and negative ranks for this example.

TABLE 14–9. Wilcoxon Signed Rank Test

Difference	Rank by Absolute Value	Positive Difference Rank	Negative Difference Rank
0			
−2	1.5		1.5
2	1.5	1.5	
3	3.5	3.5	
3	3.5	3.5	
−4	6.5		6.5
−4	6.5		6.5
4	6.5	6.5	
4	6.5	6.5	
−5	9.5		9.5
5	9.5	9.5	
−6	11.5		11.5
6	11.5	11.5	
7	13.5	13.5	
−7	13.5		13.5
−8	16		16.0
8	16	16.0	
8	16	16.0	
9	18	18.0	
10	19	19.0	
11	20.5	20.5	
11	20.5	20.5	
13	22.0	22.0	
14	23.5	23.5	
14	23.5	23.5	
15	25	25.0	
17	26	26.0	
18	27	27.0	
29	28	28.0	
35	29	29.0	
Σ signed ranks		370	65

As is the case with the Mann-Whitney procedures for analyzing differences between independent samples, the ranked information is transformed into a z score. The computer-generated z score and probability for this example are 3.298 and .001, respectively. This probability being less than our alpha of .05, we conclude that there is a significant difference between three-week and six-week ROM.

To determine the clinical significance of the difference, we examine the median of the difference between the two samples. The median difference for this example is 6.5°. This seems a fairly modest gain for a three-week period. Once again, we should temper our statistical conclusion with a statement about the relatively small size of the median difference. Wilcoxon signed rank test results might be reported in a journal article as follows:

DATA ANALYSIS

The Wilcoxon signed rank procedure was used to analyze the difference in range of motion (ROM) scores from three weeks to six weeks. This nonparametric test was selected because the distribution of the difference scores was positively skewed and did not meet parametric assumptions. A nondirectional test was performed with alpha set at .05.

RESULTS

The median difference between three-week and six-week ROM was 6.5°, with a range from −8° to +35°. A positive difference indicates an improvement over time. This difference was statistically significant (z = 3.298, p = .001).

DISCUSSION

Although the difference in ROM between the three-week and six-week measurements was statistically significant, the clinical importance of a median 6.5° change over three weeks must be questioned, particularly because so few subjects were close to the mechanical flexion limits of their prostheses. Because we had anticipated much larger changes, we conclude that the postoperative progress of these subjects, although statistically significant, is limited.

McNemar Test

The McNemar test is the nominal-data analogue to the paired-*t* test and the Wilcoxon signed rank test. The McNemar test can only be used to analyze 2 × 2 contingency tables, and thus its usefulness is limited. Suppose we want to determine whether there is a predictable change in ROM from three weeks to six weeks and are interested not in absolute range scores, but only in whether patients have greater than or less than 90° of motion. Our hypotheses are as follows:

H_0: The proportion of patients with less than 90° of motion at three weeks postoperatively is identical to the proportion of patients with less than 90° of motion at six weeks postoperatively.

H_1: The population proportions are not equal at the two time intervals.

To perform the McNemar test, we generate a 2 × 2 table of frequencies, as shown in Table 14–10. Each subject is represented only once in the table. For example, a subject who had less than 90° of motion at three weeks and still had less than 90° of motion at six weeks is one of the 20 individuals indicated in the upper left corner of the table. If the proportion of patients in each category stays the same from three weeks to six weeks, we would expect that (a) some patients will not change categories (upper left and lower right cells) and (b) the number of patients who change categories will be evenly distributed between those moving from less than to greater than 90° and those moving from greater than to less than 90° (lower left and upper right cells). Table 14–10 shows that 23 patients did not change ROM categories, 6 improved from less than to greater than 90°, and only 1 had a decline in motion from greater than to less than 90°.

The probability of such an occurrence, if in fact there is no difference in proportions, is

TABLE 14–10. McNemar Test

	Six-Week Range of Motion	
Three-Week Range of Motion	***Limited Progress (<90°)***	***Normal Progress (≥90°)***
Limited progress (<90°)	20	6
Normal progress (≥ 90°)	1	3

.1250, as generated by the computer program. Thus, we conclude that the change in proportions from three weeks to six weeks is not significant. Clinically, a change of categories in only 7 of 30 patients seems to indicate minimal effectiveness of the intervention over the three-week time span. Thus, the statistical conclusion of an insignificant difference in proportions concurs with our clinical impression. Our McNemar test might be reported in a journal article as follows:

DATA ANALYSIS

To determine whether there was a significant change in range of motion (ROM) from three weeks to six weeks postoperatively, we compared the proportion of patients with less than 90° of motion (limited progress) or greater than or equal to 90° of motion (normal progress) at three weeks and six weeks. Because the three-week and six-week categories are repeated measures, we made the comparison with a McNemar test, setting alpha at .05.

RESULTS

Twenty-three of 30 subjects did not change ROM categories over the time span studied: 20 had limited motion at both occasions, and 3 had acceptable ROM at both occasions. Of the 7 subjects who changed ROM categories over the three-week time span, 6 moved from the limited- to the normal-progress category, and 1 moved from the normal- to the limited-progress category. This change in proportions was not statistically significant (p = .1250).

Literature Examples

Brooks and associates used paired-t tests to determine whether there were significant differences in quadriceps torque production between neuromuscular electrical simulation with longitudinal versus transverse electrode placement.[18] Griffin and colleagues used a Wilcoxon signed rank test to determine whether there was a significant change in hand volume from the time that patients with chronic hand edema entered the clinic to after they rested for 10 minutes with the hand elevated.[19]

Falahee and associates studied the effectiveness of resection arthroplasty as a salvage procedure for failed total knee arthroplasties.[20] Although they did not use the McNemar test, their data on gait restrictions could be analyzed with this test. They assessed the level of gait restriction for patients before and after surgery with a five-point scale from "no restriction" to "unable to walk." The scale could be collapsed into two categories, for example, "moderate to no restriction" and "severe restriction." Once collapsed, the gait results can be concisely summarized: 17 patients had moderate to no restriction both before and after surgery, 5 patients had severe restrictions both before and after surgery, 3 improved from severe restrictions, and 1 declined from a moderate restriction.

Although a good example of the use of the McNemar statistic was not located in the physical therapy literature, the test is presented because of the reported abuse of the chi-square test when a McNemar test is more appropriate.[3(p216)] The chi-square test assumes independent samples; the McNemar test is designed for use with dependent samples, as in Falahee and associates' before- and after-surgery study.

Differences Between Two or More Dependent Samples

We wish now to determine whether patients show a pattern of ROM improvement from three weeks postoperatively, to six weeks postoperatively, to six months postoperatively. Our hypotheses for such a question are as follows:

H_0: $\mu_{\text{3-week ROM}} = \mu_{\text{6-week ROM}} = \mu_{\text{6-month ROM}}$

H_1: At least one population mean does not equal another population mean.

We set alpha at .05. The samples are dependent because each subject is measured three times. Table 14–11 shows the stem-and-leaf displays for the ROM scores at all three time periods; none are symmetrical. Additional assumptions about the variances and covariances of the measures must be met, but a full discussion of these is beyond the scope of this text. The parametric test of differences between more than two dependent means is the repeated measures ANOVA. The corresponding nonparametric test is Friedman's ANOVA.

TABLE 14–11. Stem-and-Leaf Displays of Range of Motion Data at Three Times

Stem	Week 3	Week 6	Month 6
2	7		
3	224		
4	0579	06	
5	0068	0568	
6	077	033577	5
7	6	0018	8
8	1111244478	00555	0345
9	1225	000004555	00555558
10			00000345555556
11			00

Repeated Measures ANOVA

Just as the one-way ANOVA is the extension of the independent *t* test from two groups to more than two groups, the repeated measures ANOVA is the extension of the paired-*t* test to more than three dependent samples. There are three different approaches to a repeated measures ANOVA: multivariate, univariate, and adjusted univariate. The assumptions for the univariate approach are more stringent than those for the multivariate approach; statistical packages provide a test (Mauchly's test of sphericity) of the assumptions to guide researchers in deciding which approach to use.[3(p169)] The univariate approach is similar to the one-way ANOVA and is discussed here.

Recall the procedure used for the paired-*t* test. We started with a group of subjects with ROM scores ranging from 32° to 95°. To determine the test statistic, we calculated the difference between the three-week and six-week measures. Taking the difference of the paired scores effectively eliminated the widespread variability between subjects in the sample and allowed us to focus on the changes within subjects with time. Like the paired-*t* test, the repeated measures ANOVA mathematically eliminates between-subjects variability to focus the analysis on within-subject variability.

Recall that the one-way ANOVA partitioned the variability in the data set into between-groups and within-group categories. The univariate repeated measures ANOVA first partitions the variability in the data set into *between-subjects* and *within-subject* categories. The within-subject variability is then subdivided into between-treatments and error (or residual) components (Table 14–12). Two *F* ratios can be generated from a repeated measures ANOVA: One is the ratio of between-subjects to within-subject variability; the other is the ratio of between-treatments to residual variability. The first ratio is sometimes reported but is not relevant to

TABLE 14–12. Summary of a Repeated Measures Analysis of Variance

Source	Sum of Squares	Degrees of Freedom	Mean Square	F	p
Between subjects	20,710.46	29	714.15	2.23	.0047
Within subject	19,244.67	60	320.74		
Between treatments	14,709.42	2	7354.71	94.06	.0001
Residual	4,535.24	58	78.19		
Total	39,955.12	89			

the research question we are addressing here. A significant between-subjects F ratio would merely tell us that there is substantial variability between individual subjects, and a nonsignificant between-subjects F ratio would tell us that subjects are fairly homogeneous. Neither result is relevant to the question of whether there are differences between *treatments*. Thus the between-treatments F ratio is the one that is relevant to our research question. It is the ratio of the between-treatments variability to the variability that is left after the variability due to differences between subjects is removed. Thus, the variability that makes up the denominator of the F ratio is called the *residual*. It is also referred to as *error* because this represents random differences in subjects due to sampling errors.

If a repeated measures ANOVA identifies a significant difference among the means, the next step is to make multiple comparisons between pairs of means to determine which time frames are significantly different from one another. The multiple-comparison procedures for repeated measures must be based on assumptions of dependence between the pairs being compared. Maxwell recommends the use of paired-t tests with a Bonferroni adjustment of alpha.[21]

In our example, a significant difference between treatments was identified: $F_{2, 58} = 94.06$, $p = .0001$. Three paired-t tests are used as the multiple comparisons to determine where the differences lie. Because three comparisons are needed, the overall alpha level of .05 becomes .017 (.05 / 3 = .017). The results of the paired-t tests are as follows: For three-week versus six-week scores, $t_{29} = 3.83$, $p = .001$; for three-week versus six-month scores, $t_{29} = 10.38$, $p = .000$; and for six-week versus six-month scores, $t_{29} = 11.51$, $p = .000$. (Note that the probability is never actually zero, but in this case it is low enough that it can be rounded off to zero.)

To determine the clinical relevance of these differences, we need to examine the means for the different time periods: three weeks — 66.4°, six weeks — 73.4°, and six months — 96.4°. As noted previously, the average 7.0° difference between Weeks 3 and 6 seems small, but the 23.0° difference between Week 6 and Month 6 seems highly important. A repeated measure ANOVA might be reported in the literature as follows:

DATA ANALYSIS

Differences in range of motion (ROM) scores at the three time periods were analyzed with a univariate approach to repeated measures analysis of variance since Mauchly's test of sphericity showed that the required assumptions were met ($p = .642$). Post hoc comparisons were made with paired-*t* tests. The alpha level for the ANOVA was set at .05; the Bonferroni correction was used to set alpha at .017 for each of the multiple comparisons.

RESULTS

The means and standard deviations for ROM scores at three weeks, six weeks, and six months, respectively, are 66.4° ± 21.4°, 73.4° ± 17.3°, and 96.4° ± 10.5°. Repeated measures ANOVA demonstrated a significant difference among the means, $F_{2,58} = 94.06$, $p = .000$. All three means were significantly different from one another at $p \leq .001$.

Friedman's ANOVA

Friedman's ANOVA is the nonparametric equivalent of the repeated measures ANOVA. Hypotheses are as follows:

- H_0: All possible rankings of the observations for any subject are equally likely.
- H_1: At least one population tends to produce larger observations than another population.[3(p245)]

Calculation is based on rankings of the repeated measures for each subject. Two different formulas can be used to calculate either a Friedman's *F* or a Friedman's chi-square. The computer-generated chi-square for this example is 48.75, and the associated probability is .0000. Because .0000 is less than our present alpha of .05, we conclude that at least one time frame is different than another. An appropriate nonparametric multiple-comparison procedure is the Wilcoxon signed rank test with a Bonferroni adjustment of the alpha level for each test. All three multiple comparisons show significant differences: For three-week ROM versus six-week ROM, $p = .001$; for three-week ROM versus six-month ROM, $p = .000$; and for six-week ROM versus six-month ROM, $p = .000$. Thus, for this example, the nonparametric and parametric results agree. These results might be written in a journal article as follows:

DATA ANALYSIS

Friedman's analysis of variance (ANOVA) was used to assess the differences in range of motion (ROM) three weeks, six weeks, and six months postoperatively. This nonparametric test was chosen because the distribution of scores at each time was not normal. Alpha was set at .05 for Friedman's ANOVA. Multiple comparisons were conducted between the paired time frames with Wilcoxon signed rank procedures with alpha set at .017 (.05 / 3 tests = .017) to compensate for alpha inflation with multiple testing.

RESULTS

The median ROM scores for each time frame are as follows: three weeks, 71.5°; six weeks, 74.5°; and six months, 100.0°. The Friedman's ANOVA revealed a significant difference among the groups, $\chi^2 = 48.75$, $p = .0000$; the post hoc analysis showed that all three groups were significantly different from one another at $p \leq .001$.

Literature Examples

Kelly and colleagues used a repeated measures ANOVA to examine differences between heart rates and oxygen saturation levels during treatment of preterm infants in three different positions.[22] Packman-Braun used a

Friedman's ANOVA to compare wrist extensor fatigue with three different duty cycles of electrical stimulation. Each subject participated in three sessions, receiving treatment with one of the three duty-cycle options at each session.[23]

Differences Between More than One Independent Variable

Now we wish to know whether there are differences in three-week ROM values between clinics and between the sexes. This particular question involves two between-subjects factors, meaning that neither factor consists of repeated measures on the same subjects. A different research question is whether ROM differences between clinics (a between-subjects factor) are consistent across time (a repeated, within-subject factor). The first research question is analyzed with a two-factor ANOVA for two between-subjects factors; the second is analyzed with a two-factor ANOVA for one between-subjects and one within-subject factor. The second analysis is sometimes referred to as a mixed-design ANOVA.

Whenever we examine the influence of more than one independent variable on a dependent variable, we must also examine whether there is an *interaction* between the independent variables. In the between-subjects example, the interaction question is whether the responses of men and women to treatment depend on the clinic at which they are treated. In the mixed design, the interaction question is whether changes across time are consistent across the clinics.

Between-Subjects Two-Way ANOVA

The statistical hypotheses are as follows:

H_0: There is no interaction between clinic and sex.

H_I: There is an interaction between clinic and sex.

H_0: $\mu_{C1} = \mu_{C2} = \mu_{C3}$

H_C: At least one clinic population mean is different from another clinic population mean.

H_0: $\mu_W = \mu_M$

H_S: The population mean for women is different from the population mean for men.

There are null and alternative hypotheses for the interaction between clinic and sex, for the main effect of clinic, and for the main effect of sex. The overall alpha level is set at .05. This particular test is known as a two-way or two-factor ANOVA because two independent variables are examined. It can also be described as a 3 × 2 ANOVA, describing the number of levels of each of the factors. Three- and four-way ANOVAs are also possible. Table 14–13 shows the data and Table 14–14 summarizes the ANOVA for this example.

Because interpretation of two-way ANOVAs depends on the interaction result, let's examine the interaction first. The *F* ratio for interaction (the Clinic × Sex row in Table

TABLE 14–13. Three-Week Range of Motion Data for Two-Factor Between-Subjects Analysis of Variance

	Sex	
Clinic	***Men***	***Women***
1	32, 67, 92, 87, 58	95, 92, 88, 84, 81
	$\bar{X}_{1M} = 67.2$	$\bar{X}_{1W} = 88.0$
2	34, 56, 45, 27, 40	76, 49, 47, 50, 67
	$\bar{X}_{2M} = 40.4$	$\bar{X}_{2W} = 57.8$
3	32, 50, 60, 84, 81	81, 84, 81, 82, 91
	$\bar{X}_{3M} = 61.4$	$\bar{X}_{3W} = 83.8$

TABLE 14–14. Summary of a Two-Factor Between-Subjects Analysis of Variance

Source	Sum of Squares	Degrees of Freedom	Mean Square	*F*	*p*
Clinic	4,631.667	2	2,315.833	9.963	.001
Sex	3,060.300	1	3,060.300	13.165	.001
Clinic × Sex	32.600	2	16.300	.070	.932
Residual	5,578.800	24	232.450		
Total	13,303.367	29			

14–14) is only .070, and the probability is .932. Because the probability exceeds the .05 alpha level we set prior to the analysis, we conclude that there is no interaction between sex and clinic. This means that men and women respond the same across the clinics. Interactions can be interpreted best if the cell means are graphed as shown in Figure 14–2.

Note that although the means for men and women are different, the pattern of response is the same across clinics: Both men and women do best at Clinic 1, slightly worse at Clinic 3, and worst at Clinic 2. The nearly parallel lines between the means of the men and women across clinics provide a visual picture of what is meant by no interaction.

Because no interaction has been identified, we now examine the main effects for clinic and sex. The main effect for clinic is determined by comparing the means of all subjects at each clinic, regardless of whether they are men or women. The main effect for sex is calculated by determining the sum of squares for men and women, regardless of the clinic at which they are treated. Analysis of the main effects depends on the assumption that

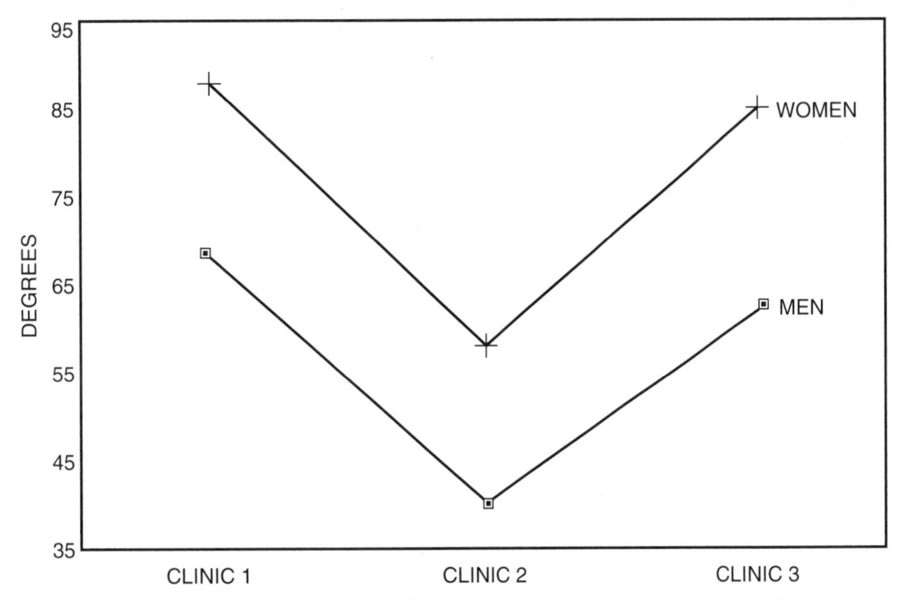

FIGURE 14–2. Parallel lines indicate no interaction between clinic and sex.

the factors do not interact and that therefore each factor can be examined independently, without concern for the other factors. In this example, the main effects for both clinic and sex are significant: $F_{2, 24} = 9.96$, $p = .001$, and $F_{1, 24} = 13.16$, $p = .001$, respectively. Because the sex variable has only two levels, we do not need to conduct post hoc testing to locate the difference. Because the clinic variable has three levels, multiple comparisons are needed, as described in the one-way ANOVA example.

To illustrate that when an interaction is present the data analysis proceeds much differently, the data above have been altered to create a significant interaction between clinic and sex. Table 14–15 shows the new data, Table 14–16 summarizes the ANOVA, and Figure 14–3 shows the modified graph of the cell means. The lines in Figure 14–3 are not parallel, indicating an interaction. Although women do better than men at Clinics 2 and 3, men do better than women at Clinic 1.

When a significant interaction is present, the main effects for the individual variables cannot be interpreted. For example, although Table 14–16 indicates that the main effect for clinic is significant, it would be erroneous for us to make any general statements about differences between clinics because these differences are not uniform across men and women. Likewise, the main effect for sex would lead us to conclude that there are no differences between men and women. However, it is clear that there are differences

TABLE 14–15. Three-Week Range of Motion Data for Two-Factor Analysis of Variance Revealing an Interaction

Clinic	Sex: *Men*	Sex: *Women*
1	95, 92, 87, 92, 88 $\overline{X}_{1M} = 90.8$	32, 67, 58, 84, 81 $\overline{X}_{1W} = 64.4$
2	34, 56, 45, 27, 40 $\overline{X}_{2M} = 40.4$	76, 49, 47, 50, 67 $\overline{X}_{2W} = 57.8$
3	32, 50, 60, 84, 81 $\overline{X}_{3M} = 61.4$	81, 84, 81, 82, 91 $\overline{X}_{3W} = 83.8$

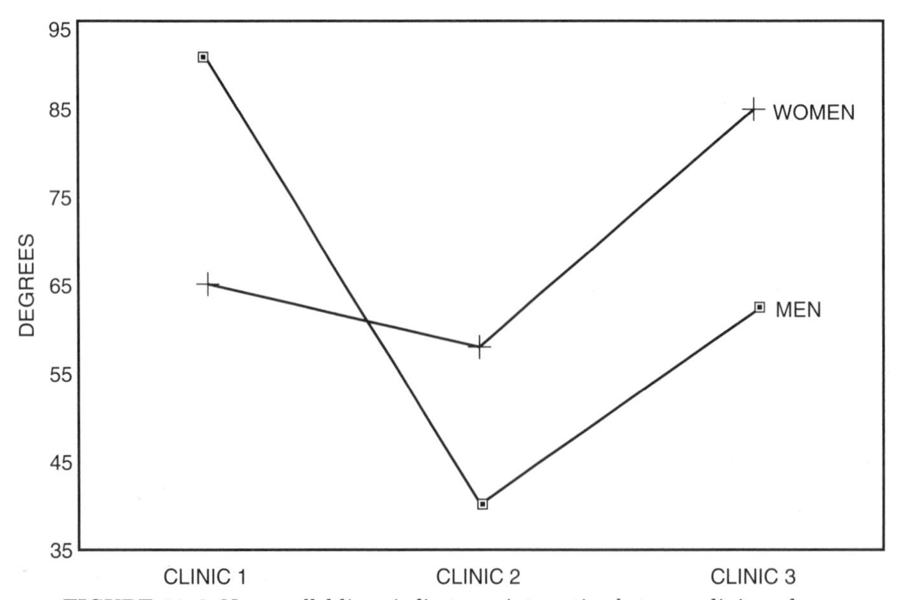

FIGURE 14–3. Nonparallel lines indicate an interaction between clinic and sex.

TABLE 14–16. Summary of a Two-Factor Analysis of Variance Revealing an Interaction with Simple Main Effects for Clinic Within Sex

Source	Sum of Squares	Degrees of Freedom	Mean Square	*F*	*p*
Clinic	4,631.66	2	2,315.83	11.301	.000
Sex	149.63	1	149.63	.730	.401
Clinic × Sex	3,604.06	2	1,802.03	8.794	.001
Clinic within sex (Women)	1,826.53	2	913.27	4.46	.023
Clinic within sex (Men)	6,409.20	2	3,204.60	15.64	.000
Residual	4,918.00	24	204.91		
Total	13,303.36	29			

between the sexes at each clinic—the opposite directions of these differences cancel out any main effect and erroneously make it appear that there are no differences between the sexes.

When a significant interaction is identified, the researcher must analyze simple main effects, rather than overall main effects. A simple main effect is one in which the differences among the levels of one factor are assessed separately for each level of the other factor. In this example, there are significant differences between clinics for the men and for the women (Table 14–16). These results might be summarized in a journal article as follows:

DATA ANALYSIS

A two-way analysis of variance was used to determine whether there were significant differences between clinics and sexes for three-week range of motion and whether there was a significant interaction between clinic and sex. Identification of a significant interaction led to further analysis of a simple main effect for clinic and post hoc analysis of significant simple main effects through the Newman–Keuls procedure. Alpha was set at .05 for each analysis.

RESULTS

As shown in Figure 14–3, there was a significant interaction between clinic and sex, $F_{2,24} = 8.794$, $p = .001$. For both the men and the women the simple main effect of clinic was significant, as shown in Table 14–16. Post hoc analysis revealed that all clinics were significantly different for the men, whereas only Clinics 2 and 3 were significantly different for the women.

Mixed-Design Two-Way ANOVA

We are now interested in determining whether there are differences in ROM across the three clinics and across the three times that measurements are taken: three weeks, six weeks, and six months. Clinic is a between-subjects factor because different subjects are measured at each clinic. Time is a within-subject factor because ROM measures are repeated on each of the subjects across the time intervals in the study. The hypotheses for our test are as follows:

H_0: There is no interaction between clinic and time.

H_I: There is an interaction between clinic and time.

H_0: $\mu_{C1} = \mu_{C2} = \mu_{C3}$

H_C: At least one clinic population mean is different from another clinic population mean.

H_0: $\mu_{3\text{-week ROM}} = \mu_{6\text{-week ROM}} = \mu_{6\text{-month ROM}}$

H_T: At least one time population mean is different from another time population mean.

Interpretation of a mixed-design ANOVA follows the same sequence of analysis as the two-factor, between-subjects ANOVA. Table 14–17 presents the means for our example, and Table 14–18 presents the *F*s and *p*s associated with each comparison. As shown in Figure 14–4, there is no interaction between clinic and time. This indicates that all the clinics had the same pattern of change across time. Because there is no interaction, the main effects for clinic and time are examined, and there is a significant effect for each. Post hoc analysis shows that all three clinics are significantly different from one another and that all three time periods are significantly different from one another.

The mixed-design ANOVA is frequently used to analyze pretest–posttest control-group designs. In the simplest design, there is a treatment factor with two levels (treatment group and control group) and a time factor with two levels (pretest and posttest). The ideal results for such a study would be for the two groups to be essentially the same at the pretest, the control group to remain unchanged at posttest, and the treatment group to be improved considerably at posttest. Figure 14–5 shows a graph of these ideal results. A significant interaction—the treatment group responded differently over time than did the control group—is illustrated. Thus, when a mixed-design two-factor ANOVA is used to analyze a pretest–posttest design, the research question is answered by examining the interaction between the group factor and the time factor. These results might be summarized in a journal article as follows:

TABLE 14–17. Mean Range of Motion over Time at Clinics 1 Through 3

Clinic	Three Weeks	Six Weeks	Six Months
1	77.6°	78.9°	100.0°
2	49.1°	58.6°	85.8°
3	72.6°	82.8°	103.3°

DATA ANALYSIS

A 3 × 3 analysis of variance with one between-subjects factor (clinic) and one within-subject factor (time) was used to analyze differences between range of motion (ROM) means at an alpha level of .05. Post hoc comparisons were made for the clinic factor, with

TABLE 14–18. Summary of Two-Factor Mixed Design Analysis of Variance

Source	Sum of Squares	Degrees of Freedom	Mean Square	*F*	*p*
Clinic	9,138.76	2	4,569.38	10.66	.000
Error	11,571.70	27	428.58		
Time	10,709.42	2	7,354.71	100.89	.000
Clinic × Time	598.64	4	149.66	2.05	.100
Error	3,936.60	54	72.90		

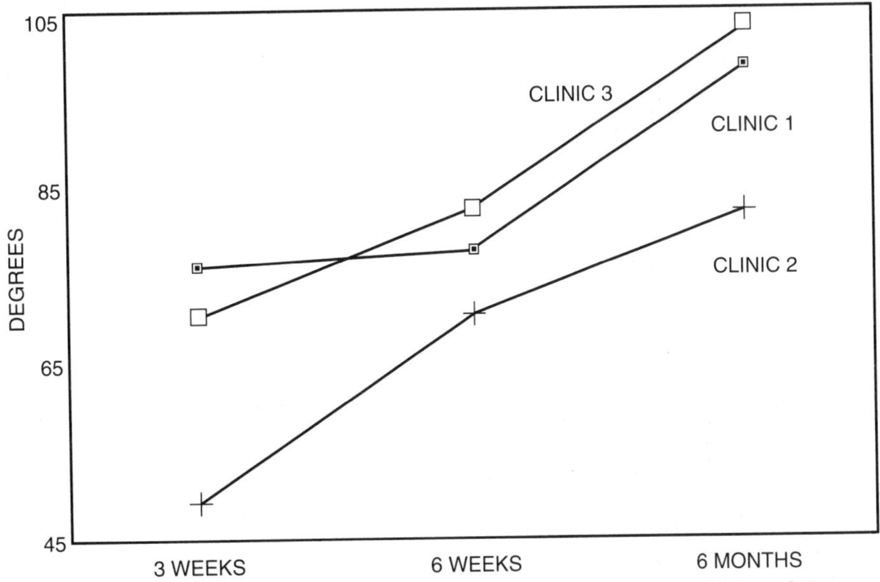

FIGURE 14–4. Nearly parallel lines indicate no interaction between clinic and time.

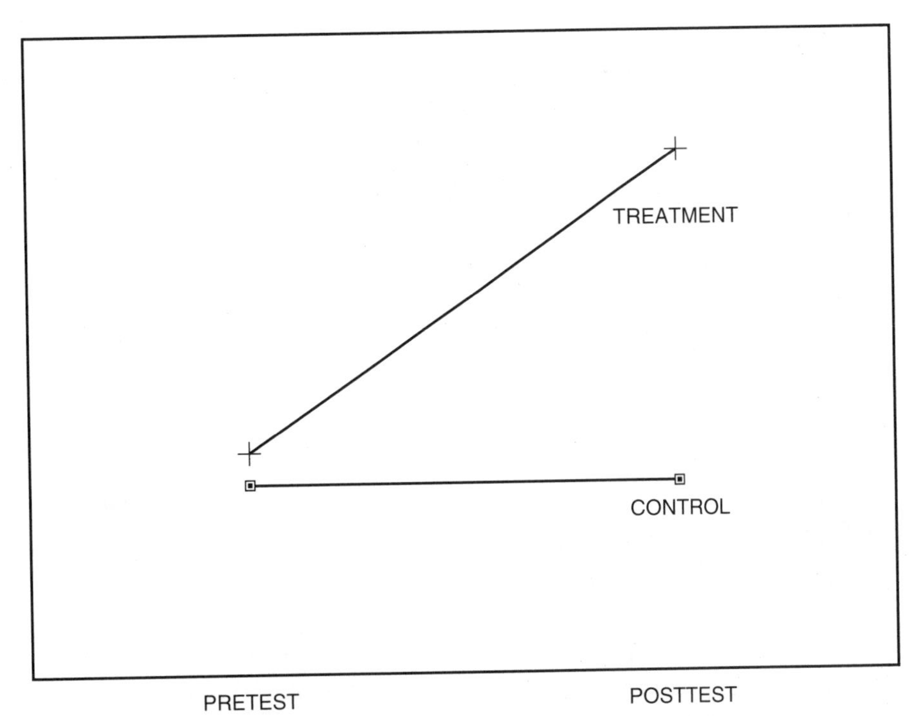

FIGURE 14–5. Ideal pretest–posttest results. The two groups are almost equal at pretest, the control group does not change at posttest, and the treatment group shows significant improvement at posttest. The nonparallel lines indicate a significant interaction between group and time.

Newman–Keuls tests at alpha = .05, and for the time factor, with paired-*t* tests at alpha = .017.

RESULTS

The mean ROM for each group at each point in time is presented in Table 14–17. There was no significant interaction between clinic and time, $F_{4,54} = 2.05$, $p = .100$. There were significant main effects for both clinic, $F_{2,27} = 10.66$, $p = .000$, and time, $F_{2,54} = 100.89$, $p = .000$. Overall means for Clinic 1 (85.5°) and Clinic 3 (86.2°) were not significantly different; Clinic 2's mean (64.5°) was significantly different from those of Clinics 1 and 3. Means for all three time periods were significantly different from one another (three-week mean = 66.4°, six-week mean = 73.4°, and six-month mean = 96.4°).

Literature Examples

Magalhaes and colleagues used three two-factor between-subjects ANOVAs to analyze their study of differences in motor coordination on three different tasks based on age and sex.[24] The age variable had five levels: 5, 6, 7, 8, and 9 years old. The sex variable had two levels: boys and girls. In this study, no interactions were found, so the main effects were interpreted for each of the analyses.

King and coworkers used a mixed-design two-factor ANOVA to test the effect of laser or placebo treatment on experimental pain threshold in a pretest–posttest control-group design.[25] One factor was group, with two levels: treatment (laser) and control (sham laser). The other factor was time, with two levels: pretest and posttest. The interaction between group and time was significant, indicating a difference in response over time for the two groups. The researchers then examined simple main effects for group and simple main effects for time.

Differences Across Several Dependent Variables

Researchers are often interested in the effects of their treatments on several different dependent variables. In our sample data set, we are now interested in whether several six-month outcomes are different between clinics: ROM, knee extensor strength, knee flexor strength, and gait velocity. One analysis approach is to run a one-way ANOVA for each dependent variable. There are two potential problems with this approach. The first is the alpha level inflation that results from conducting multiple tests. The second is the possibility that although no single variable exhibits significant differences across clinics, small, consistent differences across several dependent variables are present. Because an ANOVA can handle only one dependent variable at a time, a cumulative effect over several dependent variables would be undetected.

Multivariate procedures solve these problems by analyzing several dependent variables simultaneously. Multivariate analyses should not be confused with multifactor analyses: The former analyze several *dependent* variables simultaneously; the latter analyze several *independent* variables simultaneously. Although the mathematical basis for multivariate testing of differences is beyond the scope of this text, the interpretation of multivariate results is simply an extension of what has already been learned about ANOVA procedures.

A multivariate analysis of variance (MANOVA) uses an omnibus test to determine whether there are significant differences on the factor of interest (in our case, clinic) when the dependent variables of interest are combined mathematically. The multivariate test statistic used most frequently is Wilks' lambda, although several others are often reported by computer statistical packages. Wilks' lambda is usually converted to an estimated *F* statistic, and the probability of this estimated *F* is determined to test the null hypothesis.[26(p387)]

If the omnibus *F* is significant, then a univariate ANOVA is conducted for each dependent variable to determine where among the dependent variables the differences lie. Once the dependent variables that are significantly different are identified, multiple-comparison procedures can be conducted to determine which levels of the independent variable are different on the dependent variables for which significant differences have been identified.

For our total knee arthroplasty example, the omnibus *F* is 3.53 and is significant at the .003 level. Table 14–19 presents univariate and post hoc results for each of the dependent variables. This analysis might be reported in a journal article as follows:

DATA ANALYSIS

Differences in six-month status across clinics were examined with a multivariate analysis of variance (MANOVA) for the following dependent variables: six-month range of motion, extension torque, flexion torque, and gait velocity. Univariate *F* tests with Newman–Keuls post hoc analyses were conducted to determine the sources of any difference identified by the MANOVA.

RESULTS

The multivariate *F* of 3.53 was significant at the .003 level. Table 14–19 shows the mean for each dependent variable for each clinic, the *F* and *p* values for the test for differences across clinics for each dependent variable, and an indication of which multiple comparisons showed significant differences between clinics. All four dependent variables were significantly different across clinics. In addition, all four dependent variables showed the same pattern of pairwise differences among clinics: None of the dependent variable means were significantly different between Clinics 1 and 3; all

TABLE 14–19. Multivariate Analysis of Variance for Four Dependent Variables

Dependent Variable	Independent Variable			Statistic		Multiple Comparisons		
	Clinic 1	*Clinic 2*	*Clinic 3*	*F*	*p*	*1/2*	*1/3*	*2/3*
Six-month range of motion (degrees)	100.0	85.8	103.3	15.63	.000	*		*
Extension torque (N•m)	135.8	105.4	142.2	4.90	.015	*		*
Flexion torque (N•m)	81.8	62.6	84.1	5.12	.013	*		*
Gait velocity (cm/s)	144.0	107.6	145.6	8.25	.002	*		*

Note: Asterisk indicates a significant difference between the means of the indicated pair of clinics.

```
were significantly different between
Clinics 1 and 2 and between Clinics 2
and 3.
```

Literature Example

Gundersen and associates used a two-way MANOVA to analyze side-to-side differences in 12 different gait measures, such as cycle time, time at which maximum knee flexion occurred, and maximum plantar flexion angle.[27] Subject was treated as one independent variable with 14 levels (there were 14 subjects). Limb was treated as a second independent variable with two levels: dominant or nondominant. Significant interactions between subject and limb were found for 10 of the 12 dependent measures. This indicates that the pattern of differences between limbs was not consistent among subjects. Some subjects had higher values for the dominant limb, others had higher values for the nondominant limb, and others exhibited no differences between limbs. The simple main effect of limb was then tested for each subject for each of the 10 variables for which a significant Limb × Subject interaction was found.

Effect of Removing an Intervening Variable

In our examples we have identified significant differences between clinics. However, scrutiny of patient characteristics at the three clinics shows that Clinic 2 has a patient population that is much older ($\overline{X}$ = 81.0 years) than the patients at Clinic 1 ($\overline{X}$ = 55.8 years) and Clinic 3 ($\overline{X}$ = 69.8 years). If younger patients tend to gain ROM faster than older patients, perhaps the age difference between the clinics, rather than differences in the quality of care, explains the difference in early ROM results.

A procedure known as analysis of covariance (ANCOVA) uses the overall relationship between a dependent variable and an intervening variable, or *covariate,* to adjust the dependent variable scores in light of the covariate scores. For example, let us reexamine the differences between clinics on the three-week ROM variable by using age as a covariate. In our example, there is a strong negative correlation between age and three-week ROM; that is, younger patients tend to have higher scores, and older patients tend to have lower scores (Figure 14–6).

An ANCOVA essentially takes each subject's three-week ROM score and adjusts it to a predicted value as if the subject's age were the same as the mean age of the sample. In our total sample of 30 patients, the mean age is 68.8 years. Thus, the three-week ROM scores of subjects who are younger than 68.8 years are reduced and those of subjects who are older than 68.8 years are increased. Once this mathematical adjustment has taken place, an ANOVA is run on the adjusted data. Figure 14–7 shows this adjustment graphically. The ANCOVA is summarized in Table 14–20. Once age is accounted for, the differences between the groups disappear — the F of 1.88 is not significant (p = .173).

The preceding example used a patient characteristic (age) as the covariate. Another typical use of an ANCOVA is to test for differences between posttest scores using pre-

TABLE 14–20. Analysis of Covariance of Three-Week Range of Motion (ROM)

Clinic	Mean Age	Actual Three-Week ROM	Adjusted Three-Week ROM[a]
1	55.8 years	77.6°	64.54°
2	81.0 years	49.1°	61.22°
3	69.8 years	72.6°	73.53°

[a]No significant differences among clinics, $F_{2,26}$ = 1.88, p = .173.

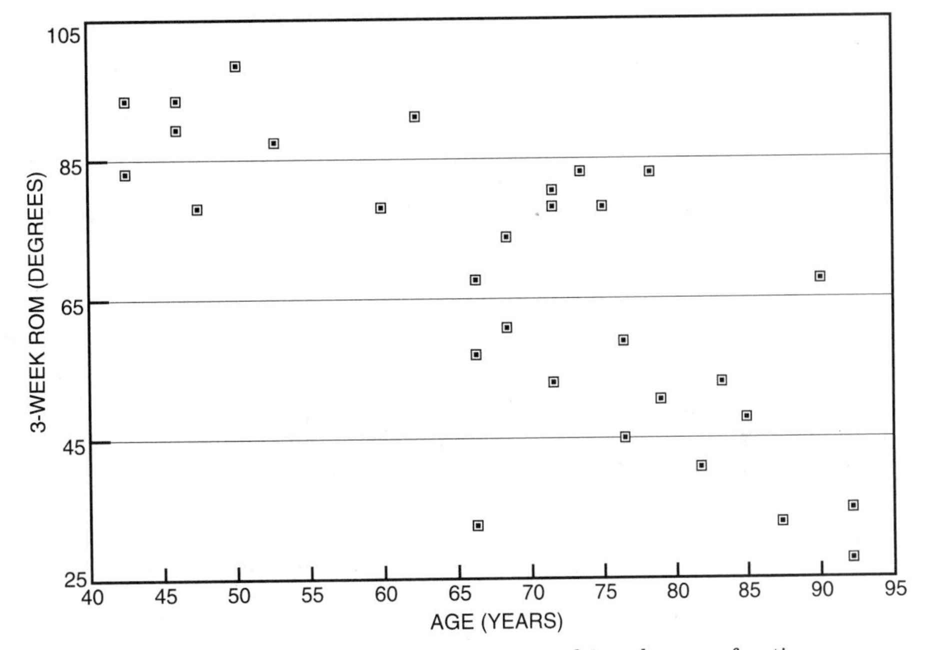

FIGURE 14–6. Relationship between age and 3-week range of motion.

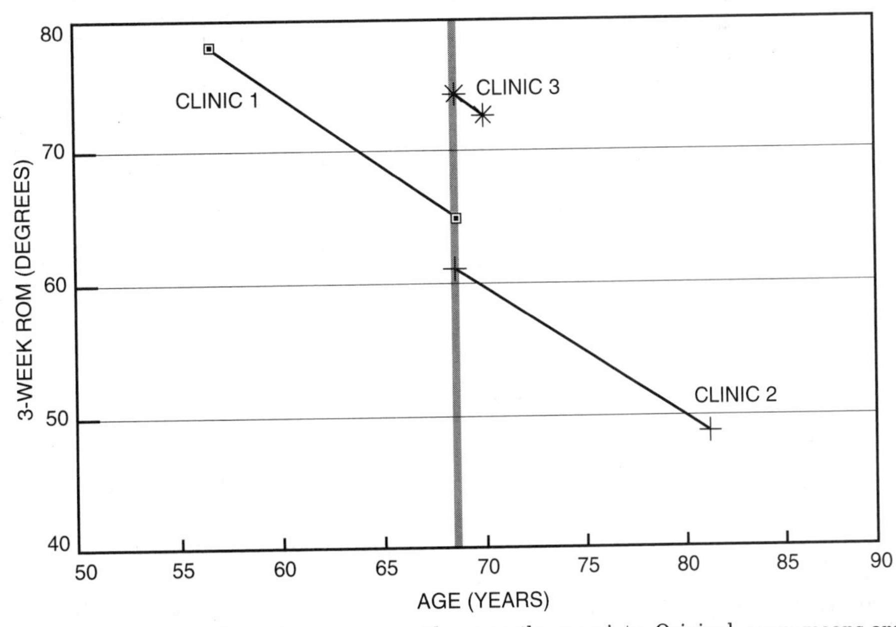

FIGURE 14–7. Analysis of covariance with age as the covariate. Original group means are adjusted to predicted values as if the mean age of each group is equal to the overall mean age of 68.8 years, represented by the vertical line.

test scores as covariates. If pretest scores between groups are significantly different, as is common in clinical research when random assignment to groups has not been possible, then posttest scores can be adjusted to mathematically eliminate the pretest differences.[12] However, it is far more preferable to have equivalent groups at the start of the study, because there are any number of assumptions that must be met before an ANCOVA can be used legitimately. The ANCOVA results in our total knee arthroplasty example might be reported in a journal article as follows:

DATA ANALYSIS

An analysis of covariance was used to determine whether there were significant differences between clinics once the effect of subject age was removed. Alpha was set at .05.

RESULTS

Table 14–20 shows the mean values for age, actual three-week range of motion (ROM), and adjusted three-week ROM across the three clinics. The difference among the adjusted means was not statistically significant.

Literature Example

Wessling and associates studied the effect of three different stretching protocols on triceps surae extensibility.[28] They used a repeated measures design in which subjects were given a different treatment at each of three different sessions. Because differences in pretreatment dorsiflexion ROM measures were found, an ANCOVA was used to adjust each subject's posttest value in light of his or her pretest value.

Analysis of Single-System Designs

Thus far, most of our analyses have been used to analyze group differences by making inferences to the populations from which the groups were drawn. This approach is not satisfactory for single-system designs, in which our interest is in whether an individual has changed over time. Let us assume that we have a patient who has extremely limited ROM 10 weeks after total knee arthroplasty. After treating the patient for 10 weeks with manual stretching and exercise, the therapist decides that more drastic measures are needed and implements a new treatment for 10 weeks, which has the results shown in Figure 14–8. It appears that the new treatment results in an improvement over the baseline, but is there any way to express this more quantitatively? Celeration lines do just this. A basic assumption of the celeration line approach is that the baseline data do not exhibit serial dependency, a phenomenon associated with the ability to predict the next point from the previous point.[29(p170)]

In celeration line analysis, a researcher compares data in different phases by generating a line or lines based on the median of subsets of data in each phase (Figure 14–9). To determine the celeration line through the baseline data, the researcher splits the data in half and splits each half in half again. The median of each of the halves is plotted on vertical lines (the points in Figure 14–9 represent these two medians). A line is drawn through these two points and is extended into the intervention area. The number of data points in the intervention phase and the number exceeding the celeration line are counted. The probability of having a certain proportion of scores above the celeration line can be generated from a table based on the binomial distribution.[29(p184)] The table indicates that in a one-tailed test at an alpha level of .05, 9 or 10 intervention-phase numbers must be

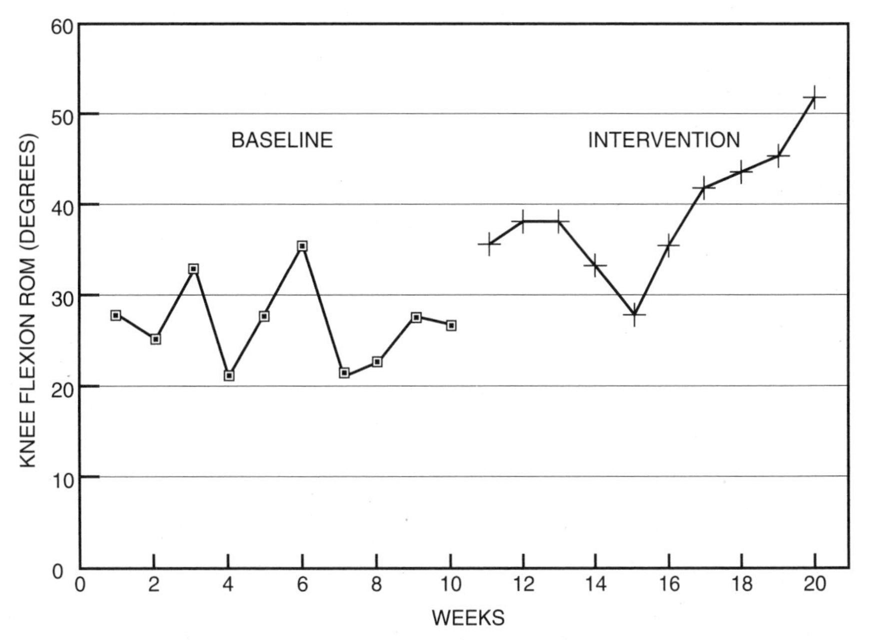

FIGURE 14–8. Single-system data.

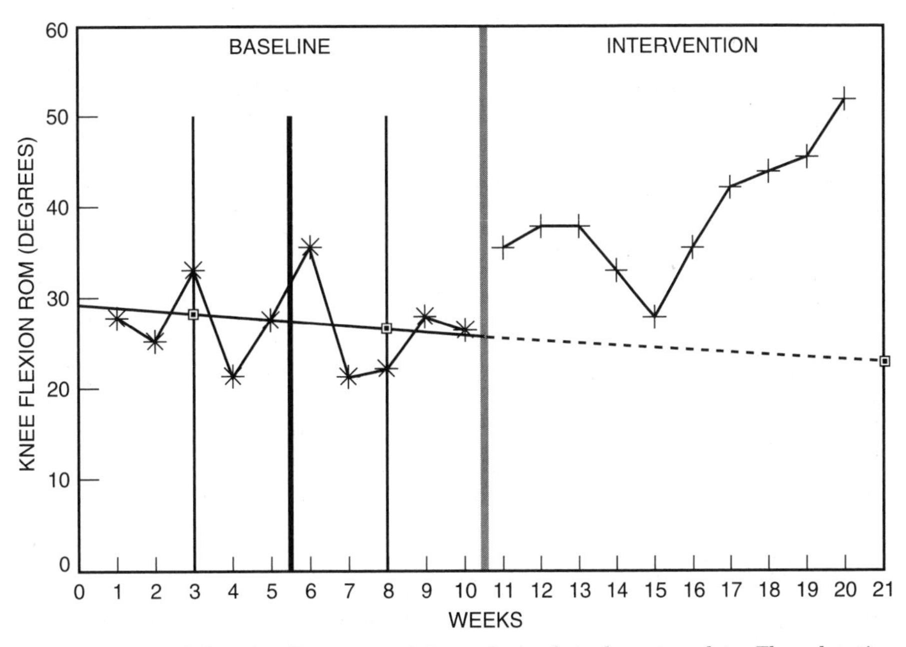

FIGURE 14–9. Celeration line approach to analysis of single-system data. The celeration line determined for the baseline phase (solid line) is extrapolated into the intervention phase (dotted line).

above the celeration line for a significant difference to have occurred. Because all 10 intervention-phase points are above the celeration line, we can conclude that significant improvement occurred during the treatment phase.

In addition to the probability results related to the extended celeration line, quantification of changes in level, trend, and slope of the data may facilitate the description of the patterns seen across time (Figure 14–10). To evaluate these changes, a researcher calculates a celeration line for each phase of the study. *Level* is the difference between the numerical value of observations in one phase and the numerical value of observations in a subsequent phase. A change in level is quantified by calculating the difference between the end of one celeration line and the beginning of the celeration line in the subsequent phase. There is a difference of +4° in level between the baseline and intervention phases of our example.

Trend is the direction of change in the pattern of results. In our example there has been a reversal of the trend: It was downward in the baseline phase and is upward in the intervention phase. Trend can be quantified by calculating the slopes of the lines. *Slope* is the amount that the Y value changes for each unit change in X. To calculate slope, we select two data points on the celeration line. The slope is the difference between the two Y values divided by the difference between the X values. In our example, the data points used to generate the baseline celeration line are (3, 28) and (8, 27). The slope is calculated as follows: $(27 - 28) / (8 - 3) = -1 / 5 = -0.2$. This means that, on average, the patient loses 0.2° of motion each week during the baseline phase. The slope of the intervention-phase celeration line is calculated simi-

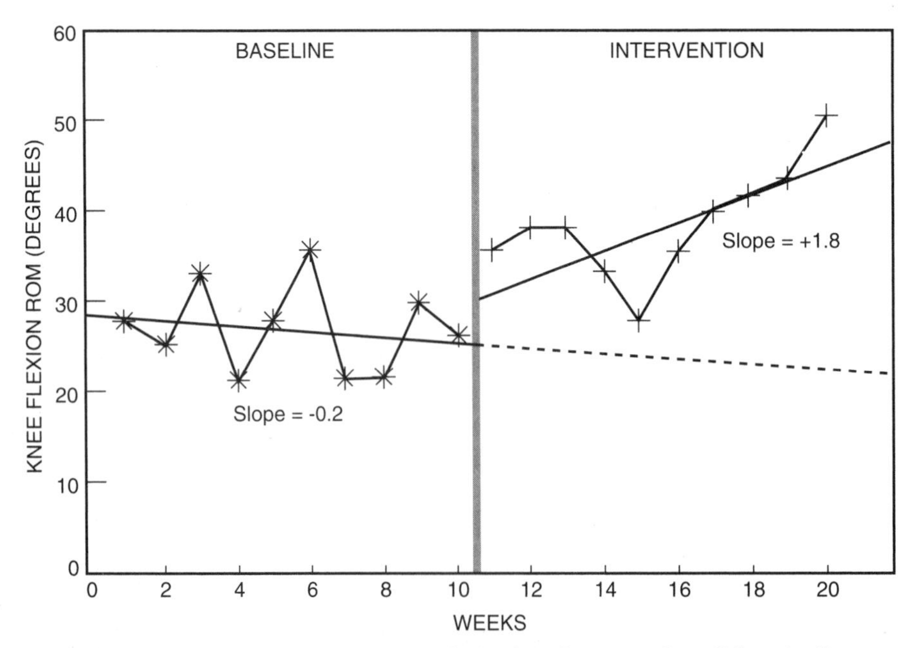

FIGURE 14–10. Level, trend, and slope analysis of single-system data. Celeration lines are calculated for each phase. There is a 4° level change, indicated by the intersections of the celeration lines in each phase with the vertical line separating the phases. There is a change in trend from downward to upward and a change in slope from −0.2 to +1.8.

larly and is +1.8. On average, the patient gained 1.8° of motion each week in the intervention phase. Thus, not only does the trend reversal indicate a positive treatment effect, but the difference in the magnitude of the slopes indicates that treatment led to a fairly rapid improvement in ROM in the intervention phase compared with the baseline phase. The results of this example analysis might be reported in a journal article as follows:

DATA ANALYSIS

Celeration lines for the baseline and intervention phases were developed using the split middle approach. Differences between phases were described through calculation of trend, slope, and level changes from phases to phase. To determine whether the difference between the baseline and intervention phase was statistically significant, we extended the celeration line for the baseline phase into the intervention phase and evaluated the distribution of scores above and below the line in the intervention phase against a tabled value based on binomial probabilities. Alpha was set at .05.

RESULTS

Figure 14–10 shows the data and celeration lines for each phase of the study. The baseline trend was downward and the intervention trend upward, as indicated by the slopes of −.2 and +1.8, respectively. The change in level, or the extent of discontinuity between the celeration lines where they intersect the vertical line separating the two phases, was +4°. All 10 data points in the intervention phase fall above the extended baseline celeration line; this indicates a statistically significant treatment effect at $p < .05$.

Literature Examples

Diamond and Ottenbacher used an extended celeration line to evaluate the results of a repeated treatment single-system study of the effects of a tone-inhibiting orthosis on the gait of an adult with hemiplegia.[30] Embrey and colleagues determined level, trend, and slope to evaluate the celeration lines generated during multiple treatment and baseline phases of a study of the effect of neurodevelopmental treatment on the gait of a child with diplegia.[31]

SUMMARY

Statistical testing of differences between samples is based on 10 steps: (1) stating the hypotheses, (2) deciding on the alpha level, (3) examining the frequency distribution and descriptive statistics to determine whether the assumptions for parametric testing are met, (4) determining whether samples are independent or dependent, (5) determining the appropriate test, (6) using the appropriate software or formulas to determine the value of a test statistic, (7) determining the degrees of freedom, (8) determining the probability of obtaining the test statistic for the given degrees of freedom if the null hypothesis is true, (9) evaluating the obtained probability against the alpha level to draw a statistical conclusion, and (10) evaluating the statistical conclusions in light of clinical knowledge.

The independent t test and Mann-Whitney

test are used to evaluate difference between two independent samples; the one-way ANOVA, Kruskal-Wallis ANOVA, and chi-square analysis can be used for two or more independent samples. The paired-*t*, Wilcoxon signed rank, and McNemar tests are used to evaluate differences between two dependent samples; the repeated measures ANOVA and Friedman's ANOVA can be used for two or more dependent samples. The basic ANOVA techniques can be extended to deal with more the one independent variable (two-factor ANOVA), more than one dependent variable (MANOVA), or an intervening variable (ANCOVA). Single-system research results can be evaluated by computing celeration lines for the data in the different phases of the study.

References

1. Brown GW, Hayden GF. Nonparametric methods: clinical applications. *Clin Pediatr.* 1985;24:490–498.
2. Siegel S, Castellan NJ. *Nonparametric Statistics for the Behavioral Sciences.* 2nd ed. New York, NY: McGraw-Hill Book Co; 1988.
3. Shott S. *Statistics for Health Professionals.* Philadelphia, Pa: WB Saunders Co; 1990.
4. Glass GV, Hopkins KD. *Statistical Methods in Education and Psychology.* 2nd ed. Englewood Cliffs, NJ: Prentice-Hall Inc; 1984.
5. Gaito J. Measurement scales and statistics: resurgence of an old misconception. *Psychol Bull.* 1980;87:564–567.
6. Nunnally JC. *Psychometric Theory.* 2nd ed. New York, NY: McGraw-Hill Book Co; 1978.
7. *SPSS^x User's Guide.* 3rd ed. Chicago, Ill: SPSS Inc; 1988.
8. Kerlinger FN. *Foundations of Behavioral Research.* 3rd ed. Fort Worth, Tex: Holt, Rinehart & Winston Inc; 1986.
9. Munro BH, Visintainer MA, Page EB. *Statistical Methods for Health Care Research.* Philadelphia, Pa: JB Lippincott; 1986.
10. Zito M, Bohannon RW. Inferential statistics in physical therapy research: a recommended core. *Journal of Physical Therapy Education.* 1990;4:13–16.
11. Wainapel SF, Kayne HL. Statistical methods in rehabilitation research. *Arch Phys Med Rehabil.* 1985;66:322–324.
12. Egger MJ, Miller JR. Testing for experimental effects in the pretest-posttest design. *Nurs Res.* 1984;33:306–312.
13. Draper V. Electromyographic biofeedback and recovery of quadriceps femoris muscle function following anterior cruciate ligament reconstruction. *Phys Ther.* 1990;70:11–17.
14. Griffin JW, Tooms RE, Mendius RA, Clifft JK, Van der Zwagg R, El-Zeky F. Efficacy of high voltage pulsed current for healing of pressure ulcers in patients with spinal cord injury. *Phys Ther.* 1991;71:433–444.
15. Weiss LW, Clark FC, Howard DG. Effects of heavy-resistance triceps surae muscle training on strength and muscularity of men and women. *Phys Ther.* 1988;68:208–213.
16. Moncur C. Perceptions of physical therapy competencies in rheumatology. *Phys Ther.* 1987;67:331–339.
17. Mayer TG, Gatchel RJ, Mayer H, Kishino ND, Keeley J, Mooney V. A prospective two-year study of functional restoration in industrial low back injury. *JAMA.* 1987;258:1763–1767.
18. Brooks ME, Smith EM, Currier DP. Effect of longitudinal versus transverse electrode placement on torque production by the quadriceps femoris muscle during neuromuscular electrical stimulation. *Journal of Orthopaedic and Sports Physical Therapy.* 1990;11:530–533.
19. Griffin JW, Newsome LS, Stralka SW, Wright PE. Reduction of chronic posttraumatic hand edema: a comparison of high voltage pulsed current, intermittent pneumatic compression, and placebo treatments. *Phys Ther.* 1990;70:279–286.
20. Falahee MH, Matthews LS, Kaufer H. Resection arthroplasty as a salvage procedure for a knee with infection after a total arthroplasty. *J Bone Joint Surg.* 1987;69A:1013–1021.
21. Maxwell SE. Pairwise multiple comparisons in repeated measures designs. *Journal of Educational Statistics.* 1980;5:269–287.
22. Kelly MK, Palisano RJ, Wolfson MR. Effects of a developmental physical therapy program on oxygen saturation and heart rate in preterm infants. *Phys Ther.* 1989;69:467–474.
23. Packman-Braun R. Relationship between functional electrical stimulation duty cycle and fatigue in wrist extensor muscles of patients with hemiparesis. *Phys Ther.* 1988;68:51–56.
24. Magalhaes LC, Koomar JA, Cermak SA. Bilateral motor coordination in 5- to 9-year-old children: a pilot study. *Am J Occup Ther.* 1989;43:437–443.
25. King CE, Clelland JA, Knowles CJ, Jackson JR. Effect of helium-neon laser auriculotherapy on experimental pain threshold. *Phys Ther.* 1990;70:24–30.
26. Tabachnick BG, Fidell LS. *Using Multivariate Statistics.* 2nd ed. New York, NY: Harper & Row; 1989.
27. Gundersen LA, Valle DR, Barr AE, Danoff JV, Stanhope SJ, Snyder-Mackler L. Bilateral analysis of the knee and ankle during gait: an examination

of the relationship between lateral dominance and symmetry. *Phys Ther.* 1989;69:640–650.
28. Wessling KC, DeVane DA, Hylton CR. Effects of static stretch and static stretch and ultrasound combined on triceps surae muscle extensibility in healthy women. *Phys Ther.* 1987;67:674–679.
29. Ottenbacher KJ. *Evaluating Clinical Change: Strategies for Occupational and Physical Therapists.* Baltimore, Md: Williams & Wilkins; 1986.
30. Diamond MF, Ottenbacher KJ. Effect of a tone-inhibiting dynamic ankle-foot orthosis on stride characteristics of an adult with hemiparesis. *Phys Ther.* 1990;70:423–430.
31. Embrey DG, Yates L, Mott DH. Effects of neurodevelopmental treatment and orthoses on knee flexion during gait: a single-subject design. *Phys Ther.* 1990;70:626–637.

CHAPTER 15

Analysis of Relationships

Researchers often wish to know the extent to which variables are related to one another. For example, in Chapter 6, a study is cited in which the relationship between bone mineral density and muscle strength was examined.[1] In Chapter 11, two studies are cited in which the reliabilities of measures were determined by documenting the relationship between scores gathered on the same individual at two or more different times and the relationship between measurements taken on the same individual by two or more therapists.[2,3]

Relationship analysis studies are generally nonexperimental, with the researcher observing different phenomena rather than manipulating groups of subjects, as is done in experimental studies. Recall from Chapter 14 that the analysis of differences centers on determining whether there are mean differences between groups or between repeated administrations of a test to a single group. In contrast, the analysis of relationships centers on determining the *association* between scores on two or more variables that are available for each individual in a single group.

This chapter introduces the major ways in which relationships among variables are analyzed. As in Chapter 14, the purpose of this chapter is not to enable readers to conduct their own statistical analyses, but to enable them to understand relationship analysis as it is presented in the physical therapy literature. Simple correlation and linear regression are presented first, followed by discussions of multiple regression techniques, the uses of relationship analysis for documenting reliability, and factor analysis.

CORRELATION

When two variables are correlated, the value an individual exhibits on one variable is related to the value he or she exhibits on another variable. The magnitude and direction of the relationship between variables are expressed mathematically as a correlation coefficient. The presence of relationships among variables does not enable researchers to draw causal inferences about the variables: Correlation is not causation. For example, although there is an obvious relationship between the amount of corn grown in a particular locale and the flatness of the land on which it is grown, reasonable people do not conclude that growing corn causes the land to become flat.[4]

This section begins with calculation of the most frequently used correlation coefficient, the Pearson product moment correlation. This is followed by discussion of alternative correlation coefficients, the assumptions that underlie correlation coefficients, the ways in which correlation coefficients are interpreted, and examples of the use of correlation from the literature.

Calculation of the Pearson Product Moment Correlation

Calculation of the Pearson product moment correlation is mathematically tedious, although relatively simple conceptually: The Pearson product moment correlation, or r, is the average of the crossproducts of the z scores for the X and Y variables. In mathematical notation,

$$r = \frac{\Sigma Z_X Z_Y}{N}$$

Suppose we are interested in determining the extent of the relationship between a functional variable such as gait velocity and a physical impairment variable such as knee flexion range of motion (ROM) in patients who have undergone total knee arthroplasty. Table 15–1 shows the calculation of the correlation between six-month ROM and gait velocity in patients at Clinic 1. In the calculation of the Pearson r value, either variable may be designated X or Y, and neither is considered independent or dependent. The X and Y scores for each subject are converted to z scores, and the product of z_X and z_Y (called the *crossproduct*) is determined for each subject. The mean of the crossproducts is the Pearson product moment correlation coefficient.

The values that r may take range from -1.0 to $+1.0$. A correlation coefficient of -1.0 indicates a perfect negative, or inverse, relationship: A higher value on one variable is associated with a lower value on the other variable. A correlation coefficient of $+1.0$ indicates a perfect positive, or direct, relationship: A higher value on one variable is associated with a higher value on the other variable. In this example $r = .76$, indicating a fairly strong direct relationship between the two variables. Figure 15–1 shows a scatterplot of the 10 pairs of scores. They fall rather loosely around an imaginary diagonal line running from the bottom left corner of the graph to the top right corner. This indicates that as ROM scores increase, so do gait velocity values.

Researchers often collect many variables within a single study and are interested in which of the variables are most related to one another. When a researcher calculates many correlation coefficients in a study, he or she usually displays them in a correlation matrix, as shown in Table 15–2. In this table, all the variables of interest are listed as both columns and rows, and the correlation between each pair of variables is presented at the intersection of the row and column of interest. For example, the Pearson r between flexion torque and extension torque is .9524 and can be found in two places on the table (the intersection of Row 2 and Column 3 and the intersection of Row 3 and Column 2). A full correlation matrix like this includes redun-

TABLE 15–1. Calculation of Pearson *r*: Relationship Between Six-Month Range of Motion and Gait Velocity at Clinic 1

Subject	X	x	Y	y	z_X	z_Y	$z_X z_Y$
01	100		165	21	0.00	1.13	0.00
02	85	−15	100	−44	−2.24	−2.37	5.31
03	100	0	130	−14	0.00	−0.75	0.00
04	105	5	170	26	0.75	1.40	1.05
05	105	5	150	6	0.75	0.32	0.24
06	95	−5	135	−9	−0.75	−0.48	0.36
07	110	10	153	9	1.49	0.48	0.72
08	100	0	145	1	0.00	0.05	0.00
09	95	−5	147	3	−0.75	0.16	−0.12
10	105	5	145	1	0.75	0.05	0.04
Σ	1,000.0		1,440.0				7.6
N	10.0		10.0				10.0
$\bar{X}$	100.0		144.0				r = .76
σ	6.71		18.60				

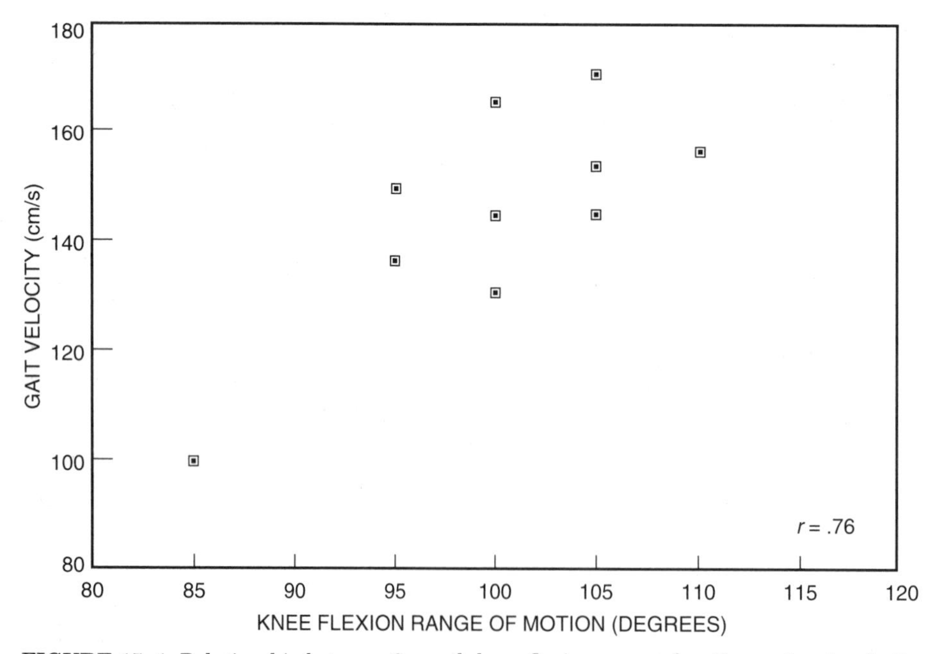

FIGURE 15–1. Relationship between 6-month knee flexion range of motion and gait velocity.

TABLE 15–2. Correlation Matrix for Six-Month Variables

	Range of Motion	Flexion Torque	Extension Torque	Gait Velocity
Range of motion	1.0000	.5610	.5947	.6399
Flexion torque	.5610	1.0000	.9524	.8921
Extension torque	.5947	.9524	1.0000	.9014
Gait velocity	.6399	.8921	.9014	1.0000

dant information because each correlation coefficient between two different variables is listed twice. It also includes unnecessary information because the correlation between each variable and itself is known (1.000), and these correlations form the diagonal. In articles, therefore, most researchers display only the nonredundant portion of the correlation matrix, which lies either above or below the diagonal.

Alternative Correlation Coefficients

Correlation coefficients other than the Pearson product moment correlation have been developed for a variety of uses beyond that of quantifying the degree of relationship between two interval or ratio variables. Several are listed in Chapter 10, where correlation is introduced as a concept related to measurement theory, and Table 15–3 lists the characteristics of several additional correlation measures.

The Spearman rho (ρ) and Kendall tau (τ) correlations are designed for use when both variables are ranked. In actuality, the Spearman rho formula is simply a shortcut version of the Pearson *r;* if the Pearson *r* is calculated for ranked data, the result will be the same as if the Spearman formula is applied.[5(p79)]

Correlation coefficients for use with nominal data are the phi (ϕ) and kappa (κ) coefficients. Phi is another shortcut version of the Pearson *r,* applicable when both variables are dichotomous, such as in determining the relationship between sex and the answer to a yes/no question.[5(p79)] Kappa, discussed in more detail in Reliability Analyses, is a reliability coefficient that can be used when nominal variables consist of more than two categories.

Correlation coefficients for more than two variables are also available. The intraclass correlation coefficients (ICCs), also discussed in Reliability Analyses, are a family of reliability coefficients that can be used when two or more repeated measures have been collected. Kappa can also be used with more than two nominal repeated measures. Partial correlation is used to assess the relationship between two variables with the effect of a

TABLE 15–3. Characteristics of Different Correlation Coefficients

Coefficient	Characteristics
Pearson product moment correlation	Two continuous variables
Spearman rho (ρ)	Two ranked variables; shortcut calculation of Pearson
Kendall tau (τ)	Two ranked variables
Phi (ϕ)	Two dichotomous variables; shortcut calculation of Pearson
Kappa (κ)	Two or more nominal variables with two or more categories; a reliability coefficient
Intraclass correlation coefficient	Two or more continuous variables; a reliability coefficient
Partial correlation	Two variables, with effects of a third held constant
Multiple correlation	More than two variables
Canonical correlation	Two sets of variables

third variable eliminated. Multiple correlation is used to assess the variability shared by three or more variables. Canonical correlation is a technique for assessing the relationships between two sets of variables.

Assumptions of the Correlation Coefficients

Calculation of the Pearson product moment and related correlation coefficients depends on three major assumptions. First, the relationships between variables are assumed to be *linear*. Analysis of a scatterplot of the data must show that the relationship forms a straight line. Curvilinear relationships (those that do not follow a straight line) may be analyzed, but this requires more advanced techniques than are discussed in this text. Figure 15–2 shows the scatterplot of our hypothetical total knee arthroplasty data showing the relationship between age and a new variable, length of acute care hospital stay postoperatively. There is an obvious relationship between variables, but it is not linear. Both the young and very old patients have short lengths of stay, possibly because the young reach their ROM goals quickly and the old are transferred to a skilled nursing facility for continued rehabilitation. Those of intermediate age stay in the hospital somewhat longer, presumably to achieve their ROM goals in the acute care hospital, without transfer to a skilled nursing facility. The Pearson r for this relationship is .3502, indicating a minimal degree of linear relationship between these two variables. If researchers rely solely on Pearson r values to guide their conclusions, they may mistakenly conclude that no relationship exists when in fact a strong *nonlinear* relationship exists.

The second assumption is *homoscedasticity*. As shown in Figure 15–3A, homoscedas-

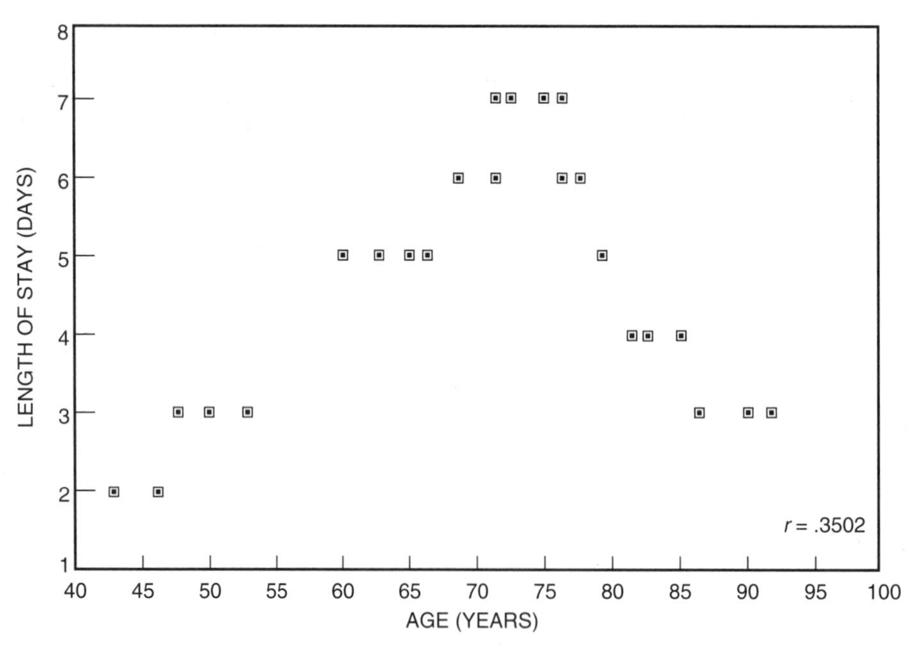

FIGURE 15–2. Relationship between age and length of stay. There is a strong nonlinear relationship between the two variables. The low r value is deceptive because it is designed to detect linear relationships only.

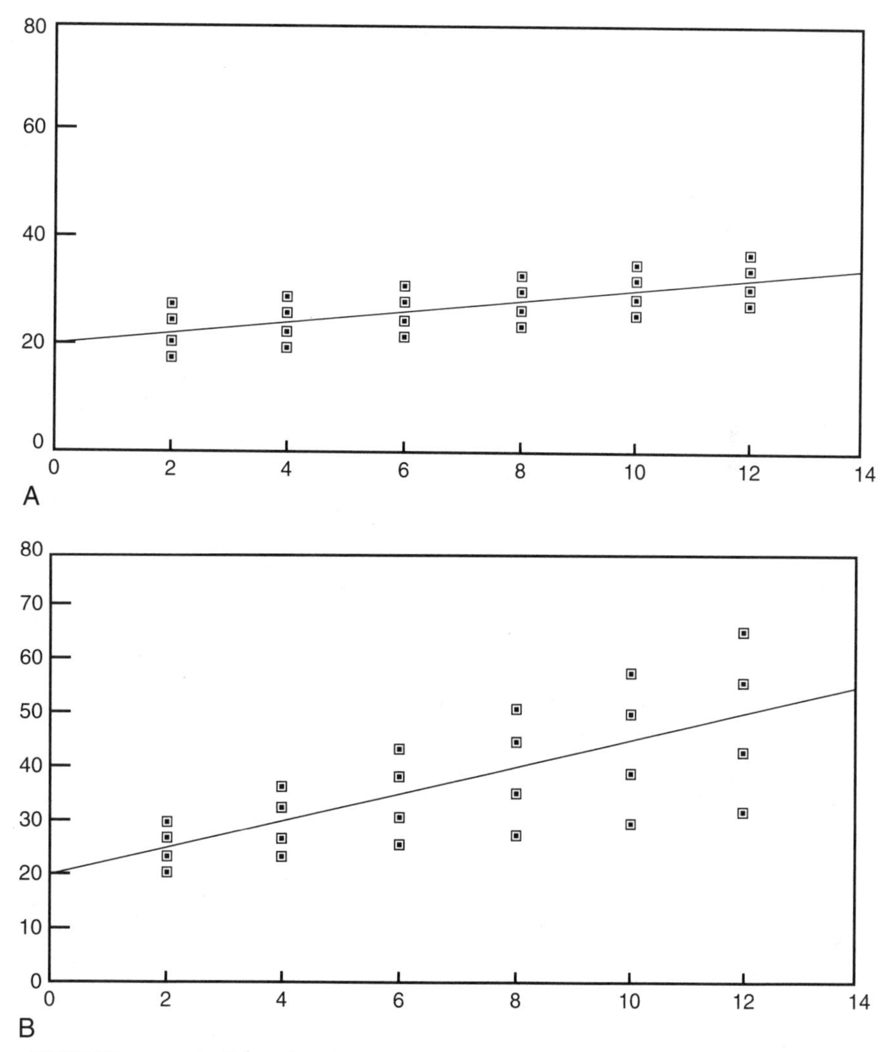

FIGURE 15–3. A. Example of homoscedasticity; the Y values are equally variable at each level of X. **B.** Example of nonhomoscedasticity; the Y values are not equally variable at each level of X.

ticity means that for each value of one variable, the other variable has equal variability. Nonhomoscedasticity is illustrated in Figure 15–3B. Because the calculation of Pearson r is based on z scores, whose calculation in turn depends on standard deviations for each variable, widely varying variances at different levels will distort the calculated value of r.

The third assumption is that both variables have enough *variability* to demonstrate a relationship. If either or both variables have a restricted range, then the correlation coefficient will be artificially low and uninterpretable. Figure 15–4A shows the scatterplot of Clinic 3's data for six-month ROM and gait velocity. There appears to be little relationship between the two, because the data cluster in the top right corner of the graph and the Pearson r is $-.2673$. However, the range of ROM values is very restricted, with all

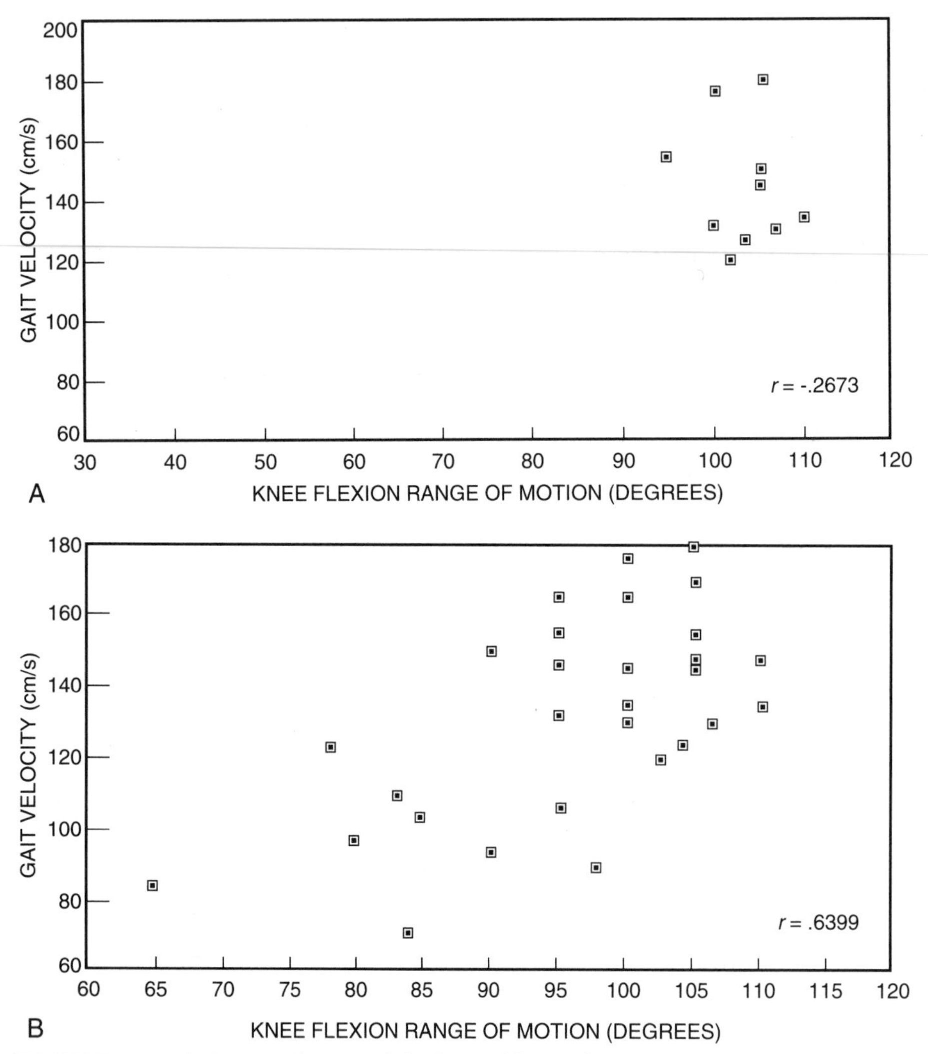

FIGURE 15–4. A. Restricted range of the X variable results in a low correlation coefficient. **B.** The addition of a broader range of X values reveals a pattern that was not apparent in **A.**

subjects showing close to full ROM of their prosthetic knees.

Figure 15–4B shows the scatterplot of six-month ROM and gait velocity for the entire sample of 30 patients. In this example each variable takes a fairly wide range of values, and the relationship between six-month ROM and gait velocity is obvious. The Pearson r for this set of data is .6399.

Thus, the restricted-range data yielded a correlation coefficient that was different in both magnitude and direction from the coefficient calculated on data with a greater range of values.

Interpretation of Correlation Coefficients

There are four major ways in which correlation coefficients are interpreted: the strength of the coefficient itself; the variance shared by the two variables, as calculated by the coefficient of determination; the statistical significance of the correlation coefficient; and the confidence intervals about the correlation coefficient. Regardless of which method is chosen, the interpretation should not be extrapolated beyond the range of the data used to generate the correlation coefficient.

Strength of the Coefficient. The first way to interpret the coefficient is to examine the strength of the relationship, which is independent of the direction (direct or inverse) of the relationship. This method of interpretation is exemplified by Munro's descriptive terms for the strength of correlation coefficients:[5(p70)]

.00–.25	little, if any correlation
.26–.49	low correlation
.50–.69	moderate correlation
.70–.89	high correlation
.90–1.00	very high correlation

Such a system of descriptors assumes that the meaningfulness of a correlation is the same regardless of the context in which it is used. This assumption is not necessarily valid. For example, if one is determining the reliability of a strength measure from one day to the next, an r of .70 may be considered unacceptably low for the purpose of documenting day-to-day changes in status. However, if one is determining the relationship between abstract constructs such as self-esteem and motivation that are difficult to measure, then a correlation of .50 may be considered very strong.

Variance Shared by the Two Variables. The second way to evaluate the importance of the correlation coefficient is to calculate what is called the *coefficient of determination.* The coefficient of determination, r^2, is the square of the correlation coefficient, r. The coefficient of determination is an indication of the percentage of variance that is shared by the two variables. For the relationship between six-month ROM and gait velocity at Clinic 1 (Table 15–1), the coefficient of determination is approximately .58 ($.76^2 = .5776$). This means that 58% of the variability within one variable can be accounted for by the other variable. The remaining 42% of the variability is due to variables not yet considered, perhaps height, leg length, pain, age, or sex. Using the coefficient of determination, we find, for example, that a "high" correlation coefficient of .70 accounts for only 49% of the variance among the variables, and a "low" correlation of .30 accounts for an even lower 9% of the variance between the variables.

Statistical Significance of the Coefficient. The third method of interpreting correlation coefficients is to statistically determine whether the coefficient calculated is significantly different from zero. In other words, we determine the probability that the calculated correlation coefficient would have occurred by chance if in fact there were no relationship between the variables. A special form of a t test is used to determine this probability. The problem with this approach is that very weak correlations may be statistically different from zero even though they are not very meaningful. This is particularly likely to occur with large samples. For example, Sellers studied the relationship between antigravity control and postural control in 107 children.[6] Correlations as low as .11 were found to be statistically different from zero at the .05 level. Although statistically significant, correlations of this magnitude probably do not describe clinically meaningful relationships.

Confidence Intervals Around the Coefficient. The fourth way to determine the meaningfulness of a correlation coefficient is to calculate a confidence interval about the correlation coefficient. To do so, a researcher converts the r values into z scores, calculates confidence intervals with the z scores, and transforms the z-score intervals back into a range of r scores. Using steps outlined by Munro, the 95% confidence interval for an r of .76 for six-month ROM and gait velocity at Clinic 1 is .17 to .94.[5(p74)] The confidence interval is very large because the sample is small and does not permit accurate estimation. Using the same procedures, the 95% confidence interval for the same r calculated for a sample of 100 subjects is approximately .65 to .83, a far smaller interval. As is the case for the confidence intervals calculated in the analysis of differences, larger samples permit more accurate estimation of true population values.

Limitation of Interpretation. A consideration common to all four interpretation methods is that the interpretation of correlation coefficients should not extend beyond the range of the original data. For example, Figure 15–5 shows the fairly strong relationship between the six-month ROM and gait velocity data (asterisks). The line showing the trend of the data is extrapolated to a ROM of 0°. At this ROM, the trend line indicates that the gait velocity would be estimated to be approximately *negative* 38 cm/s, an impossible figure! Rather than being a linear relationship throughout the ROM, it is likely that the relationship becomes curvilinear as ROM becomes closer to 0°, with gait velocity bottoming out at some low level (crosses). Knowing that the relationship between ROM and gait velocity is strong and linear in the top half of the usual values does not permit us to extrapolate these conclusions to values outside the ranges encountered in the original data collection. A full interpretation of the correlation between six-month ROM and gait

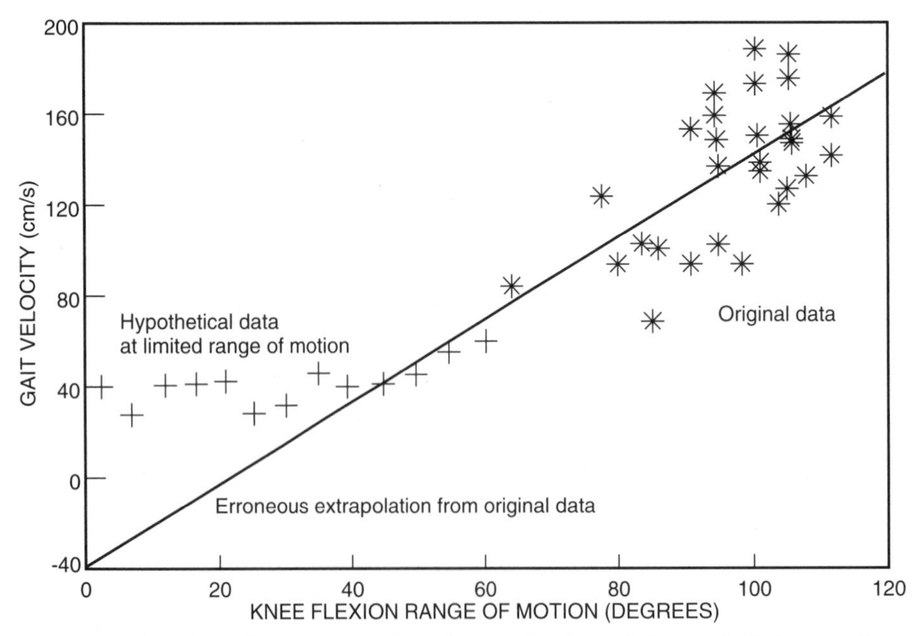

FIGURE 15–5. Extending interpretation of regression beyond the original data results in invalid conclusions. Original data (asterisks) extrapolated past the X and Y values predict that patients with no flexion range of motion will have a negative gait velocity. Crosses indicate the more likely relationship between the two variables in their lower ranges.

velocity might be written in a journal article as follows:

DATA ANALYSIS

A Pearson product moment correlation (r) was used to quantify the relationship between six-month range of motion (ROM) and gait velocity for the sample of 30 subjects. Interpretation of the coefficient was through significance testing at the 5% level, calculation of r^2, and construction of a 95% confidence interval around the correlation coefficient.

RESULTS

The Pearson r between six-month ROM and gait velocity was .6399. This was significantly different from zero at a level of $p < .01$. The coefficient of determination (r^2) was .41, indicating that about 40% of the variability in gait velocity can be attributed to differences in six-month ROM. The 95% confidence interval for r was .365–.812.

DISCUSSION

The moderate correlation of approximately .64 between six-month ROM and gait velocity seems important clinically because it provides evidence that those patients with less physical impairment (i.e., those with good ROM) also have less functional disability, as measured by gait velocity. The confidence interval for r is large, because of the moderate sample size within this study. On the basis of the strength of the correlation found in this study, we recommend further data collection on a larger sample to provide a more accurate estimation of the true relationship between these two variables.

Literature Examples

In a study by Bohannon and a study by DiFabio and Badke, relationships between variables were examined to determine whether measures of physical characteristics were related to performance of functional tasks in patients with hemiplegia.[7, 8] Bohannon compared the strength of seven different lower extremity muscle groups with gait velocity and cadence using Pearson product moment correlations and interpreted the correlations using significance testing and coefficients of determination. DiFabio and Badke compared scores on the Sensory Organization Test with various lower extremity subscores of the Fugl-Meyer Sensorimotor Assessment Test, a performance-based assessment. They used the Spearman rho rank-order correlation coefficient and interpreted correlations using significance testing.

LINEAR REGRESSION

Correlational techniques, as discussed above, are used to describe the relationships among two or more variables. When the researcher's purpose extends beyond description of relationships to include prediction of future characteristics from previously collected data, then the statistical analysis extends from correlation to regression techniques.

Suppose we wish to predict a patient's eventual gait velocity on the basis of an early postoperative indicator such as three-week ROM. The Pearson product moment correlation between these two variables is .5545, indicating a moderate degree of correlation in which 31% of the variability in gait velocity (r^2 = .3075) can be accounted for by variability in three-week ROM. Unlike correlation techniques, regression techniques require that variables be defined as independent or dependent. In this example, the independent variable is three-week ROM and is used to predict the dependent variable, gait velocity.

Figure 15–6 shows a scatterplot of three-week ROM and gait velocity scores, with a line showing the best fit between these two variables. This line is generated by using the data to solve the general equation for a straight line:

$$Y = bX + a$$

where b is the slope of the line and a is the intercept (that is, the Y value at the point at which the line intersects the Y axis). The slope, b, is found by multiplying the Pearson r value by the ratio of the standard deviation of Y to the standard deviation of X [$b = r(s_Y/s_X)$]. The intercept, a, is found by subtracting the product of the slope and the mean of X from the mean of Y ($a = \overline{Y} - b\overline{X}$). As with most statistical analyses today, computer programs can generate regression equations quickly and easily without the need for hand calculations. The formula for the regression line of gait velocity on three-week ROM is $Y = .75X + 82.56$. Although this equation defines the best-fitting line through the data, most of the points do not fall precisely on the line. The vertical distance from each point to the line is known as the *residual,* and the mean of the residuals is zero. The standard deviation of the residuals is known as the *standard error of the estimate* (SEE).

Once the regression equation is generated, it can be used to predict the gait velocity of future patients by solving for Y (gait velocity)

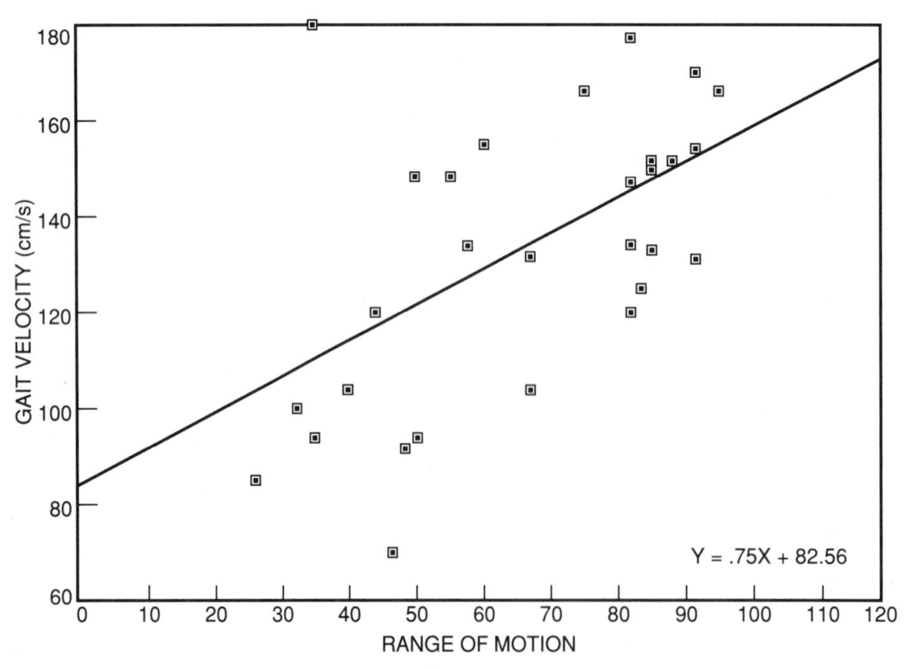

FIGURE 15–6. Regression of gait velocity on 3-week knee flexion range of motion.

on the basis of the patient's X (three-week ROM) score. For example, suppose that a patient has 70° of ROM three weeks postoperatively. The predicted gait velocity for this patient is 135.06 cm/s [135.06 = .75(70) + 82.56]. Because we know that this prediction is unlikely to be precise, we can provide additional useful information by generating a confidence interval around the predicted value. The confidence interval around the predicted value is created by using the SEE. A 95% confidence interval, for example, is created by adding and subtracting 1.96 SEEs from the regression line, as shown graphically in Figure 15–7. In this example, the SEE generated by the computer is 24.54 cm/s and the 95% confidence interval would be found by adding and subtracting 48.09 cm/s to and from the predicted Y value. For patients with three-week ROM of 70°, we therefore are 95% certain that their gait velocity at six months will be between 86.96 and 183.16 cm/s. Ideally, the dependent variable is highly correlated with the independent variable, resulting in small residuals, a small SEE, and a more precise prediction.

The statistical significance of a regression equation is usually determined with an *F* test to evaluate whether r^2, the amount of variance in Y predicted by X, is significantly different from zero. As is the case with statistical testing of the correlation coefficient using a *t* test, r^2 may be statistically different from zero without being terribly meaningful. In our example, the r^2 of .3075 is significantly different from zero at $p = .0015$. Despite this statistical significance, we know that the 95% confidence interval for predicting a single score is quite large and may not allow for clinically useful prediction. For instance, the gait velocity needed to cross most streets safely is approximately 130 cm/s.[9] The range of the confidence interval is great enough that for most patients we could not predict

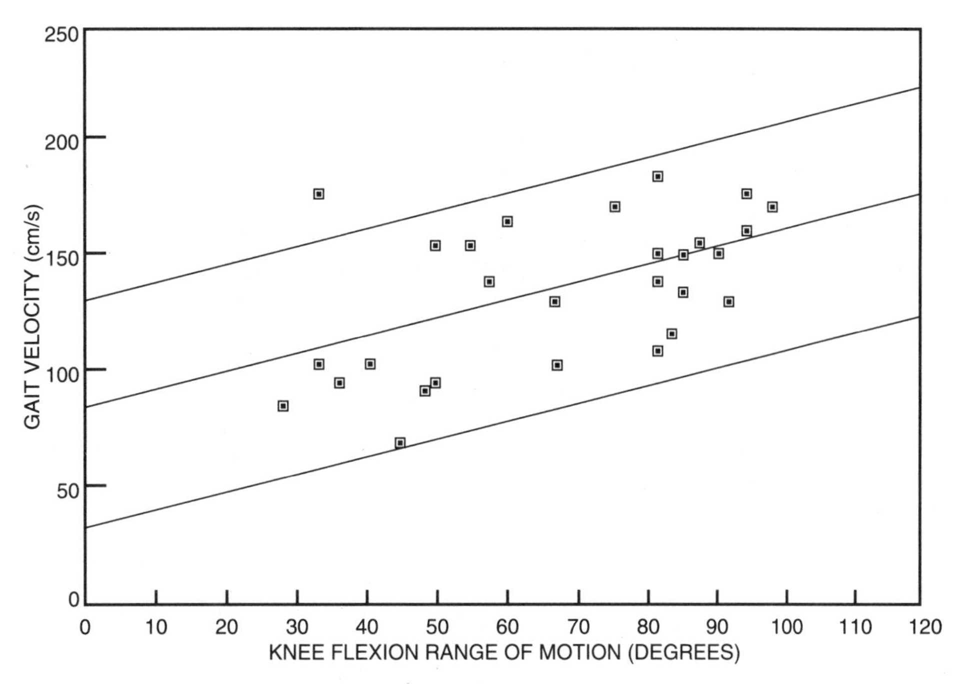

FIGURE 15–7. 95% confidence intervals around the predicted gait velocity.

whether their eventual velocity would enable them to be community ambulators. This reflects the fact that there is only a moderate correlation between the two variables in question.

In practice, then, this regression equation would not likely be perceived to be very useful, and the researchers would search for additional independent variables that would allow for more precise prediction of the dependent variable. When more than one variable is used to predict another variable, the simple linear regression technique is extended to multiple regression.

MULTIPLE REGRESSION

Because the prediction of gait velocity from three-week ROM is not precise enough to be useful clinically, the next logical step is to add an additional variable or variables to the equation to determine whether the prediction can be made more precise. For example, suppose we add patients' age to the equation. The general prediction equation for multiple regression is

$$Y = b_1X_1 + b_2X_2 + b_iX_i + a$$

For each independent variable there is a corresponding slope, which is referred to in multiple regression as a *b-weight.* For the entire equation there is one intercept, which is referred to as the constant. The computer-generated regression equation for three-week ROM and age as predictors of gait velocity is

$$\text{(velocity)} = .04\ \text{(three-week ROM)} - 1.41\ \text{(age)} + 227.04$$

A 65-year-old patient with 70° of motion three-weeks postoperatively would be predicted to have a gait velocity of 138.19 cm/s six months postoperatively:

$$138.19 = .04(70) - 1.41(65) + 227.04$$

The correlation between all the independent variables and the dependent variable in a multiple regression equation is represented by R, to distinguish it from r, the correlation between the two variables in a simple linear regression equation. For this equation the multiple correlation, R, is .77483 and the R^2 is .55477. This means that the combination of three-week ROM and age accounts for 55% of the variability in gait velocity. Recall that three-week ROM alone accounted for only 30% of the variability in gait velocity. The addition of age to the equation has greatly improved its predictability.

Variable Entry in Multiple Regression

When performing a multiple regression, researchers often specify various decision rules to guide the computer in generating the regression equation. The rules are generally constructed so that the method of variable entry maximizes the accuracy of predictions while minimizing the number of variables in the equation. Variables are retained in the equation if they improve the R^2 by a specified amount or if they are associated with a probability of some specified amount.

In a forward regression strategy, a researcher adds one variable at a time and stops when additional variables do not contribute the preset amount. In a backward regression strategy, the researcher begins with all the possible variables of interest in the equation and deletes them one at a time if their presence does not contribute the preset amount. A stepwise regression strategy combines forward and backward procedures to generate the equation. If any of these strategies were used in our example, the age variable would be entered first, and the three-week ROM variable would not be entered because it contributes so little beyond that of age. For example, the R^2 associated with age alone is .55432; for age and three-week ROM combined, it is only .55477, an increase of only .00045. This means that the addition of three-week ROM to the equation adds only .045% of additional predictability for gait velocity. Clinically, this means that if our interest is primarily in predicting gait velocity, we can eliminate the possibly inconvenient and expensive measurement of three-week ROM and substitute the inexpensive, easily obtained age value.

Interpretation of the Multiple Regression Equation

The meaningfulness of the multiple regression equation can be assessed in several ways. First, an F test of R^2 can be conducted to determine whether it is significantly different from zero. For our example the computer-generated significance of the F test is .0000, indicating that there is a very low probability that the R^2 of .55477 was obtained by chance.

The second way to assess the meaningfulness of a multiple regression equation is to generate a confidence interval. The computer-generated SEE for the multiple regression equation is 20.03 cm/s, and a 95% confidence interval would add and subtract 39.27 cm/s to the predicted Y value [$\pm$ 1.96 (SEE)]. Thus, we could be 95% certain that our 65-year-old patient with 70° of knee flexion three weeks postoperatively would have a six-month gait velocity of 98.92 to 177.46 cm/s. Because a greater proportion of the variability in gait velocity is accounted for by the multiple regression compared with the simple regression, this interval is somewhat narrower than the one generated for the simple linear regression of gait velocity on three-week ROM.

A third way to evaluate the regression equation is to determine the relative contribution of each of the variables to the equation. This can be done by either conducting a t test of the contribution of each variable or dividing the R^2 into the components attributable to each variable. This division is done through beta(β)-weights, which are standardized versions of b-weights. The beta-weight for each variable is multiplied by the correlation coefficient between that variable and the dependent variable. For our example, the mathematical notation is

$$R^2 = (\beta_{\text{3-week ROM}})(r_{\text{3-week ROM, velocity}}) + (\beta_{\text{age}})(r_{\text{age, velocity}})$$

Using computer-generated beta-weights and correlation coefficients, we find the following:

$$\begin{aligned} .5547 &= (.0305)(.5545) + (-.7224)(-.7445) \\ &= .0169 + .5378 \end{aligned}$$

This means that of the 55% of the variability in gait velocity predicted by the equation, almost 54% is due to the relationship between age and gait velocity and less than 2% is due to the relationship between three-week ROM and velocity. The t tests of the contribution of variables yield significance levels of .8711 for three-week ROM and .0006 for age. Both the division of R^2 and the t tests indicate that age is a much more important predictor of gait velocity than is three-week ROM.

Recall that in the simple linear regression of gait velocity on three-week ROM, the ROM variable accounted for approximately 31% of the variability in gait scores. How is it that it now accounts for only 2% of that variability? The answer can be found in an examination of the interrelationships among all three variables. The Venn diagrams in Figure 15–8 illustrate this principle. Independently, three-week ROM accounts for about 31% of the variability in gait velocity, as shown in Figure 15–8A. Independently, age accounts for about 55% of the variability in gait velocity, as shown in Figure 15–8B. In addition, age and three-week ROM are highly related,

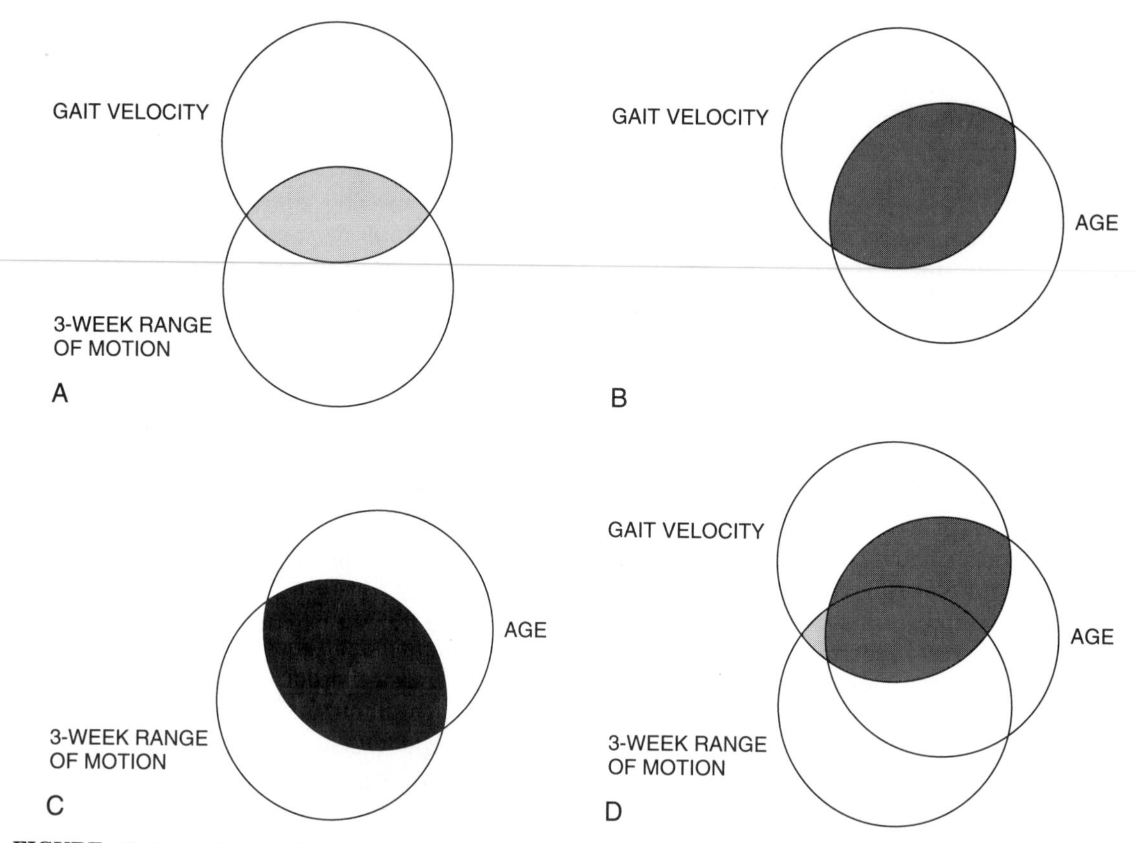

FIGURE 15–8. A. Relationship between gait velocity and 3-week range of motion. **B.** Relationship between gait velocity and age. **C.** Relationship between 3-week range of motion and age. **D.** Relationship of both age and 3-week range of motion to gait velocity. Most of the variability in gait velocity accounted for by 3-week range of motion is also accounted for by age.

with one variable accounting for approximately 53% ($r_{\text{age, 3-week ROM}} = -.7253$) of the variability in the other, as shown in Figure 15–8C. When all three are examined together, almost all of the variability in velocity that is accounted for by three-week ROM is also accounted for by the relationship between age and velocity. Thus, in the regression of gait velocity on both age and three-week ROM, the latter assumes much less importance than when it is the sole variable used to predict gait velocity. The results of this multiple regression analysis might be written up in a journal article as follows:

DATA ANALYSIS

Simple linear regression of gait velocity on three-week range of motion (ROM) was used initially to test whether early ROM status could be used to predict eventual function as measured by gait velocity. Multiple regression was used to add the variable of age to the prediction equation when three-week ROM proved to be an inadequate independent predictor. The significance of each variable was determined with a t test, the significance of R^2 was determined with an F test, and alpha was set at .05. In addition, confidence intervals around the predicted Y value were generated.

RESULTS

For the simple regression of gait velocity on three-week ROM, the r was only .5545. Although significantly different from zero (p = .0015), this means that only 30.75% of the variance in gait velocity was accounted for by three-week ROM. The 95% confidence interval around the predicted gait velocity score for a given individual would require that 48.09 cm/s be added to and subtracted from the predicted score.

To enhance predictability, a multiple regression equation was developed to predict gait velocity from both three-week ROM and age. The equation developed from the two predictor variables was Velocity = .04 (three-week ROM) − 1.41 (age) + 227.04. The R^2 for this equation was .5547 and was significant at p = .0000. The contribution of age was .5378 and significant at p = .0006; the contribution of three-week ROM was only .0169 and was not significant at p = .8711. For this equation, the 95% confidence interval around the predicted gait velocity score for a given individual would require that 39.27 cm/s be added to and subtracted from the predicted score.

DISCUSSION

The simple regression of gait velocity on three-week ROM did not confirm the clinical observation that early ROM status is a good predictor of eventual gait outcome. When age was added to the equation, prediction of gait velocity improved. However, the very strong relationship between age and gait velocity meant that the contribution of three-week ROM to prediction of gait velocity became insignificant. Thus, for this group of patients, eventual gait velocity can be predicted almost as well by age alone as by the combination of age and three-week ROM.

Literature Example

Gross and associates used stepwise multiple regression to develop prediction equations for normal knee torque production.[10] They believed that using sound limb torque to generate a torque goal for an injured leg would be inaccurate because the sound limb torque may be reduced as a result of reduced activity following the injury. As a part of their study, therefore, they tried to predict knee torque on the basis of variables that would not likely be affected by disuse: age, height, weight, and sex. Their criterion for retention of a variable within the equation was that it be significant at the .15 level. They found that they could predict between 61% and 76% of the variability in knee torque on the basis of these variables.

RELIABILITY ANALYSES

A specialized type of relationship analysis is used to assess the reliability of a measure.

As discussed in Chapter 10, there are two major classes of reliability measures: those that document relative reliability and those that document absolute reliability. It is the measures of relative reliability that depend on correlational techniques. In some instances, the correlational technique does not provide all of the desired reliability information, and regression or difference analysis techniques are used to supplement the correlational technique. Three techniques used for reliability analysis are presented here: the Pearson product moment correlation with regression and difference analysis extensions, the intraclass correlation coefficients, and the kappa correlations.

Pearson Product Moment Correlation with Extensions

The Pearson product moment correlation is a measure of relative reliability: A high, positive Pearson value indicates that high scores on one measure are associated with high scores on another measure and that low scores on one measure are associated with low scores on another measure. When we compare two different variables, such as three-week ROM and gait velocity, the strength of the relationship is the only information we desire, so the Pearson correlation is ideal.

When we are comparing paired measurements for the purpose of determining their reliability, however, we are concerned with both the relationship between the two measures and the magnitude of the differences between the two measures. These two forms of reliability are called *relative reliability* and *absolute reliability* (also *association* and *concordance*), respectively. Alone, the Pearson product moment correlation is not a complete tool for documenting reliability because it assesses association and not concordance.

There are three strategies used by physical therapy researchers to supplement the information gained from the Pearson correlation coefficient: paired-*t* test, slope and intercept documentation, and determination of the standard error of measurement. They are all demonstrated in this section using a data sample representing repeated measures of three-week ROM made by Therapists A and B at Clinic 3, as shown in Table 15–4. Therapist B consistently rates subjects higher than Therapist A—in fact, an average of 10.8° higher. The subject who scores highest for Therapist A also scores highest for Therapist B, even though the actual ROM scores differ

TABLE 15–4. Reliability Data for Three-Week Range of Motion Measurements by Therapists A and B

Subject	Therapist A	Therapist B	Difference (B − A)
01	32	38	6
02	50	64	14
03	60	73	13
04	84	90	6
05	81	87	6
06	81	93	12
07	84	94	10
08	81	98	17
09	82	98	16
10	91	99	8
Σ	726.0	834.0	108.0
$\bar{X}$	72.6	83.4	10.8

on the basis of which therapist took the measure. Thus, the relative reliability is high, with a Pearson r of .977. However, to assume that the scores are interchangeable would clearly be incorrect given the 10.8° difference between therapist measures.

The first way to extend the reliability analysis beyond the Pearson measure of relative reliability is to conduct a paired-t test on the data. For our data, t is 8.11, with an associated probability of .000. This means that there is a very small chance that the difference between therapists scores occurred by chance, so we conclude that there is a significant difference between the scores of Therapist A and Therapist B. The scores from the two therapists are highly associated but lack concordance.

The second way to extend the reliability analysis beyond the Pearson measure is to generate a regression equation for the data and document the slope and intercept. If a measure is absolutely reliable, the slope will be close to 1.0 and the intercept will be close to 0.0.[11] In Figure 15–9, the dotted line represents perfect concordance between the two repeated measures, with a slope of 1.0 and an intercept of zero. The solid line represents a proportionate bias on the part of Rater 2. The intercept is still zero, but the slope exceeds 1.0. In Figure 15–10, the dotted line again represents perfect concordance between the two repeated measures, with a slope of 1.0 and an intercept of zero. The solid line represents an additive bias on the part of Rater 2, with scores consistently 5 points higher than Rater 1. The slope of this regression line is still 1.0, but the intercept is now 5.0.

For the Therapist A and B data, the slope is 1.0156 and the intercept is 9.666, as shown in Figure 15–11. This indicates the presence of a largely additive bias on the part of one of the therapists.

The third way to add to the usefulness of the Pearson product moment correlation for documenting reliability is to also report the

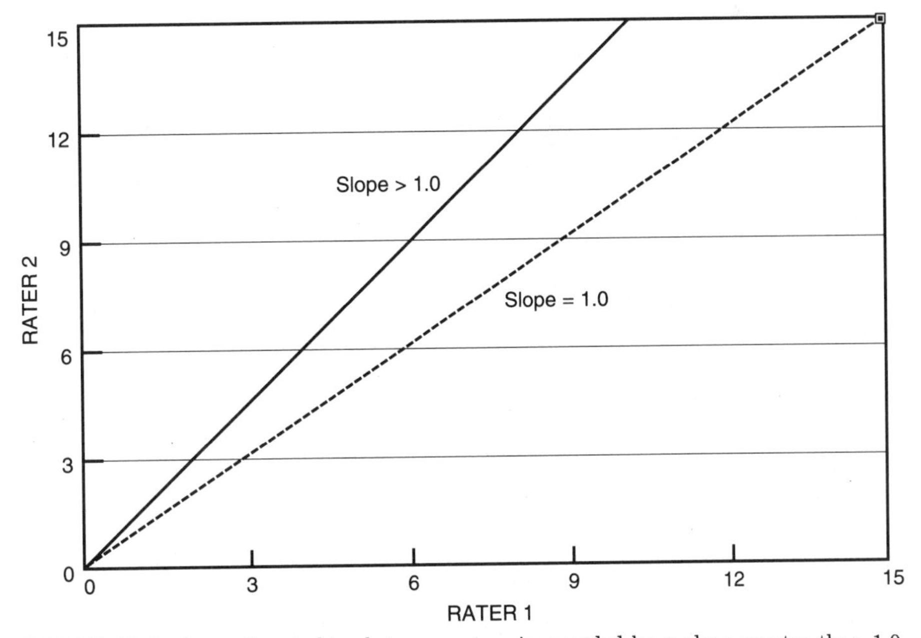

FIGURE 15–9. Proportionate bias between raters is revealed by a slope greater than 1.0. Dotted line represents perfect agreement with a slope of 1.0 and an intercept of 0.0.

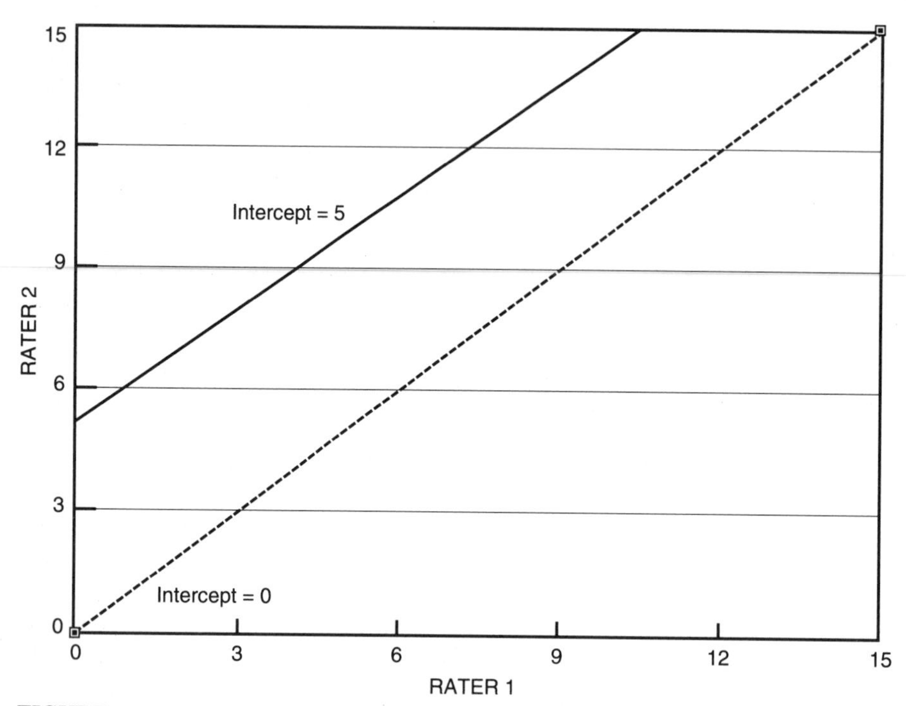

FIGURE 15–10. Additive bias between raters is revealed by an intercept equal to 5.0. Dotted line represents perfect agreement with a slope of 1.0 and an intercept of 0.0.

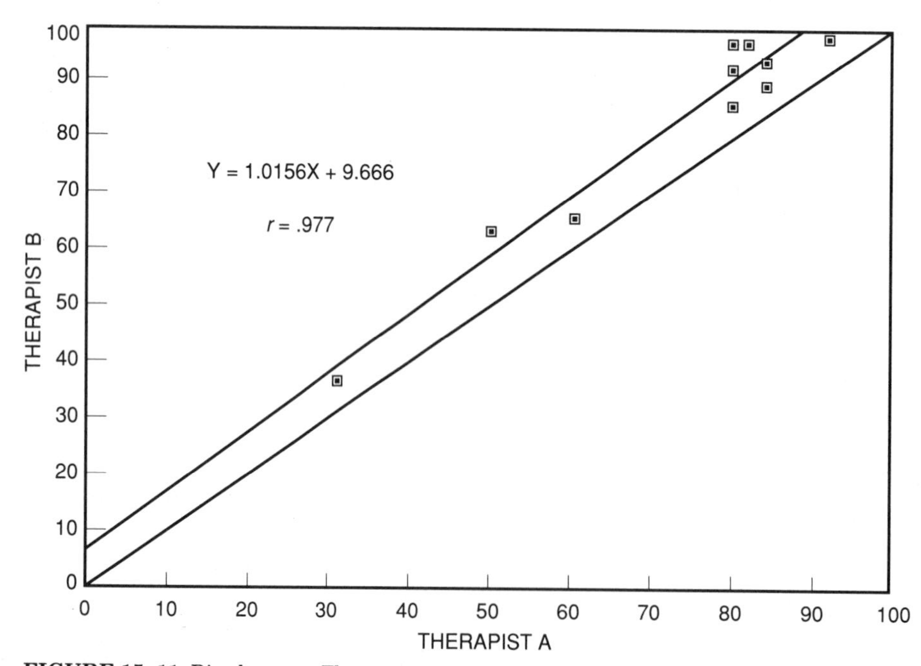

FIGURE 15–11. Bias between Therapist A and Therapist B. There is almost no proportionate bias (slope = 1.0156), but there is a large additive bias (intercept = 9.666°).

standard error of measurement for the paired data. Using the formula presented in Chapter 10, we find that the standard error of measurement for this data is 2.96, meaning that a 95% confidence interval would be ±5.8° (2.96 × 1.96), permitting us to be 95% confident that repeated measures would fall within 11.6° of one another.

The results of an extended Pearson reliability analysis might be written up as follows. However, readers should recognize that researchers would probably not use all three extensions in a single study. Any one of these extensions in this case would be sufficient to cast doubt on the absolute reliability of the measures.

DATA ANALYSIS

To assess the association between the two therapists' scores, the Pearson product moment correlation was calculated. The concordance of the scores was assessed by calculation of the slope and intercept of the regression equation of one therapist's scores on the other, determination of the standard error of measurement (SEM), and calculation of a paired-*t* test.

RESULTS

The Pearson *r* was found to be .977, indicating a high degree of association between the scores of the two therapists. However, the slope was 1.02 and the intercept was 9.67. The SEM was ±5.8°. The paired-*t* test revealed that the 10.8° mean difference between therapist scores was statistically significant at the .000 level.

DISCUSSION

Despite the high degree of association between the measures taken by Therapist A and Therapist B, the absolute difference between scores means that the interrater reliability is too low to permit viewing the measures by the two therapists as interchangeable.

Intraclass Correlation Coefficients

The ICCs are a family of coefficients that allow comparison of two or more repeated measures. The technique depends on repeated measures analysis of variance (ANOVA). There are at least six different ICC formulas, and much discussion has transpired in the physical therapy literature about which one to use when.[12, 13] Table 15–5 provides two of the formulas and indications for their use, based on the work of Shrout and Fleiss.[14] In addition to being able to handle more than two repeated measures, the ICC is said by some to be a better measure than the Pearson *r* because it accounts for absolute as well as relative reliability. Delitto and Strube believe that the ICCs take into account "level" differences, but are not true measures of concordance.[11] Thus, researchers who report reliability on the basis of an ICC should still report the results of an absolute reliability indicator such as the SEM or the repeated measures ANOVA.

For our example of the interrater reliability between Therapists A and B at Clinic 3, the ICC (2,1) may be most appropriate because the two therapists in question were selected from a larger group of therapists at the clinic, both measured each patient, and the results are to be generalized to other randomly selected judges rather than just applied to the two therapists in question.

TABLE 15–5. Calculations of Intraclass Correlation Coefficients (ICCs)

Source of Variation	Degrees of Freedom	Mean Square (MS)
Between subjects	N* − 1	Between subjects (BMS)
Within subject	N (K† − 1)	Within subject (WMS)
Between judges	K − 1	Between judges (JMS)
Error	(N − 1)(K − 1)	Error (EMS)

Formula	Appropriate Use
$\text{ICC (1,1)} = \dfrac{\text{BMS} - \text{WMS}}{\text{BMS} + (\text{K} - 1)\text{WMS}}$.	Each subject is rated by different randomly selected judges.
$\text{ICC (2,1)} = \dfrac{\text{BMS} - \text{EMS}}{\text{BMS} + (\text{K} - 1)\text{EMS} + \dfrac{\text{K(JMS} - \text{EMS)}}{\text{N}}}$.	Each subject is rated by the same randomly selected judges.

*Subjects.
†Judges.

Table 15–6 shows the ICC (2,1) calculation to be .854. This is less than the .977 that was calculated with the Pearson product moment correlation, but it still would generally be interpreted to be a fairly high level of correlation. Thus, it is useful to examine the results of a repeated measure ANOVA, which shows that there is a significant difference between the measures of the two therapists, $F_{1,9} = 65.7$, $p = .000$. Using the repeated measures ANOVA results with an ICC is analogous to using a paired-*t* test to extend the results of a Pearson product moment correlation reliability analysis.

Although this example of an ICC used only two raters to compare the results with those found with the Pearson product moment correlation analysis in the previous section, the ICC, like the ANOVA it is based on, extends easily to accommodate more than two raters.

TABLE 15–6. ICC (2,1) Calculation for Three-Week Range of Motion for Therapists A and B

Source of Variation	Degrees of Freedom	Mean Square (MS)	*F*	*p*
Between subjects	9	734.78 (BMS)		
Within subjects	10	66.30 (WMS)		
Between judges	1	583.20 (JMS)	65.7	.000
Error	9	8.87 (EMS)		

$$\text{ICC (2,1)} = \frac{\text{BMS} - \text{EMS}}{\text{BMS} + (\text{K} - 1)\text{EMS} + \dfrac{\text{K}^{\dagger}(\text{JMS} - \text{EMS})}{\text{N}^{*}}}.$$

$$\text{ICC (2,1)} = \frac{734.78 - 8.87}{734.78 + (2 - 1)8.87 + \dfrac{(2)(583.20 - 8.87)}{10}} = .854.$$

*Subjects.
†Judges.

When only two raters are present, the researcher has a choice between the Pearson and an ICC; when three or more raters measure each subject, an ICC must be used.

Watkins and associates studied intertester reliability of measurements of knee ROM.[2] Fourteen different raters were involved in the study, with each subject being measured by a randomly selected pair of raters. The ICC (1,1) they used for analysis seems appropriate for their design, in which raters for each subject were selected randomly.

Diamond and associates studied intertester reliability of diabetic foot evaluation.[15] In this study, only two raters were involved; each measured every subject. Thus, the ICC (2,1) they used seems appropriate because their design meets the criterion that each subject be assessed by the same raters.

Kappa

Kappa is a reliability coefficient designed for use with nominal data. Suppose that we wanted to determine whether Therapists A and B at Clinic 3 agreed with each other on the stair-climbing ability of their patients. Table 15–7 shows the cross-tabulation of the data of Therapists A and B. For 6 of the 10 patients, the therapists gave identical scores. For 4 of the 10 patients, the therapists differed by one category. The simplest way to express the degree of concordance between the therapists' observations is to calculate the percentage of patients on whose ability the two therapists agreed completely. For this example, the percent agreement is 60. However, because there are only a few nominal categories, there is a high probability that some of the agreements occurred by chance. The kappa correlation coefficient adjusts the percent agreement figure to account for chance agreements, as shown in the formula at the bottom of Table 15–7.[16] The kappa for this example is .3939.

Kappa can also be weighted to account for the seriousness of the discrepancy.[17] Consider one disagreement in which one rater scores the patient as a 5 in stair climbing (recipro-

TABLE 15–7. Kappa Correlation Calculation

	Therapist A				
Therapist B	***5***	***4***	***3***	***2***	***Total***
5	2 (.20) [.12]	1			3 (.30)
4	2	3 (.30) [.20]			5 (.50)
3			1 (.10) [.02]		1 (.10)
2			1		1 (.10)
Total	4 (.40)	4 (.40)	2 (.20)		10 (1.0)

$$\kappa = \frac{p_o - p_c}{1 - p_c} = \frac{.60 - .34}{1 - .34} = .3939.$$

p_0 = sum of the observed probabilities in perfect agreement = .60
p_c = sum of the chance probabilities for perfect agreement = .34

Note: Numbers are the number of observations in the cell. Numbers in parentheses are the proportion of observations in the cell. Numbers in brackets are the proportion of observations expected by chance in the cell. The proportion expected by chance is calculated by multiplying the marginal proportion (total row or column) for the corresponding row and column.

cal, no railing) and the other scores the patient as a 4 (reciprocal, with rail). Contrast this with a disagreement between a 4 and a 3 (one at a time, with or without rail). Some therapists might believe that disagreement on the use of a rail is a less serious reliability problem than disagreement about whether the patient can maneuver the stairs reciprocally. A weighted kappa allows the researcher to establish different weights for different disagreements, as described by Cohen.[18] In addition to occurring in weighted and nonweighted forms, kappa can be extended to more than two raters.[18]

Aweida and Kelsey studied the reliability of physical therapists in auscultating tape-recorded lung sounds.[19] Because of the nominal nature of lung sound classification, they used kappa to determine reliability. The percent correct was 47. Once chance agreements were accounted for, a kappa of .22 was found. Landis and Koch described this level of reliability, as determined by kappa, to be fair.[20] Aweida and Kelsey's study is an example of an investigation in which weighted kappa might have been used instead of or in addition to kappa. For example, a disagreement between a high-pitched wheeze and a low-pitched wheeze seems less serious than a disagreement between a pleural rub and a vesicular breath sound.

FACTOR ANALYSIS

Factor analysis is a tool whereby correlational techniques are used to discover which of many variables cluster together as a related unit, separate from other, unrelated clusters. It is a data reduction technique in which many variables are grouped into a smaller number of related groups.

Factor analysis is generally done for one of three reasons: test development, theory development, or theory testing. In test development, factor analysis is often used to help reduce a great number of items into a smaller number. Factor analysis groups items that are related to one another, and the test developer can then select certain questions from each factor for inclusion in the final version of the test. In theory development, factor analysis is used to examine the underlying structure of a set of variables about which the researcher has not developed a conceptual framework. The factors that emerge are then examined and named by the researcher, who then develops hypotheses about interrelationships among the factors. In theory testing, items thought to be representative of certain constructs are factor analyzed to determine whether the items load as hypothesized.

In our sample data set, 12 different pieces of data are recorded for each patient at six months postoperatively:

- one ROM measure
- two muscle strength measures
- four deformity measures
- four activities of daily living (ADL) measures
- one gait velocity measure.

A theoretical grouping of these variables might be according to impairment and disability, as defined by the World Health Organization.[21] The impairment variables relate to abnormal structures and would include the ROM measure, the strength measures, and the deformity measures. The disability variables relate to abnormal performance of activities and in this example would include the ADL measures and gait velocity. Researchers might hypothesize that if impairment and disability are truly different constructs, then a factor analysis of the 12 variables would yield one factor that consists of the impairment variables and one factor that consists of the disability variables.

The result of a factor analysis of these 12 variables is presented here. The mathematical basis of factor analysis has been presented well by others and is therefore omitted so that emphasis may be placed on interpretation rather than calculation.[22] In brief, the steps in a factor analysis are as follows:

1. A group of variables is analyzed for interrelationships.
2. The number of important underlying factors is determined by reviewing eigenvalues associated with each factor.
3. Factors are extracted.
4. The factor solution is rotated to maximize differences between the factors.
5. Rotated factor loadings are examined to determine a simple structure.
6. The resulting factors are interpreted.

Let's examine these steps in sequence for the 12 six-month variables. First, a correlation matrix is developed, as shown in Table 15–8. In this example, the matrix has been set up so that the theorized impairment and disability variables are close to one another. If we examine the last five columns of the matrix, which consists of the theorized impairment variables, we find that they are all fairly highly correlated with the ROM and strength variables (Rows 1 through 3) and with the other impairment variables (Rows 8 through 11). They are minimally correlated with the deformity variables (Rows 4 through 7). Although we can visually detect some patterns within the relationships among variables, the matrix is far too complex for simple visual analysis; hence the need for a mathematical tool like factor analysis.

The second step of a factor analysis is to determine the number of factors in the solution. Initially, the variables in the factor analysis problem are used to create the same number of factors. Each factor has an associated eigenvalue, which is related to the percentage of variability within the data set that can be accounted for by the factor. Some factors will account for very little variance and are therefore eliminated from the analysis. One convention for determining the number of factors in the solution is that only factors with eigenvalues of greater than 1.0 are retained. Another method is the scree method, which examines the pattern of eigenvalues graphically.[22(p635)] When a researcher is testing a theory, the number of factors he or she retains may simply be the number of theorized factors.

The factor analysis of our 12 variables shows that three factors had eigenvalues

TABLE 15–8. Correlation Matrix for 12-Variable Factor Analysis

	F	E	DFC	DVV	DML	DAP	V	ADW	AAD	ASC	ARC
M6R	.56	.59	−.17	−.23	.11	−.15	.63	.68	.70	.71	.65
F		.95	−.19	.19	.04	−.05	.89	.72	.69	.75	.81
E			−.13	.24	.03	−.09	.90	.70	.65	.75	.79
DFC				.46	.45	.14	−.22	−.34	−.26	−.21	−.24
DVV					.27	−.01	.17	−.10	−.19	−.01	.02
DML						.45	−.07	−.16	−.10	−.12	.02
DAP							−.17	−.06	.02	−.17	.12
V								.80	.75	.82	.85
ADW									.83	.78	.81
AAD										.83	.81
ASC											.82

Note: M6R = six-month range of motion, F = flexion torque, E = extension torque, DFC = deformity—flexion contracture, DVV = deformity—varus/valgus angulation, DML = deformity—mediolateral instability, DAP = deformity—anteroposterior instability, V = gait velocity, ADW = activities of daily living (ADL)—distance walked, AAD = ADL—assistive device, ASC = ADL—stair climbing, and ARC = ADL—rising from chair.

greater than 1.0; the scree method would retain either two or three factors, and our theoretical model predicted two factors. For the purpose of this example, then, two factors are selected for extraction, the third step in factor analysis. Terms that describe different extraction techniques are *principal components extraction, image factoring,* and *alpha factoring,* among others.

The fourth step in factor analysis is to rotate the factors. In essence, rotation can be thought of as resetting the zero point within the factor analysis. Doing so maximizes the appearance of differences between factors. Terms that describe different types of rotation techniques are *orthogonal, oblique, varimax,* and *quartimax,* among others. Once rotation has occurred, one speaks in terms of "factor loadings" rather than "correlation." A factor loading is essentially the correlation between each variable within a factor and the entire factor. Table 15–9 shows the rotated factor loadings determined by the factor analysis.

The fifth step in factor analysis is to determine, if possible, a simple structure for the factors. A simple structure is developed when each variable is associated with only one factor. To determine a simple structure, the researcher decides to retain in each factor only those variables that loaded above some arbitrary point, often .30. In our example, if factor loadings above .30 are retained, the flexion contracture variable remains in both factors because its loading on Factor I is −.305 and its loading on Factor II is .71. Thus, to obtain a simple structure for this analysis, we need to adopt a more restrictive criterion for variable retention. If we adopt a criterion of .35, then a simple structure is created.

TABLE 15–9. Rotated Factor Loadings

Variable	Factor I	Factor II
V	.94	.10
ARC	.92	.12
ASC	.91	−.03
ADW	.89	−.12
F	.89	.20
E	.88	.24
AAD	.88	−.09
M6R	.76	−.05
DML	−.07	.77
DFC	−.30	.71
DVV	−.00	.71
DAP	−.10	.44
% of variance accounted for	53.7	16.6

Note: V = gait velocity, ARC = activities of daily living (ADL)—rising from chair, ASC = ADL—stair climbing, ADW = ADL—distance walked, F = flexion torque, E = extensor torque, AAD = ADL—assistive device, M6R = six-month range of motion, DML = deformity—mediolateral instability, DFC = deformity—flexion contracture, DVV = deformity—varus/valgus angulation, and DAP = deformity—anteroposterior instability.

The final step in factor analysis is to name and interpret the factors. This is done according to the variables that were retained in each factor and is highly subjective. Researchers often name the factors in a manner consistent with the theoretical underpinnings of the study. Factor II in our solution consists of the four deformity variables and could be named "Anatomic Impairment." This name lets the reader know that Factor I consists of a subgroup of the hypothesized construct of impairment. Factor I is more difficult to name, because it consists of a combination of functional, strength, and ROM variables. A name consistent with the theoretical underpinnings would be "Physiological Impairment and Disability." Once the factors are named, the implications of the factors are discussed by the researcher. The following is the interpretation of this factor analysis as it might be written in a journal article:

DATA ANALYSIS

Factor analysis with principal components extraction and orthogonal varimax rotation was used to test whether variables loaded as predicted on two theorized factors. A simple structure was developed by including in each factor only those variables with rotated factor loadings higher than .35.

RESULTS

Table 1 shows the rotated factor loadings for the two-factor solution. The first factor included all the activities of daily living (ADL) variables, as well as the gait velocity, range of motion (ROM), and torque variables. The second factor included all the deformity variables. Factor I was labeled Physiological Impairment and Disability and accounted for 53.7% of the variance; Factor II was labeled Anatomic Impairment and accounted for 16.6% of the variance.

DISCUSSION

Our results do not fully support the hypothesized distinction between impairment and disability because some of the impairment variables loaded with the disability variables. However, the impairment variables did split among the two factors according to a physiological/anatomic distinction. The solely anatomic impairment variables (the four measures of deformity) all loaded together and were separate from the other eight variables. This indicates that the actual anatomic alignment of the knees was not related to eventual functional recovery. The variables that are more representative of physiological function than anatomic structure (flexion and extension torque and flexion ROM) loaded with the disability variables of ADL status and gait velocity. These results suggest that the constructs of impairment and disability, as defined by the World Health Organization, are not completely valid for patients who have had total knee arthroplasty.

Table 1. Rotated Factor Loadings.

	Factor	
Variable	*I Physiological Impairment and Disability*	*II Anatomic Impairment*
Gait velocity	.94	
ADL[a]—rising from chair	.92	
ADL—stair climbing	.91	
ADL—distance walked	.89	
Flexion torque	.89	
Extension torque	.88	
ADL—assistive device	.88	
Six-month range of motion	.76	
Deformity—mediolateral instability		.77
Deformity—flexion contracture		.71
Deformity—varus/valgus angulation		.71
Deformity—anteroposterior instability		.44

[a]Activities of daily living.

Geden and Taylor used factor analysis to examine the underlying constructs of the Self-as-Carer Inventory.[23] The self-as-carer construct has been hypothesized to consist of an intellectual component related to making judgments about self-care activities and an action component related to actually being able to perform self-care activities. The purpose of Geden and Taylor's study was to determine whether underlying factors associated with the inventory were consistent with the components of the construct of self-care. Thus the study served to (a) validate whether the instrument was consistent with the theory and (b) show whether the components of the theory itself could be supported by responses on the instrument. The analysis identified four factors, which Geden and Taylor named Knowledge of Self, Judgment and Decisions, Self-Monitoring, and Physical Skills. The authors believed that the first two factors fit well with the hypothesized intellectual component of self-care and the last two fit well with the action component.

SUMMARY

Relationship analysis is useful for description, prediction, reliability assessment, and theory development and testing. Correlational techniques describe relationships but cannot be used to draw causal conclusions about the variables. The meaningfulness of correlation coefficients can be determined with absolute descriptors, the coefficient of determination, significance testing, or calculation of confidence intervals. Simple and multiple linear regressions use correlational techniques to make predictions about scores on one variable based on scores on one or more other variables. Relationship analysis performed to document reliability demands that correlational techniques account for both association and concordance between repeated measures. Factor analysis is a correlational technique that is used to determine which of many variables cluster together as a related unit separate from other, unrelated clusters.

References

1. Sinaki M, Offord KP. Physical activity in postmenopausal women: effect on back muscle strength and bone mineral density of the spine. *Arch Phys Med Rehabil.* 1988;69:277–280.
2. Watkins MA, Riddle DL, Lamb RL, Personius WJ. Reliability of goniometric measurements and visual estimates of knee range of motion obtained in a clinical setting. *Phys Ther.* 1991;71:90–96.
3. Mayerson NH, Milano RA. Goniometric reliability in physical medicine. *Arch Phys Med Rehabil.* 1984;65:92–94.
4. Swartz HM, Flood AB. The corntinental theory of flat and depressed areas: on the relationship between corn and topography. *Journal of Irreproducible Results.* 1990;35(5):16–17, 19.
5. Munro BH, Visintainer MA, Page EB. *Statistical Methods for Health Care Research.* Philadelphia, Pa: J.B. Lippincott Co; 1986.
6. Sellers JS. Relationship between antigravity control and postural control in young children. *Phys Ther.* 1988;68:486–490.
7. Bohannon RW. Strength of lower limb related to gait velocity and cadence in stroke patients. *Physiotherapy Canada.* 1986;38:204–206.
8. DiFabio RP, Badke MB. Relationship of sensory organization to balance function in patients with hemiplegia. *Phys Ther.* 1990;70:542–548.
9. Lerner-Frankiel MB, Vargas S, Brown M, Krusell L, Schoneberger W. Functional community ambulation: what are your criteria? *Clinical Management.* 1986;6(2):12–15.
10. Gross MT, McGrain P, Demillo N, Plyer L. Relationship between multiple predictor variables and normal knee torque production. *Phys Ther.* 1989;69:54–62.
11. Delitto A, Strube MJ. Reliability in the clinical setting. *Research Section Newsletter.* 1991;24(1):2–8.
12. Riddle DL, Finucane SD, Rothstein JM, Walker ML. Authors' response. *Phys Ther.* 1989;69:192–194.
13. Krebs DE. Intraclass correlation coefficients: use and calculation. *Phys Ther.* 1984;64:1581–1589.
14. Shrout PE, Fleiss JL. Intraclass correlations: uses in assessing rater reliability. *Psychol Bull.* 1979;86:420–428.
15. Diamond JE, Mueller MJ, Delitto A, Sinacore DR. Reliability of a diabetic foot evaluation. *Phys Ther.* 1989;69:797–802.
16. Cohen J. A coefficient of agreement for nominal scales. *Educational and Psychological Measurement.* 1960;20:37–46.

17. Cohen J. Weighted kappa: nominal scale agreement with provision for scaled disagreement or partial credit. *Psychol Bull.* 1968;70:213–220.
18. Fleiss JL. Measuring nominal scale agreement among many raters. *Psychol Bull.* 1971;76:378–382.
19. Aweida D, Kelsey CJ. Accuracy and reliability of physical therapists in auscultating tape recorded lung sounds. *Physiotherapy Canada.* 1991;42:279–282.
20. Landis JR, Koch GG. The measurement of observer agreement for categorical data. *Biometrics.* 1977; 33:159–174.
21. Jette AM. Diagnosis and classification by physical therapists: a special communication. *Phys Ther.* 1989;69:967–969.
22. Tabachnick BG, Fidell LS. *Using Multivariate Statistics.* 2nd ed. New York, NY: Harper & Row; 1989.
23. Geden E, Taylor S. Construct and empirical validity of the self-as-carer inventory. *Nurs Res.* 1991;40:47–50.

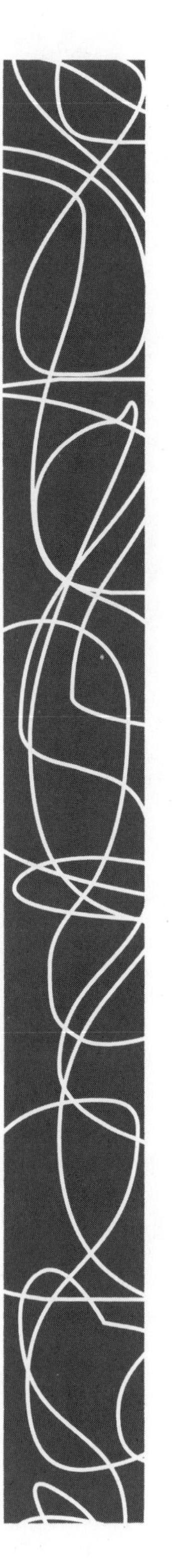

SECTION FIVE

BEING A RESEARCH CONSUMER

CHAPTER 16

Locating the Literature

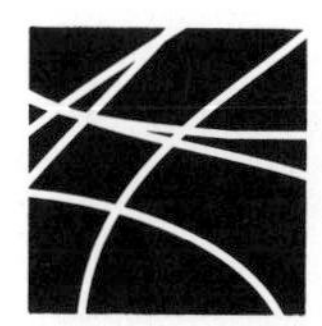

Becoming an educated consumer of research literature is a goal for many students and professionals. The first 15 chapters presented the principles needed to become educated about performing research. This chapter and the next are devoted to guidelines for becoming a consumer of research. Strategies for locating the literature are presented in this chapter, and strategies for reviewing and critiquing that literature are offered in Chapter 17.

To make advantageous use of research, one needs to know the different types of information that are available to physical therapy clinicians and researchers and in which of two broad categories of literature that information can be found. After a brief discussion of these preliminaries, this chapter details strategies for performing a focused, short-term literature search and for maintaining an ongoing search of the literature for material related to a topic of interest. Finally, suggestions are given for obtaining copies of literature items that are not in one's local library. Throughout the chapter, different search strategies are illustrated with a sample search of the literature on the use of continuous passive motion (CPM) in patients who have undergone total knee arthroplasty.

TYPES OF INFORMATION

The basic goal of any literature review is to discover what is known about a certain topic. Accomplishing this goal depends on at least four types of information about the topic: theory, facts, opinions, and methods. Some references provide primarily one type of information; others contain many different types of information. The physical therapy clinician who is interested in treating patients with CPM will likely want to know theories about how CPM works, factual information about protocols and results from other clinics, the opinions of therapists and surgeons about future directions for the clinical use of CPM, and the methods that others have used to measure the results of CPM use. The physical therapist who is planning to conduct research in the area of CPM use after total knee arthroplasty needs to place the topic of CPM into a conceptual context and to know the facts of previous investigations of CPM, the opinions of other researchers about important areas still in need of study, and the methods others have used to measure and analyze data in previous studies.

TYPES OF PROFESSIONAL LITERATURE

The literature is divided broadly into primary and secondary sources. Primary sources are those in which the authors are providing the original report of research they have conducted. Commonly encountered primary sources include journal articles describing original research, theses and dissertations, and conference abstracts and proceedings. Secondary sources of information are those in which the authors summarize their own work or the work of others. Book chapters and journal articles that review the literature are considered secondary sources. Secondary sources are useful because they organize the literature for the reader and provide a ready list of primary sources on the topic of interest. However, practitioners who wish to make their own judgments about the credibility of the research must read the primary literature.

FOCUSED LITERATURE SEARCH

Physical therapy practitioners may wish to conduct a focused literature search to help them plan new programs, evaluate existing programs, or develop research protocols. The focused search is conducted over a short period of time to meet a specific information need. In addition to their own books and journals collected over the years, practitioners initiating such a literature search have an array of tools and strategies at their disposal. Five different categories of search tools are described in this section: the catalog of library holdings, single-journal indexes, multiple-journal indexes, dissertation and thesis indexes, and conference proceedings indexes. In addition, how to use an identified article to find other citations is explained.

Practitioners who use the library should also make use of a human resource: their librarian. Librarians are educated in the art and science of retrieving information, and practitioners should not hesitate to ask for their assistance as they plan their literature searches.

Catalog of Library Holdings

The catalog of library holdings indexes books, conference proceedings published as books, and dissertations and theses that are held by the library. Today, the catalog of holdings is as likely to be an on-line computerized catalog as it is a card catalog. Libraries with either type of catalog use subject headings provided by the Library of Congress (Library of Congress Subject Headings) or the National Library of Medicine (Medical Subject Headings, or MeSH). A thesaurus of these subject headings should be available in the library to help the practitioner determine the terms under which the desired information is likely to be found.

A limitation of the catalog of holdings is that the sources it reveals are only as good as the collection of the particular library. However, even identification of a few key resources may lead to many others by examination of the references contained in each source. Table 16–1 shows how the identification of two references, a book and a collection of conference proceedings, from library holdings at the University of Indianapolis led to two relevant chapters containing more than 40 unique citations and three important references cited in both chapters.

TABLE 16–1. Use of Catalog of Library Holdings to Identify Literature Related to Continuous Passive Motion in Patients After Total Knee Arthroplasty

- Library of Congress subject headings
  - Knee—surgery
  - Artificial knee
  - Arthroplasty
- Medical subject headings
  - Knee prosthesis
  - Arthroplasty
- Resources identified under these headings
  - Hungerford DS, Krackow KA, Kenna RV, eds. *Total Knee Arthroplasty: A Comprehensive Approach.* Baltimore, Md: Williams & Wilkins; 1983.
  - Rand JA, Dorr LD, eds. *Total Arthroplasty of the Knee: Proceedings of the Knee Society, 1985–86.* Rockville, Md: Aspen Publishers Inc; 1987.
- Relevant chapters in the resources
  - Coutts RD, Toth C, Kaita JH. The role of continuous passive motion in the rehabilitation of the total knee patient. In Hungerford DS, Krackow KA, Kenna RV, eds. *Total Knee Arthroplasty: A Comprehensive Approach.* Baltimore, Md: Williams & Wilkins; 1983. (Chapter contains 33 references.)
  - Goll SR, Lotke PA, Ecker ML. Failure of continuous passive motion as prophylaxis against deep venous thrombosis after total knee arthroplasty. In Rand JA, Dorr LD, eds. *Total Arthroplasty of the Knee: Proceedings of the Knee Society, 1985–86.* Rockville, Md: Aspen Publishers Inc; 1987. (Chapter contains 12 references.)
- References common to both chapters
  - Salter RB, Simmonds DF, Malcolm BW, et al. The effects of continuous passive motion on the healing of articular cartilage defects—an experimental investigation in rabbits. *J Bone Joint Surg.* 1975;57A:570–571.
  - Salter RB, Simmonds DF, Malcolm BW, et al. The biological effect of continuous passive motion on the healing of full-thickness defects in articular cartilage: an experimental investigation in the rabbit. *J Bone Joint Surg.* 1980;62A:1232–1251.
  - Salter RB, Bell RS, Keeley FW. The protective effect of continuous passive motion on living articular cartilage in acute septic arthritis: an experimental investigation in the rabbit. *Clin Orthop.* 1981;159:223–247.

Single-Journal Indexes

Many professionals receive one or more journals regularly either as a benefit of belonging to a professional association or by subscribing to a journal of particular interest. One's own journals are a convenient starting point for a literature search. Most journals publish an annual subject and author index in the last issue of each volume. *Physical Therapy*, for example, publishes its annual index in the back of each December issue. Thus, readers with an interest in a particular topic can easily identify any pertinent citations from the journals in their own collection. Even if a professional decides not to retain all the journals he or she receives, this ready source of citations can be maintained by keeping at least the annual indexes from each journal. Some journals, including *Physical Therapy*, also publish cumulated indexes over several years.[1] Table 16–2 shows references on CPM that were identified through a review of the annual indexes of *Physical Therapy* for the last five years.

Multiple-Journal Indexes

There are several different indexes to multiple journals within the health sciences. Most of these indexes exist as books and in computerized form on compact discs or on-line systems. Not long ago, most computer searches of the literature were performed by librarians from key words supplied by patrons. Today, many forms of the computerized databases are user-friendly and designed to be used by the patrons themselves. Whether one is conducting the search on a computer or in a hard copy of the index, two basic search steps must be taken.

First, an entry point for the search needs

TABLE 16–2. Search Results from *Physical Therapy* Annual Indexes, 1986–1990

Subject headings
- Knee
- Exercise—range of motion

References identified
- Basso DM, Knapp L. Comparison of two continuous passive motion protocols for patients with total knee implants. *Phys Ther.* 1987;67:360–363. (Contains 25 references.)
- Gose JC. Continuous passive motion in the postoperative treatment of patients with total knee replacement: a retrospective study. *Phys Ther.* 1987;67:39–42. (Contains 9 references.)
- Stap LJ, Woodfin PM. Continuous passive motion in the treatment of knee flexion contractures: a case report. *Phys Ther.* 1986;66:1720–1722. (Contains 12 references.)

to be identified. The user develops a list of relevant terms that define the limits of the search. These user-generated terms are then checked against the thesaurus of terms available for each index. Many computerized systems can determine whether a user-generated term corresponds to a term used to index articles in the database. Using either the computerized thesaurus or the hard-copy list of subject headings, the practitioner can identify narrower terms, broader terms, or subheadings that may refine or expand the scope of the search. This search strategy is known as *controlled-vocabulary searching.*

If a topic is new or very specialized, the terms that best describe the topic may not be used to index articles in the database. For a practitioner using a hard copy of the index, the only alternative is to use a less specific term and accept that many articles listed under that heading will not be relevant to the topic of the search. The practitioner using a computerized system has a much better alternative—searching for the specific term in the article's title or abstract. This search strategy is known as *free-word searching.*

The second step in the index search is to use the identified terms to scan the desired period of time. The extent of the search depends on both its purpose and the number of citations identified. A clinician planning a new program may scan the last 3 years of the index; a researcher who wishes to trace the history of a particular procedure may scan 20 years of an index.

If a hard-copy search is being conducted, the researcher must carefully hand- or photocopy relevant citations from the indexes. If a computer database is being used, the citations and abstracts of articles can be printed out. When a set of citations is identified by key words, there are usually some irrelevant references. With a computer database one can browse through the identified citations and mark for printing out only those of interest.

The major databases of interest to physical therapists are the Index Medicus or its computer cousin Medline, the Cumulative Index of Nursing and Allied Health Literature (CINAHL), and the Physiotherapy Index; each is described below. Table 16–3 lists journals relevant to physical therapy[2, 3] and indicates which are indexed by each of these three databases.

Index Medicus. The Index Medicus is a comprehensive medically oriented index compiled by the National Library of Medicine through its Medical Literature and Retrieval System (MEDLARS). It exists in hard-copy form and as a computer database called Medline. The Medline database, one of several MEDLARS databases, actually includes not only the Index Medicus, but also the Index of Dental Literature, and the International Nursing Index. The entries in the database are indexed according to the MeSH of the National Library of Medicine. Unfortunately, MeSH terms related to physical therapy are not always as specific as might be desired, as shown in Table 16–4.

There are several products related to Index Medicus that make the database affordable to individuals who do not have ready access

TABLE 16–3. Databases That Index Journals of Interest to Physical Therapists

Journal*	Database		
	IM†	*CINAHL*‡	*PI*§
Acta Orthop Scand	x		x
Am J Occup Ther	x	x	x
Am J Phys Med Rehabil	x	x	x
Am J Physiol	x		
Am J Public Health	x	x	
Am J Sports Med	x	x	x
Am Rev Resp Dis	x		x
Arch Phys Med Rehabil	x	x	x
Australian Journal of Physiotherapy			x
Brain Inj	x		
Chest	x	x	x
Clin Orthop	x		x
Clinical Management		x	x
Dev Med Child Neurol	x		x
Electromyogr Clin Neurophysiol	x		
Geriatrics	x	x	x
Gerontologist	x	x	
J Allied Health	x	x	
J Appl Physiol	x		x
J Biomech	x		x
J Bone Joint Surg [Am]	x		x
J Burn Care Rehabil	x	x	x
J Gerontol	x		
J Hand Surgery [Am]	x		
J Neurosurg	x		
J Pediatr Orthop		x	
J Rehabil Res Dev	x		x
J Rheumatol	x		
JAMA	x	x	x
Journal of Head Trauma Rehabilitation		x	x
Journal of Medical Education			
Journal of Orthopaedic and Sports Physical Therapy		x	x
Journal of Physical Therapy Education		x	x
Journal of Rehabilitation		x	x
Med Sci Sport Exerc	x		x
Muscle Nerve	x		x
N Engl J Med	x	x	x
New Zealand Journal of Physiotherapy			x
Occupational Therapy Journal of Research		x	x
Orthop Clin North Am	x		
Orthopedics	x		
Orthotics and Prosthetics			x
Pain	x	x	x
Pediatrics	x		
Percept Mot Skills	x		
Physician and Sportsmedicine		x	x
Phys Ther	x	x	x
Physical and Occupational Therapy in Geriatrics		x	x
Physical and Occupational Therapy in Pediatrics		x	x
Physiotherapy		x	x
Physiotherapy Canada		x	x
Prosthet Orthot Int	x		x
Research Quarterly for Exercise and Sport			x
Scand J Rehabil Med	x		x
Spine	x		x

*To be consistent with the Manual of Style of the American Medical Association, the Index Medicus abbreviation is given for journals indexed in that database; the full name is given for journals that Index Medicus does not include.
†Index Medicus.
‡Cumulative Index of Nursing and Allied Health Literature.
§Physiotherapy Index.

TABLE 16–4. Comparison of MeSH* and CINAHL† Terms Related to Physical Therapy

MeSH	CINAHL
Physical therapy	Physical therapy
Balneology	Baths
Ammotherapy	Drainage, postural
Baths	Electrotherapy
Baths, Finnish	Cardioversion
Mud therapy	Defibrillation
Drainage, postural	Electrical stimulation
Electrical stimulation therapy	Electroconvulsive therapy
Electroacupuncture	Iontophoresis
Transcutaneous electrical nerve stimulation	Functional training
Exercise therapy	Gait training
Breathing exercise	Hydrotherapy
Motion therapy, continuous passive	Hyperthermia, induced
Hydrotherapy	Diathermy
Hyperthermia, induced	Ultrasonic therapy
Diathermy	Infrared therapy
Short-wave therapy	Joint mobilization
Ultrasonic therapy	Massage
Massage	Muscle strengthening
Photochemotherapy	Oral stimulation
Hematoporphyrin photoradiation	Photochemotherapy
PUVA therapy	Phototherapy
Phototherapy	Prosthetic fitting
Heliotherapy	Therapeutic exercise
Ultraviolet therapy	Aerobic exercise
Thalassotherapy	Breathing exercise
	Conditioning, cardiopulmonary
	Isokinetic exercises
	Isometric exercises
	Kegel exercises
	Motion therapy, continuous passive
	Neuromuscular facilitation
	Ultraviolet therapy

*National Library of Medicine Medical Subject Headings.
†Cumulative Index of Nursing and Allied Health Literature.

to it through a library. For example, the *Physical Fitness/Sports Medicine Index*, is a quarterly publication of the President's Council on Physical Fitness and Sports that contains MEDLARS citations of interest to those involved with fitness and sport.[4] Another useful product is Grateful Med, a software package that can link a Macintosh or IBM personal computer to the Medline database via a modem.[5] In addition, Medline searches are available for a fee through the American Physical Therapy Association.[6]

Cumulative Index of Nursing and Allied Health Literature. The CINAHL was developed in 1956 to meet the needs of nonphysician health care practitioners. As illustrated in Table 16–3, many of the journals of interest to nurses and allied health professionals are not indexed in Index Medicus or Medline. CINAHL provides a means to gain access to these journals. For example, both the *Journal of Orthopaedic and Sports Physical Therapy* and the *Journal of Physical Therapy Education* are not indexed in Index Medicus or Medline but are indexed in CINAHL. In addition to journals, CINAHL indexes books of interest to nurses and other health professionals and nursing dissertations. The CINAHL indexing terms are based on MeSH, but provide for greater specificity in the terms related to each profession represented in the index. Table 16–4 shows the MeSH and CINAHL terms used for physical therapy.[7, 8] Online searches of CINAHL are available for a fee from the American Physical Therapy Association.[6]

Physiotherapy Index. This affordable index is published by the Medical Information Service of the British Library.[9] Like CINAHL, it was developed because Medline does not index enough journals of interest to physical therapists. It is published monthly, with a cumulative annual index.

Dissertations and Theses

The research that students undertake as a requirement for completion of a master's or doctoral degree often is not published in the literature or is published several years after the master's thesis or doctoral dissertation has been filed with the university where the degree was completed. Most doctoral programs and some master's degree programs require that students file a copy of the thesis or dissertation with University Microfilms International. This body produces two indexes of these works: Dissertation Abstracts International and Master's Abstracts. As indicated by the title of the indexes, abstracts of the research are included in the database.

Unfortunately, because there are more master's theses in physical therapy than there are doctoral dissertations, and because not all master's degree programs require students to file their thesis with University Microfilms, using this source to identify relevant research undertaken as part of an academic program of study in physical therapy is not always fruitful. Two other sources help to fill this gap, however. *Physical Therapy* solicits and publishes a list of theses and dissertations completed each year, providing the names of the individuals who wrote them, the advisors involved, and the schools at which they were written.[10] The *Journal of Allied Health* also solicits information for and publishes an annual index of theses and dissertations completed in a broad group of health professions, including physical therapy.[11] Scanning these two indexes for the last few years yielded two different master's theses on CPM: the effects of CPM and immobilization on displaced intraarticular fractures and the effect of ice and CPM on the total knee arthroplasty.[12, 13]

Conference Proceedings

As with dissertations and theses, research papers presented at conferences may not make it to the journal literature for several years, if at all. Access to abstracts of papers presented at conferences can often be obtained by reviewing the conference issue of journals of a particular society or association. For example, *Physical Therapy*, the American Physical Therapy Association's journal, prints abstracts of presentations given at the Association's annual conference as a separate supplement to the journal.[14]

A broader source of conference proceedings is the Index of Scientific and Technical Proceedings (ISTP). Published proceedings of selected conferences are indexed. The index is organized by conference sponsor, location, paper authors, geographic location of the authors, and organizational affiliation of the authors. Depending on one's interest and the information available, any of these items of information might be the starting point of a search of conference proceedings. For example, our review of the library holdings at the University of Indianapolis, shown in Table 16–1, identified R. B. Salter as an important author of studies on CPM. By looking up his name in the author index of the 1990 ISTP, we can determine whether he has presented any recent papers on the topic. A review of Salter's work in the 1990 ISTP and a review of the American Physical Therapy Association's conference abstracts of 1991 for papers on CPM identified two relevant papers: "The Biological Concept of Continuous Passive Motion of Synovial Joints—The 1st 18 Years of Basic Research and Its Clinical Application" and "Continuous Passive Motion: A Controlled Clinical Trial."[15, 16]

Single Article

In addition to the five search tools just described, a single relevant journal article citation can be used in several different ways to identify other sources of information. It is possible to use a single article to work both backward and forward through the literature. To work backward, one examines the reference list of the article and identifies relevant citations. This strategy can also be used with the reference lists of book chapters, conference proceedings, and dissertations and theses. The disadvantage of using this strategy is that it identifies only citations that are older than the source itself.

There are two ways of working forward in the literature from a particular article. The first is to find the Medline or CINAHL citation for the article and determine the subject headings under which it is indexed. Use of these terms in a prospective search is likely to yield related articles. Some journals assist readers with this effort by printing in the article the key words that describe it.

The second way to work forward through the literature from a single article is to use the Science Citation Index or its computer form, Scisearch. This index lists sources that have used a particular article as a reference. Table 16–5 shows an example of how this index works. A key citation is used to begin the forward search: Let's use Salter's 1981 article on CPM because it was cited in many of the articles we have identified thus far in our CPM literature search. The 1990 citation section of the Science Citation Index indicated that seven articles published in 1990 cited Salter's 1981 article. The citation section provides abbreviated information about the sources. In Table 16–5, for example, the abbreviations mean that Salter's work, among others, was cited by D. P. Johnson in an article published in the 72nd volume of the American edition of the *Journal of Bone and Joint Surgery*, in 1990, beginning on page 421. The complete citation is found by consulting the source section of the Science Citation Index, as shown at the bottom of Table 16–5. The full title in the source section helps the practitioner determine whether the article is relevant to the search at hand. The source index also indicates the number of references contained in the source, another indication of the potential value of the article.

TABLE 16–5. Sample Use of Science Citation Index

Citation Index listing				
Salter RB. Clin Orthop. 1981.				
Johnson DP	J Bone–Am V	72A	421	90
Katz K	Act Orthop Scand	61	161	90
Maloney MJ	Clin Orthop		162	90
. . .				

Sample Source Index listing
Johnson DP. The effect of continuous passive motion on wound-healing and joint mobility after knee arthroplasty. J Bone–Am V. 1990;72A:421–426. (20 R)

Figure 16–1 summarizes the way in which the search tools and single-article strategies interrelate. Search tools, represented by the five-piece arch, are used to identify literature items. The literature items, represented as pieces of a circle, can then be used to identify other literature items. Practitioners conducting literature searches frequently use several strategies to identify all the literature of interest. When the citations identified by these different strategies become redundant, then the searcher can be confident that the most important references have been found.

ONGOING LITERATURE SEARCH

Regular consumers of the literature generally have developed strategies that enable them to identify articles of interest on a routine basis. Because of the enormous volume of clinical literature, practitioners must accept that they cannot remain up to date in all areas of their profession. Thus, the first element of an ongoing search strategy is to identify the specific topics in which one is most interested. Once these topics are selected, the basic strategies used for ongoing searches are single-journal contents scanning, multiple-journal contents scanning, and focused index scanning.

Single-Journal Contents Scanning

The journals that arrive in a professional's mailbox each month can be a tremendous asset to the regular literature consumer. The

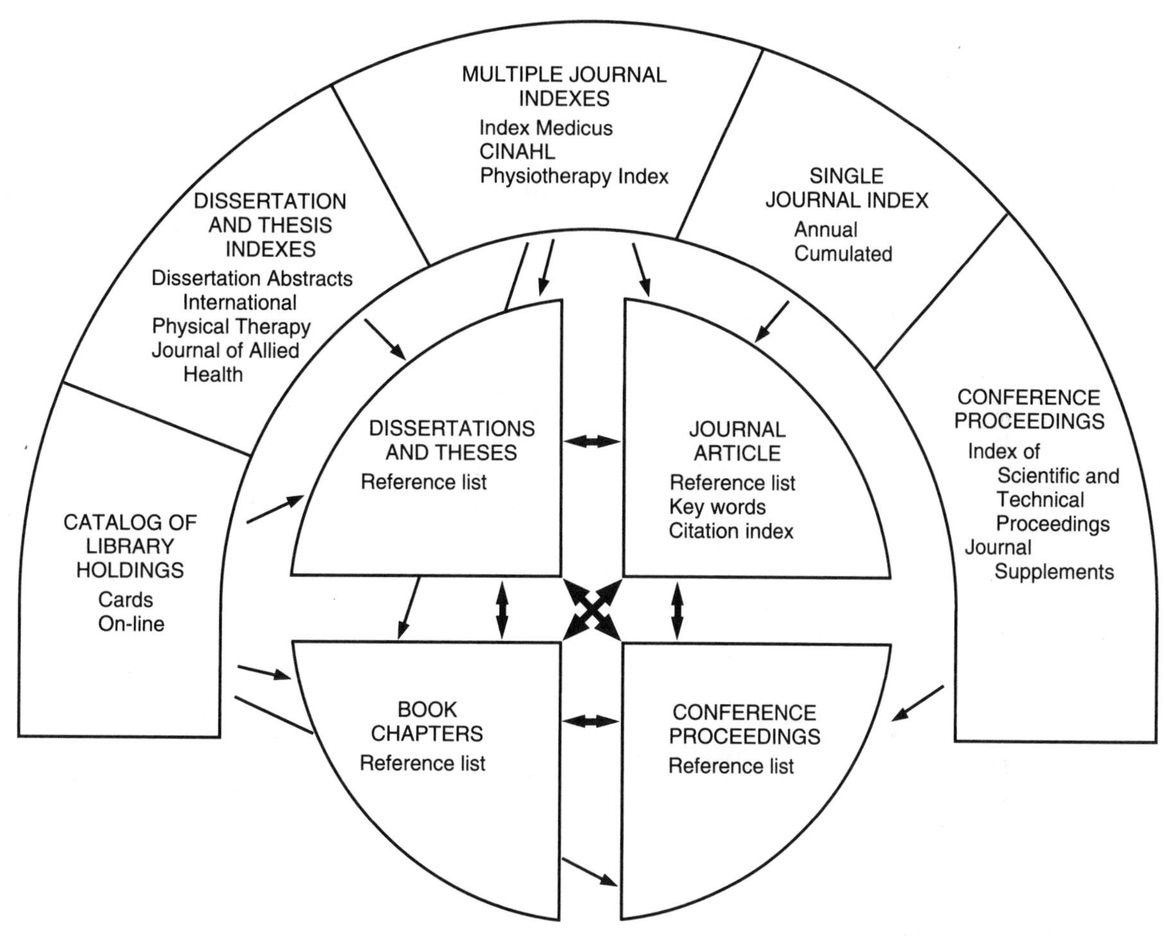

FIGURE 16–1. Relationship among search tools and types of professional literature. The search tools shown in the arch are used to identify relevant citations of the different literature types, as noted by the arrows. Once a citation is identified, its reference list can be used to identify other citations, as noted by the arrows between the pieces of the literature circle. For journal articles, additional indexing and key word strategies can be used to identify other citations.

most obvious resources in each journal are the articles in each issue. For a broadly ranging discipline like physical therapy, a general-interest journal such as *Physical Therapy* or *Physiotherapy Canada* may contain relatively few articles within the particular interest area of a reader. However, the regular reader of the literature should not limit his or her scanning to the articles portion of the journal's table of contents. Most journals publish book reviews and abstracts of relevant articles published in other journals. Both of these sections of the journal can point the reader to areas of interest not addressed in the present issue. In a book review it is often indicated whether the particular title being reviewed provides a thorough reference list, helpful information to the reader interested in acquiring other related citations.

Multiple-Journal Contents Scanning

Scanning the table of contents of several journals of interest is a second excellent way of keeping up with the literature outside the journals that one receives personally. Some libraries even provide a service in which the tables of contents of requested journals are sent to patrons when the journal arrives each month. This allows the consumer to scan the contents conveniently, marking for later review any articles that seem of interest. Literature consumers new to contents scanning may select a fairly large number of journals for initial scanning and reduce the number as it becomes apparent over time which journals most frequently publish articles in their area of interest.

Another way to scan new journal tables of contents is provided by a publication called *Current Contents*. Different versions of this publication, such as *Current Contents: Life Sciences* or *Current Contents: Clinical Medicine*, compile and publish tables of contents from journals relevant to the version. As is the case with some of the other search tools, a strong orientation to medicine reduces the usefulness of this tool to those with interests in rehabilitation.

Focused Index Scanning

Regular scanning of relevant indexes can be accomplished through regular visits to the library or with subscriptions to affordable focused indexes such as the Physiotherapy Index, Physical Fitness/Sports Medicine Index, or Grateful Med, described earlier in the chapter. The combination of focused index scanning, multiple-journal contents scanning, and single-journal contents scanning provides the literature consumer with a solid base of literature in specific areas of interest.

OBTAINING LITERATURE ITEMS

If one's local library does not have a desired item, it can generally be obtained through one of four strategies: interlibrary loan, reprint from the author, purchase of the journal from the publisher, or use of one's network of professional colleagues. Interlibrary loan arrangements give the patron of one library access to the resources of many other libraries. The patron requests the item, and the librarian uses a computer network to determine the libraries which have the item. When a journal article is requested, the lending library usually furnishes a photocopy, often for a fee to cover photocopying and mailing.

Reprints were a common form of journal article transmission until the advent of the photocopier. The system still exists, although it is not used frequently. Authors can usually request reprints of their articles, for a fee, at the time of publication. If they order the reprints they will have a ready supply to mail out if they receive requests. Today, many authors do not buy their own reprints because they realize that interested readers will simply photocopy the item themselves. Most authors are willing to send a photocopy of an article if the requesting party describes how efforts to obtain the article through interlibrary loan were unsuccessful. The probability of obtaining a photocopy from an author rises if a self-addressed, stamped envelope is enclosed to make the process as easy as possible for the author. Many reprints can also be obtained from University Microfilms International.

Back issues of journals can often be purchased from the publisher. If requests for an item through interlibrary loan have been unsuccessful, and if the author cannot be located, the most expedient way to obtain the citation may be to purchase the entire issue. If a potentially important citation still eludes you, turn to your network of professional colleagues for assistance. Colleagues with an interest in the topic may have the needed article and are often willing to share their resources to foster the growth of others with that interest.

SUMMARY

Literature searches are undertaken to obtain information about the theory, facts, opinions, and methods related to a particular area within a discipline. Primary literature sources include journal articles, dissertations and theses, and conference proceedings. Literature search tools include catalogs of library holdings, single- and multiple-journal indexes, dissertation and thesis abstracts, and conference proceedings indexes. Many of the search tools exist in either hard copy or on-line form. Regular readers of the literature often scan the table of contents of one or more journals to identify articles of interest. Once identified, literature items can be obtained through local library holdings, interlibrary loans, requests from authors, purchase from the publisher, or one's network of colleagues.

References

1. *65-Year Index to Physical Therapy*. Alexandria, Va: American Physical Therapy Association; 1987.
2. Davis AM, Findley TW. Research in physical medicine and rehabilitation. X. Information resources. *Am J Phys Med Rehabil*. 1990;69:266–278.
3. Bohannon RW, Gibson DF. Citation analysis of *Physical Therapy*: a special communication. *Phys Ther*. 1986;66:540–541.
4. *Physical Fitness/Sports Medicine*. President's Council on Physical Fitness and Sports, 450 Fifth Street, NW, Washington, DC 20001. Annual subscription rate, $9.00 (1991).
5. Grateful Med. US Department of Commerce, National Technical Information Service, 5285 Port Royal Road, Springfield, VA 22161. IBM and Macintosh versions available for $29.95 + $3.00 handling (1991). Additional fee for connect time; averages $3.00 to $5.00 per search. Information: 800-638-8480.
6. American Physical Therapy Association Online Services. 1111 North Fairfax Street, Alexandria, VA 22314–1488. 800-999-APTA.
7. Medical Subject Headings. Supplement to Index Medicus. 1991;31.
8. Headings. Cumulative Index of Nursing and Allied Health Literature. 1990;35B:256–257.
9. *Physiotherapy Index*. Medical Information Service, British Library, Document Supply Centre, Boston Spa, Wetherby, West Yorkshire, LS23 7BQ. Approximately $90.00 annually (1991).
10. Theses and dissertations. *Phys Ther*. 1991;71:85.
11. Index of graduate theses and projects in allied health. *J Allied Health*. 1990;19:412.
12. Steptoe DM. The effects of continuous passive motion and immobilization on displaced intraarticular fractures: an experimental investigation in the sheep knee joint. MAppSci thesis. Perth, Western Australia, Australia: Curtin University of Technology; 1989.
13. Walsh CM. The effect of ice and continuous passive motion on the total knee arthroplasty. Master's thesis. Philadelphia, Pa: Temple University; 1989.
14. Abstracts of papers accepted for presentation at the 66th Annual Conference of the American Physical Therapy Association. *Phys Ther*. 1991;71:S1–S137.
15. Salter RB. The biological concept of continuous passive motion of synovial joints—the 1st 18 years of basic research and its clinical application. 4th Bristol-Myers/Zimmer Orthopaedic Symposium on Articular Cartilage and Knee Joint Functions: Basic Science and Arthroscopy, Chicago, Ill, Nov 11–13, 1988. Proceedings published as: Ewing JW, ed. Articular Cartilage and Knee Joint Function. Bristol-Myers/Zimmer Orthopaedic Symposium Series. New York, NY: Raven Press; 1990.
16. McInnes J, Larson MG, Daltroy LH, Brown T, Fossel AH, Eaton MH, Shulman-Kirwan B, Steindorf S, Poss R, Liang MH. Continuous passive motion: a controlled clinical trial. 66th Annual Conference of the American Physical Therapy Association, Boston, Mass, June 23–27, 1991.

CHAPTER 17

Evaluating the Literature

Critical evaluation of the literature is a necessary part of any research endeavor. If research is to make good its claim of improving patient care, researchers must study relevant clinical problems and clinicians must conduct their practices in light of relevant research results. To be effective users of the literature, practitioners must evaluate research reports before applying the results, just as they ought to evaluate new treatment methods before adopting them. Critique of the literature may take the form of informal observations or formal reviews published in journals or presented at conferences. Because there are two important levels of formal literature review—isolated reviews of single studies and integrative reviews of several conceptually related studies—this chapter is divided into a major section on each level. First, however, the elements of a research article and a few general guidelines for writing about published research are listed.

ELEMENTS OF A RESEARCH ARTICLE

Table 17–1 lists and describes the elements of a research article. The components encountered first are the journal article title and abstract. Following these is the body of the article, which typically consists of introduction, methods, results, discussion, conclusions, and references sections. Several sections may contain tables, which consist of rows and columns of numbers or words; figures may also be included, which are photographs, diagrams, or graphs that illustrate important concepts or results within the study. Occasionally, an article contains an appendix of information that may be useful to readers but is too detailed for inclusion in the body of the report. Several authors pro-

TABLE 17–1. Elements of a Research Article

Element	Characteristics
Title	Is concise, yet descriptive. Identifies major variables studied. Provides clues about whether the purpose of the research is description, relationship analysis, or difference analysis through use of phrases such as "characteristics of," "relationship between," or "effects of," respectively.
Abstract	Briefly summarizes research purpose, methods, and results. Depending on journal, is usually 150–300 words. Does not include summary of related literature or significant discussion of the limitations and implications of the research.
Introduction	Sets the stage for the presentation of the research. Usually does *not* have a heading; sometimes is subdivided into Problem, Purpose, or Literature Review sections. Whether subdivided or not, defines the broad problem that underlies the study, states the specific purposes of the study, and places the problem and purposes into the theoretical context of previous work. Often presents null or research hypotheses. Occasionally contains tables or figures.
Method	Describes the conduct of the study. Usually is subdivided into Subjects, Instruments, Procedures, and Data Analysis sections. Often refers to methods or procedures used by others as the basis for the present study. Often contains figures showing equipment used.
Results	Presents the results without comment on their meaning. Often is subdivided into sections corresponding to the variables studied. Is often brief because much of the information is contained in tables and figures.
Discussion	Presents the authors' interpretation of their results, along with their assessment of study limitations and directions for future research. Often refers to previous work that is related to the findings of the study. May be subdivided into Limitations, Clinical Relevance, and Future Research sections.
Conclusions	Concisely restates the important findings of the research. Presents a conclusion for each individual purpose outlined in the introduction.
References	Lists references cited in the text of the article. Occasionally is followed by a bibliography that lists relevant work that is not cited in the article.
Appendix	If included, follows the references. Typically includes survey instruments or detailed treatment protocols.

vide useful descriptions of the elements of research articles.[1–3]

GUIDELINES FOR WRITING ABOUT PUBLISHED RESEARCH

Readers who formalize their reviews in writing or through oral presentation to others should follow three basic style guidelines:

1. Discuss the study in the past tense,
2. Clearly distinguish between your own opinions and those of the authors, and
3. Qualify generalizations so they are not erroneously attributed to anyone.

Table 17–2 presents examples of inappropriate and appropriate wording to illustrate each of the three stylistic guidelines.

EVALUATION OF SINGLE STUDIES

Single research studies should be evaluated from two major perspectives: trustworthiness and utility. *Trustworthiness* relates to whether sources of invalidity have been as well controlled as is practical, whether authors openly acknowledge the limitations of the study, and whether the conclusions drawn are defensible in light of the methods used in the study. In Chapters 7 and 13, more than 20 sources of invalidity within research studies are identified. Armed with a list of these

TABLE 17–2. Style Guidelines for Reviewing Published Research

Inappropriate Wording	Appropriate Wording
Basso and Knapp state that there is no difference in outcome between patients who receive CPM 5 versus 20 hours per day.[4] (This wording implies that the authors still hold this belief.)	*Basso and Knapp found no differences in outcome between patients who received 5 versus 20 hours of CPM daily.*[4] (This wording makes it clear that the authors' statements relate to the particular study under discussion.)
Use of CPM after total knee arthroplasty is a useful adjunct to conventional physical therapy. (This wording does not make it clear whether this is the conclusion of the review author or the author of the study.)	*Based on their research, Wasilewski and colleagues concluded that CPM was a useful adjunct to conventional physical therapy.*[5] (This wording clearly attributes the statement to the study authors.)
Patients with greater knee range of motion have better functional outcomes after surgery. (This wording implies that this relationship between range of motion and functional outcome is well established.)	*Therapists and surgeons often assume that patients with greater knee range of motion have better functional outcomes after surgery.* (This wording makes it clear that the relationship between range of motion and functional outcome is an unsubstantiated assumption.)

potential problems, readers of the research literature can easily become overly critical and conclude that all studies are hopelessly flawed and offer nothing of value to the practitioner. However, as we have seen in Chapters 7 and 13, there are no perfect studies because of the reciprocal nature of many of the threats to validity. In many instances, when a researcher controls one source of invalidity, another one rears its ugly head. Thus, there is no absolute standard of trustworthiness to which every study can be held. However, because trustworthiness focuses on the design and interpretation of studies themselves, different readers can be expected to identify common areas of concern related to the trustworthiness of a study.

In contrast, the *utility* of a study relates to the usefulness of its results to a particular practitioner. Unlike the assessment of trustworthiness, the assessment of utility may vary widely among readers. The results of a well-controlled study of a narrowly defined patient population may be highly trustworthy, but of low utility to a practitioner who sees a different patient population. Conversely, a first study of a given phenomenon may be highly useful despite several methodological flaws.

When evaluating the literature, readers must balance legitimate criticisms with a realistic sense of the compromises that all researchers must make in designing and implementing a study. Several authors have presented guidelines for evaluating the research literature.[6, 7] Examples of research evaluations by experienced consumers of the literature can be found as commentaries to published reports in several journals, particularly in *Physical Therapy* in the 1990s.[8] Although different evaluators of the literature structure their commentaries differently, they all assess the same basic aspects of research articles.

In this section, a six-step sequence for evaluating the literature is presented to help novice evaluators structure their critiques. The first steps emphasize classification and description of the research in order to place it in the larger context of research as a vast and varied enterprise. The middle steps emphasize identification of threats to the validity of the research. The final steps involve assessing the place the research has in both the existing literature and one's own practice. Appendix D provides a set of questions to help readers structure their critiques.

To further assist readers embarking on a

review of a study, a written critique of a study, Gose's investigation of continuous passive motion (CPM) for patients after total knee arthroplasty, is developed step by step as each of the six critique steps is presented.[9] The abstract of Gose's report reads,

> The purpose of this study was to evaluate the effects of adding three 1-hour sessions of continuous passive motion (CPM) each day to the entire postoperative program of patients who received a total knee replacement (TKR). A retrospective chart review was completed for 55 patients (8 with bilateral involvement, totalling 63 knees) who received a TKR between 1981 and 1984. The data analysis compared the following variables for 32 patients who received CPM and 23 patients who received no CPM: the length of hospital stay (LOS), the number of postoperative days (PODs) before discharge, the frequency of postoperative complications, and the knee range of motion at discharge. The CPM groups showed significant decreases in the frequency of complication ($p < .05$), the LOS ($p < .01$), and in the number of PODs ($p < .001$). No difference was demonstrated in the ROM of the two groups. These results support the use of postoperative applications of CPM, but not as strongly as those reported from studies that used longer periods of CPM. Further research is indicated to delineate the minimum dosage of CPM needed to obtain the maximum beneficial effects.[9(p39)]

Step 1: Classify the Research and Variables

Classification of the research and variables provides an immediate sense of where the individual piece of research belongs in the literature. The information needed to classify the research is found in the abstract, introduction, and methods sections of a journal article. If the reviewer determines that the research is experimental, then it should come as no surprise if the authors make causal statements about their results; if the reviewer determines that the research is nonexperimental, then the reader's expectations about causal statements should change. If the dependent variables of interest are range-of-motion (ROM) measures, then the reviewer should expect clean, easily understood results; if the dependent measures relate to patterns of interaction between therapists and patients, then the reviewer should expect complexity and depth. We might summarize this first evaluative step for Gose's CPM study as follows:

> Gose's study of the effects of continuous passive motion (CPM) on rehabilitation after total knee arthroplasty is an example of a retrospective analysis of differences between groups. The study had one independent variable, treatment, with two levels: usual postoperative therapy and postoperative therapy supplemented with CPM. The type of treatment received by each subject was not actively manipulated, but rather was apparently determined by physician prescription.
>
> There were five dependent variables: total length of stay in the acute care hospital, number of postoperative days in the acute care hospital, frequency of postoperative complications, knee flexion range of motion (ROM) at discharge, and knee extension ROM at discharge. All data

were gathered through retrospective chart review.

Step 2: Compare Purposes and Conclusions

Any piece of research needs to be assessed in light of the contribution it was designed to make to the profession. It is not fair to fault a study for not accomplishing a purpose that it was never designed to meet. Before reading the methods, results, and discussion sections of an article, it is often useful to compare the purposes, which may be found in the introduction, and the conclusions. This comparison serves two purposes. First, it provides an indication of whether or not the study is internally consistent. Purposes without conclusions, or conclusions without purposes, should alert the reader to look for the points at which the study strays from its original intents.

Knowing the study conclusions also provides guidance for the critique of the methods, results, and discussion. If the conclusions indicate that statistically significant relationships or differences were identified, then the reader knows to evaluate the remainder of the article with an eye to how well the researcher controlled for alternative explanations for the results and whether the statistical results are clinically important. If the conclusions do not indicate any statistically significant results, then the reader knows to evaluate the study with respect to power and the clinical importance of the results. With regard to Gose's study, we might write up this second step of our critique as follows:

The purpose of this study was clearly stated at the end of the introduction section of the paper: to compare the effects of adding three 1-hour daily sessions of CPM to a postoperative total knee arthroplasty rehabilitation program. The effects measured related to both the physical status of the patient (flexion and extension ROM and frequency of complications) and the cost-effectiveness of care (total length of stay and length of postoperative stay).

The conclusions were consistent with the purpose. There were significant differences between the CPM and non-CPM groups for three of the five dependent measures: length of stay, number of days of postoperative hospitalization, and frequency of postoperative complications. There were no significant differences between groups on the two ROM variables, knee flexion and extension.

Step 3: Describe Design and Control Elements

In the third step of the evaluation process, the reviewer completes the description of the study elements and begins to make judgments about the adequacy of the research design. The design of the study is identified so that the sequence of measurement and manipulation (if present) is clear to the reader of the review. This identification can be done in any of the three ways introduced in Chapter 5:

- Making a diagram of the design
- Using symbols such as Campbell and Stanley's Os and Xs
- Using descriptive terms.

The research design alone does not indicate

the trustworthiness of the study. For example, a "strong" design such as a pretest–posttest control-group design may not yield trustworthy information if the independent variable is not implemented consistently for subjects in the treatment group. Thus, a critical reader of the literature needs to determine both the design of the study and the level of control the researchers exerted over implementation of the independent variable, selection and assignment of subjects, extraneous variables related to the setting or subjects, measurement, and information. The third step in our review of Gose's CPM study can be written as follows:

> As noted previously, data for this study were collected retrospectively, with group membership determined by the postoperative rehabilitation program each patient happened to have undergone. This study was therefore of a nonexperimental, ex post facto nature with nonequivalent treatment and control groups. Because all dependent variables were collected at the completion of either rehabilitation program, the study followed a posttest-only design.
>
> The nonexperimental, retrospective nature of data collection means that many design control elements were absent. The implementation of the independent variable took place in the hospital setting and would be expected to vary accordingly. The author did not indicate the proportion of patients who received all of the intended CPM sessions. Because he later discussed how the intended dosage of CPM in this study differs from that reported in other studies, it seems important to know if the actual dosage received by the patients was equal to, greater than, or less than the indicated dosage.
>
> The selection and assignment of subjects to groups were accomplished through chart review to determine, first, whether subjects met general inclusion criteria and, second, whether they had undergone traditional or CPM-added rehabilitation. The basic inclusion criteria were having undergone a total knee arthroplasty between 1981 and 1984 at one hospital, having had ROM values recorded at admission and discharge, and having accomplished certain rehabilitation tasks by Postoperative Days 2 and 7. The nature of these criteria are such that patients with complications severe enough to impede the rehabilitation process were excluded from the study. Thus, the frequency of postoperative complications indicated in this study was likely less than the number of actual complications that occur after total knee arthroplasty.
>
> Assignment of subjects to group was accomplished simply by identification of which type of rehabilitation they had undergone. The author did not indicate what factors might have led one patient to receive CPM-added rehabilitation and another patient to receive traditional rehabilitation. If, for example, certain surgeons prescribed CPM-added rehabilitation and others prescribed traditional

rehabilitation, then the effects of the type of rehabilitation would be confounded by surgeon.

If the traditional rehabilitation group had their surgery and rehabilitation in 1981 and 1982 and the CPM-added group received care in 1983 and 1984, then the effects of type of rehabilitation would be confounded with any general changes in surgical technique, knee prosthesis design, hospital staffing patterns, and the like that may have differed between the two time periods.

Because of the retrospective design, extraneous variables such as disease severity and medication received postoperatively were not controlled. In addition, there was no control over ROM measurements taken and no indication of how many different therapists recorded ROM values in the study.

Step 4: Identify Threats to Validity

Once the type of research has been defined, the purposes and conclusions reviewed, and the design and control elements outlined, the reviewer is able to examine the threats to the validity of the study. This step involves not only assessing the threats to validity but also evaluating the extent to which the authors identify the study's limitations themselves.

As described in Chapter 7, the threats to validity can be divided into construct, internal, statistical conclusion, and external validity. Not all of the types of validity are applicable to all types of research studies. Table 17–3 lists four types of research (descriptive, relationship analysis, difference analysis, and methodological research) and indicates which of the four types of validity are applicable to each type of research. For example, we know that internal validity relates to whether a particular independent variable can be considered the cause of differences between groups within a study. Descriptive and relationship analysis studies do not involve analysis of differences, so the internal validity concerns are not applicable. Our analysis of the validity of Gose's CPM study might be written as follows:

CONSTRUCT VALIDITY CONCERNS

The major construct validity concerns in Gose's study are construct underrepresentation and interaction of different treatments. The variables studied were a combination of cost-effectiveness variables related to length of stay and patient-oriented variables such as frequency of complications and knee ROM. These variables did not, however, represent a full range of outcomes for patients

TABLE 17–3. Evaluation of Validity by Research Type

Descriptive Research	Relationship Analysis	Difference Analysis	Methodological Research
Construct External	Construct External Statistical conclusion	Construct External Statistical conclusion Internal	Construct External Statistical conclusion

after total knee arthroplasty. It would have been nice if functional measures such as ambulation or stair-climbing ability had been measured. Presumably, this information would have been as available from the medical record as the ROM data were. In addition to underrepresentation of the dependent variables, the author acknowledged that the independent variable was also underrepresented: the dosage of CPM in this study was low compared with the dosage in other studies. A more complete, prospective study would assess several different dosages of CPM to determine the minimum level needed to obtain desired results.

The interaction of different treatments is always a concern with a retrospective study such as this one. We have no way of knowing, for example, whether the CPM treatments, which were administered by nursing staff, consisted of mechanical application of the unit with minimal interpersonal contact between nurse and patient or took the form of relaxed interchanges that provided an opportunity for education and discussion. If the latter was the case, then this study may have actually been assessing the effects of a combined program of CPM, education, and attention, rather than the isolated addition of CPM to the treatment regimen. The author acknowledged the possibility that differences between groups may be related to factors other than the use of CPM.

INTERNAL VALIDITY CONCERNS

The major internal validity concerns in this study are assignment, mortality, diffusion of treatment, compensatory equalization of treatments, and compensatory rivalry or resentful demoralization of subjects. Very little information was given about why a particular patient received either the CPM-added rehabilitation or the non-CPM regimen. As noted earlier, if group membership was confounded with surgeon or time frame, it would be difficult to conclude that differences between groups were related solely to the differences in their rehabilitation regimens.

Regarding the threat of mortality to internal validity, we have no way of knowing how many potential subjects in each group were not included in the study because they developed serious complications that prevented them from meeting the inclusion criteria of supervised ambulation on Postoperative Day 2 and progressive ambulation by Postoperative Day 7.

A third threat to internal validity comes from having patients from both groups being treated at the same time. It is plausible that members of each group were hospital roommates, and if the roommate in the CPM group extolled the virtues of this new device, perhaps the roommate in the non-CPM group compensated by moving her knee more frequently. If the therapists believed that CPM was beneficial, they could have become upset when some physicians did not prescribe it and compensated by increasing the number of ROM repetitions they included for their patients who were not receiving CPM. Because the author did not clearly indicate whether the two regimens were in effect simultaneously or sequentially, we cannot speculate about the likelihood that these internal validity threats actually occurred.

STATISTICAL CONCLUSION VALIDITY CONCERNS

No concerns about statistical conclusion validity seem warranted. The sample sizes were reasonable (32 and 23); there was only one statistical test performed per dependent variable; the homogeneity-of-variance assumptions seem to have been met; the statistically significant results seem clinically important (for example, the CPM group had an average postoperative length of stay approximately 3.5 days shorter than the non-CPM group); and the statistically insignificant results seem clinically insignificant (the difference in the mean ROM values between groups was only 1.0° for both knee flexion and extension).

EXTERNAL VALIDITY CONCERNS

The study has strong external validity. The subjects seem representative of typical patients who receive total knee arthroplasties: elderly females with osteoarthritis. Therapists who work with a more predominantly rheumatoid arthritic group might find differences in patient response based on the systemic nature of rheumatoid arthritis. In addition, the retrospective nature of the study means that the treatment was implemented as it occurs in the clinical setting, with all its attendant inconsistencies. Thus, despite possible inconsistencies in application of the treatment, a clinically important reduction in length of stay was found. The study would have been strengthened by documentation of the CPM dosage delivered.

External validity is somewhat limited, however, by the 10 years that have elapsed from the beginning of the study to the present time. Length of stay in hospitals has been reduced in response to changes in federal reimbursement policies; although the CPM group's length of stay was significantly less in this study than the non-CPM group's, both lengths of stay are longer than is typical today, irrespective of the nature of the rehabilitation regimen. This issue was well addressed by the author in the discussion.

Step 5: Place the Study in the Context of Other Research

In the fifth and sixth steps of evaluation, the reviewer assesses the utility of the research.

First, the reviewer determines how much new information the study adds to what is already known about a topic. Even though only a single study is being critiqued, the question of utility cannot be answered in isolation. For example, if a treatment has consistently been shown to be effective in tightly controlled settings with high internal validity, another well-controlled study may not add much to our knowledge about that treatment. In such a case what is needed is a study conducted in a realistic clinical setting, where control is difficult. Similarly, a small one-group study of a previously unstudied area might be an important addition to the physical therapy literature, whereas the same design applied to a well-studied topic may add very little.

The best assessments of the context in which a particular study belongs are made by reviewers who have extensive knowledge of the literature on the topic. Knowledgeable reviewers can assess whether the authors of a research report have adequately reviewed and interpreted the literature they cite. Reviewers without this knowledge must rely on the authors' descriptions of the literature. Our review of the place Gose's CPM study has in the literature, based on the author's report of the related literature, might be written as follows:

> Despite the previously noted limitations of Gose's study, this work appears to add to our understanding of the role of CPM in the rehabilitation of patients after total knee arthroplasty. The author indicates that previous studies of 20-hour-a-day CPM protocols have found shorter lengths of stay, lower frequencies of postoperative complications, and greater early knee ROM in CPM groups compared with non-CPM groups. This study assessed the effectiveness of three 1-hour CPM treatments daily, a far lower dosage than that assessed previously, and provides preliminary evidence that a low dosage of CPM can reduce the length of stay and frequency of complications in a typical group of elderly arthritic patients receiving total knee replacement.

Step 6: Evaluate the Personal Utility of the Study

As the final step in any research critique, the reviewer determines whether the study has meaning for his or her own practice. Whereas the determination of the trustworthiness of a research article will be somewhat consistent across reviewers, the question of personal utility will be answered differently by different reviewers. Hypothetically, we might write our assessment of the personal utility of Gose's CPM study as follows:

> The results of this study have some potential application for the setting in which we work. In our setting, we follow a 20-hour-a-day regimen of CPM with excellent early ROM and relatively short stays. However, we believe that using such a high dosage of CPM keeps the patient in bed too much and inhibits the development of effective quadriceps femoris muscle power and the development of more functional skills such as walking at a relatively normal velocity and for longer distances.
>
> Although this study provides only partial support for the effectiveness of a very low dosage of CPM, it

challenges our assumption that we must administer CPM in very high dosages to realize its benefits. On the basis of the results of this study as well as our own dissatisfaction with some aspects of high dosages of CPM, we plan to implement and assess a trial of medium dosages of CPM in our patients who have had total knee arthroplasty.

The evaluation of personal utility is a very concrete way to conclude a review of a single research study. This ending is a reminder that the first five evaluative steps are not mere intellectual exercises, but are the means by which each reader decides whether and how to use the results of a study within his or her own practice.

CONCEPTUAL REVIEW OF THE LITERATURE

In a conceptual review of the literature, the reviewer evaluates several related studies to (a) synthesize their results into a summary of what is and is not known about the topic, (b) identify areas of controversy within the literature, and (c) develop questions that need further research. Although there are mathematical ways to synthesize the results of several related studies (see Chapter 6 for a brief discussion of meta-analysis), the focus in this section is on the conceptual synthesis that practitioners might undertake to help guide treatment or identify areas in need of further study.[10] A six-step sequence for conducting a conceptual review is presented below. Brief examples based on several studies of CPM use after total knee arthroplasty are given to illustrate some of the steps.[4, 5, 9, 11–13]

Step 1: Determine the Purpose of the Review

Just as any research that involves the collection of new data should have a clearly stated purpose, so should a conceptual review of the literature. Common reasons for performing a conceptual review of the literature are

- to guide treatment decisions in one's own clinic
- to provide a basis for determining whether one's own treatment outcomes are consistent with those of others
- to determine how others measure success for particular types of patients
- to develop a research agenda in the area reviewed.

Step 2: Conduct a Literature Search

Using the techniques outlined in Chapter 16, the reader must obtain a relatively complete set of articles on the topic. Which articles are selected obviously depends on the purpose for doing the review. If one is interested in how to document progress after total knee arthroplasty, then studies that involve functional assessment of patients with any type of knee pathology may be relevant; if one's interest is solely in post-TKA treatment regimens, then such articles are not relevant.

Step 3: Identify the Designs and Constructs of the Studies

Both the nature of the studies and the nature of the variables under study must be examined carefully. What designs were used to study the topic? Was the independent variable implemented differently in different studies? What dependent measures were used consistently? Table 17–4 lists the designs and

TABLE 17–4. Constructs of Continuous Passive Motion (CPM) after Total Knee Arthroplasty Investigated in Six Studies

Constructs	Primary Author
Design elements	
Data collection	
Retrospective	Gose,[9] Wasilewski[5]
Prospective	Basso,[4] Goll,[11] Johnson,[12] Maloney[13]
Group assignment	
Existing groups	Basso, Gose
Successive cohorts	Maloney, Wasilewski
Random	Goll, Johnson
Comparisons	
CPM with immobilization	Goll, Johnson, Maloney, Wasilewski
CPM with standard care	Gose
Different CPM protocols	Basso
Implementation of CPM	
Dosage	
20 or more hours	Basso, Johnson, Maloney, Wasilewski
5 hours	Basso
3 hours	Gose
Time of first application	
Recovery room	Basso, Goll, Johnson, Maloney, Wasilewski
2nd postoperative day	Basso
3rd postoperative day	Gose
Removal of CPM treatment	
7th postoperative day	Johnson, Maloney
12th postoperative day	Goll
Discontinued when 90° active assistive motion attained	Wasilewski
Initial range of motion (ROM)	
0–30° or 35°	Goll, Gose, Maloney
0–40°	Johnson
0–60°	Wasilewski
Progression of ROM	
5°/day	Basso
5–10°/day	Goll, Gose
10°/day	Johnson, Wasilewski
As tolerated	Maloney
No progression for 3 days	Johnson
Measurement of outcomes	
Cost measures	
Length of stay	Basso, Goll, Gose, Johnson, Maloney, Wasilewski
Postoperative days	Gose
Number of physical therapy treatments	Basso
Motion measures	
Flexion ROM	Basso, Gose, Maloney
Extension ROM	Basso, Goll, Gose, Maloney
Extensor lag	Johnson, Wasilewski
ROM arc	Basso, Goll, Johnson, Maloney, Wasilewski
Need for manipulation under anesthesia	Goll, Gose, Wasilewski
Pain measures	
Visual analog scale	Basso
Pain scale	Maloney
Analgesic use	Wasilewski

Table continued on following page

TABLE 17–4. Constructs of Continuous Passive Motion (CPM) after Total Knee Arthroplasty Investigated in Six Studies *Continued*

Constructs	Primary Author
Functional measures	
Brigham and Women's knee rating scale	Wasilewski
Modified Harris scale	Maloney
Thromboembolic factors	
Deep vein thrombosis	Goll, Gose, Wasilewski
Superficial thrombosis	Gose
Pulmonary emboli	Goll, Gose, Maloney, Wasilewski
Wound healing factors	
Oxygen tension	Johnson
Wound complications	Goll, Johnson, Maloney, Wasilewski
Miscellaneous factors	
Edema and effusion	Basso, Gose
Blood transfused	Maloney
Buttock pressure sore	Johnson
Deep knee infection	Gose, Maloney
Peroneal nerve palsy	Gose
Urinary tract infection	Gose
Length of follow-up	
Through discharge	Basso, Goll, Gose, Johnson, Maloney, Wasilewski
1 year postoperative	Johnson, Maloney
2 years postoperative	Maloney
>2 years	Maloney
Unspecified "follow-up"	Wasilewski

variables of interest identified by examination of six studies of CPM use after total knee arthroplasty. This review reveals that there are at least five important considerations in planning a program of CPM: when CPM is applied, how long CPM is used daily, what starting ROM is, how much ROM increases, and when CPM is discontinued. It also shows that the most frequently used measures of success are length of stay and ROM and that most researchers have examined only discharge outcome in patients who received CPM versus those who were treated with some type of postoperative immobilization.

Step 4: Determine the Utility of the Individual Studies

After the constructs studied have been specified, it is necessary to evaluate each study individually to determine the validity of its results and conclusions. This evaluation follows the guidelines presented in Evaluation of Single Studies.

Step 5: Make Comparisons Across Studies

Once each study has been examined independently, the reviewer compares results across the studies. In our example review of six studies of CPM after total knee arthroplasty, we see that several investigators have examined thromboembolic phenomena after total knee arthroplasty to determine whether patients who received CPM had fewer thromboembolic complications than those who did not. Wasilewski and colleagues retrospectively identified a decreased incidence of thromboembolic phenomena with an aggressive CPM program compared with a program of postoperative knee immobilization.[5] However, in both Goll and associates' prospective study of an aggressive CPM program and Gose's retrospective study of a far less aggressive CPM program, essentially no differences in the frequency of thromboembolic complications were found between CPM and comparison groups.[9, 11] Thus the research reviewed does not provide a clear picture of the relationship between CPM use and thromboembolic complications. Similar comparisons across studies would be made for each of the factors of interest (i.e., pain, function, and wound healing) we identified earlier in the review.

Step 6: Specify Problems That Need Further Study

By following the previous steps we have identified the types of designs used to study CPM after total knee arthroplasty and have identified points of consensus and controversy in the literature. On the basis of this limited literature review, we might conclude that the following types of studies are needed to enhance our understanding of the phenomenon: comparison of different CPM protocols, assessment of functional outcomes, long-term follow-up studies, and further study of the relationship between CPM use and thromboembolic complications.

SUMMARY

The major elements of a research article are the title; abstract; introduction, methods, results, discussion, conclusions, and references sections; and, sometimes, an appendix. When writing about previously published work, reviewers should use the past tense and should make clear whether statements are their own or the opinions of the authors whose study they are reviewing. Reviewers of single studies should classify the research and its variables, compare the purposes and conclusions, outline the design and control elements, determine the threats to the validity of the study, place the study in the context of previous work, and assess the study's utility for their personal practice. When doing a conceptual review of several related studies, the reviewer should identify the purpose of the review, conduct an appropriate literature search, identify the studies' designs and the variables examined within the studies, assess each study individually, compare results across studies for consistencies and inconsistencies, and determine what aspects of the topic require further study.

References

1. Domholdt EA, Malone TR. Evaluating research literature: the educated clinician. *Phys Ther.* 1985;65:487–491.
2. Braddom CL. A framework for writing and/or evaluating research papers. *Am J Phys Med Rehabil.* 1990;70:S169-S171.
3. Bailey DM. *Research for the Health Professional: A Practical Guide.* Philadelphia, Pa: FA Davis Co; 1991. Chapter 11.
4. Basso DM, Knapp L. Comparison of two continuous passive motion protocols for patients with total knee implants. *Phys Ther.* 1987;67:360–363.
5. Wasilewski SA, Woods LC, Torgerson WR, Healy WL. Value of continuous passive motion in total knee arthroplasty. *Orthopedics.* 1990;13:291–295.
6. Gay LR. *Educational Research: Competencies for Analysis and Application.* 3rd ed. New York, NY: Macmillan Publishing Co; 1987. Chapter 17.
7. Polit DF, Hungler BP. *Nursing Research: Principles and Methods.* 3rd ed. Philadelphia, Pa: JB Lippincott Co; 1987. Chapter 26.
8. Rothstein JM. Commenting on commentaries. *Phys Ther.* 1991;71:431–432.
9. Gose JC. Continuous passive motion in the postoperative treatment of patients with total knee replacement: a retrospective study. *Phys Ther.* 1987;67:39–42.
10. Findley TW. Research in physical medicine and rehabilitation II: the conceptual review of the literature or how to read more articles than you ever want to see in your entire life. *Am J Phys Med Rehabil.* 1989;68:97–102.
11. Goll SR, Lotke PA, Ecker ML. Failure of continuous

passive motion as prophylaxis against deep venous thrombosis after total knee arthroplasty. In: Rand JA, Dorr LD, eds. *Total Arthroplasty of the Knee: Proceedings of the Knee Society, 1985–1986*. Rockville, Md: Aspen Publishers Inc; 1987.
12. Johnson DP. The effect of continuous passive motion on wound-healing and joint mobility after knee arthroplasty. *J Bone Joint Surg*. 1990;72[A]:421–426.
13. Maloney WJ, Schurman DJ, Hangen D, Goodman SB, Edworthy S, Bloch DA. The influence of continuous passive motion on outcome in total knee arthroplasty. *Clin Orthop*. 1990;256:162–168.

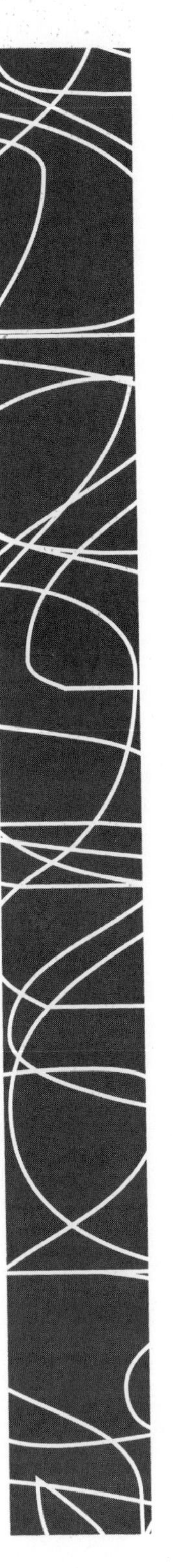

SECTION SIX

IMPLEMENTING RESEARCH

CHAPTER 18

Preliminary Research Steps

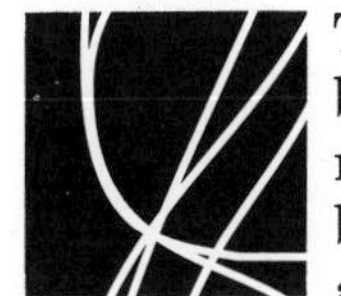

The physical therapist who is beginning a research project must complete three basic steps before collecting any data. First, a research plan, or proposal, must be prepared and submitted for approval through appropriate academic or administrative channels. Second, the researcher must seek the approval of human or animal subjects protection committees, if appropriate. Third, the researcher must secure the funds needed to implement the study. This chapter provides guidelines for each of these steps.

PROPOSAL PREPARATION

The research proposal is a blueprint for the conduct of a research study. The proposal is also the mechanism by which the researcher sells the study idea to those individuals who are in a position to approve and fund it. Thus, the proposal must be written in a fashion that makes the purpose and methods of the study intelligible to those outside the researcher's sphere of interest. In this section of the chapter, general guidelines for proposal preparation are given, followed by specific suggestions related to each basic element of a research proposal. Detailed suggestions for proposal preparation have been provided by others.[1,2]

General Proposal Guidelines

Ideas with merit may never get to the implementation stage if the proposal does not meet the technical standards of the agency to which it is submitted, if the language is confusing, or if the appearance of the document makes it difficult to read. Thus researchers need to prepare their proposal in the format, style, and appearance preferred by the agency to which they are submitting it. Whether one is submitting the proposal to a doctoral thesis committee, to an institutional review board for assessment of whether the proposal contains adequate safeguards for the human subjects involved in the research, or to a foundation for funding, there will be guidelines to follow for preparation of the proposal. If there is a page limit, do not exceed it. If you are required to submit one original and three copies, do not submit an original and two copies. If the proposal must be in someone's office by a certain date, do not simply mail the proposal on that date. In short, follow the directions of the group to whom the proposal will be submitted.

The proposal may need to be modified to meet different needs at different times. The format that students must use for the proposal they submit to their research advisors will likely differ from the format required for submission of the proposal to the human subjects review committee, and the format required for foundation funding will probably differ from the other two formats. Access to word-processing equipment facilitates making whatever changes in the proposal are necessary at different points in the preparation process.

The proposal must be well organized and contain clear, concise language appropriate for the individuals who will be reviewing it. A proposal submitted to one's academic advisors can be written with the assumption that the audience has basic knowledge of the area of study; a proposal submitted to a family-run philanthropic foundation must be written so that lay individuals can grasp the essential elements and importance of the proposal. The appearance of the document must both invite the reader and convey the investigator's competence. Misspellings convey the message that the proposal writer does not pay attention to details and may make the reviewer wonder whether adequate attention would be paid to the details of the research. Cramped type, narrow margins, draft-quality print, and poor photocopying all make the document difficult to read. Attractive documents have a good balance between text and white space, achieved through adequate margins, lots of headings for skimming, and numbered or bulleted lists.

Elements of the Research Proposal

In many ways, the elements of a research proposal are similar to those of a research article. In fact, a good proposal can serve as the outline for the first draft of a research article. Table 18–1 outlines the typical sections of a proposal.

Title. The proposal title should be concise yet precise, and should mention the most important variables under study. When seeking funding for a study, researchers may include in the title of their study words similar to those listed as priorities by the funding agency. For example, if an agency lists the funding of research related to Down's syndrome as one of its priorities, researchers studying children with hypotonia (including some with Down's syndrome) might do well to title their proposal "Assessment of Children with Down's Syndrome and Other Hypotonic Conditions" rather than "Assessment of Children with Hypotonia."

Investigators. The names, credentials, and institutional affiliations of the investigators should be given. If cooperating institutions with whom the researchers are not formally affiliated will be involved in the research, they should be specified here. A curriculum vitae, or scholar's resumé, of each investigator is often included in an appendix to the proposal.

Problem Statement. The problem statement

TABLE 18–1. Components of a Research Proposal

- Title
  - Key words
  - Variables of interest
- Investigators
  - Names and credentials
  - Affiliation
  - Curricula vitae in appendix
- Abstract
- Problem
  - Based in the work of the profession
  - Backed up with literature
- Purposes
  - Specific objectives of the study
  - Researcher hypotheses about results
- Methods
  - Subject selection and assignment
    - Procedures
    - Provisions for confidentiality
  - Procedures
    - Justified by literature
    - Detailed enough to assess benefits and risks
    - Qualifications of investigators or others to perform procedures
    - Provisions for protection of subjects during testing or treatment
    - Reference to informed consent form in appendix, if appropriate
  - Data analysis
    - Based on best-case scenario
    - May include contingency plans
- References
- Dissemination
  - Conferences at which presentations may be given
  - Journal to which results will be submitted first
  - Other means by which results may be disseminated to the communities of interest
- Budget
  - Personnel, salaries, and benefits
  - Supplies
  - Equipment
  - Mailing, printing, etc.
  - Subject stipends
  - Data analysis
  - Presentation and publication preparation
  - Presentation travel
- Work plan
  - All phases, from implementation to dissemination
- Appendices
  - Curricula vitae of investigators
  - Informed consent form
  - Very detailed procedures

in a research proposal is generated and placed in the context of related literature. A persuasive paragraph or two are needed to convince the prospective sponsors of the study's importance. The problems need to be consistent with the goals and mission of the institution at which the research will be performed and with the purposes for which an agency is making funds available.

Purposes. The purposes section of a proposal enumerates how the problem will be approached in the study. If there are several purposes, they should be listed in a logical sequence according to factors such as importance, underlying concepts, or timing. The format of the purposes varies depending on the type of research being proposed. For example, if the research is exploratory in nature, the purposes may take the form of questions, as in the following statement:

> The purpose of this study is to answer four questions:
>
> 1. To what extent do physical therapy students feel isolated from the clinical environment during their first year of study?
> 2. What difficulties do newly licensed physical therapists experience in making the transition from student to professional?
> 3. Does participation in a program in which students are matched with clinician advisors decrease

feelings of isolation from the clinic?

4. Does participation in the clinician advisor program ease the transition from student to professional?

If the research is in a more developed area, then more formalized hypotheses may be appropriate.

Methods. The methods section of a research proposal should include information on subject selection, procedures, and data analysis. Description of the sample must include the source of subjects for the study; the sample size anticipated; the methods of assigning subjects to groups, if appropriate; and the means by which the informed consent of the subjects will be obtained, if appropriate. A copy of the informed consent document should be included as an appendix to the proposal (guidelines for writing informed consent statements are presented later in this chapter).

Procedures should be discussed in detail, with reference to the literature that provides justification for the choice of procedures. Any independent and dependent variables should be clearly defined. The means by which extraneous variables are controlled should be noted, and the reasons for leaving any extraneous variables uncontrolled should be given.

The data analysis procedures in the proposal are usually based on a best-case scenario, but may include contingency plans for nonnormal data or if the number of anticipated subjects does not materialize. There should be a data analysis element for every research hypothesis or question. If statistical consultants have been used to develop the data analysis section of the proposal or will be available to assist with data analysis, this should be indicated here.

Dissemination. Readers of the proposal will want to know how the researchers will disseminate the study findings. Conference presentation and journal article publications are the most common means of dissemination (see Chapter 20).

Budget. There are costs associated with any research project. If a project is self-funded by the researcher or internally funded by an organization, these costs are frequently hidden because the individuals doing the research are donating their time or the institution in which the research is being conducted simply does not actually calculate the loss of revenue from the decreased clinical productivity of the individuals involved. Externally funded projects require detailed budgets that account for both the direct and indirect costs of the research. Direct costs include equipment, supplies, computer time, salaries and benefits of individuals with dedicated time to the project, and the like. Indirect costs include administrative costs, overhead, salaries, and benefits of individuals peripherally involved with the study. See Funding for more detailed information on developing a budget for the research project.

Work Plan. The work plan details when tasks will be accomplished and who will accomplish them. All phases from planning through implementation and dissemination need to be included in the work plan. Researchers need to be realistic in estimating the amount of time needed to accomplish the project, making sure that adequate slack is included to manage unforeseen complications. Time constraints on students or considerations of the clinic may dictate that certain events happen at certain times. When this is the case, the researchers should develop the work plan by proceeding backward from a set date to ensure that all necessary preliminary tasks are accomplished. Table 18–2 shows a work plan developed for a study required for

TABLE 18–2. Work Plan for a Graduate Research Project

Task	Time Frame	Task	Time Frame
Submit first draft to advisor	Nov 1, 1991	Arrange for photography for presentation and publication, to be done at April data collection session	Mar 15, 1992
Finish revisions to first draft	Nov 30, 1991	Collect data at amputee clinic	Apr 2, 1992
Advisor approves proposal for degree requirements	Dec 5, 1991	Enter data into computer program	Apr 12, 1992
Submit approved proposal to physical therapy (PT) director at hospital	Dec 8, 1991	Analyze data	Apr 28, 1992
PT director and amputee clinic medical director review proposal and make suggestions or approve	Jan 6, 1992	Submit first draft of academic paper to advisor	June 6, 1992
Make protocol revisions if necessary	Jan 15, 1992	Submit second draft of paper to advisor	Aug 12, 1992
Submit institutional review board (IRB) materials for university approval	Jan 20, 1992	Develop presentation script and submit to advisor	Sept 8, 1992
University IRB holds meeting	Jan 31, 1992	Advisor approves presentation script	Oct 4, 1992
Build measuring device and test with researchers	Jan 31, 1992	Generate presentation slides	Oct 21, 1992
Submit IRB materials for hospital approval	Feb 2, 1992	Submit abstract for presentation at conference	Nov 2, 1992
Hospital IRB holds meeting	Feb 18, 1992	Oral presentation to faculty	Nov 11, 1992
Reserve video equipment for pilot and test days	Feb 20, 1992	Submit third draft of paper to advisor	Nov 27, 1992
Develop data collection forms	Feb 20, 1992	Submit final draft of paper to advisor	Dec 1, 1992
Pilot test with 1 or 2 patients	Mar 1, 1992	File approved copies of paper with university	Dec 7, 1992
Revise forms and photocopy for data collection	Mar 3, 1992	Revise academic paper for journal publication	Jan 31, 1993
Collect data at amputee clinic	Mar 5, 1992	Submit for publication	Feb 15, 1993

completion of an entry-level master's degree in physical therapy. In this example, data collection will occur at an amputee clinic held only once a month. The work plan therefore revolves around the set dates on which the clinic is held.

Appendices. In the appendices, the researcher provides detailed information that may be required by reviewers of the proposal but is not required for a basic understanding of what the proposal entails. Common items include the curricula vitae of the investigators, informed consent forms, and very detailed procedures such as diagrams of specific exercises and progression of repetitions for an exercise study.

Once the proposal is prepared, it requires approval, sometimes from individuals at several different levels. Student proposals require the approval of research advisors and committees. Clinical research proposals require administrative approval at one or more levels in an organization. Proposals for studies using human or animal subjects require approval by human or animal subject protection committees. The procedures for obtaining academic and administrative approval vary widely from institution to institution and are not discussed further. In contrast, the procedure for obtaining approval from human subjects protection committees tends to be similar at most institutions.

HUMAN SUBJECTS PROTECTION

Researchers in physical therapy must undertake many procedures to ensure the protection of the human subjects they use in their studies. Researchers who use animal subjects must submit their proposals for approval from comparable animal subjects protection committees.

To protect their subjects from mental and physical harm, researchers must

- Design sound studies in which dangers to subjects are minimized
- Secure the informed consent of participants
- Implement the research with care and consideration for participants' safety.

Review committees are the mechanisms by which the design and informed consent elements of subject safety are ensured. At many institutions, such a committee is called the *institutional review board* (IRB). Federal regulations since 1971 have specified that research conducted with government funds be subject to review by a committee concerned with the rights and welfare of participants. In addition, most scientific journals today require evidence that research with animal or human subjects has undergone a review, irrespective of the funding source of the research.

Although procedures vary from institution to institution, many IRBs base their work on federal guidelines. Consequently, most of the guidelines presented here are based on the guidelines of the federal government. These guidelines have been well summarized by several authors.[3–5]

Institutional Review Boards

Federal regulations specify that an IRB be composed of at least five members with varying backgrounds representative of the type of research conducted at the university: Individuals of different sexes and races should be represented, at least one member must have a nonscientific background, and one member should be unaffiliated with the institution. This composition is designed to ensure that a closely knit group of scientists does not make the decisions about their own or their colleagues' projects.

The purpose of the IRB is to review research conducted under the auspices of the institution to ensure that the rights of human subjects are protected. These rights are protected when research designs minimize risks to subjects, when subject selection and assignment are equitable, when researchers have made provisions for the confidentiality of information, and when subjects are provided with the information they need to make an informed decision about whether to participate in the research. The IRB accomplishes its purpose through regular meetings during which it reviews written proposals submitted in a format specified by the IRB.

Levels of Review

IRBs typically have three levels of review of research projects: exempt, expedited, and full. Research that is *exempt* from review includes

- Research that involves normal educational practices
- Survey or interview procedures that do not involve sensitive areas of behavior and in which responses are recorded in such a way that they cannot be attributed to a particular individual
- Observations of public behavior
- Study of existing data.

Although federal regulations indicate that such research is exempt from review by the IRB, institutions may require researchers to submit materials (such as a proposal or questionnaires) to the IRB so that the members can determine whether the research fits the exempt category. An exempt study in physical therapy might involve retrospective chart review or opinion assessment through a mailed questionnaire.

Expedited reviews are permitted for studies that involve minimal risks to subjects. Such procedures include

- Collection of hair, nails, or external secretions
- Recording of noninvasive data
- Study of small amounts of blood through venipuncture
- Study of the effects of moderate exercise in healthy volunteers.

Expedited reviews sometimes may be accomplished by a single committee member. Expedited studies in physical therapy might involve measuring range of motion in a patient group or assessing strength gains following an exercise program using normal subjects.

The IRB conducts a *full* review of

- Research projects that involve more risks than those identified for exempt or expedited review
- Studies of lower-risk procedures in children or the mentally ill who are unable to provide meaningful consent.

Examples of physical therapy studies that would require full review include assessment of the fitness level of patients with cardiovascular disease or a trial of a new exercise program in children with cerebral palsy.

Informed Consent

In the context of research, informed consent refers to an interaction between the researcher and potential participant. The researcher provides the potential subject with the information he or she needs to make an informed decision about whether to participate in the research. The potential subject then makes his or her decision and communicates it to the researcher, usually by either signing or declining to sign a written consent form.

Consent forms must be written in language that is understandable to the individuals who will be giving consent. The typical reading level of participants should be considered, as should visual acuity and native language. A copy of the consent form itself should be provided to the subject. Table 18–3 lists the elements of an informed consent statement, and Figure 18–1 presents a sample consent

TABLE 18–3. Elements of a Consent Form

Statement that the study constitutes research
Explanation of study's purposes
Explanation of basis of subject selection and duration of subject involvement
Explanation of provisions for subject confidentiality
Description of procedures, with experimental procedures identified
Description of risks and discomforts
Description of potential benefits to subjects and others
Description of alternative treatments, if available
Statement of whether compensation is available for injuries
Name of person to contact if questions or injuries arise
Statement emphasizing that participation is voluntary
Statement that the subject has the right to withdraw from the study at any time
Statement of disclosure of information gained in the study that might influence subject's willingness to continue participation
Explanation of payment arrangements, if applicable
Consent statement
Date line
Subject's signature line
Investigator's signature line
Investigator's institutional affiliation and telephone number

University of Anytown
1256 Holt Road
Department of Physical Therapy

Anytown, Indiana 46234
(317) 555-4300

CONSENT TO PARTICIPATE IN A RESEARCH STUDY

TITLE OF STUDY: Comparison of Integrated Electromyographic Activity and Strength Measures in the Supraspinatus Muscle in Two Positions.

You are invited to participate in a research study which measures the electrical activity and strength of the supraspinatus muscle, which is located in the back of the shoulder. You have been invited to participate based on the assumption that you have a shoulder which is free of injury or disability. Your participation would require attendance at a single measurement session lasting approximately one hour.

Prior to your participation, an investigator will take a brief medical history to determine whether you have had previous shoulder problems which would make you ineligible to participate. Weight, height, age, and sex will also be recorded. You will be assigned a subject number so that your name will not be associated with any of the findings of this study.

The research procedure consists of measurement of muscle electrical activity and strength in two positions. The electrical activity of your supraspinatus muscle will be measured by an experienced electromyographer. He will insert a 27-gauge sterile needle containing two fine wire electrodes into your muscle. After positioning the wires, the needle will be removed and the wires will remain in place for testing in both positions. The wires will be removed on completion of data collection in both positions.

Strength will be measured with a hand-held dynamometer, which is a stationary device held by the researcher and placed at the back of your wrist. You will be asked to use your shoulder muscles to push against the device as hard as you can. This will be repeated three times in each of the two positions.

In the first position you will be seated, with your arm straight in front of you with your thumb pointing down. In the second position you will lie on your stomach with your arm out straight in front of you and with your thumb pointing up.

PAGE 1 of 2 __________ (Participant's Initials)

FIGURE 18–1. Example of a consent form.

CONSENT TO PARTICIPATE IN A RESEARCH STUDY (Continued)

TITLE OF STUDY: Comparison of Integrated Electromyographic Activity and Strength Measures in the Supraspinatus Muscle in Two Positions.

The risks of participation in this study include muscle fatigue or soreness from exercise, temporary discomfort from needle insertion, infection from the needle electrode, bleeding from needle insertion, and a small risk of puncture of the chest cavity which could lead to pain, difficulty breathing, and would require medical attention. To protect from infection, sterile needles and electrodes will be used and will be disposed of after each use. To protect from the risk of chest cavity puncture, the electromyographer will use needle placement designed to minimize this risk. If muscle soreness occurs, you will be instructed in procedures to minimize discomfort. No compensation is available for injuries resulting from participation in this research.

By determining the position in which the supraspinatus muscle is most effective, the results of this research may benefit patients and athletes who wish to strengthen their shoulder muscles.

If you have questions about this research or need to report an injury related to your participation in this research, contact xxxxx at (xxx) xxx-xxxx. Your participation in this research is voluntary, and your decision whether or not to participate will not affect your standing at this institution. If you elect to participate in the study, you have the right to withdraw from the study at any time without affecting your standing at the institution. You will receive a copy of this form.

CONSENT

I, ______________________________, voluntarily consent to participate in this research study as described above. I have had a chance to ask questions of the researcher, and have had any questions answered to my satisfaction.

____
Subject Signature

____
Researcher Signature

____
Date

PAGE 2 of 2

FIGURE 18–1 *Continued*

form document. Consent forms may not contain exculpatory language, that is, language that asks subjects to waive any of their legal rights or releases the investigator or institution from liability for negligent acts associated with the research project. Ideally, the form is contained on a single sheet of paper, with front and back sides used as needed. If more pages are needed, they should be numbered "1 of 3," "2 of 3," and the like so that subjects are assured that all the needed information has been received.

The researcher should keep the signed consent forms in a secure location. The length of time the forms are retained depends on the nature and length of the research and on the latency and duration of foreseeable complications related to the research procedures. Researchers should recognize that the signed consent form is usually the only point at which each subject's name is linked to the study. Therefore secure storage of signed consent forms is an important part of maintaining subjects' confidentiality.

There are two general situations in which consent forms are not appropriate. The first is the collection of data via a mailed survey. In this case, the elements of informed consent should be contained within the cover letter written by the researcher to the potential respondent, and return of the questionnaire by the respondent is taken as evidence of consent. The second situation is a study that is of a sensitive nature and signed consent forms would be a means by which the study participants could be identified. In this situation, informed consent should be obtained verbally.

FUNDING

Conducting research is a costly affair. The challenge for researchers is to find funding to support their research interests. Funds generally come from one of four sources: institutions, corporations, foundations, or the government. A review of the first nine months of *Physical Therapy* in 1991 showed that approximately 55% of published research reports were apparently internally funded by the institutions at which they were conducted, 9% were funded by corporations, 11% were funded by foundations, and 25% were funded by government sources.

The small proportion of studies funded externally is evidence of the infancy of physical therapy research. To aid researchers who try to fund studies externally, this section of the chapter presents a typical budget for a research study and then discusses the peculiarities of the four funding sources.

Budget

Table 18–4 presents a budget for a descriptive study that would require data collection by two physical therapists and support services from an aide and one secretary. Personnel costs are determined by estimating the proportion of time each individual would be involved in the study, multiplying the salary by that proportion, and adding a reasonable percentage for benefits. Equipment costs should be estimated, including service and repair costs if appropriate. Consultants are individuals who are not employed by the sponsoring institution, but are engaged on a daily or hourly basis to fulfill a special need of the research project. Statistical, computer, and engineering consultants are examples. The cost of disseminating the results of the research includes the cost of manuscript preparation, the cost of creating photographs and graphs, the cost of slide presentations, and the cost of traveling to conferences to present the research. The overhead costs covering the use of existing facilities is often figured as a percentage of the direct costs. This percentage is often specified by either the funding agency

TABLE 18–4. Research Project Budget

Item	Explanation	Cost
PERSONNEL		
Joyce McWain, PT Principal Investigator	10% time for 1 year, Benefits 20% of salary, Annual salary $42,000.	$ 5040
Randall Myers, PT Coinvestigator	5% time for 6 months, Benefits 20% of salary, Annual salary $42,000.	$ 1260
Ben Riley PT Aide	5% time for 6 months, Benefits 20% of salary, Annual salary $16,000.	$ 480
Sally Knapp Secretary	5% time for 6 months, Benefits 20% of salary, Annual salary $18,000.	$ 540
EQUIPMENT		
Hand-held dynamometers	Two at $600 each	$ 1200
CONSULTANTS		
Statistician	20 hours at $40/hour	$ 800
DISSEMINATION		
Photocopying	1000 pages at $.05 per page	$ 50
Photography	Black and whites, $100 Slides, 40 at $10 each	$ 500
Travel	Principal investigator and coinvestigator to annual conference, $1300 each	$ 2600
OVERHEAD	8% of $12470	$ 998
TOTAL		$13,468

or the institution in which the research is conducted.

Institution Funding

As already mentioned, much of physical therapy research is funded by the institution in which it is conducted. Department managers who believe in research as an essential element of professionalism may allow staff to conduct limited amounts of research on work time. However, because research time does not produce revenue like patient care does, even the most research-oriented managers have difficulty releasing therapists from patient care to perform research. If the study budgeted in Table 18–4 was funded internally, the therapists might be able to reduce expenditures by doing the clerical work and data collection on their own time and by using their prebudgeted continuing education money for conference travel.

Corporation Funding

A corporation may fund a research project directly through its operating funds or indirectly through a grant from a foundation associated with the company, discussed next.

When a corporation provides research funds through direct giving, it is usually to support activities directly related to the corporation's function. For example, equipment manufacturers may be willing to provide equipment for and pay the salaries of researchers who are conducting studies that showcase their products. Some manufacturers are willing to loan equipment for the duration of a project; many students, who typically conduct research on a shoestring budget, have obtained loaner equipment simply by writing a letter of inquiry to the manufacturer or a local sales representative.

Researchers who accept funds directly from corporations need to be sure they understand who has control of the data and its dissemination. A corporation may wish to retain ownership of the data so that it has the prerogative of not releasing any data that are not favorable toward their product. Researchers who contact companies for support must decide whether they are willing to accept such terms, should the company request them.

Foundation Funding

Foundations are private entities that distribute funds according to the priorities set by their donors or their board of trustees. There are many types of foundations; how to identify those that may be interested in your proposal and how to apply for funds from a foundation are discussed below.

Types of Foundations. Foundations that provide research grants can be broadly divided into independent, company-sponsored, and community foundations. The funds of an independent foundation usually come from a single source, such as a family, an individual, or a group of individuals. Independent foundations give grants in fields specified by the few individuals who administer the fund; giving is often limited to the local geographic region in which the fund is located. The major independent foundation that supports physical therapy research is the Foundation for Physical Therapy. This foundation is associated with the American Physical Therapy Association but is not sponsored by them. Donors are those with interests in the physical therapy community, for example, individual physical therapists, equipment manufacturers and vendors, academic programs of physical therapy, and private physical therapy practices.

A company-sponsored foundation is an independent entity that is funded by contributions from a company. Although the foundation is independent from the corporation, it tends to give grants in fields related to the company's products or customers. Giving is often limited to the geographic region or regions in which the company is located.

Community foundations are publicly supported by funds derived from many donors. The mission of a community foundation is to meet the needs of its locale; thus the projects it funds must be directly related to the welfare of the community.

Identifying Foundations. Large institutions supported by several grant agencies have grants administration officers who can help researchers identify appropriate funding sources. The Foundation Center, a nonprofit organization, publishes comprehensive references that can also help researchers identify foundations that fund studies in their area of interest.[6–8] These references are available in most university or public libraries. The information provided for each foundation includes the size of the fund, the amount given annually, the names of agencies to whom funds were given, and the types of projects funded (scholarships, construction of new facilities, education, or research). Several specialized indexes focus on funding projects in health or health-related areas such as aging.[9, 10]

Applying for Foundation Funds. The procedure for applying for foundation funds varies greatly from foundation to foundation. Funding decisions in independent foundations may rest with a very few individuals. Consequently, applying for funds is relatively informal. A letter of inquiry describing the research in general terms should be sent to the foundation. Ways in which the research meets the goals of the foundation should be emphasized. The reply from the foundation will indicate whether the idea is appealing to them and will ask for additional information if it is. The additional information required is likely to be fairly brief and can be assembled in a format determined by the researcher.

Corporate-sponsored foundations often have more formalized grant application procedures. However, the letter of inquiry is still the first means by which the researcher contacts the foundation. If the general area of the research is within the scope of the foundation's activities, the foundation will respond with directions for formal application for funds.

Government Funding

The federal government is a major provider of research grants in the United States. Table 18–5 lists the government agencies that provide funding for health sciences research.[11] Several references provide detailed information about the grant programs of the federal government.[12–14] The sources of government funds for studies published in *Physical Therapy* in 1991, in decreasing order of frequency, were as follows:

- National Institutes of Health
- Maternal and Child Health
- National Institute for Disability and Rehabilitation Research
- Department of Education
- Veterans Administration

The procedure for obtaining federal grant funding is far more formal than that for obtaining foundation funding. First, the grant funds must be made available. To do this, Congress must both authorize the grant-funding program and then, in a separate legislative step, appropriate funds for the program. Administration of appropriated funds is delegated to a large grants administration bureaucracy in Washington, DC. When funds are appropriated for a grant program, notice is placed in the *Federal Register*, the daily federal government news publication. Once notice is placed in the register, application materials can be released to potential grant recipients. Applications are highly formalized, and grant applicants must certify that they are in compliance with a variety of federal regulations related to nondiscrimination and protection of human subjects. Although the process is formalized, the individuals who direct the various grant programs are available to discuss the application process with grant writers.

The awarding of federal grants is usually accomplished by a peer review committee. Experienced researchers are assembled to review the submitted proposals and make recommendations about their disposition. Often

TABLE 18–5. Federal Government Funding Sources for Health Research*

Agency
Department of Health and Human Services
Administration on Aging
Agency for Health Care Policy and Research
Centers for Disease Control
Maternal and Child Health
National Institute for Occupational Safety and Health
National Institutes of Health
National Heart, Lung, and Blood Institute
National Institute of Arthritis and Musculoskeletal and Skin Diseases
National Institute of Child Health and Human Development
National Institute of Neurological Disorders and Stroke
National Institute on Aging
National Science Foundation
Department of Education
National Institute for Disability and Rehabilitation Research
Veterans Administration

*Compiled from information presented in *Capturing Research Dollars: Strategies for Physical Therapy Researchers.* Workshop notebook. Alexandria, Va: American Physical Therapy Association; 1991:2–2 to 2–4.

only one or two reviewers read the entire proposal; the rest of the committee members read only the abstract of the study and hear the primary reviewers' descriptions and evaluations of the program. It is therefore imperative that the abstract of the grant proposal accurately reflect the scope of the project for which funding is sought. Detailed guidelines for preparation of federal research grant proposals are available.[1, 15]

Federal grant proposals will have one of three outcomes: approval with funding, approval without funding, or disapproval. A proposal is disapproved if the study does not meet the purpose of the grant or its design is not acceptable. Proposals that meet the technical requirements are approved and given a certain priority level. Only those with the highest priority level are funded.

SUMMARY

A research proposal is a blueprint for a study, specifying the investigators, research problem, purposes, methods, references, methods of dissemination of results, budget, and work plan. Research proposals must be approved by facility administrators, an academic committee, or an IRB. The role of the IRB is to ensure that the investigators have put into place procedures needed to safeguard the rights of their subjects. Research proposals are also used to secure funding for the study. Major sources of funding include institutions, corporations, foundations, and the government. Increasing levels of formalization of the grant application and award process are exerted as the research moves from institutional funding to government funding. Many private foundations and government agencies sponsor research that is of interest to physical therapists.

References

1. Krathwohl DR. *How to Prepare a Research Proposal.* 3rd ed. Syracuse, NY: Syracuse University Press; 1988.
2. Brink PJ, Wood MJ. *Basic Steps in Planning Nursing Research: From Question to Proposal.* Boston, Mass: Jones & Bartlett Publishers; 1988.
3. Appelbaum PS, Lidz DW, Meisel A. *Informed Consent: Legal Theory and Clinical Practice.* New York, NY: Oxford University Press; 1987.
4. Greenwald RA, Ryan MK, Mulvihill JE, eds. *Human Subjects Research: A Handbook for Institutional Review Boards.* New York, NY: Plenum Press; 1982.
5. Levine RJ. *Ethics and Regulation of Clinical Research.* 2nd ed. Baltimore, Md: Urban & Schwarzenberg; 1986.
6. *The Foundation Grants Index.* 19th ed. New York, NY: Foundation Center; 1990.
7. *National Data Book of Foundations.* 14th ed. New York, NY: Foundation Center; 1990.
8. *Corporate Foundation Profiles.* 5th ed. New York, NY: Foundation Center; 1988.
9. *National Guide to Funding in Aging.* New York, NY: The Foundation Center; 1989.
10. *National Guide to Funding in Health.* New York, NY: Foundation Center; 1988.
11. *Capturing Grant Dollars: Strategies for Physical Therapy Researchers.* Workshop notebook. Alexandria, Va: American Physical Therapy Association; 1991.
12. *Catalog of Federal Domestic Assistance.* Washington, DC: US Government Printing Office.
13. *Annual Register of Grant Support.* Chicago, Ill: Marquis Academic Media; 1992.
14. *Directory of Research Grants.* Phoenix, Ariz: Oryx Press; 1992.
15. Reif-Lehrer L. *Writing a Successful Grant Application.* 2nd ed. Boston, Mass: Jones & Bartlett Publishers; 1989.

CHAPTER 19

Project Implementation

Obtaining Subjects
Inpatient recruitment
Outpatient recruitment
Recruitment of the lay public
Recruitment of subjects for survey research
Data Collection Tools
Biophysiological instruments
Interviews
Questionnaires
Data Collection
Biophysiological data collection
Interview data collection
Questionnaire data collection
Data Analysis
Data coding
Data entry
Statistical analysis

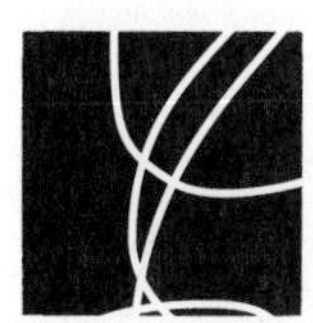

After obtaining approval and funding for a proposal, the researcher is ready to implement the project. This chapter presents guidelines for implementing all phases of a research project, from subject selection to data analysis. Methods of obtaining subjects are discussed first, followed by the development and use of research instrumentation, including biophysiological measurement tools, interviews, and questionnaires. Tips for managing data collection and recording are then presented, and the chapter ends with suggestions for data analysis, including guidelines for using computer statistical programs and statistical consultants. Additional guidelines for these steps may be found in a series of articles published in the *American Journal of Physical Medicine and Rehabilitation.*[1–3]

OBTAINING SUBJECTS

The time and effort required to obtain research subjects are often far greater than the researcher anticipates. For example, assume that we wish to implement a study of elderly patients who have undergone total knee arthroplasty. We plan to study two groups who undergo different inpatient and outpatient postoperative rehabilitation. Measurement of certain outcomes will be taken at discharge, three months postoperatively, and six months postoperatively. If we know that 100 such surgeries are performed in a six-month period at our facility, we may assume that there will be no difficulty obtaining two study groups of 40 subjects each for our study. Table 19–1 shows, however, several ways in which the number of available subjects will be far fewer than the 100 patients who undergo the surgery. If the scenario in Table 19–1 were realized, we would be faced with a situation in which fewer than 20 subjects were avail-

TABLE 19–1. Eventual Sample from a Potential 100 Patients

Reason for Participation or Nonparticipation	Number	Number Remaining
Total knee arthroplasties performed in six months	100	100
Young patient with hemophilia	3	97
Patient with perioperative complications	5	92
Patient lives more than 60 miles away or has received outpatient physical therapy at another clinic	10	82
Patient's surgeon does not wish to participate	12	70
Patient does not consent to be in study	10	60
Patient does not complete outpatient physical therapy	12	48
Patient dies before six-month visit	2	46
Patient moves or cannot be located to schedule six-month appointment	4	42
Patient does not come to the scheduled six-month follow-up appointment	6	36

able per group during the six months in which subjects were to be recruited.

Researchers need to plan their subject recruitment strategy carefully to ensure an adequate number of subjects. Different strategies are appropriate when recruiting inpatients, outpatients, or the general public. In all cases, recruitment of subjects should take place after an institutional review board has approved both the conduct of the study and the procedures to be used for ensuring the informed consent of participants.

Inpatient Recruitment

In the inpatient setting, the admitting physician is clearly in control of the care that the patient receives while in the hospital. Thus, securing inpatients for study requires careful work with the medical staff of the institution. In fact, the best way to secure subjects for study is to invite key physicians to collaborate with you in the entire research endeavor. Typically, the chain of command for securing permission to use particular inpatients proceeds from the medical director of rehabilitation services, to the chief physician of the particular service, to the individual admitting physician.

After securing the permission of the admitting physician, the researcher contacts subjects directly to secure their informed consent. As with all subject recruitment methods, patients must be approached in a manner that conveys that regardless of whether they choose to participate, their care will not be prejudiced. The physical therapist and physician should determine together the best procedure for securing patient consent: The physician may mention the study to the patients first and indicate that the therapist will be around with details; the therapist may accompany the physicians on rounds so that they can jointly present the study to patients, assuring them that the different professionals are working together on the research endeavor; or the therapist may present the study first, giving patients the opportunity to discuss the study later with the physician before consenting.

Outpatient Recruitment

Outpatient recruitment is somewhat easier than inpatient recruitment because permission of the patient's physician is not always necessary. If a descriptive, correlational, or methodological study is being conducted that does not involve any procedures contraindicated by the current orders of the patient, the researcher can feel free to proceed without obtaining the individual physician's consent. As is the case with inpatients, it is wise to inform the physicians of the ongoing project, so that they will not be alarmed if patients tell them that they have participated in a research study.

After the study, it is courteous to send the physicians of subjects who participated a summary of the study results, along with your assessment of how the results will allow you to serve their patients better in the future. Alternatively, collaboration with physicians may prove rewarding for both physicians and therapists while having the added benefit of providing therapists with easier access to some subjects.

If the research protocol requires a departure from a physician's orders, then permission must be sought and gained from both the physician and the patient, as described in Inpatient Recruitment. Again, collaboration or communication with the physicians about the study results may make them more willing to have their patients participate in future studies.

Recruitment of patients who have completed their course of treatment requires careful consideration of the confidentiality of their medical records. Consider a case where a university-based researcher contacts a clinic to request access to patient records to identify subjects who meet certain inclusion criteria. The clinic, being interested in the project, agrees to participate in the study and provides the researcher with the names and addresses of patients with the particular diagnosis. Patients would have good reason to be concerned about breaches of confidentiality if they received a letter from an unknown researcher requesting their participation in a study based on the fact that they had had a certain surgery and were seen for treatment at a certain clinic. A procedure that protects patient privacy may involve having a clinic employee—who already has access to the clinic records—write a letter to eligible patients explaining the study and asking for their permission to release their name and address to the researcher. A form letter (and stamped return envelope) on which patients indicate their willingness to have their name released to the investigator can be included with the letter.

Recruitment of the Lay Public

When a study requires the participation of the lay public rather than patients, researchers are challenged by the need to balance their desire for convenient access to a particular group of subjects with their hope that results will be generalizable beyond the particular sample studied. In the past, this balance has often been lacking: Use of physical therapy students as a convenient source of subjects has limited the generalizability of many studies to young, healthy women, who make up the majority of physical therapy students.

Groups that consist of individuals with a wide range of educational, racial, and socioeconomic characteristics are desirable for many studies. If one works in a large organization, recruiting subjects from employees at all levels—from upper administration to maintenance staff—often provides the sort of variety that is desired.

Researchers who require specific types of subjects need to be creative in identifying existing groups from which to recruit. Examples of groups that may yield good subject pools for certain populations include churches, senior citizen or retirement centers, apartment complexes, health clubs, day care centers, and youth or adult sport leagues. For example, if one wished to study balance in the well elderly, subjects might be found in church groups, senior bowling leagues, residential retirement centers, or senior citizen centers with daytime programs. The choice of which group to use would depend on the contact the researcher has with members of the groups and how seriously biased the group membership is in light of the particular research question. For instance, if a researcher's great-aunt bowls three days a week in a senior league, she might be able to recruit plenty of subjects for a balance study. However, if the researcher believes that the senior bowlers would be biased in the direction of better balance than most of the well elderly, the bowling league may not be a good choice, no matter how easy it would be to obtain subjects from the group.

Once a researcher has determined that a particular group is suitable for study, the appropriate administrative approval is needed—be it from the director of personnel, the manager of the bowling alley, the pastor of the church, or the administrator of the retirement center. When seeking such approval, the researcher needs to prepare a brief version of the study proposal, written in terms understandable to the person whose approval is sought. A blank consent form should be included along with documentation of the institutional review board approval. To gain administrative approval, the researcher will need to convince the official that the study has value; that participation in the study will not greatly disrupt the facility's routine; that subjects are at minimal risk of harm and will be treated with dignity and respect; and, if appropriate, that subjects may enjoy participation and the interaction with others that it affords.

Once administrative approval has been given to recruit subjects from a particular facility, the researcher needs to make initial contact with potential subjects. This may be done by discussing the study at a group meeting, writing letters to particular potential subjects, or posting flyers in areas frequented by the members of the desired group. Whatever the format, this initial information should include the purpose of the study, the actual activities in which the subject would be participating, the time commitment required to participate, and the means by which interested parties can contact the researcher.

Recruitment of Subjects for Survey Research

When survey research is accomplished through interview, the researcher must contact the subjects to determine their willingness to participate. One way is a letter of introduction, with a return postcard on which subjects indicate their willingness to participate and the means by which the researcher should set up the interview. Another way is a telephone call to prospective subjects in which the purpose of the study and the nature of participation that is desired are described and an interview is scheduled if the potential subject agrees to participate.

When the survey data are collected through a mailed questionnaire, potential subjects can often be identified from the mailing lists of various groups. Mailing labels of member addresses are available from sources such as professional associations. For example, if one is interested in physical therapists' opinions on a certain topic, then purchasing mailing labels from the American Physical Therapy Association or state physical therapist licensing agencies may be indicated. Some groups that sell mailing labels will not do so until they have had an opportunity to inspect a copy of the material to be sent.

Once the individuals to whom a questionnaire will be sent are identified, it is the researcher's job to sell them on the idea of completing the questionnaire. The cover letter that accompanies the survey is the sales tool. It must be attractive, be brief but complete, and provide potential respondents with a good reason to complete the study. Figures 19–1 and 19–2 provide two examples of cover letters annotated with comments on their good and bad points. Suggestions for construction of the survey instrument itself are included in the next section.

October 8, 1991

(A) Dear Program Director:

(B) We are students in the master's degree program in physical therapy at the University of Anytown. For our research project we are studying the content of physical therapy
(C) curriculums in geriatrics to determine whether enough attention is paid to geriatrics education for physical therapists. Please complete this survey and return it to us
(D) at the following address by October 15, 1991:

University of Anytown
(E) 1256 Holt Road
Anytown, IN 46234

(F) Thank you for your participation. If you would like a summary of the results, please write your name and address on the last page of the survey.

Sincerely,

(G)

(H) Jodi Beeker — Physical Therapy Student

Jonathon Mills — Physical Therapy Student

FIGURE 19–1. Example of a poor cover letter for a questionnaire. (A) There is no personalization of greeting to potential respondents. (B) When the first sentence indicates that the researchers are students, potential respondents may assume that the research is being done only because it is required. (C) The second sentence indicates a bias on the part of the researchers. (D) Because of the early return date, the potential respondents might not receive the questionnaire until 1 or 2 days before the deadline. (E) The researchers have obviously not included a self-addressed, stamped return envelope and are asking potential respondents to bear part of the cost of the study. (F) The mechanism for respondents to indicate their interest in the study results destroys the anonymity of the questionnaire. (G) Lack of signatures (or photocopied signatures) indicates an impersonal approach to potential respondents. (H) There is no way, other than through the mail, to contact the student researchers if the potential respondent has questions about the study.

(A) **University of Anytown**
1256 Holt Road
Department of Physical Therapy

Anytown, Indiana 46234
(317) 555-4300

October 8, 1991

Elizabeth Domholdt, PT, EdD
Dean, Krannert Graduate School of Physical Therapy
University of Indianapolis
1400 E. Hanna Avenue
Indianapolis, IN 46227

(B) Dear Dr. Domholdt:

(C) We are requesting your participation in a survey of physical therapy programs in the United States to determine the characteristics of geriatric education within physical therapy curriculums. We know that directors of physical therapy education programs are faced with dilemmas about the breadth and depth of content that should be included in today's overcrowded physical therapy curriculums. We believe that a compilation of information about geriatrics curriculum content will be helpful to physical therapy (D) educators as they determine the amount of emphasis they wish to place on geriatric education within their own curriculums.

(E) In pilot testing, the enclosed questionnaire took an average of less than 10 minutes to complete. We would greatly appreciate your time in completing the questionnaire and (F) returning it in the enclosed envelope by **November 8, 1991**. If you would like a copy of the results, please complete the enclosed postcard and return it separately from the (G) questionnaire.

Thank you in advance for your consideration. If you have any questions or concerns about the study, please feel free to contact any of us at the address or telephone numbers listed.

Sincerely,

(H) Jodi Beeker — Jon Mills — Jan Woolery

Jodi Beeker	Jon Mills	Jan Woolery, PT, PhD
PT Student	PT Student	Associate Professor
(I) (317) 555-4321	(317) 555-6789	(317) 555-4378

FIGURE 19–2. Example of a good cover letter for a questionnaire. (A) Letterhead paper is used to indicate affiliation of the researchers. (B) The greeting is personalized. (C) Introductory paragraph is neutral on the subject matter. (D) The last sentence of the introductory paragraph indicates the usefulness of findings; this provides a reason for completing the questionnaire. (E) The time required of respondents is indicated. (F) The return date gives respondents a few weeks to reply. (G) The mechanism for obtaining survey results does not violate the anonymity of responses. (H) Signing each cover letter individually provides a personal touch. (I) Telephone numbers for students and the name and telephone number of a responsible faculty member provide a mechanism by which potential respondents can contact them about the survey.

DATA COLLECTION TOOLS

The three major classes of data collection tools used by physical therapists are biophysiological instruments, interviews, and questionnaires. Chapter 12 presents basic information about many different types of measuring tools appropriate for use by physical therapy researchers. This section provides specific suggestions for the use or development of the three classes of data collection tools.

Biophysiological Instruments

Physical therapists who use biophysiological measuring equipment in their studies often prefer to use existing tools rather than developing new ones. If appropriate equipment is not available, an engineer, carpenter, or electrician may be able to help the physical therapist fabricate a device that will meet the needs of the study.

When using existing instrumentation, the researcher must be familiar with both the manufacturer's instructions for use of the equipment and the protocols that other researchers have followed with the equipment. From this information, decisions can be made about the procedures for data collection. Although a general procedure for data collection will have been developed for the research proposal, very detailed procedural guidelines should be established and written down so that they can be implemented uniformly within the study. For example, a procedure such as height measurement seems simple and would not require detailed description in a proposal. However, before data collection is begun, the specific procedure for taking the height measurement should be developed: Will the measurement be taken with subjects barefoot, stocking-footed, or in shoes? Will subjects be instructed to stand comfortably or stand tall? Should the head be comfortably erect or in military axial extension? Written standardization procedures are particularly important if more than one researcher will be measuring subjects.

Accuracy checks of the equipment should be conducted, if necessary. Goniometer scales can be checked against known angles, scales can be checked against known weights, and calibration of equipment can be accomplished according to manufacturer's instructions. In some instances, the researcher may wish to have an engineer or manufacturer's technician give the equipment a mechanical or electrical checkout to determine that it is operating properly before data are collected.

Interviews

Physical therapists who use interviews to collect data generally ask questions that they have developed themselves. The researcher must decide whether structured, semistructured, or unstructured interviews are appropriate based on the nature of information desired.

A *structured interview* is essentially an oral administration of a written questionnaire. When a surveyor stops you in the shopping mall to determine whether you have purchased a certain brand of facial tissue within the last six weeks, he or she is using a structured interview. The surveyor asks the same questions of everyone and does not deviate from the wording in the question. Structured interviews are most appropriate when relatively factual information is sought.

Semistructured interviews are based on predeveloped questions, but the format permits the interviewer to clarify questions to help the subject provide more information for the study. Semistructured interviews are appropriate when information of a somewhat abstract nature is sought.

Unstructured interviewing is used frequently by researchers who have adopted the qualitative research paradigm for a particular study. In an unstructured interview, the researcher has a general idea of the topics that should be covered during the interview. However, the order and way in which the topics are covered are left to the interviewer as he or she interacts with subjects. Unstructured interviews are particularly appropriate when the purpose of the research is to determine the opinions and beliefs of the subjects.

Whichever style of interviewing is used, the researcher must consider several common concerns. First, the interviewer's vocabulary must match that of the individuals being interviewed. Second, interviewers must be sensitive to the meaning of specific words that they use. For example, if interviewing therapists who are members of racial or ethnic groups about their experiences as minority professionals, the interviewers should determine subjects' preferences for identifying terms such as *black* versus *African-American, American Indian* versus *Native American,* and *Latino* versus *Hispanic*.

Third, interviewers must do what they can to establish rapport and make the interviewee comfortable. Friendly chit-chat and social conventions such as talking about the weather, taking coats, offering coffee or soft drinks, and the like can all be used to place the subject at ease in the research situation. The interviewees' comfort may be enhanced if the interview takes place on their turf—their office, their home, or a public place of their choosing.

Fourth, interviewers must ensure that subjects give their informed consent to participate in the interview. The interviewer should specify the purposes of the study, emphasize the provisions for confidentiality of responses, and make it clear that the subject can terminate the interview at any time. If the researcher is going to audio- or video-tape the interview, the subject needs additional assurances about the provisions for confidentiality of the recorded information. In survey research conducted using interviews, the primary risk to the subject is often the breach of confidentiality; informed consent is therefore often accomplished verbally rather than in writing so there is no written record of the names of those who participated in the study.

Questionnaires

Researchers who use a questionnaire as their data collection tool may use a standardized instrument, a modification of a standardized instrument, or a new instrument they design themselves. Because many survey research topics require unique information, researchers frequently develop their own questionnaire for use in a particular study. There are five basic steps to questionnaire development: drafting, expert review, first revision, pilot test, and final revision.

Drafting

The first step in developing a questionnaire is to draft items for consideration for inclusion in the questionnaire. Different types of items are discussed in Chapter 12. Before writing any items, the researcher needs to reexamine the purposes of the study and outline the major sections the questionnaire needs to include to answer the questions under study. Researchers seem to have an almost irresistible urge to ask questions because they seem interesting, without knowing how the answers will be used. This lengthens the questionnaire and may decrease the number of subjects who respond. Several authors have provided specific suggestions for questionnaire design and format.[4–6]

Even for the first draft, the researcher must begin to consider issues of format and comprehensibility. The items in a questionnaire are often divided into topical groups to break the questionnaire into more easily digestible parts. In addition, because different topics may require items with different formats, the section headings provide for a transition between different types of items. Some recommend that easier items be placed first on the questionnaire, with more difficult items presented later. The thought behind this is that the easy initial questions will get respondents interested in the questionnaire so that they will follow through with the more difficult questions that come later. For similar reasons, some recommend that demographic questions come last. It is thought that completing the demographic questions first will either bore respondents or offend them with questions about sensitive areas such as salary.

The readability of the type used in the questionnaire is important. The smallest readable type is generally considered to be 10-point type. Twelve-point type is more readable and is probably preferable for most questionnaires. If the population is expected to have difficulty with vision or if reading skills are likely to be low, 14-point type may be useful. The drawback of larger type is that the questionnaire physically becomes longer.

The type style is also important; researchers should not use atypical styles that may be difficult to read. With the widespread availability of personal computers and low-cost desktop publishing services, any researcher should be able to produce an attractive, inviting questionnaire at a reasonable cost.

A second aspect of readability is the reading level required to understand the questionnaire. College-educated researchers are so accustomed to reading and writing that they forget that their writing is likely to be at an academic level that many will not be able to comprehend easily. To increase readability, researchers should write clearly and avoid jargon.

The instructions on how to complete the survey also must be extremely clear and specific (for example, "Check one box," "Circle as many items as apply," and "Write in your age in years at your last birthday"). If the same format of questions is used throughout a questionnaire, the instructions need be given only once. If the format of questions changes from item to item, instructions should be provided for each item.

Researchers designing questionnaires must decide whether to include space for data coding on the questionnaire itself. Data coding is used to turn answers to questions into numbers suitable for analysis. Figure 19–3 shows an example of a questionnaire page with a data-coding column completed.[7] Some researchers do not like to include a data-coding column on questionnaires because they believe it is distracting to the respondent and takes up unnecessary space.

The researcher must also consider format and printing decisions such as the color of paper, the size and arrangement of pages, and the amount of white space on the questionnaire. The color of paper should be fairly light to ensure good readability. Good-quality paper should be used because it is the first means by which the potential respondent determines whether the questionnaire is worth responding to. One format that has been recommended is a booklet.[6] A four-page questionnaire could be made by printing on both sides of a single sheet of 11″ × 17″ paper and folding it in half to make an 8½″ × 11″ booklet. One benefit of such a booklet is that because multiple sheets of paper are not needed, none will inadvertently get separated from one another. Another benefit is that the familiar booklet form should lead to fewer skipped questions; if single pages are printed front and back and stapled together, the reverse side of one sheet may be omitted by some respondents. The booklet may also have the appearance of being more professional, thereby increasing the return rate for the study.

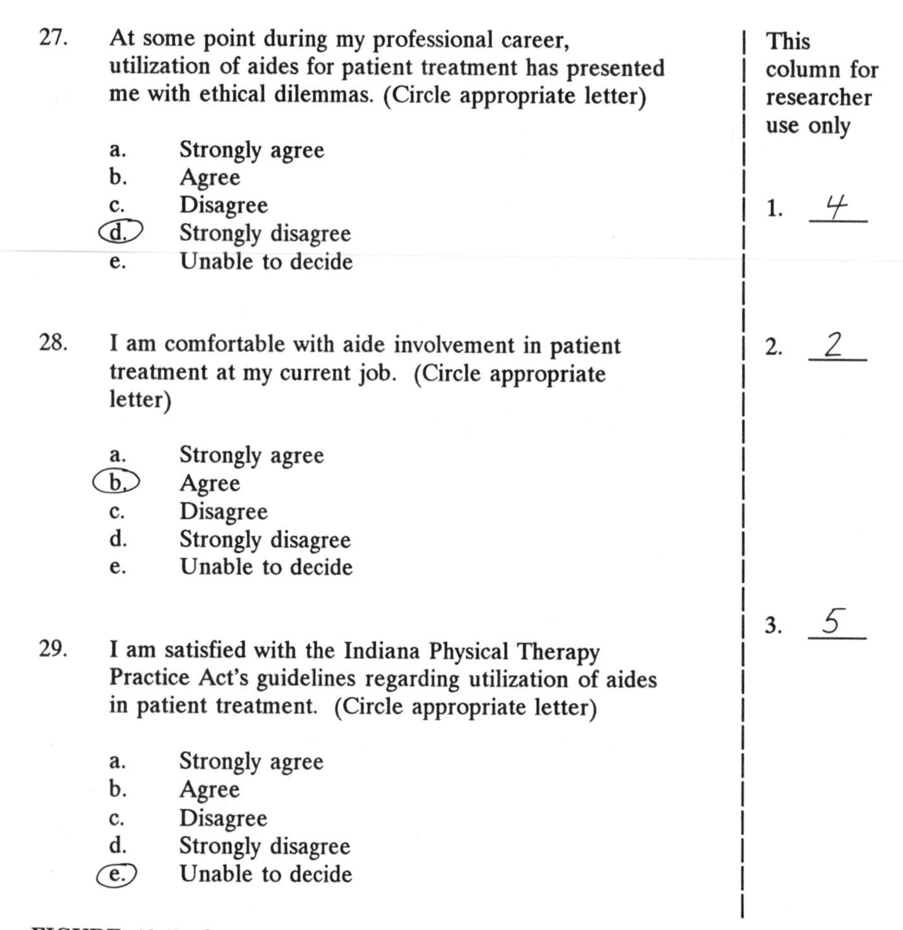

27. At some point during my professional career, utilization of aides for patient treatment has presented me with ethical dilemmas. (Circle appropriate letter)

a. Strongly agree
b. Agree
c. Disagree
d. Strongly disagree
e. Unable to decide

28. I am comfortable with aide involvement in patient treatment at my current job. (Circle appropriate letter)

a. Strongly agree
b. Agree
c. Disagree
d. Strongly disagree
e. Unable to decide

29. I am satisfied with the Indiana Physical Therapy Practice Act's guidelines regarding utilization of aides in patient treatment. (Circle appropriate letter)

a. Strongly agree
b. Agree
c. Disagree
d. Strongly disagree
e. Unable to decide

This column for researcher use only

1. 4

2. 2

3. 5

FIGURE 19–3. Questionnaire excerpt, with coding column. The circled letters are converted to numbers before data entry.

Expert Review

Once the draft is written the researcher needs to undertake the second step in questionnaire development: subjecting the questionnaire to review by a colleague knowledgeable about the topic under study. This is essentially a check for content validity. Did the colleague think that all the important elements of the constructs under study were addressed? Were questions understandable? Were terms defined satisfactorily? In addition to providing feedback on the content of the questionnaire, a colleague can also assess the format of the questionnaire.

First Revision

After the expert review, the researcher makes revisions in the questionnaire based on the expert's feedback. If the colleague you selected made no recommendations for change, you probably need to find another more critical colleague to review your work.

Pilot Test

The next step is to pilot test the instrument on the types of subjects who will complete the questionnaire. When pilot testing, it is useful to have subjects indicate the time it took them to complete the questionnaire. The final item on the pilot questionnaire should be a request for the subjects to review the questionnaire and write any comments they might have about the nature and format of the items.

When the pilot surveys are returned, the researcher should determine the return rate of the questionnaires and look for troublesome response patterns. For example, if only 40% of the pilot subjects return questionnaires, then the researcher should not expect a better return rate from actual subjects. The researcher should attempt to determine the reasons for nonresponse to the pilot survey so that corrective measures can be taken on the final questionnaire.

Patterns to be looked for among responses to the pilot testing are missing responses, lack of range in responses, and many "other" responses or extraneous comments. For example, if one used several Likert-scale items and one was always answered "strongly agree," this may mean the item was worded so positively that no reasonable person would ever disagree with the statement. Rewording should create an item that is more likely to elicit a range of responses. Assume that the purpose of a survey is to determine physical therapists' attitudes toward long-term care of the elderly. An item worded "Quality long-term care for the elderly is an important component of the health care system in the United States" would be difficult to disagree with. Rewording the item to read "Funding for long-term care of the elderly should take priority over funding for public education" requires the respondent to make choices between funding priorities and would likely elicit a greater range of responses.

An item repeatedly left unanswered may indicate that placement of the item on the page is a problem, the item is so sensitive that people do not wish to answer it, or the item is so complicated that it takes too much energy to answer it. A multiple-choice item frequently responded to with "other" may indicate that the choices given were too limited.

Final Revision

Rewording of items, elimination of items, addition of items, or revision of the questionnaire format may all be indicated by the results of the pilot study. If a great many problems were identified in the pilot study, the researcher may wish to retest the questionnaire on a small group of subjects before investing the money and time in the final questionnaire.

DATA COLLECTION

When collecting data, the researcher needs to take steps to ensure quality and completeness. Although specific suggestions for data collection are provided in the following sections, all researchers must consider the overriding concern of the safety of data that have been collected. Briefcases get lost, cars get stolen, hard disks crash, dogs chew, and buildings can be destroyed by fires or floods. Given the many possible disasters that can threaten one's data, it makes sense to maintain backup copies of the information one has collected. If the data are collected and stored on computer disk, make a backup copy of the disk. If the data are collected on handwritten forms, either make copies of the completed forms or transfer the information to a data file soon after collecting it.

The two copies of the data should be stored in two different locations; it does no good to have two copies of the data if both are in the same file that was stored directly under the pipe that burst. If several researchers collaborate with one another, then different researchers should probably keep the data in different locations. If there is a single investigator, one copy can be kept at work or school and one at home.

Biophysiological Data Collection

Specific considerations for biophysiological data collection include subject identification, design of data collection forms, pilot study, and scheduling of subjects and personnel.

Subject Identification

When each subject enters the trial, he or she should be assigned a number and, if appropriate, a study group according to one of the plans developed in Chapter 8. A master list specifying each subject's name, address, and phone number; study identification number; and group membership should be maintained. If data recorders and subjects are blind to group membership, generally only one researcher has access to the master list. This researcher should keep the master list in a secure location where other researchers will not accidentally come across the information; a second copy should be kept separately from the original copy.

Data Recording Forms

Researchers must design forms for data collection. Today, the form may be a pen-and-paper form or one that is filled out directly on the computer. The form should contain space for each subject's identification number but not name, to ensure confidentiality of the information. The order of items on the form should be carefully considered to coincide with the order in which the information will be collected. Adequate space should be left for a readable response to the information.

In general, the information should be collected at the highest measurement level possible. For example, adult ages should be recorded as age at last birthday. Even if the researcher plans to categorize subjects into age groups, such as those younger than 60 and those 60 and older, it is wise to collect the information as actual age and then code it into groups. In this way, if a later research question requires actual age, that information is available. If just the group membership (<60 or ≥ 60) is recorded originally, then there is no way to later determine subjects' actual ages.

If data require coding (for example, conversion of letters into numbers and collapse of actual ages into age groups) for analysis, the form should be designed to facilitate the coding process. Figure 19–4 shows a completed data collection form with space for data coding for the hypothetical total knee arthroplasty study described in the statistics chapters of this text. The blank spaces on the right-hand side of the form are for the pieces of information that will be entered in the computer data file (see Tables 13–1 and 13–2). Some information such as the date and the name of the therapist collecting the data may not be relevant to the final data set, but may be useful to have if there is a question about a piece of information. For two of the deformity variables, actual angular value is reduced to a category; however, there is room on the form for both the actual value and the code that corresponds to the category in which the angular value belongs.

Pilot Study

A pilot study is crucial to the smooth running of a research trial. In a pilot study, the researchers go through a dress-rehearsal of the research study, using a few volunteers similar to those who will participate in the study. The pilot study allows the researchers to take care of small glitches in the procedure

TOTAL KNEE ARTHROPLASTY REHABILITATION STUDY

BACKGROUND INFORMATION

Case Number (CN) 1 5

Clinic Attended (CL)
1 = Community Hospital
2 = Memorial Hospital
3 = Religious Hospital
2

Patient Sex (SEX)
0 = Male
1 = Female
1

Patient Age in years at last birthday (AGE) 6 8

Type of Prosthesis (PRO)
1 = Total condylar
2 = Posterior stabilizer
3 = Flat tibial plateau
2

Miscellaneous Information
Surgeon Bennett
Side of Surgery (R)
Date of Surgery 2-12-92
Diagnosis OA

THREE WEEK POSTOPERATIVE DATA

Date 3-5-92

Three-week ROM, degrees (W3R) 0 7 6
Therapist BD

SIX WEEK POSTOPERATIVE DATA

Date 3-25-92

Therapist BD

Six-week ROM, degrees (W6R) 0 7 0

SIX MONTH POSTOPERATIVE DATA

Date 8-15-92

Six-month ROM, degrees (M6R) 0 9 5

Six-month Extension Torque, N•m (E) 1 7 0

OVER

FIGURE 19–4. Data collection form, with coding column.
Illustration continued on following page

Six-Month Flexion Torque, N•m (F) 1 0 2

Gait Velocity, cm/s (V) 1 6 5

Flexion Contracture at Six Months (DFC)

Value 8°

1 = >15 degrees
(2 =) 6 to 15 degrees
3 = 0 to 5 degrees

2

Varus/Valgus Angulation in Stance (DVV)

Value 4° varus

1 = > 10 degrees valgus
2 = > 5 degrees varus or 6 to 10 degrees valgus
(3 =) 5 degrees varus to 5 degrees valgus

3

Mediolateral Stability (DML)
1 = Marked instability
(2 =) Moderate instability
3 = Stable

2

Anteroposterior Stability with Knee at 90° Flexion (DAP)
1 = Marked instability
(2 =) Moderate instability
3 = Stable

2

Distance Walked (ADW)
5 = Unlimited
(4 =) 4 to 6 blocks
3 = 2 to 3 blocks
2 = Indoors only
1 = Transfers only

4

Assistive Device (AAD)
5 = None
4 = Cane outside
(3 =) Cane full time
2 = Two canes, crutches
1 = Walker or unable

3

Stair Climbing (ASC)
(5 =) Reciprocal, no rail
4 = Reciprocal, with rail
3 = One at a time, with or without rail
2 = One at a time, with rail and assistive device
1 = Unable to climb stairs

5

Rising from Chair (ARC)
(5 =) No arm assistance
4 = Single arm assistance
3 = Difficult with two arm assistance
2 = Needs assistance of another
1 = Unable to rise

5

FIGURE 19–4 *Continued*

and reveals the little details that need attending to: How long does it actually take to collect the data? Is the planned sequence cumbersome? Is another assistant needed for one part of the study? How much paper is used for the computer printout, and is there enough available to complete the study? Is an extension cord or extra batteries needed to power your equipment? Should office supplies be handy?

Scheduling of Subjects and Personnel

The pilot study allows the researcher to make educated guesses about how the data collection will proceed. Subjects in the actual study should expect the researcher to provide a realistic estimate of the time it will take to complete their participation. Subjects may not mind participating in a study that requires five hours of data collection as long as they know up front that this is the time that will be involved. Subjects will understandably be upset and may withdraw from participation if they are initially led to believe that data collection will require one hour and are still waiting to finish after three hours.

Adequate personnel need to be available for data collection. The types of tasks that need to be accomplished are greeting subjects as they arrive, explaining the study and securing informed consent, phoning subjects who have not arrived as expected, gathering background information and screening subjects to ensure that they meet inclusion criteria, preparing subjects for data collection, collecting the actual data, spotting subjects for safety, and thanking subjects for their assistance. In some studies, one researcher could handle all these tasks; in others, five or six researchers might be required.

Interview Data Collection

The data collection procedure in an interview study is often somewhat simpler than that in a study using biophysiological instruments because the interviewer and subject are in a one-on-one situation. If the interviews take place on the subjects' turf, the interviewer needs to be prompt. If the interviews are being conducted at, for example, the interviewer's office, then a receptionist should be available to greet arriving subjects or take calls from subjects who will be late or unable to make their appointment. The interviewer needs to be prepared with an adequate supply of paper and working pens and pencils. If the interviews are to be recorded, the interviewer needs to be familiar with the recording equipment and ensure that the supply of tapes and batteries is adequate to meet the needs of the day.

Questionnaire Data Collection

The data collection process in a study using a mailed questionnaire involves an intense mailing effort and then a wait for returns. Before stuffing the envelopes, the researcher must decide whether to include a mechanism for follow-up of nonrespondents. To do so, the researcher numbers the master list of subjects and in the envelope going to each subject places a return envelope or postcard with that subject's number on it. When the questionnaire is returned, the number is marked on the master list as returned, and the return envelope is discarded, maintaining the confidentiality of the subject responses to the questionnaire.

A postcard system for follow-up maintains even greater anonymity. A numbered postcard is included with the questionnaire packet, and the subject is instructed to mail the postcard and questionnaire back separately so that the questionnaire and subject number will never be directly linked as they are if the return envelope is coded. The disadvantages of the postcard system are that it increases mailing and printing costs and subjects may forget to mail the postcard.

If the return rate is lower than desired by a week to 10 days after the first responses were due, a second mailing to nonrespondents should be done. This follow-up packet should contain a new cover letter and a duplicate copy of the questionnaire. It is often appropriate to differentiate between first and second returns so that one can check to see whether there is a difference of opinions between those who initially responded and those who required a second prodding. This can be done by using a different-colored questionnaire for the follow-up mailing or by making an inconspicuous mark on all the questionnaires sent with the second mailing. If the first respondents were positive and the second respondents somewhat more negative on the issues studied, this is an indication that overall opinion may not be as positive as that of the initial respondents.

DATA ANALYSIS

The ease with which the data analysis is accomplished depends greatly on whether the researcher has (a) written a well-developed proposal with a sound plan for data analysis and (b) collected data carefully with an eye to the analysis stage. In discussing data analysis, this section presumes that a computer statistical package and a statistical consultant are available. For all but the smallest data sets, both are necessary. After a discussion of the roles of computers and consultants, suggestions are provided for the three steps of data analysis: data coding, data entry, and statistical analysis.

Many computer statistical packages are available for use on personal or mainframe computers. Three widely used statistical packages are Statistical Package for the Social Sciences (SPSS), Statistical Analysis System (SAS), and Biomedical Data Processing (BMDP); all three are available in mainframe or personal computer versions. In addition, many other programs are available.[8] The basic procedure for all of the computer statistical packages is that the variables of interest are defined, the data are coded numerically and entered into a data file, and then the analyses are run.

Statistical consultants should be used in several different ways. First, they can be consulted during the planning stages of a project to help determine whether the planned design can be analyzed in a way that will answer the research question. Second, they can help the researcher determine the sample size needed to obtain statistically significant results given certain assumptions about the size of differences between groups and the extent of variability within groups. Third, they can provide access to and are knowledgeable about statistical software. Fourth, they can check any analysis the researcher might have done on his or her own. Finally, they can review the written report of a research project to ensure that what the researcher has written about the statistical analysis is in fact what was done.

Before working with statistical consultants, the researcher must have a clear idea of the purposes of his or her research. A list of proposed variables and the values they may take is essential because statistical decisions will be based in part on the measurement characteristics of the data. Consultants may also wish to review published reports of studies similar to the one being planned so they can see the type of analysis that is the norm in the discipline or for a particular journal.

The researcher and consultant must be clear about who will do which tasks associated with the analysis. Will the consultant enter data, run the analysis, prepare summary tables, and summarize the results for the researcher? Or will the researcher enter the data, receive a stack of printouts, and contact the consultant only if there are any questions? Because the consultant will likely work for an hourly fee, the researcher should ask the consultant for an estimate of the number of hours that will be required for the level of involvement desired.

Data Coding

The first step of data analysis is to develop a coding scheme for the data. Table 13–1 shows the coding scheme for our hypothetical total knee arthroplasty data. Figure 19–4 shows how the coding scheme is translated into a form that encourages simultaneous data collection and coding.

Responses that are letters or descriptors (a, b, c, and d on multiple-choice items; "strongly agree," "agree," "neutral," "disagree," and "strongly disagree" for Likert-type items) are generally converted into numbers for data analysis. Some statistical programs permit the researcher to enter the letter and convert it to a number; others require that numbers be entered.

The researcher needs to decide how to handle missing data points. One option is to simply leave them as blanks in the data set. In other instances, the researcher may want frequency counts of missing data or may wish to analyze a subgroup of individuals who did not respond to a certain question. In these cases, missing data need to be given their own code. The number 9 or 99 is often used as the code for missing data.

Some questionnaire items may permit multiple responses. For example, a multiple-choice item may ask respondents to indicate all the choices that apply to their situation. Coding of multiple responses is often best accomplished by converting the single item into several yes/no items. Assume that in our coding system a yes response is coded 1 and a no response is coded 0. The response for a respondent who checked a, c, and e out of a through f responses for a multiple-answer item would be coded as follows: A = 1, B = 0, C = 1, D = 0, E = 1, and F = 0.

Once the coding scheme is accomplished, the researcher should go through the data and convert it to codes as necessary. Although some researchers may be able to sit in front of the computer with raw data and simultaneously code and enter it, most will have a more accurate data set, and will save time in the long run, if they perform coding and entering separately. After the data have been coded initially, the codes need to be rechecked and corrected by either the original coder or another member of the research team.

Data Entry

Once the data are coded, they need to be entered into the computer for analysis. In many instances, the data file can be created through a word-processing or spreadsheet program and then transferred into a format that can be used by the statistical software.

Although the actual procedures for data entry vary from package to package, the basic structure of a data file is that the variables are represented by columns and the subjects by rows. Table 13–2 shows the data file for our hypothetical study of patients with total knee arthroplasty.

When data have already been coded before they are entered, the researcher can enter data quickly without needing to think about what the numbers actually mean. Some researchers find that data entry goes more quickly if one person reads the numbers aloud and another enters them.

After data entry, the data set needs to be edited against the data-coding sheets. Once again, this process may go more quickly if one member of the team reads the coding numbers aloud while the other checks the computer data printout. Only after the data set is edited, or "cleaned," is the researcher ready to run the statistical analyses that will answer the research questions.

Statistical Analysis

Too often, investigators test their research hypotheses without first gaining a sense of the character of the data set. The first statistical procedure done should be running frequencies and descriptive data for each variable within the data set as a whole. In doing so, the researcher can get a sense of the distribution, means and standard deviations, and frequencies of the variables overall. If there are very extreme values for some variables, the researcher should recheck them against the original data sheets for accuracy. If the person collecting the data thought there might be an irregularity, it may be noted on the original data collection sheet. Extreme values are known as *outliers* and may sometimes be deleted from a data set with justification. A statistical consultant can help the researcher decide when it is reasonable to delete outliers.

Next, the researcher should divide the total sample into groups, if appropriate to the study purposes. For example, after the descriptive information about the total knee arthroplasty sample has been examined, frequencies, means, and standard deviations for each of the clinics under study should be run. This tells the researcher whether data are normally distributed and whether there is homogeneity of variance within the subgroups of interest. This information is essential to determining whether the assumptions for parametric testing are met. If they are not, then the researcher adopts the nonparametric contingency plan for the variables that have not met parametric assumptions.

Only after the data have been examined as noted above can the statistical tests of interest be conducted. Many of the programs have a dizzying array of options from which to choose for a given statistical test. If uncertain about which options are appropriate, the researcher should use the services of a statistical consultant.

SUMMARY

Implementation of a research project requires attention to detail at every step of the process. Recruitment of subjects involves consideration of physician consent, subject consent, administrative approval, and generalizability of research findings. Researchers must be familiar with procedures for use of biophysiological data collection tools, and the tools themselves must be checked for accuracy. Researchers who develop interview items or questionnaires must carefully consider the nature of their subjects and plan interviews or questionnaires that will elicit subjects' cooperation. Data analysis for all but the smallest data sets requires the use of a computer statistical package and a statistical consultant.

References

1. Findley TW, Stineman MG. Research in physical medicine and rehabilitation: V. data entry and early exploratory data analysis. *Am J Phys Med Rehabil.* 1989;68:240–251.
2. Findley TW, Daum MC, Macedo JA. Research in physical medicine and rehabilitation: VI. research project management. *Am J Phys Med Rehabil.* 1989;68:288–299.
3. Findley TW, Daum MC, Stineman MG. Research in physical medicine and rehabilitation: VII. the role of the principle investigator. *Am J Phys Med Rehabil.* 1990;69:39–45.
4. Michels E. *Using and Understanding Surveys: An Introductory Manual.* Alexandria, Va: American Physical Therapy Association; 1985.
5. Sudman S. *Asking Questions.* San Francisco, Calif: Jossey-Bass Publishers; 1982.
6. Dillman DA. *Mail and Telephone Surveys: The Total Design Method.* New York, NY: Wiley; 1978.
7. Bashi HL. Use of unlicensed support personnel for patient treatment in physical therapy. Master's research project. Indianapolis, Ind: University of Indianapolis; 1990.
8. Raskin R. Statistical software for the PC: testing for significance. *PC Magazine.* 1989;8(5):103–116.

CHAPTER 20

Publishing and Presenting Research

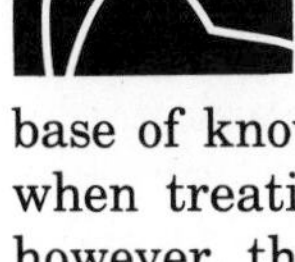

The culmination of the research endeavor is the dissemination of the results of the research. When made public, research can fulfill its goal of adding to the base of knowledge on which clinicians draw when treating patients. This is not to say, however, that all research that is conducted should be disseminated. Some research is so flawed that valid conclusions cannot be drawn from the results. Given this caveat, once an investigator has obtained results that have something to add to the body of knowledge, he or she needs to find the appropriate way to disseminate the results. There are two main mechanisms for doing so: publication and conference presentation.

The purposes of this chapter are to describe the publication and presentation process and to present guidelines for developing effective publications and presentations. Complete guidelines for manuscript preparation, a complete manuscript, and a presentation script and slides are provided in Appendixes E through G, respectively.

PUBLICATION OF RESEARCH

The main vehicle for publication of research results is the journal article. This section differentiates between types of publications and journals; discusses the peer review process, authorship, and acknowledgment issues in publication; and presents a variety of language and usage issues that arise when writing about research.

Types of Publications

Professional publications usually fall into one of three categories: journals, magazines, and newsletters. Newsletters present news of interest to subscribers. They may occasionally highlight important research findings but do not report original research. The *Progress Report* of the American Physical Therapy Association is an example of a newsletter.

Magazines are publications with full-length articles about general topics of interest to professionals. Some magazine articles may refer to original research, but they do not ordinarily report original research. Articles on practice management, overviews of patient care for certain groups, and discussions of professional issues are appropriate topics for a professional magazine, exemplified by *Clinical Management*, a professional magazine published by the American Physical Therapy Association.

Journals have as their primary purpose the reporting of original research findings in a defined area. Although original research publication is the primary focus of a journal, this does not preclude a journal from publishing scholarly review articles, editorials, or the news of a professional association. *Physical Therapy* is the journal of the American Physical Therapy Association.

There are two types of journals: peer reviewed or not peer reviewed. In considering a manuscript submitted for publication, editors of peer-reviewed, or *refereed,* journals contact professionals who are knowledgeable about the content area of a manuscript to determine whether the manuscript has scientific rigor and significantly adds to knowledge in the discipline to merit publication. The final decision about whether a paper is published is made by an editor who is a scholar within the discipline. Publication decisions for non-peer-reviewed, or *nonrefereed,* journals may be made by individuals who are professional editors rather than scholars within the discipline. A journal's peer review status may be mentioned in its instructions to authors and can be found in *The Serials Directory* in the reference section of the library.[1]

Peer Review Process

The personnel involved in the peer review process include the journal editor, an editorial board chaired by the editor, and manuscript reviewers. All of these individuals are scholars or practitioners in the discipline. The journal editor is appointed by the managing body that publishes the journal; the editorial board is usually appointed by the editor, with the consent of the managing body that publishes the journal; the editorial board establishes qualifications for being a manuscript reviewer and accepts applications from interested professionals. For most journals, these three positions are voluntary; however, the editor of larger journals may receive a stipend or honorarium.

When a manuscript is submitted to a peer-reviewed journal for consideration for publication, a chain of events is triggered. The editor or staff reviews the manuscript to see if it meets the journal's technical requirements (length, reference style, etc.) and fits the general mission of the journal. If either of these conditions is not met, the manuscript is returned to the authors without further review. If the manuscript meets the technical and mission criteria, then it is retained for further review.

The manuscript is usually assigned for review to one editorial board member and one or more manuscript reviewers. The board and manuscript reviewers are selected on the basis of their area of expertise in the profession or their knowledge of the research methods used by the authors. The board member and reviewers critique the manuscript to determine the soundness of the research design, the importance and usefulness of the research in light of other literature and the needs of practitioners, and the clarity and readability of the manuscript.

The manuscript reviewers summarize their opinions of the manuscript to the editorial board member and indicate whether they believe it merits publication. The editorial board member synthesizes his or her opinion with the input from the various reviewers and renders an opinion about the paper to the editor.

On the basis of the information from the editorial board member and reviewers, the editor makes a decision about publication of the manuscript. A manuscript can have one of four fates: acceptance, provisional acceptance pending revision, rejection with suggestion to rewrite, or rejection without suggestion to rewrite. Very few manuscripts are accepted for publication without revisions; most that are published were accepted provisionally pending revision. This decision is made when the content and structure of the study seem sound and useful to the profession, but the article format needs to be polished. A rejection with a suggestion to rewrite usually means that the topic is important to the profession, but the article as written is too incomplete or disorganized to be able to permit judgment about the credibility of the research. A rejection without a suggestion to rewrite usually means that the topic is simply not a high priority for the journal or that the research methods are too flawed to permit valid conclusions.

As might be inferred by the process just described, peer review is time consuming. Several months may elapse between submission and a first decision about the manuscript. Author revisions may take several more months, as will final editing of the manuscript by the journal staff. Moreover, because many journals have a backlog of articles waiting to be published, publication of an accepted paper may be delayed several more months. It is not uncommon for more than a year to elapse between submission of a manuscript and its eventual publication.

Authorship and Acknowledgment

Today, many journal articles are cowritten by multiple researchers. In addition to the authors, there are often individuals who have contributed to the study and deserve acknowledgment at the conclusion of the article. Because authorship and acknowledgment involve prestige and recognition, there are often controversies about who should be an author, in what order the authors should be presented, and who should be acknowledged.

The International Committee of Medical Journal Editors has published guidelines to help researchers make such decisions.[2] For an investigator to be listed as an author of a journal article, the committee believes that the following requirements should be met:

- Contribution to the intellectual development or analysis of the project
- Participation in the writing or editing of the intellectual content of the paper
- Approval of the version of the study that is to be published.

Mere collection of data does not meet these requirements, nor does holding an administrative post at the facility at which the research was conducted.

The order in which the authors' names are listed should reflect the relative strength of the contributions they have made to the project. This order should be discussed when tasks are being divided among the researchers in the early stages of a project. The order may change somewhat as the project progresses; before submission of the paper for publication, the authors should negotiate among themselves what the final order will be.

Authors should acknowledge individuals who have made significant contributions to the project but do not qualify to be listed as coauthors. Such contributors include those who collected or analyzed some of the data, colleagues who loaned facilities or equipment, or peers who provided critical review of early drafts of the manuscript. All acknowledged individuals should receive a copy of the manuscript and give their permission to be named.

Multiple Publication

Most journals require authors to disclose prior publication and will not accept for consideration papers that have been published in full elsewhere. In fact, most journals require that authors assign the copyright of an article to them when they submit it for publication, meaning that the authors give up the right to submit the paper elsewhere while it is being reviewed. If the first journal to which an article is submitted does not accept the manuscript for publication, the copyright reverts back to the authors, who may then submit it to another journal.

Style Issues

The research article is a specialized form of writing. Its hallmarks are precision, conciseness, and consistency. The novelist uses words to paint pictures and uses different words to convey similar meanings in different contexts. Creative use of language makes novels enjoyable—it makes research articles infuriating if several different terms are used to represent the same construct.

Each journal publishes its own instructions for authors. These instructions typically specify the types of articles accepted for review, the editorial process, the format that the manuscript should take, the reference style to use, procedures for manuscript submission, and the style manual that should be used to prepare the paper.

A style manual is a document of technical information for authors. The style manual for *Physical Therapy* is the American Medical Association's *Manual of Style*; for the *American Journal of Occupational Therapy*, it is the *Publication Manual of the American Psychological Association*.[3, 4] In addition, there are several good references that provide general guidelines for scientific and medical writing.[2, 5, 6] Style manuals specify such things as when numbers are presented as numerals (for example, 227) and when they are written out (two hundred twenty-seven), what levels of headings and subheadings to use, how to present mathematical symbols, how to set up tables, how to cite literature in the text of an article, and what format to follow for the reference list at the end of the article. They also present useful writing-style and grammar suggestions, including how to differentiate among confusing terms (for example, *affect* and *effect*), when to use certain punctuation marks, and how to avoid exclusionary language so that sexist and racial stereotypes are not unconsciously adopted. Table 20–1 presents style problems that commonly appear in the papers of physical therapy students. This table can be used to help writers eliminate these mistakes from their papers, but it is no substitute for frequent reference to a style manual.

A set of style guidelines not included in many style manuals relates to references about people with disabilities.[7] Because physical therapists frequently write about such individuals, they should pay close attention to the implications of the words they use to refer to this population. Table 20–2 presents a set of guidelines for writing about people with disabilities.

TABLE 20–1. Common Style Problems in Student Manuscripts

Problem	Example of Problem	Corrected Text
Abbreviation is used without being identified at the first use.	*Rupture of the ACL is a common problem for athletes in contact sports. The ACL is a primary stabilizer of the knee.*	*Rupture of the anterior cruciate ligament (ACL) is a common. . . . The ACL is a primary stabilizer of the knee.*
Sentence begins with a numeral.	*224 responses were received.*	*Two hundred twenty-four responses were received.* or *Responses were received from 224 patients.*
Abbreviations of units of measurement are inconsistent or nonstandard. (Standard units do not have to be spelled out the first time they are used.)	*Velocity was measured in centimeters per sec, with the younger group walking at a pace of 180 cm/sec.*	*Velocity was measured in cm/s, with the younger group walking at a pace of 180 cm/s.*
Language includes jargon or informal terms understood by only a single group of professionals.	*The subjects completed 20 reps of quad sets.*	*The subjects completed 20 repetitions of a quadriceps femoris muscle setting exercise.*
Quotation marks are not used properly with punctuation. Closing quotation marks go outside periods and commas and inside semicolons and colons.	*Boswell has stated that "complacency rules when a profession does not control its own destiny".*	*Boswell has stated that "complacency rules when a profession does not control its own destiny."*
Author refers to him- or herself in the third person; the first person is now preferred, even in scientific writing.	*This author believes that Mayberry overstated the clinical applicability of his findings.*	*I believe that Mayberry overstated the clinical applicability of his findings.*
Comparative terms are used, but no comparison is made.	*Johnson found an increase in strength of the middle deltoid muscle.*	*Johnson found an increase in strength of the middle deltoid after completion of the exercise program.*
Exclusionary terms are used, or constructions to avoid them are too awkward.	*The therapist should not let his emotions cloud his judgments.* or *The therapist should not let his/her emotions cloud his/her judgment.*	*Therapists should not let their emotions cloud their judgments.* or *Emotions should not cloud the judgments of therapists.*
Male or *female* is used as a noun, rather than an adjective.	*We studied 50 females.*	*We studied 50 female patients.* or *We studied 50 women.*
Author unnecessarily hyphenates compound words	*The post-test scores for the non-injured leg were . . .*	*The posttest scores for the noninjured leg were . . .*

TABLE 20–2. Guidelines for Writing about People with Disabilities.*

Sensational or Negative Portrayal	Straightforward, Positive Portrayal
Traumatic brain injury patient [focuses on the injury rather than the person]	*Individual with a traumatic brain injury* [focuses on the person rather than the injury; use *patient* only if the person is, in fact, undergoing medical treatment]
Physically challenged [euphemisms imply that disabilities cannot be dealt with in a straightforward manner]	*Person with a disability* [puts the person first, then the disability; acknowledges the disability directly]
Special children [attempts to glorify differences]	*Children with disabilities* [straightforward portrayal]
Wheelchair-bound [evokes a confined image contrary to the active role of many people who use wheelchairs]	*Uses a wheelchair* [describes the wheelchair as the tool that it is]
Suffers from multiple sclerosis [sensationalizes the disease]	*Has multiple sclerosis* [states the disease matter-of-factly]

*Adapted from *Guidelines for Reporting and Writing About People with Disabilities.* 3rd ed. Lawrence, Kan: Research and Training Center on Independent Living, Institute for Life Span Studies, University of Kansas; 1990.

Components of a Research Article

The components of a research article are as follows:

- title and title page
- abstract
- introduction
- methods
- results
- discussion
- conclusions
- acknowledgments
- references
- tables
- figures

Appendix E provides a numbered list of guidelines for the preparation of each section; Appendix F contains a complete journal article manuscript, annotated with numbers that correspond to the items in Appendix E.

PRESENTATION OF RESEARCH

Presentation is the second major format by which research results are disseminated. Many professional associations hold meetings at which research presentations are made. The process of selecting a paper for presentation usually involves submission of an abstract of the study. Some associations use peer review to select abstracts for presentation; others accept any abstracts that meet the technical guidelines and can be accommodated within the conference schedule. Some associations specify that abstracts must be of studies that have not been presented previously. Because conference presentations are less permanent and less accessible than publications, multiple presentation of the same study is acceptable if each presentation is targeted to a different audience. Thus, researchers may feel comfortable presenting the results of their study at both a local and a national meeting of an association or at meetings of different types of professionals. For example, a study related to the roles of physical therapists and athletic trainers in the clinical setting might be appropriate for presentation at a conference of physical therapists and at a conference for athletic trainers.

There are two major formats for conference presentations: platform presentations and poster presentations. Each is described and illustrated below.

Platform Presentations

A platform presentation is made by a researcher to an audience of peers attending the conference. The presentation time is usually short—anywhere from 8 minutes to 20 minutes is common. Researchers are usually expected to show slides during the presentation. A suggested sequence for development of a research presentation is presented below. Appendix G provides a script and slides for a presentation of the manuscript presented in Appendix F.

1. Complete the Manuscript. The manuscript provides the complete picture of the study to be described in the presentation. Being able to look at a complete manuscript can help the presenter decide which elements are essential and which can be deleted for the presentation. In addition, because most research presentations follow the same sequence as a journal article, the full manuscript provides a ready-made outline for the presentation.

2. Edit the Manuscript to Presentation Length. Examine each paragraph to determine whether it is essential to an understanding of the presentation. A guideline for developing the script for presentation is to spend approximately

10% of the allotted time establishing the problem and context of the study,

20% of the time describing the methods,

30% of the time presenting the results,

30% of the time discussing the results, and

10% of the time summarizing the conclusions.

The introduction section of the paper can be shortened by deleting many specific references to the related literature and developing the problem conceptually. The methods sections can be shortened by eliminating detail about measurement procedures and minimizing technical information about the instruments used. Remember that a presentation audience is interested in simply understanding your methods, not in replicating them in a future study.

Whereas research papers often include separate instruments and procedures sections, a presentation may flow more smoothly if the two are combined. Similarly, some repetition may be eliminated if the data analysis, results, and some parts of the discussion sections of the presentation are integrated. Conclusions should be clear and concise, reiterating the central message of the study.

Once the first edit has been done, read the text aloud, time the delivery, and note phrases that are awkward or seem too formal for your audience. Edit the script as needed for length and smooth delivery.

3. Divide the Script into Segments. A general guideline for preparation of a slide presentation is to have each slide displayed for between 10 and 20 seconds. This requires that the researcher divide the script into small "sound bites" that can be illustrated with a slide. Varying the length of the segments helps maintain audience interest.

4. Design the Slides. For each text segment, decide whether it is best illustrated with text, a table, a photograph, a drawing, or a graph. Most conferences are set up for horizontal projection of slides, so the presenter should design slides in a horizontal format. Some studies are best illustrated with dual projection, that is, projection of two slides side by side. Studies best suited for dual projection are those that present a great deal of visual information that needs to be reinforced by text. For example, a presentation of a study of different specific exercise techniques might benefit from photographs of the exercise displayed on one side and text about the exercise on the other. Because not all conferences can accommodate dual projection, you should confirm that this equipment is available before planning an elaborate dual slide presentation.

Slides of text should generally contain no more than 10 lines of text and no more than six words per line. The style should be telegraphic, using phrases rather than complete sentences. The text in the slide should not exactly repeat the script of the presentation; audiences do not like to have slides read to them. Use of upper- and lowercase letters is thought to be more readable than using all capital letters; simple sans serif type faces are preferred.

Slides of tables of information should contain no more than three columns and no more than seven rows. Use of data tables as they appear in the manuscript is rarely suitable, because they contain far more information than can be absorbed in 10 to 20 seconds. Graphs are often more effective than tables in a slide presentation.

Slides of photographs should be clear enough that the audience can locate the item of interest quickly. Photographers should strive for an uncluttered background that contrasts well with the subject. Sometimes photographs are simply not the best way to get a visual message across. For example, a line diagram of a particular piece of equipment may be able to focus attention on the relevant portion of the instrument; an illustration of an anatomical part may be more effective than a photograph.

Slides of graphs should be used to illustrate the relationships between different numbers within the data set. Pie charts show proportions well, bar graphs effectively illustrate differences in quantities between groups, and line graphs are ideal for illustrating change across time. Because the slide will be displayed for a limited time, the graph should be as simple and clear as possible. Labels should be large enough to read; words should be kept to a minimum.

5. Produce the Slides. Larger hospital and university settings have media services departments that can help researchers design and produce slides. Researchers who do not have access to such a resource can use commercial slide production services, which are available in any large city, or buy commercially available graphics software to design the slides and send them via modem to a production center.[8] Presenters who cannot afford computer graphics can use any number of lower technology alternatives that produce serviceable slides.[9, 10]

6. Practice the Complete Presentation. Once the slides have been produced, the researcher needs to practice delivering the text in coordination with the slides. Often, the text needs to be reedited to help integrate the slides with the text. Figure 20–1 shows a graph and the text that highlights its important points.

The final practice is the time to decide on the format of the written materials that you will use to make the presentation. Some presenters like to use 3″ × 5″ cards on which the text for each slide and a diagram of the slide are written. Others like to use standard-sized paper on which (a) the text is written in paragraph form and markings are inserted

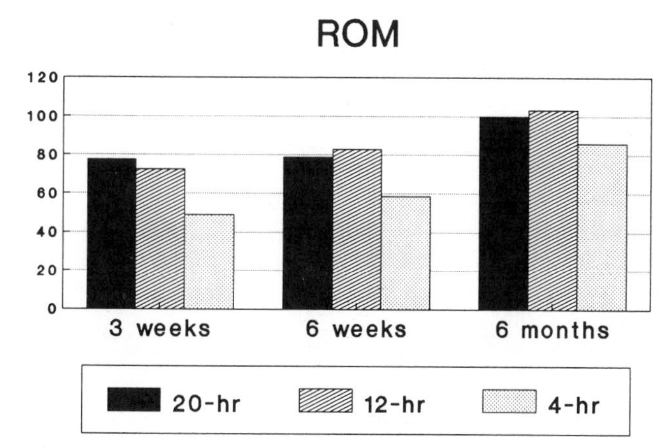

Slide 25.

This slide shows the nearly equal ROM scores for the 20-hr and 12-hr groups, illustrated by the solid and hatched bars; and the low three-week, six-week, and six-month range of motion values for the 4-hr groups, represented by the dotted bars. Even at six months postoperatively, the 4-hr group has not achieved an average flexion range of motion of 90 degrees.

FIGURE 20–1. Example of slide and text for a platform presentation. Text highlights important features of the graph shown in the slide.

to indicate when to change the slide or (b) two columns are printed, one listing the diagrams of the slides and the other listing the text that accompanies each slide. Appendix G shows the text and slides for a presentation of the hypothetical paper provided in Appendix F.

Poster Presentations

Poster presentations are a common feature at conferences and are becoming increasingly accepted as a means of dissemination of scientific information. A poster session consists of a collection of large posters describing research studies. The posters are generally displayed for several hours, and presenters are required to be with their posters for a certain portion of the display time. The advantages of a poster session over a platform presentation are (a) conference attendees can view the posters when they have time and (b) the researcher has more opportunity to interact with interested colleagues.

The space available for the posters is generally about 4′ × 8′. Some presenters have professionally produced posters that they unroll from a tube and tack up onto the board. Most, however, will post a series of miniposters that are easily transported. Researchers who prepare posters should ensure that the type is readable from a distance of two to three feet and that the sequence in which the posters should be examined is clear.[10, 11] Figure 20–2 shows a schematic diagram of a poster.

SUMMARY

Research results are disseminated through either publication or presentation. Publication of research results in journals is a formal process guided by peer review. Journal articles usually follow a standard sequence: introduction, methods, results, discussion, and conclusions. Presentation of research usually occurs at conferences through a platform talk with accompanying slides or through a poster session in which the researcher can interact with conference attendees less formally than in the platform format. Presentations usually follow the same sequence as journal articles.

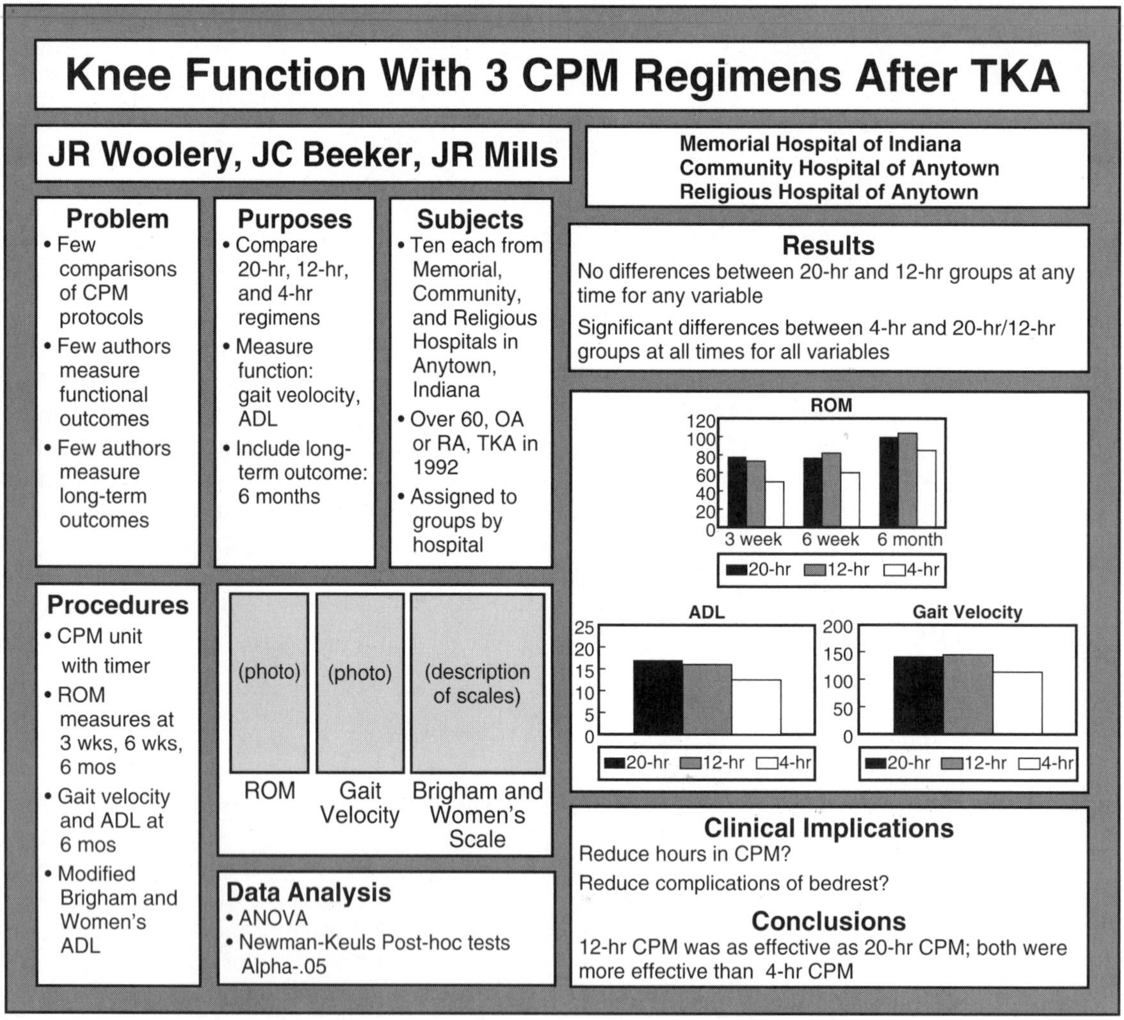

Knee Function With 3 CPM Regimens After TKA

JR Woolery, JC Beeker, JR Mills

Memorial Hospital of Indiana
Community Hospital of Anytown
Religious Hospital of Anytown

Problem
- Few comparisons of CPM protocols
- Few authors measure functional outcomes
- Few authors measure long-term outcomes

Purposes
- Compare 20-hr, 12-hr, and 4-hr regimens
- Measure function: gait veolocity, ADL
- Include long-term outcome: 6 months

Subjects
- Ten each from Memorial, Community, and Religious Hospitals in Anytown, Indiana
- Over 60, OA or RA, TKA in 1992
- Assigned to groups by hospital

Procedures
- CPM unit with timer
- ROM measures at 3 wks, 6 wks, 6 mos
- Gait velocity and ADL at 6 mos
- Modified Brigham and Women's ADL

(photo) (photo) (description of scales)
ROM | Gait Velocity | Brigham and Women's Scale

Data Analysis
- ANOVA
- Newman-Keuls Post-hoc tests Alpha-.05

Results
No differences between 20-hr and 12-hr groups at any time for any variable
Significant differences between 4-hr and 20-hr/12-hr groups at all times for all variables

ROM
120 100 80 60 40 20 0
3 week 6 week 6 month
20-hr 12-hr 4-hr

ADL
25 20 15 10 5 0
20-hr 12-hr 4-hr

Gait Velocity
200 150 100 50 0
20-hr 12-hr 4-hr

Clinical Implications
Reduce hours in CPM?
Reduce complications of bedrest?

Conclusions
12-hr CPM was as effective as 20-hr CPM; both were more effective than 4-hr CPM

FIGURE 20–2. Schematic diagram for a poster presentation.

References

1. *The Serials Directory*. 5th ed. Birmingham, Ala: EBSCO Industries Inc; 1991.
2. International Committee of Medical Journal Editors. Uniform requirements for manuscripts submitted to biomedical journals. *Ann Intern Med*. 1988;108:258–265.
3. American Medical Association. *Manual of Style*. 8th ed. Baltimore, Md: Williams & Wilkins; 1989.
4. *Publication Manual of the American Psychological Association*. 3rd ed. Washington, DC: American Psychological Association; 1983.
5. Huth EJ. *How to Write and Publish Papers in the Medical Sciences*. 2nd ed. Baltimore, Md: Williams & Wilkins; 1990.
6. Day RA. *How to Write and Publish a Scientific Paper*. 3rd ed. Phoenix, Ariz: Oryx Press; 1988.
7. *Guidelines for Reporting and Writing About People with Disabilities*. 3rd ed. Lawrence, Kan: Research and Training Center on Independent Living, Bureau of Child Research, University of Kansas; 1990.
8. Simone L. Presentation graphics. *PC Magazine*. 1991;10(10):107–192.
9. Craik RL, Krebs DE. *Handbook for APTA Oral and Poster Presentations*. Alexandria, Va: American Physical Therapy Association; 1985.
10. Reynolds L, Simmonds D. *Presentation of Data in Science*. Boston, Mass: Martinus Nijhoff Publishers; 1983.
11. Committee on Research. *Research Presentations at Annual Conference: Guidelines for Poster Presenters*. Alexandria, Va: American Physical Therapy Association; 1985.

Appendix A

Integrity in Physical Therapy Research*

Preamble

The American Physical Therapy Association (APTA) and its physical therapist members are committed to encouraging and improving research in physical therapy. This commitment is grounded in the Association's Object and Functions, as set out in its Bylaws. The Association and the profession are also committed to maintaining and promoting professional ethics in physical therapy, and this commitment is grounded in the *Code of Ethics* which is binding on all physical therapist members of the APTA.

A concern for integrity in research follows quite naturally from the dual commitment to research and professional ethics. Integrity in research requires that the research be humane and both professionally and scientifically acceptable. Essential to integrity in physical therapy research are certain considerations addressed in this document.

The number of physical therapists who design, conduct, and report, or otherwise engage in, research is growing. Many of these physical therapists, as well as the students who are learning to do research and their mentors, may not have ready access to guidance or advice on the considerations that are essential to integrity in physical therapy research. This document was developed to satisfy that need.

The Association's Committee on Research consulted and reviewed a number of published and unpublished resources, including laws, regulations, consent forms, and guides, during the period 1981 to 1985 when the work on the document was done. The work was assisted by extensive written comments received in response to a first draft circulated in 1983, by oral comments received at a hearing on a second draft in 1984, and through a continuing exchange of ideas with the Association's Judicial Committee.

Purpose and Use

The statements in this document are offered as considerations for physical therapists who design, conduct, and report, or otherwise engage in, research. Individual and collective attention to these considerations will help assure integrity in physical therapy research.

The statements are not to be considered inclusive of all of the situations to which they might apply. Developments within and outside physical therapy, including societal trends and changes in law and regulation, will require that the statements be continuously reviewed and modified as warranted. Additional statements will be developed as needed to address situations not now addressed in this document.

No attempt was made to include or append detailed information from, or examples of, the materials which were reviewed in developing this document. The uses of and responses to this document will be reviewed to determine at a later date the need for including or appending detailed information and examples.

The statements in this document are not intended to codify, explain, modify, or replace, in whole or in part, any of the ethical principles in the Association's *Code of Ethics* or any of the interpretations in the *Guide for Professional Conduct* issued by the Association's Judicial Committee.

I. THE RIGHT, PRIVACY, AND WELL-BEING OF RESEARCH SUBJECTS
   A. *Rights of Subjects*
      1. Physical therapists should ensure that the participation of human subjects in research is voluntary, free of coercion and deception, and based on an understanding by the subjects, or their legally authorized representatives, of the nature of the research and its expected benefits and risks.
         a. Legally effective informed consent should be obtained in writing from human subjects, or their legally authorized representatives, before the subjects participate in research.
         b. Human subjects, or their legally authorized representatives, should be assured in writing of the right to withdraw consent or to discontinue participation in research at any time without prejudice of any kind to the subjects.
         c. Human subjects, or their legally authorized representatives, should not be made to waive or appear to waive

*American Physical Therapy Association, Board of Directors. Approved 3/85; amended 11/87. Reprinted with permission of the American Physical Therapy Association, IIII North Fairfax Street, Alexandria, VA 22314.

any of the subjects' legal rights, or to release or appear to release the investigator, the sponsoring or funding agency, or the institution or any of its agents from liability for negligence.

d. Human subjects, or their legally authorized representatives, should be informed as to whether any compensation or treatment is available to the subjects if any physical injury results from the research.

2. Physical therapists should ensure that animal subjects used in research are treated humanely and, if sacrifice is necessary, are killed in a humane manner.

B. *Confidentiality and Privacy*

1. Physical therapists should ensure that data and observations obtained on human subjects who participate in research are recorded, stored, and reported in ways that protect the individual and personal identity of the subjects.

a. The information furnished to human subjects, or their legally authorized representatives, at the time that informed consent is obtained should include statement of the extent to which the confidentiality of data and observations on individual subjects will be maintained.

b. In situations where patients participate as human subjects in research, consideration may be given to releasing data and observations which reveal the identity of individual subjects to specified persons for purposes of real or potential benefit to the subjects. The subjects, or their legally authorized representatives, should be informed of and consent to such release before any release is made.

c. Signed release for the publication or exhibition, or other scientific or educational use, of photographic or other recorded images of human subjects who participate in research should be obtained from the subjects or their legally authorized representatives.

2. In situations where research procedures require the simultaneous presence of more than one human subject, or one or more groups of human subjects, physical therapists should ensure that the individual subjects have the maximum possible privacy during their participation.

C. *Risk to Subjects*

1. Physical therapists should identify and reduce as far as is possible the risk of physical, psychological, or social harm to research subjects.

a. Proposals of research requiring the application of experimental procedures or the imposition of experimental conditions should be submitted to institutional review boards or similar review bodies for independent assessment of the expected risk of physical, psychological, or social harm to research subjects.

b. The use of experimental procedures or conditions should be suspended if research subjects incur physical, psychological, or social harm to an extent or in a form which exceeds or deviates from the expected risk of harm. A full report on the procedures or conditions used, and the resultant harm observed, should be submitted for study by the appropriate review body. The use of the procedures or conditions should be resumed only if the appropriate review body approves the resumption.

D. *Well-being of Subjects*

1. Physical therapists should be guided at all times by concern for the physical, psychological, and social well-being of research subjects.

2. Research conducted by physical therapists on live animals should be done only in facilities that comply with the Code of Federal Regulations, Title 9, Subchapter A—Animal Welfare, and that either are accredited by the American Association for Accreditation of Laboratory Animal Care or have institutional committees which review animal facilities and practices for compliance with the National Institutes of Health *Guide for the Care and Use of Laboratory Animals,* and that comply with pertinent local laws and regulations governing the housing, care, and feeding of animals.

II. OBSERVANCE OF THE LAWS AND REGULATIONS GOVERNING RESEARCH

A. *Laws and Regulations*

Physical therapists who engage in research on human subjects who are patients should comply with the laws and regulations governing the practice of physical therapy in the jurisdiction in which the research is done on those subjects.

B. *Institutional Requirements*

Physical therapists should comply with the requirements governing the approval and conduct of research within the institutional or organizational settings in which they engage in research. If there are no requirements governing the approval and conduct of research within the institutional or organizational setting, the physical therapist should make every effort to assist in developing and implementing such requirements.

III. MAINTENANCE AND PROMOTION OF PROFESSIONAL AND SCIENTIFIC ACCEPTABILITY IN RESEARCH

A. *Honesty*

1. Physical therapists should ensure that truthful statements and descriptions of the required information are contained in research proposals submitted to institutional review boards, funding agencies, and others for approval.

2. Physical therapists should adhere to the purposes and methods of approved research projects.

a. Deviations from the purposes and methods of approved research projects should be avoided except when made in accordance with the policies and procedures of the approving bodies or persons.

3. Physical therapists should ensure that research reports provide truthful statements of the work done and the findings obtained in their research.

a. The deliberate misrepresentation or falsification of results, the suppression of findings, and the presentation of another's work as one's own should be avoided.
b. Every effort should be made to avoid the bias that can occur in the interpretation of research results when financial support of any kind, before, during, or after the research is done, is received from any party that may stand to gain financially from the results of the research.

B. *Openness*
1. Physical therapists should make every effort to report their research and research results to the appropriate professional or scientific community.
2. Physical therapists should make every effort to honor the requests of their professional and scientific colleagues for access to the data obtained in research. The purposes of such requests and the uses to which the data will be put should be mutually agreed in writing. The individual and personal identity of human subjects should be fully protected when access to data is provided.
3. Physical therapists should identify publicly any potential conflict of interest that might compromise, or might be perceived as compromising, the interpretation of their research and research results.

C. *Credibility*
1. Physical therapists should recognize that ensuring the credibility of research and research findings is an obligation to be assumed in exchange for the trust and cooperation of research subjects, the support of involved institutions and agencies, and the expected attention and consideration of the professional and scientific community.
2. Physical therapists should base their studies on a thorough knowledge and consideration of the pertinent professional and scientific literature.
3. Physical therapists should make every effort to ensure the legitimate and logically correct choice of research design and data analysis, the avoidance of bias in selection or assignment of subjects, and the professionally skillful performance of appropriate treatment methods and reliable measurement procedures for their studies.
   a. In the course of designing their studies and preparing research protocols and proposals, physical therapists should seek the constructive criticism of their professional and scientific colleagues.
   b. The advice of a competent consultant should be sought if there is any question or doubt about the choice of research design and data analysis for a study. This advice should extend to the presentation and interpretation of results when the study is completed.

D. *Accuracy*

Physical therapists should make every effort to ensure that research reports contain descriptions, findings, and references that are free from error.

E. *Thoroughness*

Physical therapists should make every effort to ensure that research reports contain information sufficient to enable constructive criticism and replication of the research and to demonstrate absence of bias in the research. Written reports of research should contain brief descriptions of the steps taken to assure the protection of the rights, confidentiality and privacy, and well-being of research subjects.

F. *Acknowledgement*
1. Physical therapists should publicly acknowledge, in the appropriate form, both the fact and the source of any financial support, consultation, or assistance received for research that is reported.
2. Physical therapists should publicly identify, in the appropriate form, the institutions or facilities where reported research was done and the affiliations of the authors of the research reports. The identities of institutions, agencies, or organizations which serve as the objects of study should be confidential unless written consent to reveal the identities is obtained from authorized officials in those institutions, agencies, or organizations.
3. When the acknowledgement of degrees held by authors of research reports is required or permitted, physical therapists should confine this acknowledgement to only their earned academic degree(s).

IV. UNETHICAL, INCOMPETENT, OR ILLEGAL ACTS IN RESEARCH

A. *Intervention*
1. Physical therapists should intervene directly in the conduct or reporting of research, for which they are responsible or in which they participate, to prevent or correct any acts which are unethical, incompetent, or illegal.
2. Physical therapists should dissociate themselves from the conduct of any research or from the preparation of any research report in which unethical, incompetent, or illegal acts occur or may occur and have not been, or are unlikely to be, prevented or corrected by direct intervention.

B. *Reporting*
1. Physical therapists should report to the appropriate institution or facility the facts regarding any acts in the conduct of research which appear to be unethical or illegal, or the facts regarding any acts in the conduct of research which appear to be incompetent and of actual or potential harm which exceeds or deviates from the expected risk of harm to research projects.
2. Physical therapists should report to the appropriate institution or facility the facts regarding any published or oral report of research which appears to be fraudulent.

C. *Investigation*
1. Physical therapists under investigation because of alleged unethical, incompetent, or illegal acts in the conduct or

reporting of research should cooperate in the investigation and accept the investigation, without recrimination or reprisal, as part of the process of the search for truth.

2. Physical therapists appointed to investigate alleged unethical, incompetent, or illegal acts in the conduct or reporting of research should be objective in exercising judgment within the scope of the inquiry, should possess the special competencies necessary to understand the research in question, and should not be associated with the person or persons under investigation.

D. *Criticism*

1. Physical therapists should comment critically, objectively, constructively, and openly on any reports of research which they consider to be professionally or scientifically unacceptable.
   a. Constructive criticism of research should be well-founded and should include suggestions for enhancing the acceptability of the research.
2. Physical therapists whose reports of research are criticized as representing research which is professionally or scientifically unacceptable should respond objectively to the criticism, and without recrimination or reprisal, as part of the process of the search for truth.

Appendix B

Random Numbers Table

From Beyer WH (ed). *Standard Mathematical Tables*. 27th ed. Boca Raton, Fla: CRC Press, Inc; 1984:555–558.

A TABLE OF 14,000 RANDOM UNITS

Line/Col.	(1)	(2)	(3)	(4)	(5)	(6)	(7)	(8)	(9)	(10)	(11)	(12)	(13)	(14)
1	10480	15011	01536	02011	81647	91646	69179	14194	62590	36207	20969	99570	91291	90700
2	22368	46573	25595	85393	30995	89198	27982	53402	93965	34095	52666	19174	39615	99505
3	24130	48360	22527	97265	76393	64809	15179	24830	49340	32081	30680	19655	63348	58629
4	42167	93093	06243	61680	07856	16376	39440	53537	71341	57004	00849	74917	97758	16379
5	37570	39975	81837	16656	06121	91782	60468	81305	49684	60672	14110	06927	01263	54613
6	77921	06907	11008	42751	27756	53498	18602	70659	90655	15053	21916	81825	44394	42880
7	99562	72905	56420	69994	98872	31016	71194	18738	44013	48840	63213	21069	10634	12952
8	96301	91977	05463	07972	18876	20922	94595	56869	69014	60045	18425	84903	42508	32307
9	89579	14342	63661	10281	17453	18103	57740	84378	25331	12566	58678	44947	05585	56941
10	85475	36857	43342	53988	53060	59533	38867	62300	08158	17983	16439	11458	18593	64952
11	28918	69578	88231	33276	70997	79936	56865	05859	90106	31595	01547	85590	91610	78188
12	63553	40961	48235	03427	49626	69445	18663	72695	52180	20847	12234	90511	33703	90322
13	09429	93969	52636	92737	88974	33488	36320	17617	30015	08272	84115	27156	30613	74952
14	10365	61129	87529	85689	48237	52267	67689	93394	01511	26358	85104	20285	29975	89868
15	07119	97336	71048	08178	77233	13916	47564	81056	97735	85977	29372	74461	28551	90707
16	51085	12765	51821	51259	77452	16308	60756	92144	49442	53900	70960	63990	75601	40719
17	02368	21382	52404	60268	89368	19885	55322	44819	01188	65255	64835	44919	05944	55157
18	01011	54092	33362	94904	31273	04146	18594	29852	71585	85030	51132	01915	92747	64951
19	52162	53916	46369	58586	23216	14513	83149	98736	23495	64350	94738	17752	35156	35749
20	07056	97628	33787	09998	42698	06691	76988	13602	51851	46104	88916	19509	25625	58104
21	48663	91245	85828	14346	09172	30168	90229	04734	59193	22178	30421	61666	99904	32812
22	54164	58492	22421	74103	47070	25306	76468	26384	58151	06646	21524	15227	96909	44592
23	32639	32363	05597	24200	13363	38005	94342	28728	35806	06912	17012	64161	18296	22851
24	29334	27001	87637	87308	58731	00256	45834	15398	46557	41135	10367	07684	36188	18510
25	02488	33062	28834	07351	19731	92420	60952	61280	50001	67658	32586	86679	50720	94953
26	81525	72295	04839	96423	24878	82651	66566	14778	76797	14780	13300	87074	79666	95725
27	29676	20591	68086	26432	46901	20849	89768	81536	86645	12659	92259	57102	80428	25280
28	00742	57392	39064	66432	84673	40027	32832	61362	98947	96067	64760	64584	96096	98253
29	05366	04213	25669	26422	44407	44048	37937	63904	45766	66134	75470	66520	34693	90449
30	91921	26418	64117	94305	26766	25940	39972	22209	71500	64568	91402	42416	07844	69618
31	00582	04711	87917	77341	42206	35126	74087	99547	81817	42607	43808	76655	62028	76630
32	00725	69884	62797	56170	86324	88072	76222	36086	84637	93161	76038	65855	77919	88006
33	69011	65797	95876	55293	18988	27354	26575	08625	40801	59920	29841	80150	12777	48501
34	25976	57948	29888	88604	67917	48708	18912	82271	65424	69774	33611	54262	85963	03547
35	09763	83473	73577	12908	30883	18317	28290	35797	05998	41688	34952	37888	38917	88050
36	91567	42595	27958	30134	04024	86385	29880	99730	55536	84855	29080	09250	79656	73211
37	17955	56349	90999	49127	20044	59931	06115	20542	18059	02008	73708	83517	36103	42791
38	46503	18584	18845	49618	02304	51038	20655	58727	28168	15475	56942	53389	20562	87338
39	92157	89634	94824	78171	84610	82834	09922	25417	44137	48413	25555	21246	35509	20468
40	14577	62765	35605	81263	39667	47358	56873	56307	61607	49518	89656	20103	77490	18062
41	98427	07523	33362	64270	01638	92477	66969	98420	04880	45585	46565	04102	46880	45709
42	34914	63976	88720	82765	34476	17032	87589	40836	32427	70002	70663	88863	77775	69348
43	70060	28277	39475	46473	23219	53416	94970	25832	69975	94884	19661	72828	00102	66794
44	53976	54914	06990	67245	68350	82948	11398	42878	80287	88267	47363	46634	06541	97809
45	76072	29515	40980	07391	58745	25774	22987	80059	39911	96189	41151	14222	60697	59583
46	90725	52210	83974	29992	65831	38857	50490	83765	55657	14361	31720	57375	56228	41546
47	64364	67412	33339	31926	14883	24413	59744	92351	97473	89286	35931	04110	23726	51900
48	08962	00358	31662	25388	61642	34072	81249	35648	56891	69352	48373	45578	78547	81788
49	95012	68379	93526	70765	10593	04542	76463	54328	02349	17247	28865	14777	62730	92277
50	15664	10493	20492	38391	91132	21999	59516	81652	27195	48223	46751	22923	32261	85653

A TABLE OF 14,000 RANDOM UNITS

Line/Col.	(1)	(2)	(3)	(4)	(5)	(6)	(7)	(8)	(9)	(10)	(11)	(12)	(13)	(14)
51	16408	81899	04153	53381	79401	21438	83035	92350	36693	31238	59649	91754	72772	02338
52	18629	81953	05520	91962	04739	13092	97662	24822	94730	06496	35090	04822	86772	98289
53	73115	35101	47498	87637	99016	71060	88824	71013	18735	20286	23153	72924	35165	43040
54	57491	16703	23167	49323	45021	33132	12544	41035	80780	45393	44812	12515	98931	91202
55	30405	83946	23792	14422	15059	45799	22716	19792	09983	74353	68668	30429	70735	25499
56	16631	35006	85900	98275	32388	52390	16815	69298	82732	38480	73817	32523	41961	44437
57	96773	20206	42559	78985	05300	22164	24369	54224	35083	19687	11052	91491	60383	19746
58	38935	64202	14349	82674	66523	44133	00697	35552	35970	19124	63318	29686	03387	59846
59	31624	76384	17403	53363	44167	64486	64758	75366	76554	31601	12614	33072	60332	92325
60	78919	19474	23632	27889	47914	02584	37680	20801	72152	39339	34806	08930	85001	87820
61	03931	33309	57047	74211	63445	17361	62825	39908	05607	91284	68833	25570	38818	46920
62	74426	33278	43972	10119	89917	15665	52872	73823	73144	88662	88970	74492	51805	99378
63	09066	00903	20795	95452	92648	45454	09552	88815	16553	51125	79375	97596	16296	66092
64	42238	12426	87025	14267	20979	04508	64535	31355	86064	29472	47689	05974	52468	16834
65	16153	08002	26504	41744	81959	65642	74240	56302	00033	67107	77510	70625	28725	34191
66	21457	40742	29820	96783	29400	21840	15035	34537	33310	06116	95240	15957	16572	06004
67	21581	57802	02050	89728	17937	37621	47075	42080	97403	48626	68995	43805	33386	21597
68	55612	78095	83197	33732	05810	24813	86902	60397	16489	03264	88525	42786	05269	92532
69	44657	66999	99324	51281	84463	60563	79312	93454	68876	25471	93911	25650	12682	73572
70	91340	84979	46949	81973	37949	61023	43997	15263	80644	43942	89203	71795	99533	50501
71	91227	21199	31935	27022	84067	05462	35216	14486	29891	68607	41867	14951	91696	85065
72	50001	38140	66321	19924	72163	09538	12151	06878	91903	18749	34405	56087	82790	70925
73	65390	05224	72958	28609	81406	39147	25549	48542	42627	45233	57202	94617	23772	07896
74	27504	96131	83944	41575	10573	08619	64482	73923	36152	05184	94142	25299	84387	34925
75	37169	94851	39117	89632	00959	16487	65536	49071	39782	17095	02330	74301	00275	48280
76	11508	70225	51111	38351	19444	66499	71945	05422	13442	78675	84081	66938	93654	59894
77	37449	30362	06694	54690	04052	53115	62757	95348	78662	11163	81651	50245	34971	52924
78	46515	70331	85922	38329	57015	15765	97161	17869	45349	61796	66345	81073	49106	79860
79	30986	81223	42416	58353	21532	30502	32305	86482	05174	07901	54339	58861	74818	46942
80	63798	64995	46583	09765	44160	78128	83991	42865	92520	83531	80377	35909	81250	54238
81	82486	84846	99254	67632	43218	50076	21361	64816	51202	88124	41870	52689	51275	83556
82	21885	32906	92431	09060	64297	51674	64126	62570	26123	05155	59194	52799	28225	85762
83	60336	98782	07408	53458	13564	59089	26445	29789	85205	41001	12535	12133	14645	23541
84	43937	46891	24010	25560	86355	33941	25786	54990	71899	15475	95434	98227	21824	19585
85	97656	63175	89303	16275	07100	92063	21942	18611	47348	20203	18534	03862	78095	50136
86	03299	01221	05418	38982	55758	92237	26759	86367	21216	98442	08303	56613	91511	75928
87	79626	06486	03574	17668	07785	76020	79924	25651	83325	88428	85076	72811	22717	50585
88	85636	68335	47539	03129	65651	11977	02510	26113	99447	68645	34327	15152	55230	93448
89	18039	14367	61337	06177	12143	46609	32989	74014	64708	00533	35398	58408	13261	47908
90	08362	15656	60627	36478	65648	16764	53412	09013	07832	41574	17639	82163	60859	75567
91	79556	29068	04142	16268	15387	12856	66227	38358	22478	73373	88732	09443	82558	05250
92	92608	82674	27072	32534	17075	27698	98204	63863	11951	34648	88022	56148	34925	57031
93	23982	25835	40055	67006	12293	02753	14827	22235	35071	99704	37543	11601	35503	85171
94	09915	96306	05908	97901	28395	14186	00821	80703	70426	75647	76310	88717	37890	40129
95	50937	33300	26695	62247	69927	76123	50842	43834	86654	70959	79725	93872	28117	19233
96	42488	78077	69882	61657	34136	79180	97526	43092	04098	73571	80799	76536	71255	64239
97	46764	86273	63003	93017	31204	36692	40202	35275	57306	55543	53203	18098	47625	88684
98	03237	45430	55417	63282	90816	17349	88298	90183	36600	78406	06216	95787	42579	90730
99	86591	81482	52667	61583	14972	90053	89534	76036	49199	43716	97548	04379	46370	28672
100	38534	01715	94964	87288	65680	43772	39560	12918	86537	62738	19636	51132	25739	56947

Table continued on following page

A TABLE OF 14,000 RANDOM UNITS

Line/Col.	(1)	(2)	(3)	(4)	(5)	(6)	(7)	(8)	(9)	(10)	(11)	(12)	(13)	(14)
101	13284	16834	74151	92027	24670	36665	00770	22878	02179	51602	07270	76517	97275	45960
102	21224	00370	30420	03883	96648	89428	41583	17564	27395	63904	41548	49197	82277	24120
103	99052	47887	81085	64933	66279	80432	65793	83287	34142	13241	30590	97760	35848	91983
104	00199	50993	98603	38452	87890	94624	69721	57484	67501	77638	44331	11257	71131	11059
105	60578	06483	28733	37867	07936	98710	98539	27186	31237	80612	44488	97819	70401	95419
106	91240	18312	17441	01929	18163	69201	31211	54288	39296	37318	65724	90401	79017	62077
107	97458	14229	12063	59611	32249	90466	33216	19358	02591	54263	88449	01912	07436	50813
108	35249	38646	34475	72417	60514	69257	12489	51924	86871	92446	36607	11458	30440	52639
109	38980	46600	11759	11900	46743	27860	77940	39298	97838	95145	32378	68038	89351	37005
110	10750	52745	38749	87365	58959	53731	89295	59062	39404	13198	59960	70408	29812	83126
111	36247	27850	73958	20673	37800	63835	71051	84724	52492	22342	78071	17456	96104	18327
112	70994	66986	99744	72438	01174	42159	11392	20724	54322	36923	70009	23233	65438	59685
113	99638	94702	11463	18148	81386	80431	90628	52506	02016	85151	88598	47821	00265	82525
114	72055	15774	43857	99805	10419	76939	25993	03544	21560	83471	43989	90770	22965	44247
115	24038	65541	85788	55835	38835	59399	13790	35112	01324	39520	76210	22467	83275	32286
116	74976	14631	35908	28221	39470	91548	12854	30166	09073	75887	36782	00268	97121	57676
117	35553	71628	70189	26436	63407	91178	90348	55359	80392	41012	36270	77786	89578	21059
118	35676	12797	51434	82976	42010	26344	92920	92155	58807	54644	58581	95331	78629	73344
119	74815	67523	72985	23183	02446	63594	98924	20633	58842	85961	07648	70164	34994	67662
120	45246	88048	65173	50989	91060	89894	36063	32819	68559	99221	49475	50558	34698	71800
121	76509	47069	86378	41797	11910	49672	88575	97966	32466	10083	54728	81972	58975	30761
122	19689	90332	04315	21358	97248	11188	39062	63312	52496	07349	79178	33692	57352	72862
123	42751	35318	97513	61537	54955	08159	00337	80778	27507	95478	21252	12746	37554	97775
124	11946	22681	45045	13964	57517	59419	58045	44067	58716	58840	45557	96345	33271	53464
125	96518	48688	20996	11090	48396	57177	83867	86464	14342	21545	46717	72364	86954	55580
126	35726	58643	76869	84622	39098	36083	72505	92265	23107	60278	05822	46760	44294	07672
127	39737	42750	48968	70536	84864	64952	38404	94317	65402	13589	01055	79044	19308	83623
128	97025	66492	56177	04049	80312	48028	26408	43591	75528	65341	49044	95495	81256	53214
129	62814	08075	09788	56350	76787	51591	54509	49295	85830	59860	30883	89660	96142	18354
130	25578	22950	15227	83291	41737	79599	96191	71845	86899	70694	24290	01551	80092	82118
131	68763	69576	88991	49662	46704	63362	56625	00481	73323	91427	15264	06969	57048	54149
132	17900	00813	64361	60725	88974	61005	99709	30666	26451	11528	44323	34778	60342	60388
133	71944	60227	63551	71109	05624	43836	58254	26160	32116	63403	35404	57146	10909	07346
134	54684	93691	85132	64399	29182	44324	14491	55226	78793	34107	30374	48429	51376	09559
135	25946	27623	11258	65204	52832	50880	22273	05554	99521	73791	85744	29276	70326	60251
136	01353	39318	44961	44972	91766	90262	56073	06606	51826	18893	83448	31915	97764	75091
137	99083	88191	27662	99113	57174	35571	99884	13951	71057	53961	61448	74909	07322	80960
138	52021	45406	37945	75234	24327	86978	22644	87779	23753	99926	63898	54886	18051	96314
139	78755	47744	43776	83098	03225	14281	83637	55984	13300	52212	58781	14905	46502	04472
140	25282	69106	59180	16257	22810	43609	12224	25643	89884	31149	85423	32581	34374	70873
141	11959	94202	02743	86847	79725	51811	12998	76844	05320	54236	53891	70226	38632	84776
142	11644	13792	98190	01424	30078	28197	55583	05197	47714	68440	22016	79204	06862	94451
143	06307	97912	68110	59812	95448	43244	31262	88880	13040	16458	43813	89416	42482	33939
144	76285	75714	89585	99296	52640	46518	55486	90754	88932	19937	57119	23251	55619	23679
145	55322	07589	39600	60866	63007	20007	66819	84164	61131	81429	60676	42807	78286	29015
146	78017	90928	90220	92503	83375	26986	74399	30885	88567	29169	72816	53357	15428	86932
147	44768	43342	20696	26331	43140	69744	82928	24988	94237	46138	77426	39039	55596	12655
148	25100	19336	14605	86603	51680	97678	24261	02464	86563	74812	60069	71674	15478	47642
149	83612	46623	62876	85197	07824	91392	58317	37726	84628	42221	10268	20692	15699	29167
150	41347	81666	82961	60413	71020	83658	02415	33322	66036	98712	46795	16308	28413	05417

A TABLE OF 14,000 RANDOM UNITS

Line/Col.	(1)	(2)	(3)	(4)	(5)	(6)	(7)	(8)	(9)	(10)	(11)	(12)	(13)	(14)
151	38128	51178	75096	13609	16110	73533	42564	59870	29399	67834	91055	89917	51096	89011
152	60950	00455	73254	96067	50717	13878	03216	78274	65863	37011	91283	33914	91303	49326
153	90524	17320	29832	96118	75792	25326	22940	24904	80523	38928	91374	55597	97567	38914
154	49897	18278	67160	39408	97056	43517	84426	59650	20247	19293	02019	14790	02852	05819
155	18494	99209	81060	19488	65596	59787	47939	91225	98768	43688	00438	05548	09443	82897
156	65373	72984	30171	37741	70203	94094	87261	30056	58124	70133	18936	02138	59372	09075
157	40653	12843	04213	70925	95360	55774	76439	61768	52817	81151	52188	31940	54273	49032
158	51638	22238	56344	44587	83231	50317	74541	07719	25472	41602	77318	15145	57515	07633
159	69742	99303	62578	83575	30337	07488	51941	84316	42067	49692	28616	29101	03013	73449
160	58012	74072	67488	74580	47992	69482	58624	17106	47538	13452	22620	24260	40155	74716
161	18348	19855	42887	08279	43206	47077	42637	45606	00011	20662	14642	49984	94509	56380
162	59614	09193	58064	29086	44385	45740	70752	05663	49081	26960	57454	99264	24142	74648
163	75688	28630	39210	52897	62748	72658	98059	67202	72789	01869	13496	14663	87645	89713
164	13941	77802	69101	70061	35460	34576	15412	81304	58757	35498	94830	75521	00603	97701
165	96656	86420	96475	86458	54463	96419	55417	41375	76886	19008	66877	35934	59801	00497
166	03363	82042	15942	14549	38324	87094	19069	67590	11087	68570	22591	65232	85915	91499
167	70366	08390	69155	25496	13240	57407	91407	49160	07379	34444	94567	66035	38918	65708
168	47870	36605	12927	16043	53257	93796	52721	73120	48025	76074	95605	67422	41646	14557
169	79504	77606	22761	30518	28373	73898	30550	76684	77366	32276	04690	61667	64798	66276
170	46967	74841	50923	15339	37755	98995	40162	89561	69199	42257	11647	47603	48779	97907
171	14558	50769	35444	59030	87516	48193	02945	00922	48189	04724	21263	20892	92955	90251
172	12440	25057	01132	38611	28135	68089	10954	10097	54243	06460	50856	65435	79377	53890
173	32293	29938	68653	10497	98919	46587	77701	99119	93165	67788	17638	23097	21468	36992
174	10640	21875	72462	77981	56550	55999	87310	69643	45124	00349	25748	00844	96831	30651
175	47615	23169	39571	56972	20628	21788	51736	33133	72696	32605	41569	76148	91544	21121
176	16948	11128	71624	72754	49084	96303	27830	45817	67867	18062	87453	17226	72904	71474
177	21258	61092	66634	70335	92448	17354	83432	49608	66520	06442	59664	20420	39201	69549
178	15072	48853	15178	30730	47481	48490	41436	25015	49932	20474	53821	51015	79841	32405
179	99154	57412	09858	65671	70655	71479	63520	31357	56968	06729	34465	70685	04184	25250
180	08759	61089	23706	32994	35426	36666	63988	98844	37533	08269	27021	45886	22835	78451
181	67323	57839	61114	62192	47547	58023	64630	34886	98777	75442	95592	06141	45096	73117
182	09255	13986	84834	20764	72206	89393	34548	93438	88730	61805	78955	18952	46436	58740
183	36304	74712	00374	10107	85061	69228	81969	92216	03568	39630	81869	52824	50937	27954
184	15884	67429	86612	47367	10242	44880	12060	44309	46629	55105	66793	93173	00480	13311
185	18745	32031	35303	08134	33925	03044	59929	95418	04917	57596	24878	61733	92834	64454
186	72934	40086	88292	65728	38300	42323	64068	98373	48971	09049	59943	36538	05976	82118
187	17626	02944	20910	57662	80181	38579	24580	90529	52303	50436	29401	57824	86039	81062
188	27117	61399	50967	41399	81636	16663	15634	79717	94696	59240	25543	97989	63306	90946
189	93995	18678	90012	63645	85701	85269	62263	68331	00389	72571	15210	20769	44686	96176
190	67392	89421	09623	80725	62620	84162	87368	29560	00519	84545	08004	24526	41252	14521
191	04910	12261	37566	80016	21245	69377	50420	85658	55263	68667	78770	04533	14513	18099
192	81453	20283	79929	59839	23875	13245	46808	74124	74703	35769	95588	21014	37078	39170
193	19480	75790	48539	23703	15537	48885	02861	86587	74539	65227	90799	58789	96257	02708
194	21456	13162	74608	81011	55512	07481	93551	72189	76261	91206	89941	15132	37738	59284
195	89406	20912	46189	76376	25538	87212	20748	12831	57166	35026	16817	79121	18929	40628
196	09866	07414	55977	16419	01101	69343	13305	94302	80703	57910	36933	57771	42546	03003
197	86541	24681	23421	13521	28000	94917	07423	57523	97234	63951	42876	46829	09781	58160
198	10414	96941	06205	72222	57167	83902	07460	69507	10600	08858	07685	44472	64220	27040
199	49942	06683	41479	58982	56288	42853	92196	20632	62045	78812	35895	51851	83534	10689
200	23995	68882	42291	23374	24299	27024	67460	94783	40937	16961	26053	78749	46704	21983

Appendix C

Table: Areas in One Tail of the Standard Normal Curve

This table shows the shaded area

z	.00	.01	.02	.03	.04	.05	.06	.07	.08	.09
0.0	.500	.496	.492	.488	.484	.480	.476	.472	.468	.464
0.1	.460	.456	.452	.448	.444	.440	.436	.433	.429	.425
0.2	.421	.417	.413	.409	.405	.401	.397	.394	.390	.386
0.3	.382	.378	.374	.371	.367	.363	.359	.356	.352	.348
0.4	.345	.341	.337	.334	.330	.326	.323	.319	.316	.312
0.5	.309	.305	.302	.298	.295	.291	.288	.284	.281	.278
0.6	.274	.271	.268	.264	.261	.258	.255	.251	.248	.245
0.7	.242	.239	.236	.233	.230	.227	.224	.221	.218	.215
0.8	.212	.209	.206	.203	.200	.198	.195	.192	.189	.187
0.9	.184	.181	.179	.176	.174	.171	.169	.166	.164	.161
1.0	.159	.156	.154	.152	.149	.147	.145	.142	.140	.138
1.1	.136	.133	.131	.129	.127	.125	.123	.121	.119	.117
1.2	.115	.113	.111	.109	.107	.106	.104	.102	.100	.099
1.3	.097	.095	.093	.092	.090	.089	.087	.085	.084	.082
1.4	.081	.079	.078	.076	.075	.074	.072	.071	.069	.068
1.5	.067	.066	.064	.063	.062	.061	.059	.058	.057	.056
1.6	.055	.054	.053	.052	.051	.049	.048	.048	.046	.046
1.7	.045	.044	.043	.042	.041	.040	.039	.038	.038	.037
1.8	.036	.035	.034	.034	.033	.032	.031	.031	.030	.029
1.9	.029	.028	.027	.027	.026	.026	.025	.024	.024	.023
2.0	.023	.022	.022	.021	.021	.020	.020	.019	.019	.018
2.1	.018	.017	.017	.017	.016	.016	.015	.015	.015	.014
2.2	.014	.014	.013	.013	.013	.012	.012	.012	.011	.011
2.3	.011	.010	.010	.010	.010	.009	.009	.009	.009	.008
2.4	.008	.008	.008	.008	.007	.007	.007	.007	.007	.006
2.5	.006	.006	.006	.006	.006	.005	.005	.005	.005	.005
2.6	.005	.005	.004	.004	.004	.004	.004	.004	.004	.004
2.7	.003	.003	.003	.003	.003	.003	.003	.003	.003	.003
2.8	.003	.002	.002	.002	.002	.002	.002	.002	.002	.002
2.9	.002	.002	.002	.002	.002	.002	.002	.001	.001	.001
3.0	.001									

Adapted from Croxton [25]. Permission sought: Colton T. *Statistics in Medicine*. Boston, Mass: Little, Brown & Co; 1974 and Croxton FE. *Elementary Statistics with Applications in Medicine*. New York, NY: Prentice-Hall; 1953.

Appendix D

Questions for Evaluating a Research Article

STEP ONE

CLASSIFICATION OF RESEARCH AND VARIABLES

- □ Was data collection prospective or retrospective? (Chapter 4)
- □ Was the purpose of the research description, relationship analysis, difference analysis, or some combination? (Chapter 4)
- □ Was the study experimental or nonexperimental? (Chapters 4 through 6)
- □ Was the study conducted according to the assumptions and methods of the quantitative, qualitative, or single-system paradigms? (Chapter 9)
- □ What were the independent variables? (Chapter 5)
- □ What were the dependent variables? (Chapter 5)

STEP TWO

ANALYSIS OF PURPOSES AND CONCLUSIONS

- □ Is there a conclusion for every purpose?
- □ Is there a purpose for every conclusion?
- □ Are there significant results that should be evaluated for possible alternative explanations and clinical importance? (Chapter 13)
- □ Are there nonsignificant results that should be evaluated for power and clinical importance? (Chapter 13)

STEP THREE

ANALYSIS OF DESIGN AND CONTROL ELEMENTS

- ☐ What was the design of the study? (Chapters 5 through 7)
- ☐ Was the independent variable implemented in a laboratory-like or clinic-like setting? (Chapter 5)
- ☐ Was selection of subjects done randomly, by cluster, by convenience, or purposively? (Chapter 8)
- ☐ Were subjects assigned to groups through individual random assignment, block assignment, systematic assignment, matched assignment, or consecutive assignment? (Chapter 8)
- ☐ Were extraneous experimental-setting variables under tight laboratory-like control or loose, clinic-like control? (Chapter 5)
- ☐ Were extraneous subject variables under laboratory-like or clinic-like control? (Chapter 5)
- ☐ What was the level of control over measurement techniques? (Chapters 5, 10, and 11)
- ☐ Was information controlled through incomplete information, subject blinding, or researcher blinding? (Chapter 5)

STEP FOUR

VALIDITY QUESTIONS

- ☐ Construct Validity (Chapter 7)

Were the variables in the study defined and implemented in meaningful ways?

Construct Underrepresentation

Were variables well developed and defined?

Were there enough levels of the independent variable? Was treatment administered as an all-or-none phenomenon or in varying levels?

Do the dependent variables provide information in all areas important to the phenomenon under study?

Was the independent variable administered at a lower intensity or in a different manner than would be typical in a clinical setting?

Experimenter Expectancies

Were the experimenter's expectations transparently obvious to subjects?

Were there differences between the construct as labeled and the construct as implemented, based on the influence of the experimenter?

Interaction of Different Treatments

What uncontrolled treatments might have interacted with the independent variable?

Interaction of Testing and Treatment

Could any of the measurements used in the study have contributed to a treatment effect?

- ☐ Internal Validity (Chapter 7)

Was the independent variable the probable cause of differences in the dependent variables?

History and Interaction of History and Assignment

What events other than implementation of the independent variable occurred during the study that might have plausibly caused changes in the dependent variable?

If any historical events took place, did the events have an equal impact on treatment and control groups?

Maturation and Interaction of Maturation and Assignment

Could changes in the dependent variable have been the result of the passage of time, rather than the implementation of the independent variable?

If a control group was present, were the same maturational influences at work for them as for the treatment group?

Testing

Is familiarity with testing procedures a likely explanation for differences in the dependent variable?

Were tests conducted with equal frequency for treatment and control groups so that any testing effects were consistent for all groups within the study?

Instrumentation and Interaction of Instrumentation and Assignment

Were instruments calibrated appropriately?

Were measurements taken under controlled environmental conditions such as temperature or humidity?

If the instrument was a human observer, what measures were taken to ensure consistency of observations?

Were instruments expected to be equally sensitive across the values expected for both the treatment and control groups?

Statistical Regression to the Mean

Were subjects selected for the study based on an extreme score on a single administration of a test?

Can improvements or declines in performance be attributed to statistical regression rather than true change?

Assignment

Were subjects assigned to groups randomly?

If not assigned randomly, what factors other than the one of interest might have influenced their assignment?

Mortality

What proportions of subjects were lost from the treatment and control groups?

Were the proportions of subjects lost equal for the treatment and control groups?

What are possible explanations for differential loss of subjects from the groups?

Diffusion or Imitation of Treatments

Were treatment and control subjects able to share information about their respective routines?

Was either the treatment or control regimen likely to have been perceived as more desirable by subjects in the other group?

Compensatory Equalization of Treatments

Were researchers aware of which subjects were in which group?

Were those implementing the treatments likely to have paid extra attention to control group subjects because of the presumed inferiority of care they received?

Compensatory Rivalry or Resentful Demoralization

Did subjects know whether they were in the treatment or control group?

Were control-group subjects likely to have either tried harder or withdrawn their efforts because they knew they were in the control group and perceived it to be a less desirable alternative than being in the treatment group?

□ Statistical Conclusion Validity (Chapter 13)

Were statistical tools used appropriately?

Low Power

Are statistically insignificant results related to small sample size, high within-group variability, or small between-groups differences?

Do statistically insignificant differences seem clinically important?

Clinical Insignificance

Are statistically significant results clinically important?

Error Rate Problems

If multiple statistical tests were performed, did the researcher set a conservative alpha level to compensate for alpha level inflation?

Are identified significant differences isolated and difficult to explain, or is there a pattern of significant differences that suggests true differences rather than Type I errors?

Violated Assumptions

Were tests used appropriately for independent and dependent samples?

Were normal-distribution and homogeneity-of-variance assumptions satisfied?

□ External Validity (Chapter 7)

To whom and under what conditions can the research results be generalized?

Selection

Were volunteers used for study? In what ways do these volunteers differ from clinical populations?

Are results from normal subjects generalized to patient populations?

Do the authors limit their conclusions to subjects similar to those studied?

Setting

To what extent did the experimental setting differ from the setting to which the researchers wish to generalize the results?

Were control elements implemented fastidiously, as in a laboratory, or pragmatically, as in a clinic?

Time

How much time elapsed between the collection of the data in the study and the present time?

Do differences in overall clinical management of patients make the studied procedures less appropriate today than when the study was implemented?

STEP FIVE

PLACE STUDY INTO LITERATURE CONTEXT

- □ Do results confirm or contradict the findings of others?
- □ Does this study correct some of the deficiencies identified in other studies?
- □ Does the study examine constructs or variables unstudied by others?
- □ How do the sample size and composition compare with those of other studies?
- □ How do the internal and external validities of this compare with those of related studies?

STEP SIX

PERSONAL UTILITY QUESTIONS

- □ Are your setting and the research setting similar enough to warrant application of the results of the research to your clinical practice?
- □ Does the study cause you to question some of the assumptions under which you have managed patients?
- □ Do the methods of this study suggest ways in which you can improve on the design of a study you are planning?

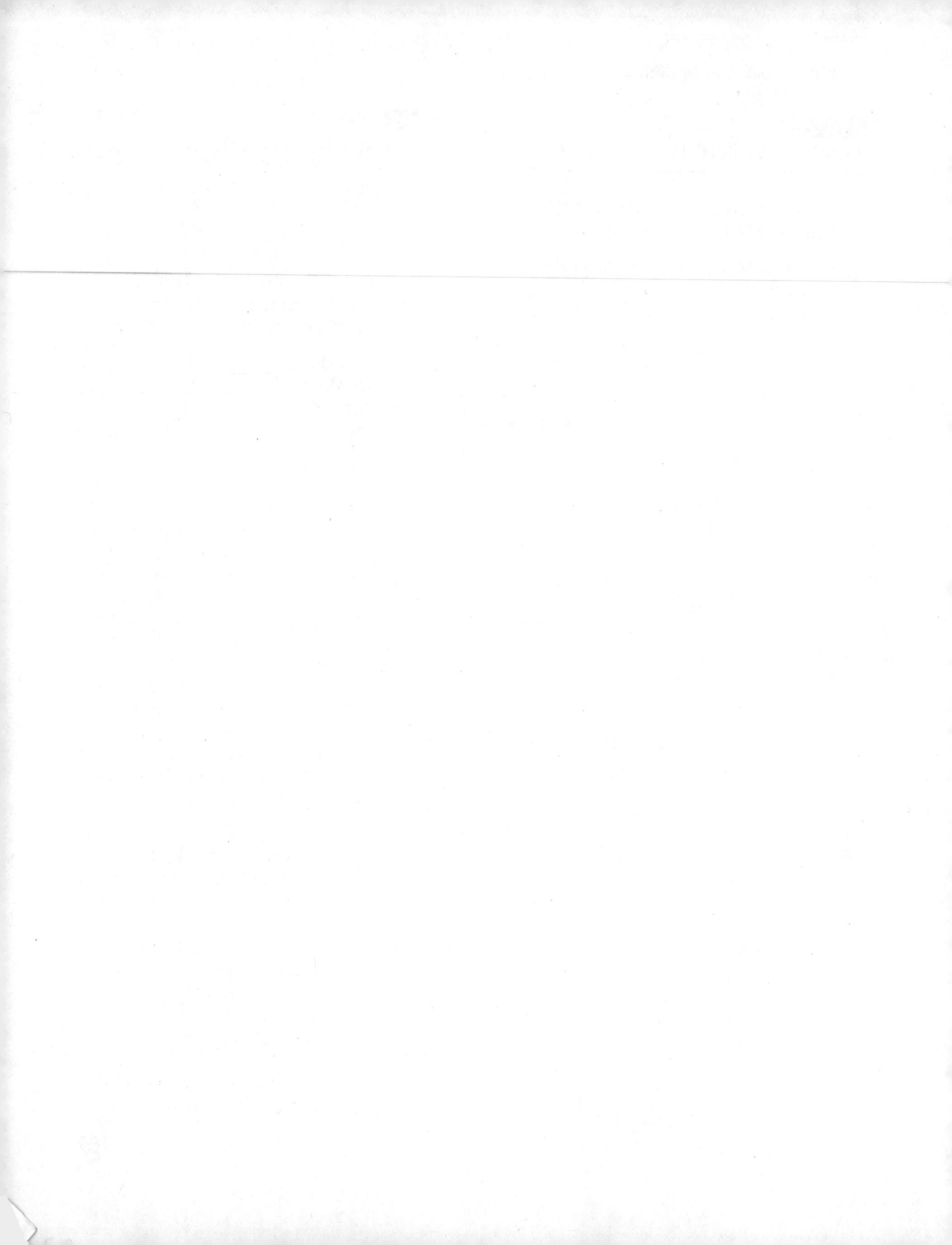

Appendix E

Guidelines for Preparing a Journal Article Manuscript

1. General Guidelines
   - 1.1 Double-space everything, including block quotes, tables, and references.
   - 1.2 Margins should be a minimum one inch; some journals will request more generous margins.
   - 1.3 Don't right justify the text or hyphenate words at the ends of lines. These adjustments may make an attractive document but hinder the editing process.
   - 1.4 Generally plan for 15 pages of text, plus title page, abstract page, tables, references, and figures. Consult journal instructions to authors for more specific length guidelines.
   - 1.5 Manuscript pagination is as follows: Title page is page 1, but is not labeled; abstract page is page 2; text begins on page 3. Tables follow the references. Each table begins on a new page, and table pages are numbered consecutively with the manuscript. The final numbered manuscript page is the one on which the figure legends are written; it starts on a separate page following the tables.
   - 1.6 Determine formats for headings and subheadings and use them consistently. One common scheme:

METHOD (First-level side heading in uppercase letters, set off from text with extra spacing above and below the heading)

Subjects (Second-level side heading, upper- and lowercase letters, set off from text with extra spacing above and below the heading)

Facility A. (Third-level side heading, indented with period following heading; leave extra space above heading, and run in text after heading)

2. Title and Title Page

2.1 Be concise, yet specific. Include important variables under study. "Knee Function after Total Knee Arthroplasty" is too concise if the study is really one of "Effect of Three Continuous Passive Motion Regimens on Knee Function Six Months After Total Knee Arthroplasty."

2.2 Titles may be descriptive (such as "Effect of Continuous Passive Motion on Knee Range of Motion After Total Knee Arthroplasty") or assertive (such as "Continuous Passive Motion Does Not Improve Knee Range of Motion After Total Knee Arthroplasty"). Some journal editors prefer the latter, which summarizes results in the title; others prefer to let readers draw their own conclusions.

2.3 Consider using terms that are indexed in the data bases interested readers are likely to search; for example, use "total knee arthroplasty" rather than "total knee replacement" because "arthroplasty" is indexed and "replacement" is not.

2.4 Refer to journal requirements for author and affiliation format because these vary widely among journals.

3. Abstract

3.1 Generally limit the abstract to less than 150 words.

3.2 Summarize the study's purpose, procedures, results, and major conclusions.

3.3 Use major indexing terms because users of computer data bases often search abstracts as well as titles.

3.4 Do not cite references or provide *p* values because these are meaningful only in the context of the study.

4. Introduction

4.1 No heading is used for the introduction; just begin the first paragraph.

4.2 In a paper of 15 pages, the introduction section is typically 2 to 3 pages.

4.3 Cite only the most relevant citations about the topic area. A journal article does not contain an exhaustive review of the literature, but rather it places the problem into the context of the literature.

4.3.1 American Medical Association (AMA)-style citations in the text use superscript numerals in sequential order.

4.3.2 If superscripts are unavailable, then the number should be enclosed in parentheses.

4.3.3 If the text refers to an author's name, the numeral follows the name directly. If the author's name is not mentioned and the entire sentence is related to the citation, the numeral goes at the end of the sentence. If the citation refers to only part of the sentence, the numeral is placed at the conclusion of that part.

4.3.4 When using a numbered reference style like the AMA, writers often cite references with the author name in parentheses in early drafts of the papers. This prevents repeated renumbering of references as the paper is edited. For the final draft, the names and parentheses are removed and the correct numbers inserted.

4.3.5 The other most frequently encountered reference style is the name–date style, in which the author's name and the date of publication are placed in parentheses within the text. Journals that follow the *Publication Manual of the American Psychological Association* use the name–date citation format.

4.4 Suggested first paragraph: Broadly state the problem, with documentation as needed.

4.5 Suggested second through fourth paragraphs, as needed: Summarize what is known about the problem, that is, what others have found out about the problem in their own research.

4.6 Suggested last paragraph: Identify the gap in the literature that needs to be filled, and then state the purpose of your research. State research hypotheses if appropriate. Identify major variables, using the names that you will use throughout the rest of the paper. If you have several purposes, place them in order of importance or in the order that they will be discussed in the rest of the paper.

5. Methods

5.1 The methods section is usually subdivided into "Subjects," "Instruments," "Procedures," and "Data Analysis."

5.2 In a paper of 15 pages, the methods section is typically 3 to 5 pages long.

5.3 Cite literature needed to justify the methods you used, or cite others' procedures if they are too lengthy to be repeated in your article.

5.4 The subjects subsection should describe inclusion and exclusion criteria, sampling and assignment methods, and source of the subjects.

5.5 The instruments subsection should describe each instrument used in data collection.

5.5.1 Present instruments in the order that you will eventually present your results. For example, if you have taken range of motion, strength, and functional measures and plan to discuss them in that order, describe the goniometers first, the dynamometers second, and the functional scale last.

5.5.2 If you developed the instrument, provide details about the instrument development process.

5.5.3 If you performed reliability or validity testing with the instruments but this was not the primary purpose of the research, present reliability or validity information here. If the research is methodological, then reliability or validity information belongs in the results section.

5.6 The procedures subsection should describe what you did in enough detail that others can replicate the study. Refer to other authors if necessary to justify your procedures.

5.6.1 If the measurement order is irrelevant, then present the procedures in the same order as you described the instruments. If the measurement order is critical, describe it.

5.6.2 Consider combining the instrument subsection with the procedures subsection if the equipment used is nontechnical and familiar to most professionals to whom the article would be of interest.

5.7 The data analysis subsection should include data reduction procedures and statistical testing for each variable.

5.7.1 If possible, present information about the data analysis in the order of variables presented earlier in the paper.

5.7.2 State the statistical package used and alpha level if appropriate.

5.7.3 If necessary, justify or clarify your use of statistical procedures with references.

6. Results

6.1 Sometimes the results section is subdivided by variables or class of variables.

6.2 Text is often short, with much of the information presented in tables and figures. Tables and figures should substitute for information in the text, not repeat it. Tables and figures are numbered separately in order of their appearance in the text (see Sections 11 and 12).

6.3 Present variables in previously established order.

6.4 Don't discuss the implications of the results here; just present the appropriate descriptive and statistical information.

6.5 In a paper of 15 pages, the results section is typically only 1 to 2 pages long, supplemented by figures and tables.

7. Discussion

7.1 The discussion is the heart of the paper, the place for interpretation of the results.

7.2 In a paper of 15 pages, the discussion is typically 3 to 4 pages long.

7.3 Additional references are often cited to place the results into a broader context.

7.4 Suggested first section: Restate the major results in terms of your original hypotheses.

7.5 Suggested second section: Examine the expected results, showing reinforcement of the theory that led you to a hypothesis that was supported.

7.6 Suggested third section: Examine the unexpected results, providing theoretical explanation through examination of related literature.

7.7 Suggested fourth section: Discuss the limitations of the study.

7.8 Suggested fifth section: Discuss the clinical implications of the findings.

7.9 Suggested sixth section: Discuss directions for future research.

8. Conclusions

8.1 Not all articles have a conclusions section. If the conclusions are not a separate section, they are addressed in the discussion.

8.2 In a paper of 15 pages, the conclusions are typically less than a page long. The conclusions are stated concisely, in the order in which the questions were posed in the purpose section of the study.

9. Acknowledgments

9.1 Each person acknowledged should have given permission to be acknowledged.

9.2 Be specific about the contribution of each person: "critical review," "manuscript preparation," or "data collection."

9.3 Place acknowledgments on a separate page so that they can be removed from the manuscript to maintain authors' anonymity when the paper is sent out for review.

10. References

10.1 Begin references on a separate page.

10.2 Remember to double-space references, with triple or quadruple spacing between references.

10.3 List only references cited in the study.

10.4 The *Manual of Style* of the AMA numbers references in the reference list in the order they are cited in text. If you are submitting to a journal that follows another style, consult their style manual and order the references appropriately.

10.5 Place references into proper format. Pay attention to punctuation, capitalization, and abbreviation of journal article title. AMA formats for the different elements of a journal article citation are as follows:

10.5.1 *Authors:* Smith DL, Riley JW, Anderson MD. There is no internal punctuation within each name; names are separated by commas; a period follows the final name.

10.5.2 *Journal article title:* Effects of prolonged sitting on attention span: a study of physical therapy students. Only the first word is capitalized unless there is a proper name within the title; the first word after a colon starts with a lowercase letter; a period follows the title.

10.5.3 *Journal name: Phys Ther.* Use the Index Medicus abbreviation for the journal name; if the journal is not indexed in Index Medicus, then spell out the name in full. The journal abbreviation or name is italicized (or underlined if an italicized font is not available), and a period follows. For a list of journals and journal abbreviations used frequently by physical therapists, see Table 16–3.

10.5.4 *Year, volume, issue and pages:* 1987;67:3002-3007. The year comes first, followed by a semicolon; the volume number comes next, followed by a colon; an issue number is required only if each issue begins with page 1 (if the issue number is necessary, it is enclosed in parentheses); the page numbers are last, followed by a period. Inclusive page numbers are listed and the full page number is repeated on each side of the hyphen.

10.6 Consult the appropriate style manual for detailed directions on specific formats for different types of references (for example, book, chapter in a book, dissertation, etc.).

11. Tables

 11.1 Tables consist of rows and columns of numbers or text.
 11.2 Vertical lines are not used in tables; use horizontal lines only.
 11.3 Tables should not repeat information in the text. If a table can be summarized in a sentence or two, then it should probably not be a table.
 11.4 Number tables (Table 1, Table 2, Table 3 . . .) according to their order in the paper. Refer to each table in the text, highlighting the most important information. If there is only one table, it is not numbered.
 11.5 Table titles should describe the specific information contained within the table; for example, "Data" is too general a title; "Mean Knee Function Variables by Clinic" is more specific.
 11.6 Each table begins on a separate page placed after the references. Tables may be continued onto additional pages.

12. Figures

 12.1 Figures are illustrative materials such as graphs, diagrams, or photographs.
 12.2 Figures should not repeat information in text or tables. They should be used only when visual information is more effective than tabular or text information.
 12.3 Figures are numbered (Figure 1, Figure 2, Figure 3 . . .) in order of their appearance in the paper. If there is only one figure, it is not numbered.
 12.4 Figure legends are listed on a separate sheet following the tables. The legend should make the figure meaningful on its own by explaining any abbreviations and describing concisely the important points being illustrated.
 12.5 The figure itself is not labeled or numbered on its face. Figures are identified on the back using lightly pencilled writing or a gummed label; be careful not to damage the figure by labeling it. When submitting a manuscript, encase the figures in cardboard to protect them.
 12.6 Identification of figures in theses or dissertations will deviate from this format. Because they are used in the format prepared by the author, rather than being typeset in a journal, figure numbers and legends must accompany the figures themselves.

References

American Medical Association. *Manual of Style.* 8th ed. Baltimore, Md: Williams & Wilkins; 1989.

Day RA. *How to Write and Publish a Scientific Paper.* 3rd ed. Phoenix, Ariz: Oryx Press; 1988.

Huth EJ. *How to Write and Publish Papers in the Medical Sciences.* 2nd ed. Baltimore, Md: Williams & Wilkins; 1990.

International Committee of Medical Journal Editors. Uniform requirements for manuscripts submitted to biomedical journals. *Ann Intern Med.* 1988;108:258–265.

Publication Manual of the American Psychological Association. 3rd ed. Washington, DC: American Psychological Association; 1983.

Appendix F

Sample Manuscript for Hypothetical Study

The following manuscript is based, with a few changes in the demographic variables, on the hypothetical data set for patients who have had total knee arthroplasty presented in Tables 13–1 and 13–2. The literature cited in the manuscript is from the conceptual review of the literature presented in Chapter 16. However, an exhaustive review of the literature related to continuous passive motion and total knee arthroplasty was not developed for use in this example. Although the individual studies are cited appropriately, readers should realize that the hypothetical problem statement may not accurately reflect the overall state of research in this area.

The eighth edition of the American Medical Association's *Manual of Style* was used to guide the preparation of the sample manuscript. Writers should consult the particular journal's instructions for authors to determine whether another style manual should be followed.

The circled numbers in the manuscript correspond to guidelines listed in Appendix E.

Effect of Three Continuous Passive Motion Regimens on Knee Function Six Months After Total Knee Arthroplasty ← (2.1)

Jan R. Woolery
Jodi C. Beeker
Jonathon V. Mills

JR Woolery, PT, PhD, is Research Therapist, Department of Physical Therapy, Memorial Hospital of Indiana, 555 Main Street, Anytown, IN 46234 (USA). Address all correspondence to Dr Woolery.

JC Beeker, PT, MS, is Senior Physical Therapist, Department of Rehabilitation Services, Community Hospital of Anytown, Anytown, IN.

JV Mills, PT, MS, is Staff Therapist, Physical Therapy Department, Religious Hospital of Anytown, Anytown, IN.

The results of this study were presented in a platform presentation at the Conference, Association, City, State, Date.

This study was approved by the institutional review boards of Memorial Hospital of Indiana, Community Hospital of Anytown, and Religious Hospital of Anytown.

2

ABSTRACT

The purpose of this study was to determine the effects of three different continuous passive motion (CPM) regimens on knee motion, strength, and function 6 months after total knee arthroplasty. Subjects at three different hospitals (n = 10 at each) received CPM for 20, 12, or 4 hours daily while inpatients. Dependent variables were knee flexion range of motion at 3 and 6 weeks postoperatively and knee flexion range of motion, gait velocity, and activities of daily living score at 6 months postoperatively. Analysis of variance and Newman-Keuls post hoc tests showed that the 20-hour and 12-hour groups scored significantly higher on all variables than did the 4-hour group. There were no significant differences between the 20-hour and 12-hour groups for any of the dependent variables.

3.1

4.1 Total knee arthroplasty is a common surgical procedure used to reduce pain and enhance function for individuals with knee impairment secondary to osteoarthritis or rheumatoid arthritis. Continuous passive motion (CPM) is used routinely to encourage early motion of the knee joint after total knee arthroplasty. Despite its widespread clinical use, the optimal CPM regimen for short-term and long-term function of patients after total knee arthroplasty has not been identified.

The first limitation in the literature is that studies on the effects of CPM for patients after total knee arthroplasty have not compared different CPM regimens. Most studies have compared a single CPM regimen of 20 hours of motion per day to immobilization or limited motion in the early postoperative period.[1–4] (4.3.1) A less aggressive regimen of 3 hours of CPM per day was studied by Gose,[5] but the comparison was still to a traditional postoperative range of motion exercise program rather than to a different dosage of CPM. Only Basso and Knapp[6] (4.3.3) have compared different CPM regimens; they found no discharge differences in knee excursion or length of stay between groups who received 20 or 5 hours of CPM per day.

The second limitation of the literature is that the dependent measures studied are only minimally related to functional outcomes. The most frequently reported dependent measures are length of stay and knee joint range of motion (ROM). Most authors have found that postoperative CPM significantly reduces length

4

of stay after total knee arthroplasty.[1-5] The ROM results are less consistent. Johnson and associates[2] and Wasilewski and colleagues[4] found that groups who received CPM had significantly greater ROM at discharge than groups who did not receive CPM. Goll and coworkers,[1] Gose,[5] and Maloney and associates[3] found no significant ROM differences between CPM and non-CPM groups at discharge. Outcomes such as activities of daily living (ADL) status or gait velocity have not been studied for patients receiving CPM after total knee arthroplasty.

The third limitation of the literature is that researchers have not examined long-term outcomes on a regular basis. In three of the six studies cited thus far, data were collected at discharge only.[1,5,6] Of the three studies that examined long-term outcomes,[2-4] only Johnson and colleagues[2] found a statistically significant difference in knee ROM between CPM and non-CPM groups one year postoperatively. (4.6)→ To fill these gaps in the literature, we decided to study long-term functional outcomes after different CPM regimens. To enable us to compare our results to others in the literature, we also collected data on short-term knee flexion ROM. Specifically, the purpose of this study was to determine whether there were differences between three dosages of CPM (20, 12, and 4 hours daily) on knee flexion ROM at three and six weeks postoperatively and on knee flexion ROM, gait velocity, and ADL score at six months postoperatively. We hypothesized that there would be no differences between the 20- and 12-hour groups at any time; that there would be differences between the 4-hour group and both the 20- and 12-hour groups at 3 and 6 weeks postoperatively, and that there would be no differences among the groups at 6 months postoperatively.

METHOD

Subjects

Subjects were patients who were at least 50 years old, had a diagnosis of either osteoarthritis or rheumatoid arthritis, and underwent total knee arthroplasty in 1992 at one of three hospitals in Anytown, Indiana: Community Hospital, Memorial Hospital, and Religious Hospital. Before beginning this study, the characteristics of patients undergoing total knee arthroplasty and the postoperative rehabilitation regimens of patients after total knee arthroplasty were compared across the three participating hospitals. All used similar regimens, which included preoperative instructions from a physical therapist; CPM application within 24 hours after surgery and maintenance of CPM approximately 20 hours daily; twice-daily physical therapy beginning within 36 hours of surgery; and weight-bearing, progression of ROM, and strengthening exercises as tolerated by the patient. The comparison showed nearly identical patient characteristics on the variables of age, sex, diagnosis, and type of prosthesis implanted. Because of the similarity of both patient characteristics and rehabilitation regimens at the three hospitals, we decided to assign the CPM protocol randomly to hospitals rather than individually to patients. Patients at Community Hospital received 20 hours of CPM per day, patients at Religious Hospital received 12 hours of CPM per day, and patients at Memorial Hospital received 4 hours of CPM per day.

The first 10 patients in 1992 who met the inclusion criteria were selected for study at each hospital.

(11.4)→Table 1 shows that the background characteristics of the subjects are nearly identical across facilities.

Instruments←(5.5.1)

CPM Units. ACME CPM (ACME Orthopedics, 123 Canyon Road, Roadrunner, AZ, 44304) units were used to deliver the CPM treatment at all three facilities.

Goniometers. ROM measurements were taken with the 12-inch, full-circle, plastic universal goniometers available at each facility.

ADL Scale. We modified the Brigham and Women's knee rating scale[7] to assess ADL (Table 2). The values for each of the four subscales (distance walked, assistive device, stair climbing, and rising from a chair) were added for each person to give a single ADL score that could range from a low of 4 to a high of 20.

Procedure

Patients underwent the postoperative rehabilitation protocol described above, with the only difference between groups being the amount of time spent in the CPM unit daily. A timer on the unit was set so that time could be monitored precisely. A buzzer sounded and the machine shut off automatically when the assigned time was complete for each day. A day was defined as the 24 hours beginning at 7:00 AM. Each morning, a physical therapist recorded the total time in the CPM unit from the previous day and reset the timer for the next day.

(5.3)

Knee flexion ROM measurements were taken with patients supine according to the procedures described by Norkin and White,[8] with values recorded to the nearest degree. The 3-week and 6-week measures were taken by the treating therapists at each hospital when patients came for their routine outpatient physical therapy visits. The 6-month measures were all taken in the physical therapy department at Community Hospital. One investigator (JRW) measured 6-month ROM for all subjects. Velocity was measured by having the subject walk at a comfortable pace across a 20-m measured distance. Each subject was timed with a stopwatch during the center 10 meters of the walk. This time was converted to cm/s for analysis. One investigator (JCB) took all the velocity measures. The modified Brigham and Women's knee function scale was administered to each subject by the third investigator (JVM). Use of an assistive device, rising from a chair, and stair climbing were actually observed and rated; distance walked was a self-report measure. All subjects completed the functional scale first, the ROM measures second, and the gait velocity measure last.

Data Analysis

Average time in CPM per day and total time in CPM across days was calculated for each subject from the timer data; means were calculated for each group. An analysis of variance (ANOVA) was used to test for differences between groups for each of following dependent variables: 3-week ROM; 6-week ROM; and 6-month ROM, gait velocity, and ADL score. The Newman-Keuls procedure was used for post hoc analysis. Alpha was set at .05 for each analysis. The Statistical Package for the Social Sciences was the software used for the data analysis.

RESULTS

Mean daily time spent in CPM was 18.6 hours for the 20-hour group, 11.4 hours for the 12-hour group, and 3.9 hours for the 4-hour group. The Figure shows

6.2 and 12.3

the total time in CPM for each patient. Table 3 shows the group means for each of the dependent variables, accompanied by the *F* and *p* values for the ANOVA. There were significant differences between groups for all variables. Post hoc analysis showed that for all variables the 20- and 12-hour groups were not statistically different from one another, but that both were significantly different from the 4-hour group.

DISCUSSION

Of our three hypotheses, two were supported: that there would be no differences between the 20- and 12-hour groups at any time and that there would be three- and six-week differences between the 4-hour group and both the 20- and 12-hour groups. Our final hypothesis--that differences between the 4-hour group and the other two groups would not be present at six months--was not supported. This is in contrast to the findings of Maloney and associates[3] and Wasilewski and colleagues,[4] who found no differences between CPM and non-CPM groups at one to two years postoperatively. Even Johnson,[2] who found significant ROM differences between CPM and non-CPM groups, found only a 9-degree difference between groups at 1 year postoperatively. This difference is much smaller than our ROM difference, which was approximately 15 degrees. This difference seems clinically important because whereas the 20- and 12-hour groups achieved mean flexion ROM (100.0

and 103.3 degrees, respectively) close to the mechanical limits of their prostheses, the mean flexion ROM of the 4-hour group was less than 90 degrees. The discrepancy between our findings and those of others may be related to the differences in the follow-up times between our patients and those reported in the literature. We studied our patients for only 6 months postoperatively; others have reported their follow-up information at 1 to 2 years postoperatively. Although we had initially believed that patient status would stabilize by six months postoperatively, we need to continue the study to determine if the differences in all variables disappear 1 year postoperatively.

Gait velocity of the 20- and 12-hour groups (144.0 and 145.6 cm/s) was well above that needed to cross a typical city street (approximately 80 cm/s).[9] The 4-hour group had an average gait velocity of only 107.6 cm/s; this is sufficient to cross many streets, but certainly well below the averages of the other two groups. (7.3)

The ADL scores of the 20- and 12-hour groups were approximately 18 and 17 of 20, respectively. This indicates minor impairment on two of the components or moderate impairment on one of the components. On contrast, the average ADL score for the 4-hour group was 11, indicating moderate to severe impairment in one or more of the ADL components.

In interpreting these results, several limitations or alternative explanations must be considered. First, because the treatments were assigned by hospital and not by patient, there may have been systematic differences between care at the hospitals that could explain the difference in results. Second, because the investigators were not blind to the group membership of the subjects, their expectations may have influenced subject performance. Third, there may be differences among groups that are important but were not measured. For example, if a greater proportion of patients in the 4-hour group live with family members who assist them in ADL, perhaps they have less incentive to achieve higher levels of function than individuals who live alone.

Despite these limitations, the results have clinical implications for facilities using CPM for patients after total knee arthroplasty. First, facilities may wish to consider changing their protocols to reduce CPM from 20 hours per day to as low as 12 hours per day. In this way, the probability of developing complications from postoperative bedrest (atelectasis, sacral pressure ulcers, cardiovascular deconditioning, and deep vein thrombosis) may be reduced. Further research must be done to see if these results can be replicated and to determine the minimum dosage of CPM necessary to achieve results similar to those seen in our group who received 12 hours of CPM per day.

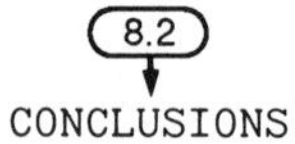

CONCLUSIONS

Patients who underwent total knee arthroplasty and received 20 hours or 12 hours of CPM per day had significantly better knee flexion ROM at 3 weeks and 6 weeks and significantly better knee flexion ROM, gait velocity, and ADL scores at 6 months postoperatively than did those who received 4 hours of CPM per day.

ACKNOWLEDGMENTS

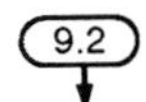

We would like to thank Ben Counter, PhD, for assistance with the statistical analysis of the study, and Ellen Redline, PT, PhD, for her critical review of an earlier draft of the manuscript.

14

REFERENCES ← 10.1

1. Goll SR, Lotke PA, Ecker ML. Failure of continuous passive motion as prophylaxis against deep venous thrombosis after total knee arthroplasty. In: Rand JA, Dorr LD, eds. *Total Arthroplasty of the Knee: Proceedings of the Knee Society, 1985–1986*. Rockville, Md: Aspen Publishers Inc; 1987.

2. Johnson DP. The effect of continuous passive motion on wound-healing and joint mobility after knee arthroplasty. *J Bone Joint Surg*. 1990;72[A]:421–426.

3. Maloney WJ, Schurman DJ, Hangen D, Goodman SB, Edworthy S, Bloch DA. The influence of continuous passive motion on outcome in total knee arthroplasty. *Clin Orthop Rel Res*. 1990;256:162–168.

4. Wasilewski SA, Woods LC, Torgerson WR, Healy WL. Value of continuous passive motion in total knee arthroplasty. *Orthopedics*. 1990;13:291–295.

5. Gose JC. Continuous passive motion in the postoperative treatment of patients with total knee replacement: a retrospective study. *Phys Ther*. 1987;67:39–42.

10.2 10.5.1 10.5.2 10.5.4 10.5.3 10.5.2

6. Basso DM, Knapp L. Comparison of two continuous passive motion protocols for patients with total knee implants. *Phys Ther*. 1987;67:360–363.

7. Ewald FC, Jacobs MA, Miegel RE, Waller PS, Poss R, Sledge CB. Kinematic total knee replacement. *J Bone Joint Surg*. 1984;66[A]:1032–1040.

8. Norkin CC, White DJ. *Measurement of Joint Motion: A Guide for Goniometry*. Philadelphia, Pa: FA Davis Co; 1985.

9. Lerner-Frankiel MB, Vargas S, Brown M, Krusell L, Schoneberger W. Functional community ambulation: what are your criteria? *Clinical Management*. 1986;6(2):12–15.

Table 1. Subject Characteristics

Variable	Hospital and Regimen		
	Community 20 hours	Religious 12 hours	Memorial 4 hours
Mean age in years	73.2	71.7	72.5
Sex			
Women (%)	50	40	60
Men (%)	50	60	40
Diagnosis			
Osteoarthritis (%)	70	80	70
Rheumatoid arthritis (%)	30	20	30
Type of Prosthesis			
Total condylar (%)	40	20	40
Posterior stabilizer (%)	40	10	30
Flat tibial plateau (%)	20	70	30

17

11.6

Table 2. Modified Brigham and Women's Knee Rating Scale

Variable	Scoring Criteria
Distance walked	5 = Unlimited
	4 = 4 to 6 blocks
	3 = 2 to 3 blocks
	2 = Indoors only
	1 = Transfers only
Assistive device	5 = None
	4 = Cane outside
	3 = Cane full time
	2 = Two canes, crutches
	1 = Walker or unable
Stair climbing	5 = Reciprocal, no rail
	4 = Reciprocal, with rail
	3 = One at a time, with or without rail
	2 = One at a time, with rail and assistive device
	1 = Unable to climb stairs

Table 2. Modified Brigham and Women's Knee Rating Scale (continued)

Variable	Scoring Criteria
Rising from a chair	5 = No arm assistance 4 = Single arm assistance 3 = Difficult with two arm assistance 2 = Needs assistance of another 1 = Unable to rise

19

Table 3. Differences Between Continuous Passive Motion (CPM) Protocols

	Hours in CPM				
Variable	20	12	4	*F*	*p*
Mean 3-week range of motion (ROM) (degrees)	77.6	72.6	49.1	7.21	.0031
Mean 6-week ROM (degrees)	78.9	82.8	58.6	8.53	.0031
Mean 6-month ROM (degrees)	100.0	103.3	85.8	15.63	.0000
Mean gait velocity (cm/s)	144.0	145.6	107.6	8.25	.0016
Mean activities of daily living (ADL) score	18.3	17.0	11.0	16.24	.0000

FIGURE LEGEND ← (12.4)

Figure. Total time in continuous passive motion for each patient.

Appendix G

Sample Platform Presentation Script with Slides

1. Effect of Three Continuous Passive Motion Regimens on Knee Function Six Months After Total Knee Arthroplasty

Jan R. Woolery
Jodi C. Beeker
Jonathon V. Mills

Good afternoon. I'm pleased to be here in Denver to present the results of our study on the effect of three different CPM regimens on knee function after total knee arthroplasty.

2. We were prompted to do this study because we found we had trouble defending our choice of CPM protocols after total knee arthroplasty.

SLIDES

Effect of Three Continuous Passive Motion Regimens on Knee Function Six Months After Total Knee Arthroplasty

Jan R. Woolery, PT, PhD
Jodi C. Beeker, PT, MS
Jonathon V. Mills, PT, MS

Memorial, Community, and Religious Hospitals, Anytown, Indiana

- **Problem**
- Method
- Results
- Discussion
- Conclusions

SLIDES	
(Photo of preoperative knee alignment)	3. As you know, total knee arthroplasty is a common surgical procedure used to reduce pain and enhance function for individuals with knee impairment secondary to osteoarthritis or rheumatoid arthritis.
(Photo of CPM in use)	4. CPM is used routinely in our facilities to encourage early motion of the knee joint after total knee arthroplasty. Despite its widespread clinical use, the optimal CPM regimen for short-term and long-term function of patients after total knee arthroplasty has not been identified.
CPM Comparisons • **20-hr CPM *versus* immobilization** Goll, Johnson, Maloney, Wasilewski • **3-hr CPM *versus* early motion** Gose	5. The first limitation in the literature is that studies on the effects of CPM for patients after total knee arthroplasty have not compared different CPM protocols but have instead compared a single CPM regimen to immobilization or limited motion in the early postoperative period.
Nonfunctional Outcomes • **Range of motion** • **Length of stay** Wasilewski, Johnson, Maloney, Basso, Gose, Goll	6. A second limitation is that studies on CPM use after total knee arthroplasty have typically reported only range of motion and length of stay outcomes, ignoring more functional outcomes such as gait velocity or ADL status.
Short-Term Outcomes Only **Discharge status** Wasilewski, Maloney, Basso	7. The third limitation of the CPM literature is that few authors have studied whether CPM has a positive effect on long-term outcomes. Most studies have documented outcomes at discharge only.

SLIDES

8. To fill these gaps in the literature, we decided to study long-term functional outcomes after different CPM regimens.

9. Specifically, our purposes were to determine whether there were differences between three dosages of CPM (20, 12, and 4 hours daily) on gait velocity, activities of daily living, and knee flexion range of motion at 3 weeks, 6 weeks, and 6 months postoperatively.

10. We hypothesized that there would be no differences between the 20-hour and 12-hour groups at any time, that there would be significant differences between the 4-hour group and both the 20-hour and 12-hour groups at 3 and 6 weeks postoperatively, and that there would be no differences between any groups at 6 months postoperatively.

11. We used a prospective experimental design to study this problem.

SLIDES

(Photo of group of patients)

12. Subjects were patients who were at least 50 years old, had a diagnosis of either osteoarthritis or rheumatoid arthritis, and underwent total knee arthroplasty in 1992 at one of three hospitals in Anytown, Indiana: Community Hospital, Memorial Hospital of Indiana, and Religious Hospital.

Regimen Assignment By Hospital

- Community: 20-hr group
- Religious: 12-hr group
- Memorial: 4-hr group

13. One regimen was randomly assigned to each hospital. Patients at Community received the 20-hour-per-day regimen, patients at Religious received the 12-hour-per-day regimen, and patients at Memorial received the 4-hour-per-day regimen. The first 10 patients who met the inclusion criteria in 1992 were selected for study at each hospital.

Subject Characteristics

20-hr Group	12-hr Group	4-hr Group
73.2 yrs	71.7 yrs	72.5 yrs
50% women	40% women	60% women
70% OA	80% OA	70% OA

14. The table shows that the mean age of subjects from the different facilities was nearly identical, as was the proportion of men and women and the proportion of patients with osteoarthritis.

Prosthesis Characteristics

20-hr Group	12-hr Group	4-hr Group
40% Condylar	20% Condylar	40% Condylar
40% Stabilizer	10% Stabilizer	30% Stabilizer
20% Flat plateau	70% Flat plateau	30% Flat plateau

15. The only operative difference between groups that we identified was that there was a higher proportion of flat plateau prostheses implanted in patients in the 12-hour group than in the 20-hour and 4-hour groups.

(Photo of timer)

16. Patients underwent our routine postoperative rehabilitation protocol, with the only difference between groups being the amount of time spent in the CPM unit daily. A timer on the unit was used to monitor time on the machine each day.

17. Knee flexion range of motion measurements were taken in the supine position with the 12-inch universal goniometers available at each facility.

18. Velocity was measured by having the subject walk at a comfortable pace across a 20-meter measured distance. Each subject was timed with a stopwatch during the center 10 meters of the walk. This time was converted to centimeters/ second for analysis.

19. We used a modified Brigham and Women's knee rating scale to assess ADLs. The scale consists of four activities scored so that a 5 is most functional and a 1 least functional. The four scores are added together to create a single ADL score, with a maximum of 20.

20. To ensure that patients had spent the appropriate amount of time in CPM, we determined the average daily time in CPM. As you can see from this slide, the intended times were very nearly met.

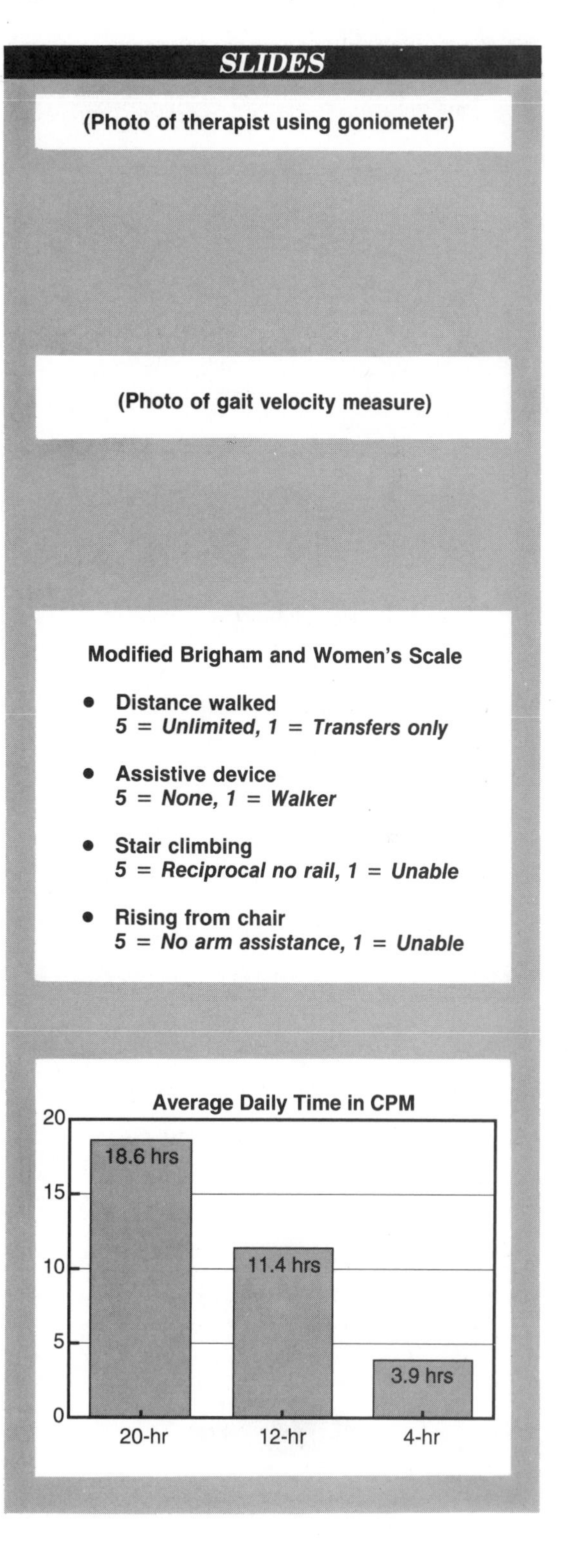

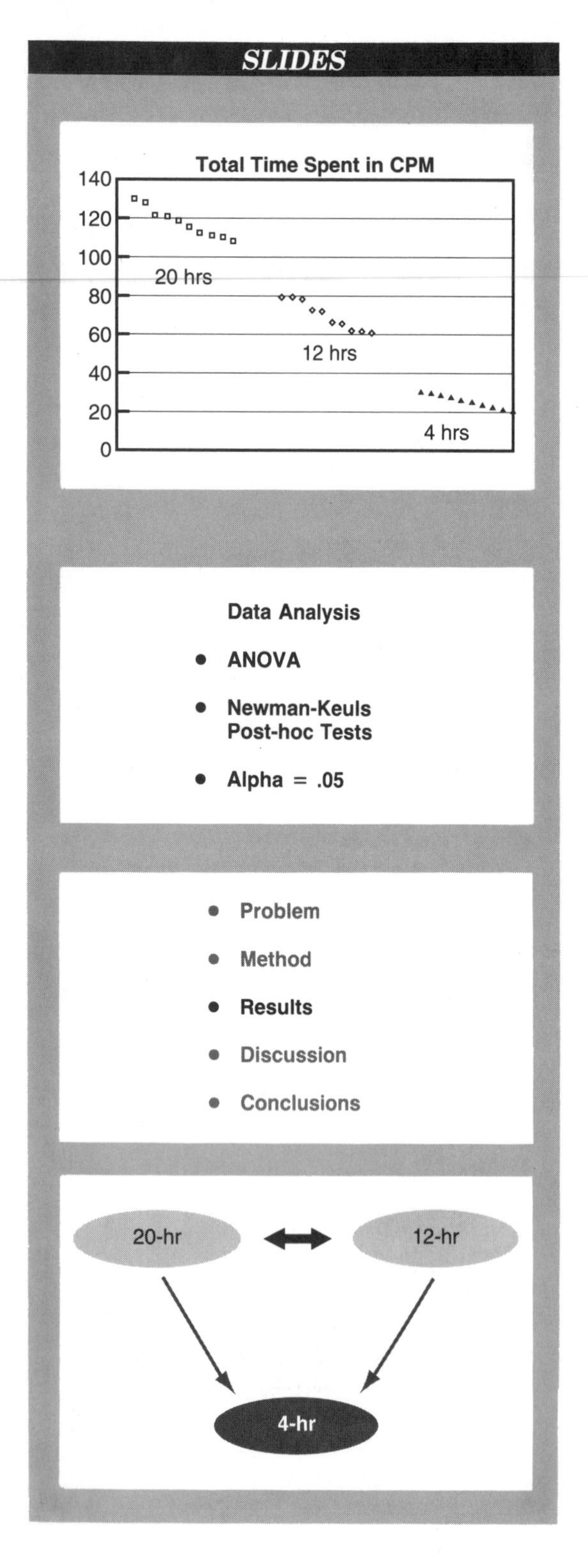

21. In addition to looking at the average daily time in CPM, we wanted to ensure that the total dosage of CPM across days was different between groups. The slide shows the total time spent in CPM for each subject, with the groups represented by the different shapes. The gaps between groups illustrate that the dosage differences we had hoped to maintain were in fact realized.

22. We used analysis of variance to test for differences between groups for each of the following dependent variables: 3-week ROM; 6-week ROM; and 6-month ROM, gait velocity, and ADL. The Newman-Keuls procedure was used for post hoc analysis. Alpha was set at .05 for each analysis.

23. Our results showed that . . .

24. No significant differences between the 20-hour and 12-hour groups were identified for any variables, as shown by the light ovals. In addition, the 4-hour group, represented by the dark oval, scored significantly lower on all variables than did either the 20-hour or 12-hour group.

25. This slide shows the nearly equal ROM scores for the 20-hour and 12-hour groups, illustrated by the dark and medium bars; and the low 3-week, 6-week, and 6-month range of motion values for the 4-hour group, represented by the white bars. Even at 6 months postoperatively, the 4-hour group had not achieved an average flexion ROM of 90 degrees.

26. This slide shows that the gait velocity for the 4-hour group was only an average of 107.6 cm/s, just a little bit faster than the velocity needed to cross a typical city street during the green light.

27. This slide shows that the ADL score for the 4-hour group was far lower than the scores of the other two groups. A score of 11 indicates moderate to severe impairment in more than one of the four ADL components measured.

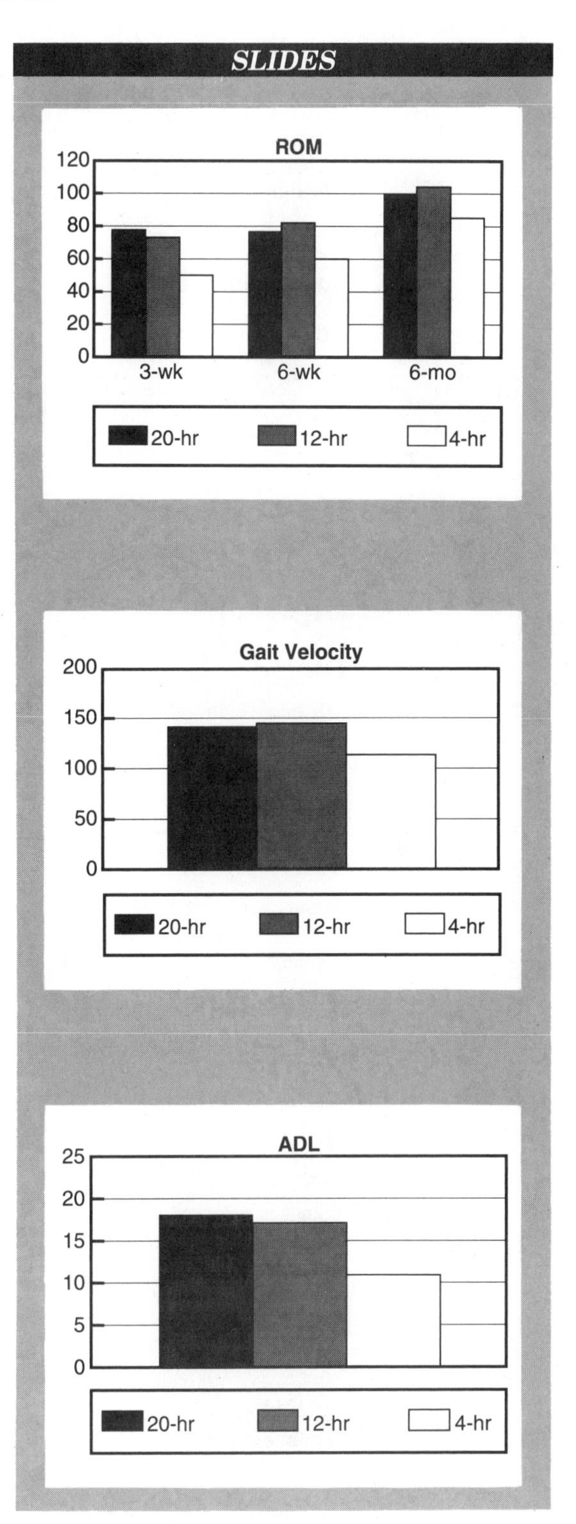

SLIDES
Problem
Method
Results
Discussion
Conclusions
Differences Between Hospitals?
Group membership known: potential influence of examiner expectations
(Photo of patient in CPM)

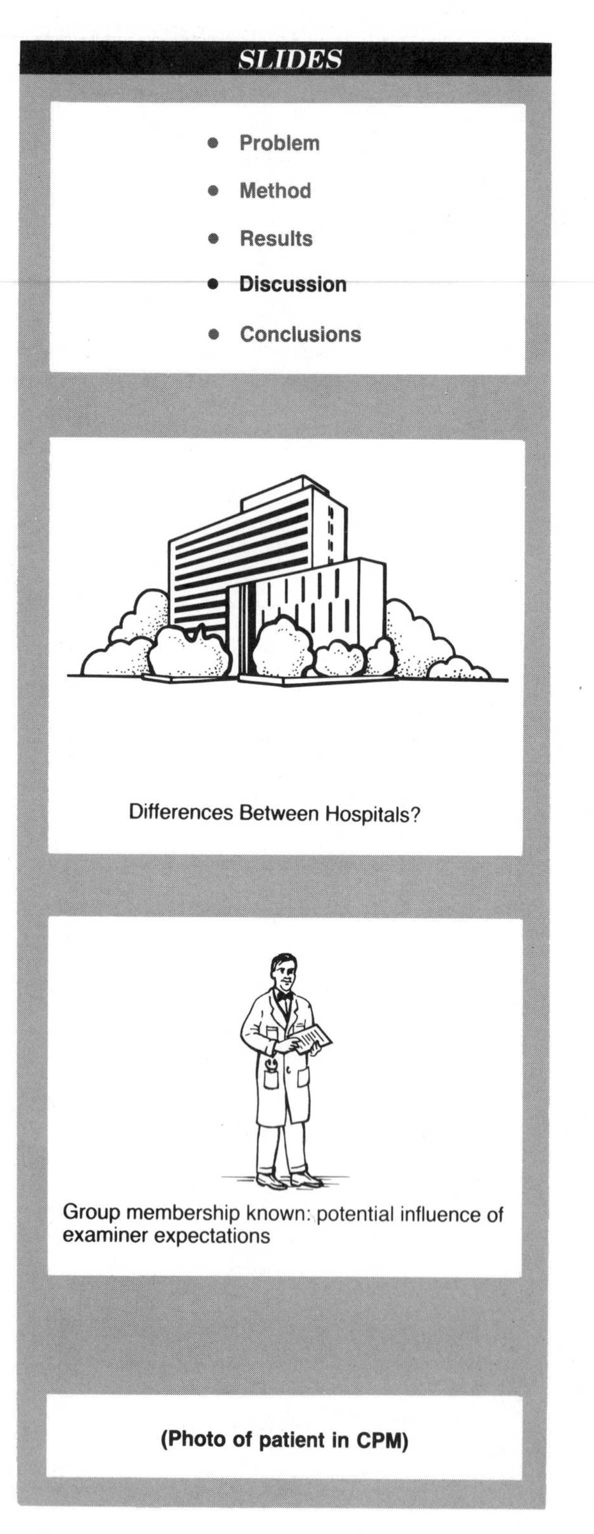

28. Discussion of these findings must, of course, include examination of the limitations of the study.

29. First, because the treatments were assigned by hospital and not by patient, there may have been systematic differences between care at the hospitals that could explain the difference in results.

30. Second, because we were not blind to the group membership of the subjects, our expectations may have influenced subject performance.

31. Despite these limitations, the results have clinical implications for facilities using CPM for patients after total knee arthroplasty.

SLIDES

32. First, facilities may wish to consider changing their protocols to reduce them from 20 hours of CPM per day to as low as 12 hours per day. In this way, the probability of patients' developing complications from postoperative bedrest—atelectasis, sacral pressure ulcers, cardiovascular deconditioning, and deep vein thrombosis—may be reduced.

> **Clinical Implications**
>
> - **Reduce hours in CPM**
> - **Reduce complications of bedrest?**

33. Further research must be done to see if these results can be replicated and to determine the minimum dosage of CPM necessary to achieve results similar to those seen in our 12-hour-per-day group.

> **Further Research**
>
> - **Replication**
> - **Minimum dosage?**

34. In conclusion, I would like to summarize our findings.

> - Problem
> - Method
> - Results
> - Discussion
> - **Conclusions**

35. First, there were no differences between the 20-hour-per-day group and the 12-hour-per-day group in 3-week range of motion, 6-week range of motion, or 6-month range of motion, gait velocity, and ADL score.

> **20-hr group = 12-hr group**
>
> **ROM**
> **(3 weeks, 6 weeks, 6 months)**
>
> **Gait velocity, ADL**
> **(6 months)**

36. Second, the 4-hour-per-day group performed significantly worse than either the 20-hour-per-day group or the 12-hour-per-day group in all variables.

> **4-hr group $<$ 20-hr group and 12-hr group**
>
> **ROM**
> **(3 weeks, 6 weeks, 6 months)**
>
> **Gait velocity, ADL**
> **(6 months)**

37. Before I take any questions, I would like to thank the patients, therapists, nurses, and orthopedic surgeons who participated in the project at

> **(Photo of research team)**

38. Community Hospital

39. Religious Hospital

40. and my own Memorial Hospital.

Glossary

A–B designs. A family of single-system designs in which baseline (A) and intervention (B) phases are alternated. Common forms are A–B, A–B–A, B–A–B, A–B–A–B.

Absolute reliability. The extent to which a score varies on repeated measurements; is quantified by the standard error of measurement.

Ad hoc theory. Descriptive theory in which a nonexhaustive list of characteristics is used to describe a phenomenon.

Alpha level. The probability of concluding that the null hypothesis is false, when in fact it is true. The alpha level is set by the researcher before data analysis; contrast this with *probability level,* which is generated by the data analysis.

Analysis of variance (ANOVA). A family of statistical tests used to analyze differences between two or more groups; based on partitioning the sum of squares into that attributable to between-groups differences and that attributable to within-group differences.

Archival data. Records or documents of the activities of individuals, institutions, or governments found in sources such as medical records, voter registration rosters, newspapers and magazines, and meeting minutes.

Assignment threat. An internal validity threat that is realized when subjects are assigned to groups in ways that do not ensure their equivalence.

Attribute variable. A variable created not by manipulation, but through division of subjects into groups based on an existing attribute such as sex or age; also called *classification variable.*

Autonomy. The moral principle that individuals should be permitted to be self-determining.

Beneficence. The moral principle that people should act to promote the welfare of others.

Beta-weight. Used to interpret multiple-regression equations by standardizing the slopes associated with each independent variable within the equation.

Between-subjects design. An experimental design in which all of the independent variables are between-subjects factors.

Between-subjects factor. An independent variable whose different levels are administered to different groups of subjects.

Bimodal distribution. A frequency distribution in which there are two modes, or most frequently occurring scores.

Block. A grouping of subjects based on a classification or attribute variable, such as age, sex, or diagnosis.

Bonferroni adjustment. Divides the total alpha level for an experiment by the number of statistical tests conducted to control for alpha level inflation.

Case-control design. An epidemiological research design in which groups of patients with and without a desired effect are compared to determine whether they have different proportions of presumed causes; contrast with *cohort design*, which proceeds from cause to effect.

Categorical theory. Descriptive theory in which the characteristics that describe a phenomenon are exhaustive.

Causal-comparative research. Nonexperimental research in which assignment to groups is based on preexisting characteristics, or attributes, of subjects; also called *ex post facto research*.

Chi-square distribution. A distribution of squared z scores; it forms the basis for chi-square tests of differences between groups when the dependent variable is in the form of a frequency or percentage.

Classification variable. A variable created not by manipulation, but through division of subjects into groups based on an existing attribute such as sex or age; also called *attribute variable*.

Coefficient of determination. The square of the correlation coefficient; indicates the percentage of variance shared by the variables.

Cohort. In general, any group. More specifically, groups that follow one another in time, as in subsequent school-year classes.

Cohort design. An epidemiological research design that works forward from cause to effect; contrast with *case control design*, which works from effect to cause.

Compensatory equalization of treatments. A threat to internal validity that is realized when a researcher who has preconceived notions about which treatment is more desirable showers attention on subjects receiving the treatment perceived to be less desirable.

Compensatory rivalry. This threat to internal validity is realized when members of one group react competitively to the perception that they are receiving a less desirable treatment than the other groups.

Concept. A phenomenon expressed in words; sometimes used as a more concrete term than *construct*.

Conceptual framework. Theory that specifies relationships between variables but does not have a deductive component; used interchangeably with *model*.

Concurrent validity. The extent to which a developing measure is comparable to a measurement standard.

Confidence interval. A range of scores around a mean; represents a specified probability that the true mean is within the range.

Construct. A property that is invented for a specific purpose; sometimes used as a more abstract term than *concept*.

Construct underrepresentation. A threat to construct validity that is realized when the independent or dependent variables are poorly developed.

Construct validity. Threats to construct validity are realized when the independent or dependent variables within a study are not well developed or are incorrectly labeled.

Content analysis. A process by which the text of archival records is reduced to quantifiable information.

Continuous variable. A variable that theoretically can be measured to finer and finer degrees.

Contrast. Comparison of two means; specifically, multiple-comparison tests conducted as part of complex analysis of variance tests.

Correlation coefficient. Mathematical expression of the degree of relationship between two or more variables; several different forms exist.

Criterion-referenced measure. A measurement framework in which each individual's performance is evaluated with respect to some absolute level of achievement.

Criterion validity. The extent to which one measure is systematically related to other measures or outcomes; subdivided into concurrent and predictive validity.

Deductive reasoning. Reasoning that proceeds from the general to the specific.

Degrees of freedom. The number of items that are free to vary. For example, the degrees of freedom for the mean is $n - 1$, meaning that if a certain mean score is desired, $n - 1$ of the values are free to fluctuate as long as one can control the final value.

Delphi technique. A survey design in which several rounds of a questionnaire are administered, each round building on information collected in previous rounds.

Dependent variable. The measured variable; used to determine the effects of the independent variable.

Descriptive theory. The least restrictive form of theory, simply describing the phenomenon of interest.

Deviation score. Calculated by subtracting the mean of a data set from each raw score.

Dichotomous variable. A variable that can take only two values, such as male/female or present/absent.

Diffusion of treatments. This threat to internal validity is realized when subjects in treatment and control groups share information about their respective treatments.

Discrete variable. A variable that can assume only distinct values. An example is a ligamentous laxity scale, which can assume values of hypomobile, normal, and hypermobile.

Epidemiology. The study of disease, injury, and health in a population. Epidemiological research documents the incidence of a disease or injury, determines causes for the disease or injury, and develops mechanisms to control the disease or injury.

Ethnographic research. Research whose purpose is to develop an in-depth picture of the culture of a particular group or unit.

Ex post facto research. Nonexperimental analysis of differences in which the independent variable is not manipulated. An example is research that examines differences between men and women on various dependent variables. Also called *causal-comparative research.*

Experimental research. Research in which at least one independent variable is subjected to controlled manipulation by the researcher.

Experimenter expectancy. A threat to construct validity that is realized when the subjects are able to guess the ways in which the experimenter wishes them to respond.

Explanatory theory. Theory that examines the *why* and *how* questions that undergird a problem.

External criticism. Concerns about the authenticity of archival records.

External validity. Concerns the issue of to whom, in what settings, and at what times the results of research can be generalized.

Facets. The factors of interest within a generalizability study; examples of facets might be raters, days, and times of measurement.

Factorial design. A design in which there are at least two independent variables, and all levels of each independent variable are crossed with all other independent variables.

***F* distribution.** A distribution of squared *t* statistics; the basis of analysis of variance.

Fisher's exact test. A modified chi-square statistic that is sometimes used if the dependent variable consists of only two categories.

Frequency distribution. A tally of the number of times each individual score is represented in a data set; can be presented visually as a histogram or a stem-and-leaf plot.

Friedman's ANOVA. The nonparametric version of the repeated measures analysis of variance.

Generalizability theory. An extension of classical measurement theory that quantifies the extent of variability on repeated measures that can be attributed to different facets of interest.

Grounded theory. A qualitative research approach that starts from an atheoretical perspective and develops theory that is grounded in the information gathered.

Heuristic. Discovering or revealing relationships that may lead to further development of a particular line of research.

Historical research. Research in which past events are documented because they are of inherent interest or because they provide a perspective that can guide decision making in the present.

History. This threat to internal validity is realized when events unrelated to the treatment of interest occur during the course of the study and cause changes in the dependent variable.

Homoscedasticity. One of the assumptions that should be met before calculating a correlation coefficient. Homoscedasticity means that for each value of one variable, the other variable has equal variability.

Hypothesis. A conjectural statement of the relationship between variables. Sometimes used interchangeably with *proposition*.

Idiographic. Pertaining to a particular case in a particular time and context; the opposite of *nomothetic*.

Independent *t* test. A parametric test of differences between two independent samples.

Independent variable. The presumed cause of a measured effect. In experimental research, at least one independent variable is manipulated by the researcher.

Informed consent. A process by which health care practitioners or investigators provide potential subjects with the information they need to make informed decisions about treatment or participation within a study. Four components are required for autonomy in making such decisions: disclosure, comprehension, voluntariness, and competence.

Instrumentation. This threat to internal validity is realized when changes in measuring tools themselves are responsible for observed changes in the dependent variable.

Interaction. A research question in which the effect of one variable is assessed to determine whether it is consistent across the different levels of a second independent variable.

Interaction of different treatments. A threat to construct validity that may be realized when treatments other than the one of interest are administered to subjects.

Internal criticism. Concerns about the neutrality of the interpretation of information found in archival records.

Internal validity. Concerns whether the independent variable is the probable cause of changes in the dependent variable.

Interrater reliability. The consistency among different judges' ratings of the same object or response. In its purest form, interrater reliability is determined by having the judges perform the ratings of one group of subjects at the same point in time.

Interval scale. Has the real-number system properties of order and distance, but lacks a meaningful origin.

Intrarater reliability. The consistency with which one rater assigns scores to a single set of responses on two or more occasions.

Kruskal-Wallis test. The nonparametric version of the one-way analysis of variance.

Level. A value of the independent variable; for example, a design in which the independent variable consists of a treatment group and a control group is said to have two levels of the independent variable.

Likert-type items. Used to assess the strength of response to a declarative statement. The most typical set of responses is "strongly agree," "agree," "undecided," "disagree," and "strongly disagree."

Mann-Whitney test. The nonparametric version of the independent *t* test.

Maturation. This threat to internal validity is realized when changes within a subject due to the passage of time occur during the course of a study and cause changes in the dependent variable.

McNemar's test. A statistical test that analyzes frequency or percentage data collected on repeated occasions.

Mean. The sum of observations divided by the number of observations.

Median. The middle score of a ranked distribution.

Meta-analysis. A means by which research results across several different studies are synthesized in a quantitative way.

Mixed design. A design in which some of the independent variables are between-subjects factors and some of the independent variables are within-subject factors; also called a *split-plot design.*

Mode. The most frequently occurring score within a distribution; if there are two modes, the distribution is called *bimodal.*

Model. A theory that specifies relationships between variables but does not have a deductive component; used interchangeably with *conceptual framework.*

Mortality. This threat to internal validity is realized when subjects are lost from the different study groups at different rates or for different reasons.

Multiple baseline design. A single-system design in which several subjects are studied after baselines of varying lengths.

Naturalistic. One term for qualitative research; refers specifically to the philosophy that qualitative researchers should study subjects in their natural setting.

Negative predictive value. The percentage of individuals identified by a test as negative who actually do not have the diagnosis.

Nested design. A design in which there are at least two independent variables, but not all levels of the independent variables are crossed.

Newman-Keuls test. A multiple comparison procedure.

Nominal scale. Has none of the properties of a real-number system; provides classification without placing any value on the categories within the classification.

Nomothetic. Relating to general or universal principles; opposite of *idiographic.*

Nondirectional. A t test hypothesis in which the researcher is open to the possibility that one mean is either greater than or less than the other mean.

Nonexperimental research. Research in which there is no manipulation of an independent variable.

Nonmaleficence. The moral principle of doing no harm.

Nonparametric tests. Statistical tests that do not rest on assumptions related to the distribution of the populations from which the samples are drawn.

Normal curve. A symmetrical, bell-shaped frequency distribution that can be defined in terms of the mean and standard deviation of a set of data.

Norm-referenced measure. A measure that judges individual performance in relation to group norms.

Null hypothesis. The statistical hypothesis that there is no difference between groups; contrast with *research hypothesis.*

Number. A numeral that has been assigned quantitative meaning.

Numeral. A symbol that does not necessarily have quantitative meaning; it is a form of naming.

Omnibus test. An overall test of a hypothesis within an analysis of variance; if the omnibus test identifies a significant difference between groups, then multiple-comparison procedures are needed to determine the location of the differences.

Operational definition. A specific description of the way in which a construct is presented or measured within a study.

Ordinal scale. Has only one of the properties of a real number system: order. Ordinal scales do not ensure that there are equal intervals between categories or ranks.

Paired t test. A statistical test that determines the difference between two paired measures.

Paradigm. A belief system researchers use to organize their discipline.

Parameter. A characteristic of a population; estimated by sample statistics.

Parametric tests. Statistical tests that rest on assumptions related to the distribution of the populations from which the samples are drawn.

Pathokinesiology. The application of anatomy and physiology to the study of abnormal human movement.

Phenomenology. A qualitative research approach whose purpose is to describe some aspect of life as it is lived by the participants.

Positive predictive value. The percentage of individuals identified by the test as positive who actually have the diagnosis.

Positivism. A research tradition that rests

on the objective measurement of reality; the traditional method of science.

Post hoc comparisons. Tests that are used to make pair-wise comparisons of means after an omnibus test has identified significant differences between more than two means.

Postpositivist. The qualitative research tradition, resting on the assumption of multiple constructed realities.

Predictive theory. A theory that is used to make predictions based on the relationships between variables.

Predictive validity. The ability of a measurement made at one point in time to predict future status.

Primary sources. Scholarly works that constitute the first documentation of the results of a study; the traditional primary source in the health sciences is the journal article, which reports the findings of original research.

Probability (*p*) level. The probability of obtaining a certain test statistic if the null hypothesis is true; the probability level is generated by the data analysis itself. Contrast with *alpha level*, which is set by the researcher.

Proposition. A statement of the relationship between concepts. Sometimes used interchangeably with *hypothesis.*

Prospective research. A research approach in which the researcher completes data collection after the research question is developed. Also used by epidemiologists as a synonym for *cohort research.*

Quasiexperimental research. A form of experimental research characterized by nonrandom assignment of subjects to groups or repeated treatments to the same group.

Questionnaire. A written self-report instrument used in survey research.

Randomized block design. A design in which the levels of at least one independent variable are randomly assigned and the levels of at least one independent variable are determined by blocks.

Randomized clinical trial. The name often given to clinical research in which subjects are randomly assigned to treatment and control groups.

Ratio scale. Exhibits all three components of a real-number system: order, distance, and origin. All the arithmetic functions of addition, subtraction, multiplication, and division can be applied to ratio scales.

Relative reliability. Exists when individual measurements within a group maintain their position within the group on repeated measurement; quantified by correlation coefficients.

Reliability. The extent to which measurements are repeatable.

Repeated measures analysis of variance. One of a family of analysis of variance techniques; used to determine differences between two or more dependent samples.

Research hypothesis. A statement that makes predictions about the expected outcome of the study; contrast with *null hypothesis.*

Resentful demoralization. This threat to internal validity is realized when members of one group react negatively to the perception that they are receiving a less desirable treatment than the other groups.

Residual. The amount of variability left unexplained after a data analysis; part of some analysis of variance and linear regression procedures.

Retrospective research. A research approach in which data are collected before the research question is developed. Also used by epidemiologists as a synonym for *case-control research.*

Reversed treatment design. A design in which the subjects or groups receive treatments that are expected to cause changes in opposite directions. This is in contrast to typical control-group designs, in which the control group is not expected to change.

Robust. Describes statistical procedures that tolerate violation of their assumptions without distortion of the probability of making a Type I error.

Sampling distribution. A distribution of sample means formed by drawing repeated samples from the same population. Ordinarily, the sample distribution is a theoretical distribution with a standard deviation estimated by dividing a single sample standard deviation by the square root of the number within the sample.

Scheffé test. A multiple-comparison procedure.

Secondary sources. Scholarly works, such as book chapters or literature reviews, that are interpretations of original sources such as journal article reports of original research.

Selection. This threat to external validity is realized when the selection process is biased because it yields subjects who are in some manner different from the population to whom researchers hope to generalize their results.

Self-report measures. These measures are the foundation of survey research; it is assumed that meaningful information can be obtained by asking the parties of interest what they know, what they believe, and how they behave.

Sensitivity. The percentage of individuals with a particular diagnosis who are correctly identified as positive by a test.

Setting. This threat to external validity is realized when peculiarities of the setting in which the research was conducted make it difficult to generalize results to other settings.

Single-system research. Research in which the unit of interest is a single person or setting, studied over time under baseline and treatment conditions.

Skewed. A distribution that is not symmetrical, that is, one with a long tail at its upper or lower end.

Slope. A characteristic of a line; the ratio of the change in Y that accompanies a change of one unit of X.

Specificity. The percentage of individuals without a particular diagnosis who are correctly identified as negative by a test.

Split-plot design. A design in which some of the independent variables are between-subjects factors and some are within-subject factors; also called a *mixed design*.

Standard deviation. The square root of the variance; expressed in the units of the original measure.

Standard error of measurement. A measure of absolute reliability; represents the standard deviation of measurement errors.

Standard error of the estimate. The standard deviation of the difference between individual data points and the regression line through them.

Standard error of the mean. The standard deviation of the sampling distribution.

Standard normal distribution. A normal distribution with a mean of 0.0 and a standard deviation of 1.0.

Statistic. A characteristic of a sample; used to estimate population parameters.

Statistical conclusion validity. Concerns whether statistical tools have been used and their results interpreted properly within a study.

Statistical regression to the mean. This threat to internal validity may be realized when subjects are selected on the basis of extreme scores on a single administration of a test.

***t* distribution.** A flattened standard normal curve; the basis for *t* tests, which are used to assess the differences between two groups or between paired data.

Testing. This threat to internal validity is realized when repeated testing itself is likely to result in changes in the dependent variable.

Test–retest reliability. The ability of a measurement to be repeated from one test occasion to another.

Theory. A body of interrelated principles that present a systematic view of phenomena; a theory is testable and tentative.

Time. This threat to external validity is realized when the results of a study are applicable to limited time frames.

Transform. Mathematical manipulation of data, usually to make it fit a normal distribution.

Trend. Related to data analysis of single-system research designs; describes whether the direction of change during a study phase is upward or downward.

Triangulation. A method of establishing reliability in qualitative research; consists of comparing responses across several different sources.

Tukey's test. A multiple-comparison procedure.

Utility. The moral principle that we should act to bring about the greatest benefit and the least harm.

Validity. The meaningfulness of test scores as they are used for specific purposes.

Variance. Conceptually, the average of the squared deviations about the mean. The *population variance* is found by dividing the sum of the squared deviations by the number within the sample; the *sample variance* is found by dividing the sum of the squared deviations by $n - 1$.

Wilcoxon rank sum test. The nonparametric version of the independent *t* test; synonymous with *Mann-Whitney test.*

Wilcoxon signed rank test. The nonparametric version of the paired *t* test.

Within-subject design. A design in which all of the factors are within-subject factors.

Within-subject factor. An independent variable whose different levels are administered to the same group of subjects. The comparison of interest is within the subject group.

Yates' correction. A correction factor sometimes used with chi-square tests in which the expected frequency in several cells is very small.

***z* score.** A deviation score divided by the standard deviation; indicates how many standard deviations the raw score is above or below the mean.

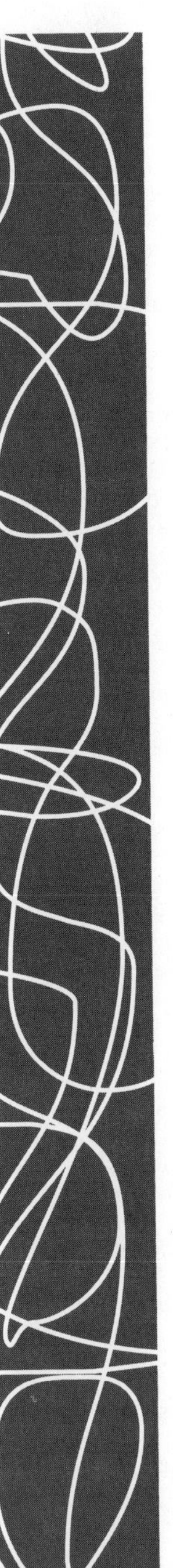

INDEX

Note: Page numbers in *italics* indicate figures; those followed by t indicate tables.

ISBN 0-7216-3611-X